FUNDAMENTALS of
HUMAN ANATOMY

[Vol. III]

FUNDAMENTALS of
HUMAN ANATOMY

[Head and Neck, Eyeball, Special Embryology, Surface and Radiological Anatomy]

[Vol. III]

Dhruba Chakraborty MS [JIPMER], FIAMS
Professor and Head, Department of Anatomy
College of Medicine and JNM Hospital
West Bengal University of Health Science

Formerly at
Kasturba Medical College, Manipal
Narayana Medical College, Nellore
Dr Pinnamanani Siddharth Academy of Medical Science, Vijaywada
International Medical University, Kualalumpur
University Sains Malaysia, Kota Bharu

Netai Chandra Chakraborty MBBS, MS, PhD, FAIMS
Ex-principal, Prof. and Head of the Dept. of Anatomy
Burdwan Medical College, Burdwan, West Bengal

New Central Book Agency (P) Ltd
LONDON
HYDERABAD ERNAKULAM BHUBANESWAR
NEW DELHI KOLKATA PUNE GUWAHATI

NCBA

REGD OFFICE

8/1 Chintamoni Das Lane, Kolkata 700 009, India

email: ncbapvtltd@eth.net

OVERSEAS

NCBA (UK) Ltd, 149 Park Avenue North, Northampton, NN3 2HY, UK

email: ncbauk@yahoo.com

EXPORT

NCBA Exports Pvt. Ltd, 212 Shahpur Jat, New Delhi 110 049

email: ncbaexports@ncbapvtltd.com

BRANCHES

2/27 Ansari Road, 1st Floor
Daryaganj, **New Delhi** 110 002
email: ncbadel@ncbapvtltd.com

House No. 3-1-315, 1st Floor
Nimboliadda, Kachiguda, **Hyderabad** 500 027
email: ncbahydb@ncbapvtltd.com

Shop Nos. 3 & 4, Vinayak Towers
681/B Budhwar Peth, Appa Balwant Chowk
Pune 411 002
email: ncbapune@ncbapvtltd.com

GSS Shopping Complex, 1st Floor
Opposite College Post Office, Convent Road
Ernakulam 682 035
0484-4021054 / 53

Shop No. 15, Bharati Towers, Ground Floor
Forest Park
Bhubaneswar 751 001
email: ncbabub@ncbapvtltd.com

Radhamayee Complex (Second Floor)
Opp. SBI, Panbazar, Jaswanta Road
Guwahati 781 001
email: ncbaguwahati@ncbapvtltd.com

FUNDAMENTALS OF HUMAN ANATOMY [Vol. III] • Dhruba Chakraborty, Netai Chandra Chakraborty

First Published: 1997
Reprinted: 2004
Reprinted: 2013
Thoroughly Revised Second Edition: 2018
Reprinted: 2019

PUBLISHER AND TYPESETTER
New Central Book Agency (P) Ltd
8/1 Chintamoni Das Lane, Kolkata 700 009

PRINTER
New Central Book Agency (P) Ltd
Web-Offset Division, Dhulagarh, Sankrail, Howrah

COVER DESIGNER
Angik, Kokata

PROOF-CHECKING
Author

PROJECT TEAM
Prabir Ghosh, Pradip Biswas and Joydeep Ghosh

ISBN: 978 81 7381 280 4

Price ₹735.00

Dedicated to

Father: Late Sudhansu Ranjan Chakraborty
Mother: Late Sadhana Chakraborty
Father-in-law: Late Prof (Dr) Netai Chandra Chakraborty

Acknowledgments

1. Late Prof Netai Chandra Chakraborty
2. Late Prof Inderbir Singh
3. Late Prof Mehdi Hassan
4. Late Prof Samar Mitra
5. Prof AK Dutta
6. Prof TS Ranganathan

CONTENTS

Chapter	Page No

Preface to the Second Edition

I have written this book to try and improve the way Human Anatomy is taught in India, a dream handed down to me by late Dr NC Chakraborty. Learning Anatomy requires easy and colourful diagrams aplenty. This book sets itself apart from the rest with its liberal use of diagrams to accompany textual descriptions.

I ackonwledge the support of Prof Ashok Sanyal, Prof Ramchandra Rao, Prof KSN Prasad, Prof Shakuntala Pai, Prof Siddique, Prof Ratna Prava, Prof Aizaz Ahmed, Prof Bhaskar Pal, Prof Kalyan Bhattacharyya, Prof Pitbaran Chakraborty, Prof BK Guha, Dr Saikat Roy and Dr Vinode Simlote.

I deeply appreciate the support of my publisher Mr Amitabha Sen and technical editor Dr Mita Sen. I am also grateful to Mr Prabir Ghosh, Mr Prosenjit Halder (artist) and Mr Ashok Swain (artist) for their valued contribution.

In addition to the people belonging to my professional circle, I would also like to thank my family, especially my wife Kajal, for putting up with my antics during the book writing process. My granddaughter Anaya, the youngest member of the clan, has been a huge source of inspiration. Thanks also to my daughter Kaushiki, son-in-law Shyamantak, son Kaustav, brother-in-law Pinak, nephew Pathikrit and mother-in- law Ivy.

I sincerely hope that students of Anatomy will find this book useful and instructive. I wish to apologize for mistakes, if any, textual or print-related, that may have crept in despite meticulous proof-reading. I request you, my reader, to write to me to point out mistakes or offer suggestions.

Dr Dhruba Chakraborty

129B, Indra Biswas Road

Kolkata 700037

Preface to the First Edition

The third volume has seen the light of the day quite late. In spite of my sincere efforts I could not complete the volume in time though there was urgent demand from both the teachers and the taught in India and abroad. I beg to be excused for this delay but would also like to point out that it was due to the fact that this volume contains different comprehensive and diverse topics as follows: Head and Neck, Upper Limb, Brain and Eyeball, their Special Embryology and Window Dissections, Surface Anatomy and Radiological Anatomy of the whole body and important appendices containing Testes and the Diaphragm (which really should have been incorporated in the volume consisting of Abdomen and Thorax).

At the outset I offer my deep respect and regard to my revered teacher Late Prof Hirendra Kumar Chatterjee for his scholarly guidance through his lectures with diagrams, particularly in Embryology. Teachers who had inspired me are Dr (Mrs) Bani Marjit of BMC, Dr (Mrs) D Basu and Dr S A Asad of RGRMC, Dr R K Guha Roy and Dr Prabir Sen of CMC, Dr Barun Banerjee of NRS, Dr D N Chowdhury of Cal NMC, Dr S K Basu and Dr Arun Kar of NBMC.

I record my deep appreciation to Mr J N Sen (Publisher) and Dr (Mrs) Mita Sen for her untiring efforts and meticulous correction of proofs, arrangement of manuscripts and index preparations etc. I also appreciate the work of the artists Mr Narayan Sur, Mr Chandan Roy and Mr Sunil Paul for the wonderful reproduction of my rough sketches. My Coauthor Dr Dhruba Chakrabarty has contributed quite a lot in this volume, particularly in the chapters on Embryology, Brain and Surface Anatomy.

Dr Chiranjoy Mukherjee, son of Dr Mongol Mukherjee, helped me a lot in the Window Dissection chapter. Dr Pinak Pani Byattacharyya, MD — Radiology (my son-in-law) and Radiologist of Duncan Glean Eagles Clinic, Calcutta, has helped me in correction, arrangement and collection of X-ray plates required for compiling the chapter on Radiological Anatomy.

I appreciate the help of my following relatives, Dr (Mrs) Kum Kum Bhattacharyya, MD (daughter), Mrs Kajal Chakrabarty, MSc (daughter), Dr Samudra Chakrabarty, Dept. of FSM of BMC (nephew) and my elder brother Mr G C Chakrabarty. I should not fail to mention the name of my beloved wife Smt Ivy Charkraborty who is my constant inspiration and who had to make many a sacrifice in domestic matters. Finally, I must mention the names of my granddaughter and grandsons. They are Kaushiki, Pathikrit, Prabudhya and Kaustav. They inspire me to draw, inadvertently, by taking and hiding my sketch pens very often. In fine I offer apologies for mistakes (textual and printing) in spite of meticulous proof reading. Readers are requested to point out the mistakes and send constructive suggestions which will be thankfully accepted.

I will be amply rewarded for my labour at this age if teachers and students derive some benefit from by painstaking endeavour.

Netai Chandra Chakraborty

11th June,

129B, Indra Biswas Road

Kolkata 700037

chapter 1

OSTEOLOGY OF HEAD AND NECK

AT A GLANCE

- *Skull as a whole—Norma verticalis; Norma occipitalis; Norma frontalis; Norma lateralis; Norma basalis; Interior of cranium; Anterior cranial fossa; Middle cranial fossa; Posterior cranial fossa*
- *Cranial bones—Occipital bone; Frontal bone; Parietal bone; Sphenoid bone; Temporal bone; Mandible; Maxilla; Zygomatic bone; Nasal bone; Ethmoid bone; Palatine bone; Inferior nasal concha; vomer; Lacrimal bone; Hyoid bone*
- *Cervical vertebrae—Atypical cervical vertebrae; Atlas, axis & seventh cervical vertebrae; Typical cervical vertebrae;*
- *Neonatal skull*

A. SKULL AS A WHOLE

TABLE 1.1:

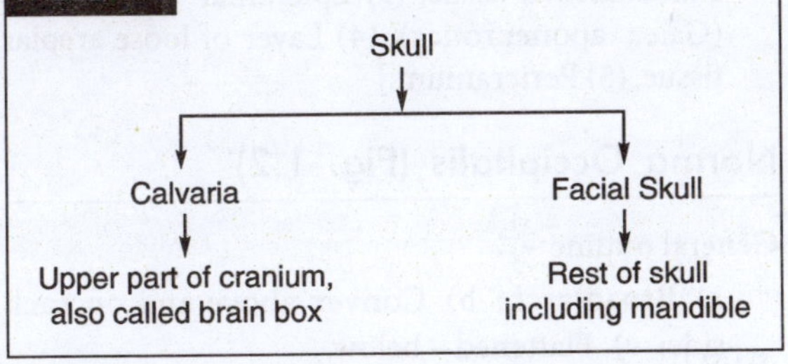

Anatomical Position

Line joining the infraorbital margin and external accoustic meatus i.e. preauricular point must be horizontal. This is also known as Reid's base line.

Frankfurt's plane – A plane is passing through lower margin of the orbit and upper margin of the external acoustic meatus.

Study of Skull

Study of skull as a whole is practically important specially for men of medicine.

This study can be done in two ways –

1. Exterior of skull (Outer aspect)
2. Interior of skull (Inner aspect)

TABLE 1.2:

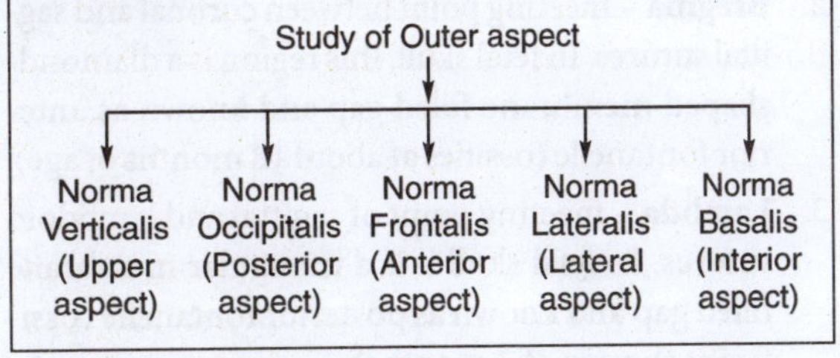

NORMA VERTICALIS

General outline – Oval, convex (shape) and wider behind than in front.

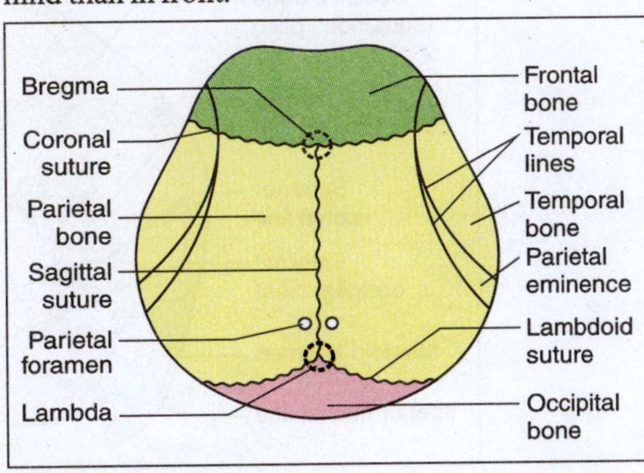

Fig. 1.1: Norma verticalis

Bones taking part (Fig. 1.1)

1. In front – upper part of the frontal bone
2. Behind – upper most part of the occipital bone
3. In the middle – one parietal bone on each side.

Sutures

1. **Coronal suture** – Transverse between anterior margins of two parietal bones and posterior margin of the frontal bone.
2. **Lambdoid** – In the posterior part and transversely, but more or less directed downwards and laterally. It is between posterior margins of two parietal bones and superior borders of squamous part of the occipital bone.
3. Sagittal suture – Between two parietal bones.

Other Features

1. **Vault** – Dome or arched roof of the skull (calvaria) is formed by four bones—squamous part of the frontal (in front) and occipital (behind) bone and two parietal bones.
2. **Bregma** – meeting point between coronal and sagittal sutures. In fetal skull, this region is a diamond-shaped membrane filled gap and known as anterior fontanelle (ossifies at about 18 months of age).
3. **Lambda** – meeting point of sagittal and lambdoid sutures. In fetal skull it is a triangular membrane filled gap and known as posterior fontanelle (ossifies at the age of 3 months).
4. **Vertex** – Position varies – usually the highest point on the sagittal suture.
5. **Parietal eminence** or **tuber** – Prominent area of maximum lateral bulging of the parietal bone at about midway between coronal and lambdoid sutures. The line joining the two eminences form the widest transverse diameter of the skull.
6. **External occipital protuberance** – Ovoid bulging where the posterior slopes of the skull meet.
7. **Parietal foramen** – At about 3 cm. in front of lambda and one on each side of sagittal suture – transmitting a) emissary vein, b) a branch of occipital artery.
8. **Temporal lines** – Begins as a single line from zygomatic process of the frontal bone and run upwards and backwards and divides over the parietal bone into superior and inferior temporal lines.

Attachments:

Superior temporal line –

– Epicranial aponeurosis

– Temporal fascia

Inferior temporal line –

– Temporalis muscle.

[Norma verticalis is covered by scalp which consists of – from outside inwards – (1) Skin, (2) Dense subcutaneous tissue, (3) Epicranial aponeurosis (Galea aponeurotica), (4) Layer of loose areolar tissue, (5) Pericranium.]

Norma Occipitalis (Fig. 1.2)

General outline –

a) Broad arch; b) Convex above and on each side; c) Flattened – below.

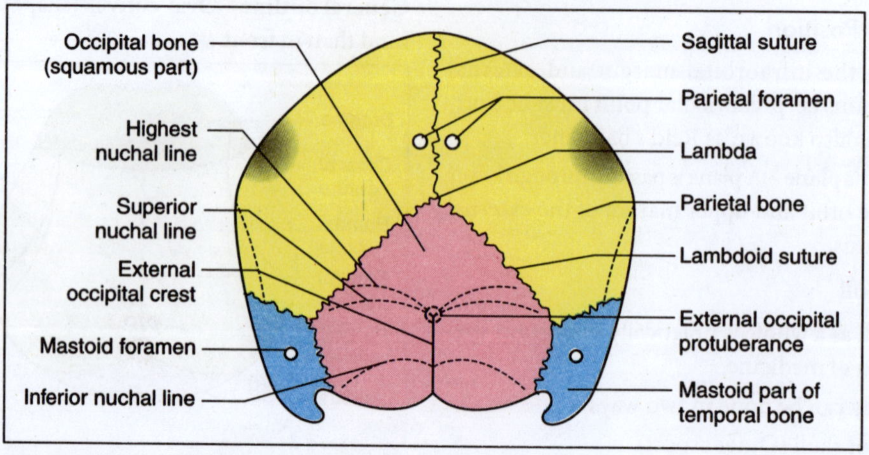

Fig. 1.2: Norma occipitalis

Bones taking part –

1. Above – Posterior parts of the parietal bone
2. Below – Squamous part of the occipital bone
3. On each side – Mastoid part of the temporal bone.

Sutures

1. Lambdoid – between occipital and two parietal bones; 2. Posterior part of sagittal – between two parietals; 3. Occipitomastoid; 4. Parietomastoid.

Other Features

1. **Lambda**
2. **Parietal foramen**
3. **External occipital protuberance** – An elevated prominence in the median plane, and is at the junctional region of head and neck. It is the most important landmark (in the midway between lambda and posterior margin of foramen magnum) in norma occipitalis.

   Inion is prominent point of external occipital protuberance [Structures attached to it – (a) origin of trapezius – from the upper part; (b) ligamentum nuchae – in the lower part].
4. **Highest nuchal lines** – A faint line extend laterally from external occipital protuberance. It is about 1 cm. above the superior nuchal line.

   Structures attached: (a) epicranial aponeurosis (medial 1/3rd); (b) origin of occipital belly of the occipitofrontalis muscle (lateral 2/3rd).
5. **Superior nuchal line** – A prominent ridge extend laterally from protuberance and below highest nuchal line.

   Structures attached: (a) origin of trapezius (medial 1/3rd); (b) insertion of the sternocleidomastoid and splenius capitis (lateral 1/3rd); (c) middle 1/3rd form the apex of the posterior triangle.
6. **Mastoid foramen** – Situated in mastoid part of temporal bone transmitting:
   a) Emissary vein; b) A branch of the occipital artery.
7. Occasionally interparietal bones – Membrane ossified squamous part of occipital when fail to fuse with the bone ossified in cartilage.

NORMA FRONTALIS (Fig. 1.3)

(Anterior aspect of skull)

General outline or shape – more or less oval and wider above than lower part.

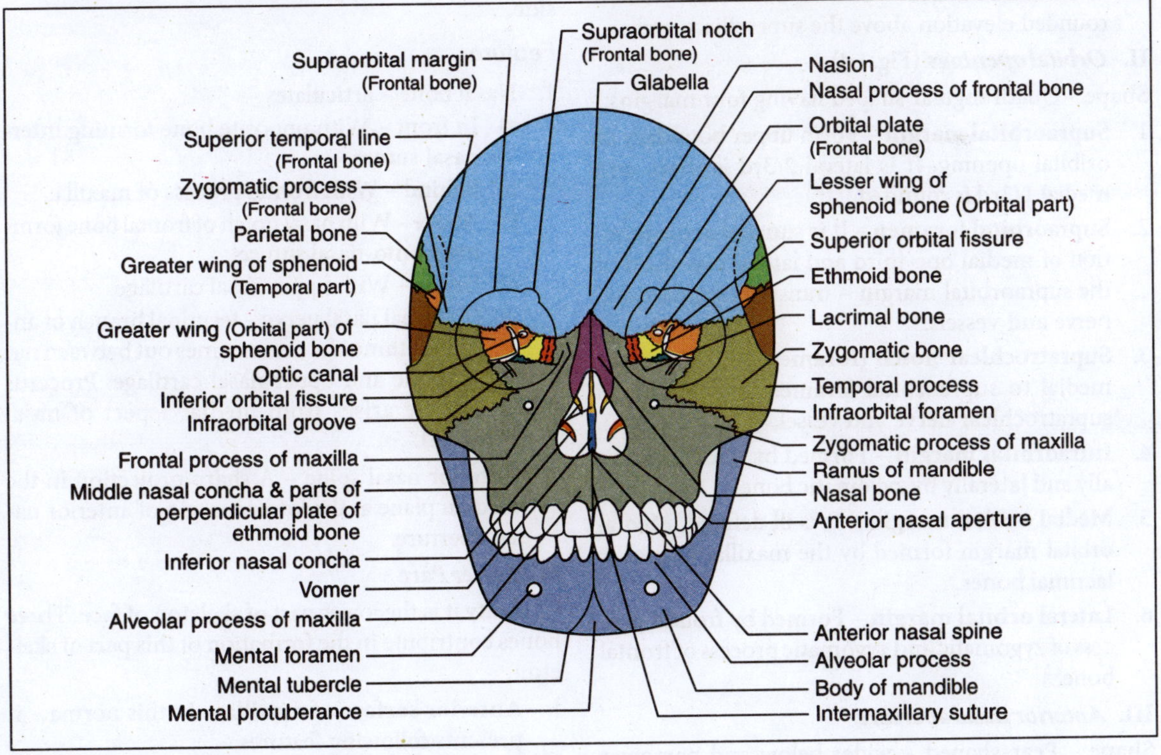

Fig. 1.3: Norma frontalis

Bones taking part:

1. Frontal bone
2. Two nasal bones
3. Zygomatic bones
4. Two maxillae
5. Mandible.

Sutures

1. Internasal; 2. Frontonasal; 3. Frontomaxillary; 4. Frontozygomatic; 5. Zygomaticomaxillary; 6. Occasionally metopic suture (Frontal) 9% cases.

Features

I. ***Upper part or frontal region:***

1. **Superciliary arch** – A curved elevation above the supraorbital margin
   a) Frontal air sinus lies deep to it
   b) Corrugator supercilli muscle takes origin from medial part of it.
2. **Glabella** – A medial elevation in between two superciliary arches.
3. **Nasion** – Meeting point of internasal and frontonasal sutures at the root of nose.
4. **Frontal eminence** – one on each side – small rounded elevation above the superciliary arch.

II. ***Orbital openings:*** (Fig. 1.4)

Shape – Quadrangular shaped having four margins.

1. **Supraorbital margin** – Form upper boundary of oribital opening. It is lateral 2/3rd is sharp and medial 1/3rd is rounded.
2. **Supraorbital foramen** – It is situated at the junction of medial one-third and lateral two-third of the supraorbital margin – transmits supraorbital nerve and vessels.
3. **Supratrochlear notch (foramen)** – It is present medial to supraorbital foramen, and transmits supratrochlear nerve and vessel.
4. **Infraorbital margin** – Formed by maxilla medially and laterally by zygomatic bone.
5. **Medial orbital margin** – It is ill defined. Medial orbital margin formed by the maxilla, frontal & lacrimal bones.
6. **Lateral orbital margin** – Formed by frontal process of zygomatic and zygomatic process of frontal bone.

III. ***Anterior nasal aperture:***

Shape – Pear-shaped – wider below and narrower above.

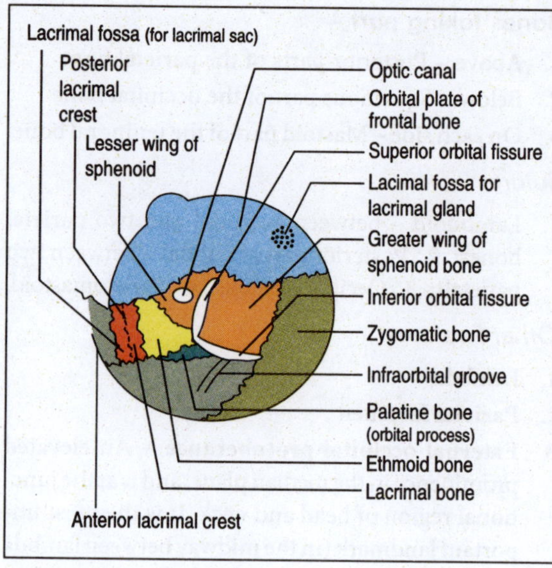

Fig. 1.4: Bones in the orbit

Formation or boundaries

Above – By lower border of the nasal bones.

Below – By nasal notch of body of the maxilla on each side.

Features

1. Nasal bone – articulates –
   a) In front – With opposite bone forming internasal suture.
   b) Behind – With frontal process of maxilla.
   c) Above – With nasal notch of frontal bone forming fronto-nasal suture.
   d) Below – With upper nasal cartilage. (External nasal nerve – terminal branch of anterior ethmoidal nerve comes out between nasal bone and upper nasal cartilage. Procerus muscle arises from medial aspect of nasal bone).
2. Anterior nasal spine – A sharp projection in the median plane at the lower margin of anterior nasal aperture.

IV. ***Lower Part:***

In reality it is the lower part of skeleton of face. Three bones contribute in the formation of this part of skeleton.

I. **Anterior surface of maxilla** – In this norma – it presents following features –

1. **Nasal notch** – medially

2. **Infraorbital foramen** – Below inferior orbital margin and transmits infraorbital vessels and nerves.
3. Anterior nasal spine.
4. **Incisive fossa** – above incisor teeth.
5. **Canine eminence** – lateral to incisive fossa.
6. **Canine fossa** – lateral to canine eminence
7. 3 Processes of maxilla: (a) Frontal, (b) Zygomatic, (c) Alveolar.
8. A number of muscles are attached in this aspect –
   a) **Orbicularis oculi** (orbital part) from frontal process of maxilla and nasal part of frontal bone.
   b) **Levator labii superioris alaeque nasi** from frontal process of the maxilla.
   c) **Levator labii superioris** – from body of maxilla between inferior orbital margin and infra orbital foramen.
   d) **Levator anguli oris** – from canine fossa.
   e) **Nasalis** and **depressor septi** – from adjoining part of nasal notch.

Besides – **Medial palpebral ligament** from frontal process of maxilla.

II. **Zygomatic bone** presents
   1. Origin of zygomaticus minor medially
   2. Origin of zygomaticus major laterally
   3. Zygomaticofacial foramen.

   Transmitting zygomaticofacial nerve branch of zygomatic, branch of maxillary nerve.

III. **Mandible** –

Features

1. Upper alveolar arch containing sockets for teeth.
2. Base or lower border.
3. In median plane of the anterior surface –
   a) Mental protuberance
   b) Symphysis menti
   c) Mental tubercle.
4. Mental foramen transmitting mental vessels and nerves.
5. Oblique line – for attachment of buccinator.

NORMA LATERALIS (Fig. 1.8)

This is the lateral view of the skull.

Bones Taking Part – 1. Frontal; 2. Parietal; 3. Occipital; 4. Temporal 5. Sphenoid (greater wing); 6. Zygomatic; 7. Maxilla; 8. Mandible; 9. Nasal

Features

I. **Temporal lines – Superior temporal line**: It starts from posterior margin of frontal process of zygo-

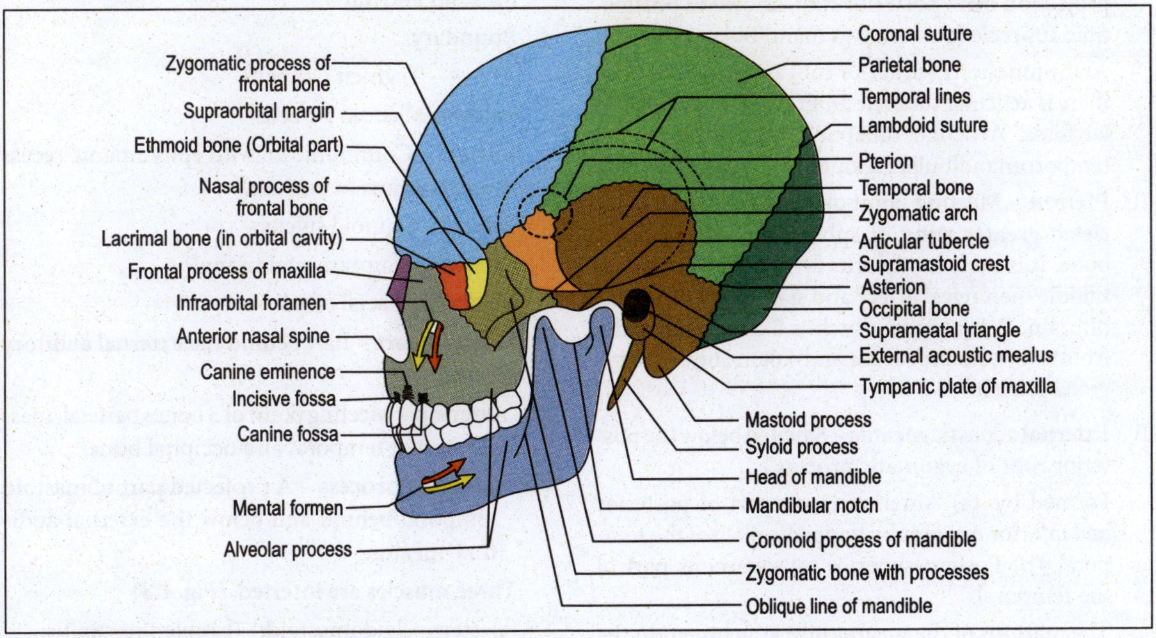

Fig. 1.5: Lateral aspect of Skull (Normal Lateralis)

matic bone, curve supero-laterally splits into superior and inferior temporal. Superior temporal line gives attachment temporal fascia.

Inferior termporal line: It runs below the superior line. Its posterior part proceeds downwards and forwards, merges with supramastoid crest to reach the posterior root of the zygomatic process. Temporalis muscle takes origin from it.

II. **Zygomatic arch** – A bar of bone horizontally disposed in front and little above the tragus of ear.

Formed by: a) Anterior one-third by temporal process of zygomatic bone, b) Posterior two-third by zygomatic process of the temporal bone.

Inner surface – Origin of the masseter muscle.

Outer surface – Subcutaneous and is crossed by the auriculotemporal nerve, superficial temporal vein and artery (behind forwards).

Upper border – Temporal fascia is attached.

Lower border – Origin of the masseter muscle.

Posterior end of zygomatic process of the temporal bone divides into anterior and posterior roots. Anterior root forms the anterior margin of mandibular fossa.

Posterior root passes lateral to the mandibular fossa and above the external acoustic meatus and continuous with supramastoid process. There is a projection from posterior root, known as postglenoid tubercle (posterior to mandibular fossa).

At the junction of anterior root and posterior root there is articular tubercle anterior to the mandibular fossa. Articular tubercle gives attachment to temporomandibular ligament.

III. **Pterion** – Meeting point of 4 bones – frontal, parietal, greater wing of sphenoid, and temporal bone. It is bony landmarks for anterior branch of middle meningeal artery and start of lateral sulcus of brain. It is a point which is 3.5cm behind the frontto-zygomatic suture and 4.0cm above the zygomatic arch.

IV. **External acoustic meatus** – Situated below the posterior root of zygomatic process.

Formed by: (a) Anterior, lower part of posterior and inferior margins by tympanic plate of the temporal, (b) Postero-superior by squamous part of the temporal.

The margins of the meatus give attachment to the cartilaginous part of the external auditory meatus.

TABLE 1.3: Zygomatic Process

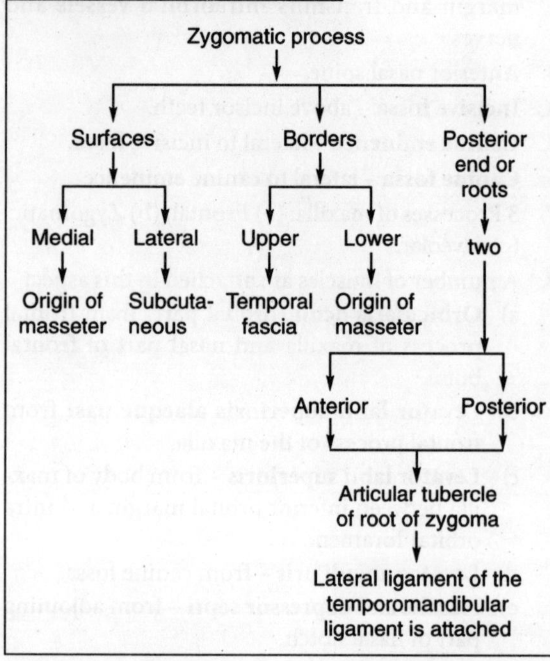

V. **Suprameatal triangle** – A small more or less triangular depression situated posterosuperior to external auditory meatus. It corresponds to tympanic (mastoid) antrum at about 1/2" depth.

Mastoid antrum –

Boundary:

Above – Tegmen tympani

Below – Mastoid air cells

Infront – Communicate with epitympanic recess through aditus to antrum.

Behind – Sigmoid sulcus

Laterally – Suprameatal triangle

Medially – Facial canal.

VI. **Mastoid part** – Part behind the external auditory meatus.

VII. **Asterion** – Meeting point of 3 bones parietal, mastoid part of temporal and occipital bone.

VIII. **Mastoid process** – A projected part of mastoid temporal behind and below the external auditory meatus.

Three muscles are inserted: (Fig. 1.8)

(a) sternocleidomastoid; (b) splenius capitis; (c) longissimus capitis.

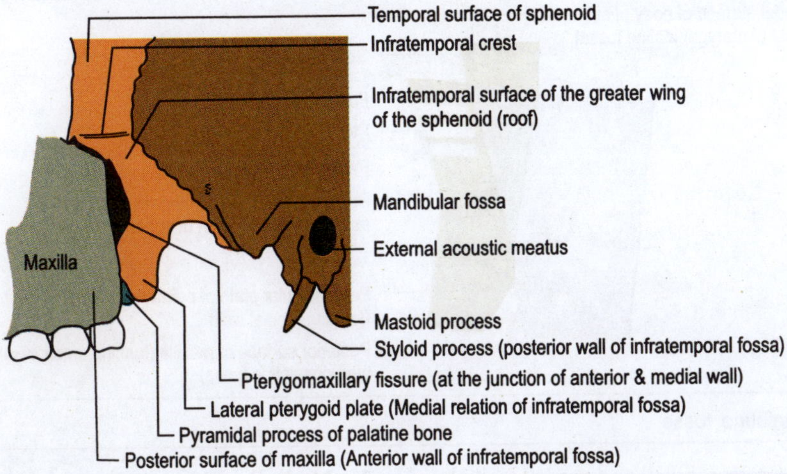

Fig. 1.6: Temporal & infratemporal fossa

IX. **Styloid process**–A bony projection from antero medial part of mastoid process. Two parts –

1. Tympanohyal (Part ensheathed by tympanic plate).
2. Stylohyal – Part freely projected – Three muscles are attached –
   a) Stylohyoid from posterior aspect near the mid-way (between the tip and base) (supplied by facial nerve).
   b) Styloglossus – from tip and anterior surface near tip (supplied by hypoglossal nerve).
   c) Stylopharyngeus – from medial surface of the base (supplied by glossopharyngeal nerve).

Two ligaments are attached –

1. Stylohyoid – To tip
2. Stylomandibular – lateral aspect. (Tip of the styloid process)

IX. **Temporal fossa** – A bony fossa situated on the lateral aspect of skull.

Boundaries

A. **Superiorly** – Temporal line in the frontal and superior temporal line in parietal.

B. **Inferiorly** –
   a) Lateral aspect – Zygomatic arch.
   b) Medial aspect – Infratemporal crest of the greater wing of the sphenoid bone.

C. **Anteriorly** –
   a) Zygomatic
   b) Parts of the frontal and the sphenoid bones.

D. **Contents** –
   a) Temporalis muscle;
   b) Deep temporal nerves;
   c) Middle temporal vessels;
   d) Zygomaticotemporal nerves.

E. **Communication** – With infratemporal fossa – through the gap deep to the zygomatic arch.

F. **Structures transmitting through the gap** *between zygomatic arch and side of skull*
   a) Tendon of the temporalis;
   b) Deep temporal vessels;
   c) Deep temporal nerves.

X. **Infratemporal fossa** – An irregular bony space situated below the middle cranial fossa of the skull, behind body of maxilla and lateral to the lateral pterygoid plate.

Boundaries (Fig. 1.6)

A. **Anterior wall** – Posterior surface of body of the maxilla.

B. **Posterior wall** – Styloid process of the temporal bone.

C. **Roof** – Greater wing of the sphenoid and a small part of squamous part of the temporal.

D. **Floor** – Open.

E. **Laterally** – Covered by lateral and medial pterygoid muscle and part of ramus of the mandible.

F. **Medially** – Lateral pterygoid plate of the sphenoid and the pyramidal process of the palatine bone. At

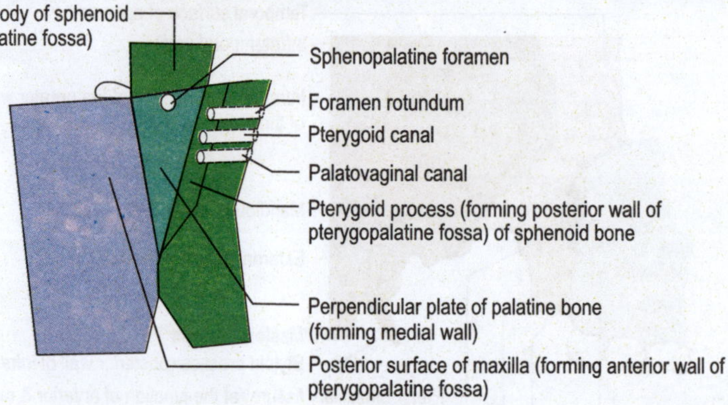

Fig. 1.7: Pterygopalatine fossa

the junction of anterior wall and medial wall, there is presence of the pterygomaxillary fissure.

XI. **Pterygopalatine fossa** – A small bony space situated deep to the pterygomaxillary fissure.

Boundaries

1. **Anteriorly** – Posterior surface of the maxilla.
2. **Posteriorly** – Root of the pterygoid processes and adjoining part of the greater wing of the sphenoid (Fig. 1.7).
3. **Medially** – Upper part of the perpendicular plate of the palatine bone with the sphenoidal and the orbital processes.
4. **Laterally** – Pterygomaxillary fissure which communicates with the infratemporal fossa.
5. **Roof** – Undersurface of body of the sphenoid bone.
6. **Floor** – Fusion of the maxilla and pterygoid processes.

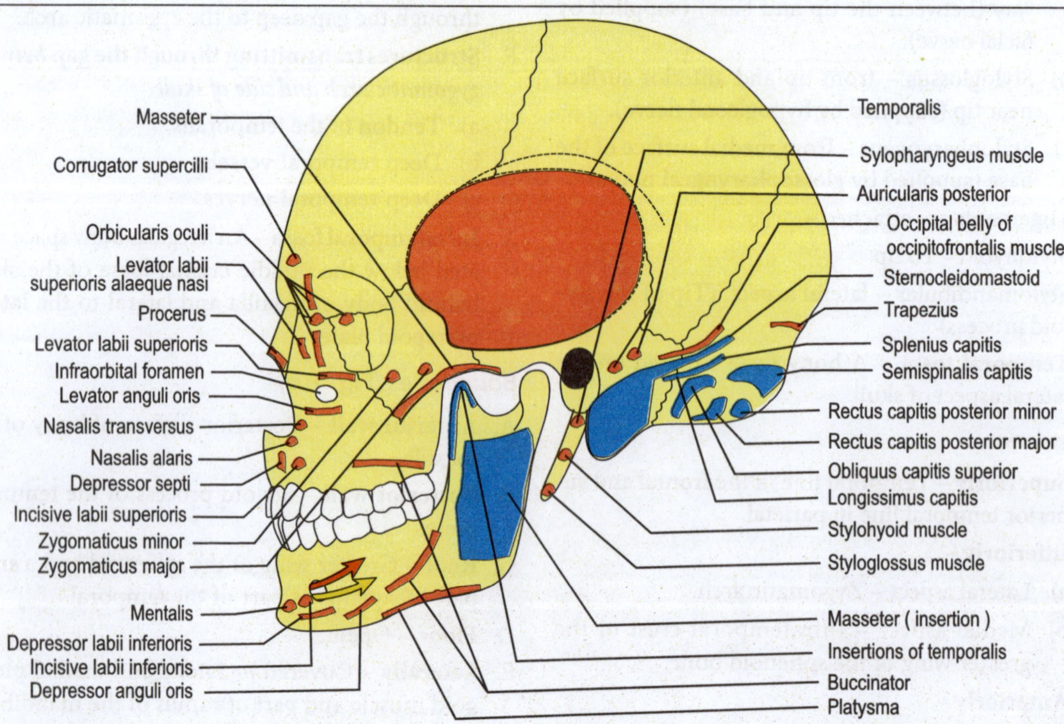

Fig. 1.8: Lateral view of skull showing the muscle attachments

NORMA BASALIS (Figs. 1.9, 1.10)

It is the inferior aspect of skull bounded by —

In front – incisor teeth

Behind – superior nuchal lines of the occipital bone

On each side –

a) Remaining teeth of the alveolar arch
b) Zygomatic arch with posterior root
c) Mastoid process and line joining it with superior nuchal line.

For the sake of description and convenience of study of this aspect – It is divided into three parts:

(1) Anterior, (2) Middle, (3) Posterior Parts.

I. ANTERIOR PART OF NORMA BASALIS

A. **Alveolar arch** – for upper teeth (Fig. 1.11)

B. **Hard palate:**

1. **Formation**
   a) Palatine processes of the maxillae forming anterior two-third
   b) Horizontal plates of the palatine bone – Posterior one-third.
2. **Sutures Present**:
   a) Intermaxillary
   b) Inter palatine;
   c) Palatomaxillary
3. **Shape** – Arched on all aspects with pits for palatine glands.
4. **Incisive fossa** – A sutural line is often found bilaterally from incisive foramen (in incisive fossa) to the junction between lateral incisor and canine. The portion of the bone in front of suture is known as **premaxilla** (which develops from **frontonasal process**).

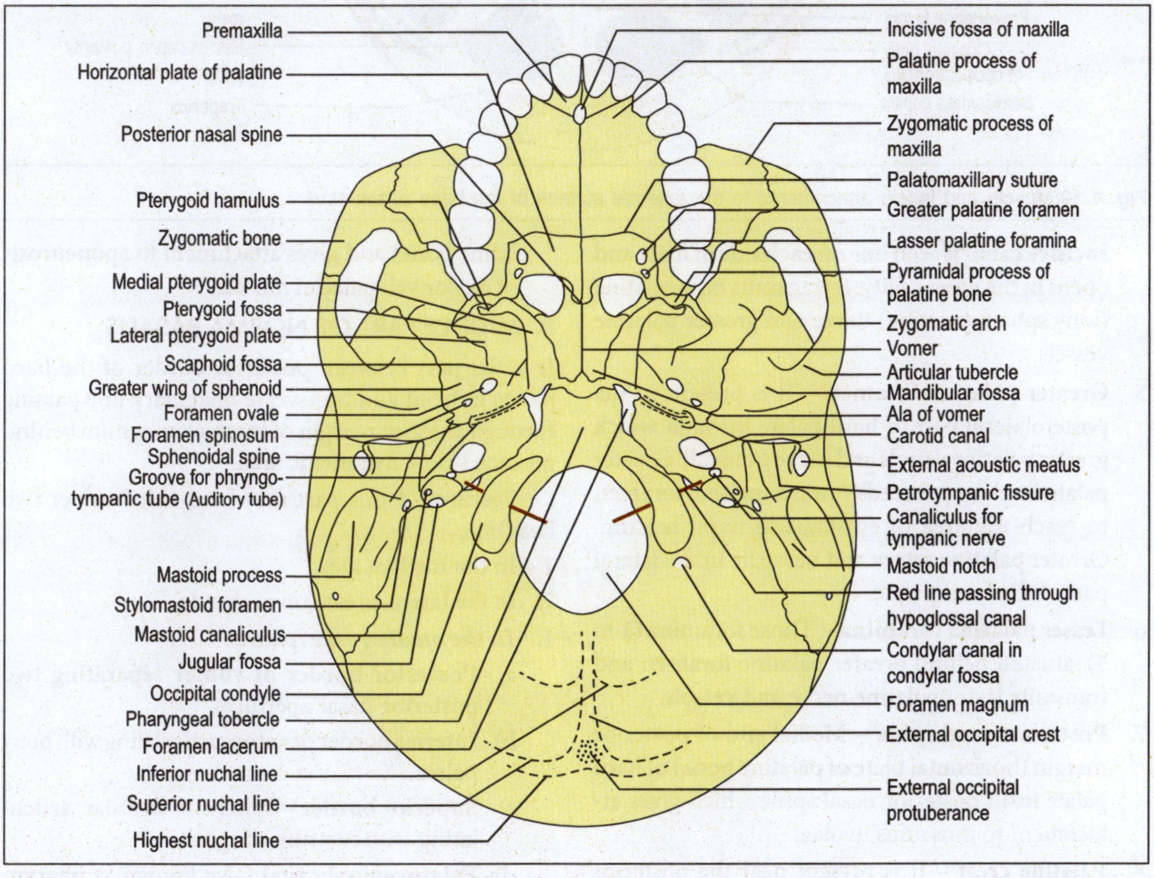

Fig. 1.9: The external surface of the base of the skull

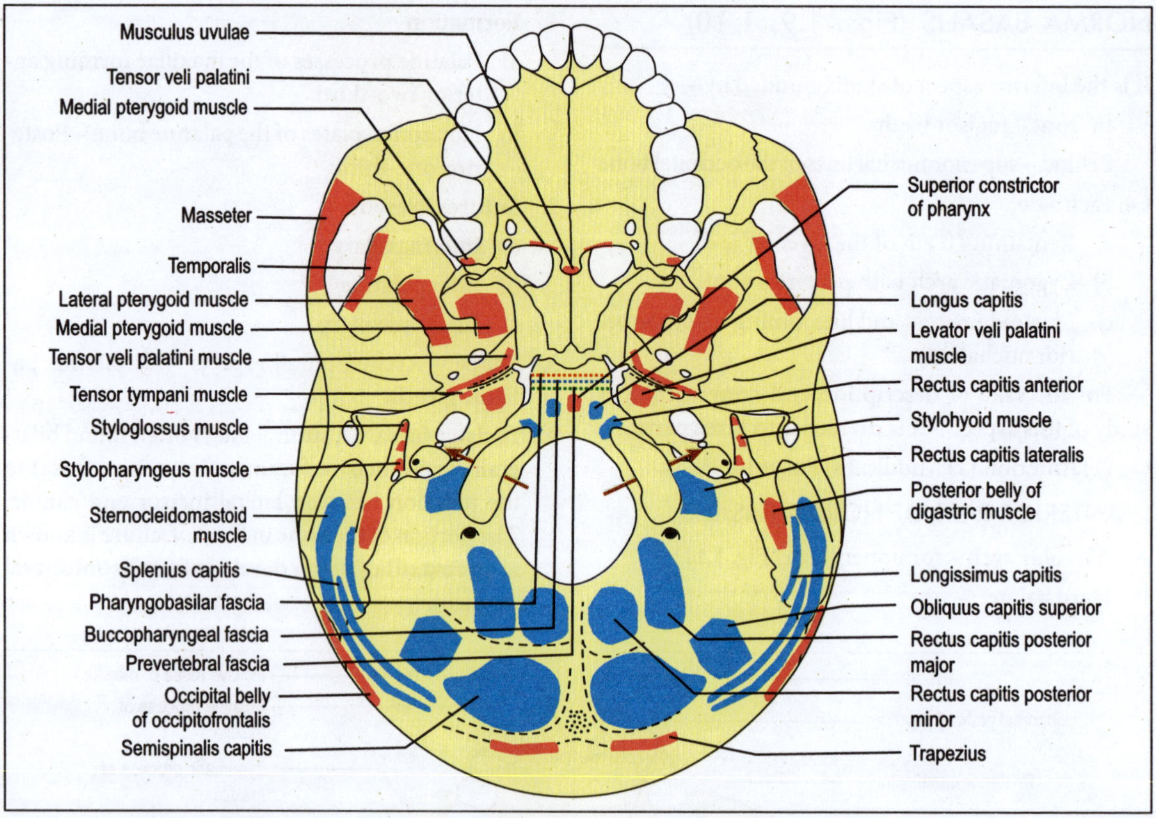

Fig. 1.10: Muscle and fascia attachments to the external surface of the base of the skull

Incisive canal is seen one on each side of fossa and opens in the nasal cavity. It transmits nasopalatine (long sphenopalatine) nerve and greater palatine vessels.

5. **Greater palatine foramen** – It is present in the posterolateral part of hard palate through which greater palatine vessels and nerve transmit. Greater palatine artery proceeds toward incisive foramen to reach the area of epistaxis in nasal septum. Greater palatine artery and nerve lie in the lateral part of the hard palate.
6. **Lesser palatine foramina** – Those foramina (1 to 3) situated behind greater palatine foramen and transmits lesser palatine nerve and vessels.
7. **Posterior nasal spine** – Medial end of posterior margin (horizontal plate of palatine bone) of hard palate form posterior nasal spine which gives attachment to musculus uvulae.
8. **Palatine crest** – It is present near the posterior margin of hard palate (horizontal plate of the palatine bone) and gives attachment to aponeurosis of tensor veli palatini muscle.

II. MIDDLE PART OF NORMA BASALIS

It is the part between posterior border of the hard palate in front and transverse imaginary line passing through anterior margin of foramen magnum behind on each side – Zygomatic arch.

Features of this part may be divided under two headings:

1. In the median area,
2. In the lateral areas (on each side),

1. ***In the median area (plane)***
   a) **Posterior border of vomer** separating two posterior nasal apertures.
   b) **Inferior border of vomer** articulating with bony palate.
   c) **Superior border** – Splits into two alae, articulating with rostrum of sphenoid.
   d) **Palatovaginal canal** (also known as pharyngeal canal) – formed by vaginal process of

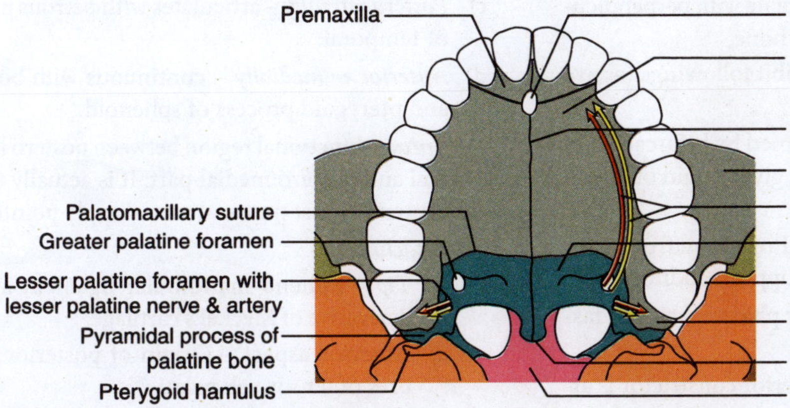

Fig. 1.11: Anterior part of the norma basalis

medial pterygoid plate with sphenoidal process of the palatine bone transmitting:

1. Pharyngeal branch of 3rd part of the maxillary artery.
2. Pharyngeal branch of the pterygopalatine ganglion.

e) **Vomerovaginal canal** – formed by ala of the vomer and vaginal process of the medial pterygoid plate.

f) **Broad bar of bone** – formed by union of body of sphenoid and basilar part of the occipital bone. It presents **pharyngeal tubercle** – In the median plane :

1. for attachment of fibrous raphe of pharynx.
2. in front – forms roof of pharynx and pharyngeal tonsil.
3. on each side – Insertion of longus capitis.
4. behind – Rectus capitis anterior.

In front of **pharyngeal tubercle** following structures are attached (before backwards):

(i) Pharyngobasilar fascia; (ii) Buccopharyngeal fascia; (iii) Prevertebral fascia.

2. ***In the lateral area***

It presents a) **Pterygoid process**; b) **Greater wing of the sphenoid**; c) **Inferior surface of petrous part** of temporal bone; d) **Squamous part of temporal bone**; and e) **Tympanic part of temporal bone.**

(a) Pterygoid process (features) (Fig. 1.26)

1. It descends perpendicularly at the junction of greater wing and body.
2. Each consist of medial and lateral plate. (Fig. 1.27)
3. **Upper parts of two plates are fused anteriorly** to form posterior wall of the pterygopalatine fossa, pierced by **anterior orifice of the pterygoid canal** which transmits:
   a) Artery of pterygoid canal (branch of 3rd part of the maxillary artery).
   b) **Nerve of pterygoid canal** – Formed by union of (i) greater petrosal nerve branch of facial nerve; (ii) deep petrosal nerve from sympathetic plexus around internal carotid artery.
4. **Pterygoid fossa** – Behind fused part of both plate, a depression, known as pterygoid fossa and **contain tensor veli palatine and medial pterygoid muscles.**
5. Pterygoid fissure – Lower ununited portions of both medial and lateral pterygoid plate forms an angular gap where pyramidal process of the palatine bone lie.

Medial pterygoid plate (Fig. 1.27)

It has two surfaces, two borders and vaginal process.

A. **Surfaces** – There are medial and lateral surface.forms lateral wall of nose and nasopharynx.
   i) **Medial surface** – Forms the lateral wall of posterior nasal aperture.
   ii) **Lateral surface** – Forms medial surface of pterygoid fossa and related to tensor veli palatini muscle.

B. **Borders** – Two borders: (i) anterior border and (ii) posterior border.

i) **Anterior border** – Articulate with perpendicular plate of the ethmoid bone.

ii) **Posterior border** – Exhibit followings (above downwards)

1. *Scaphoid fossa* – Formed by bifurcation of posterior border and gives origin of tensor veli palati muscle.
2. *Processus tubarius* – Projection from midpoint of this border supports auditory tube.
3. Whole of this border pharyngobasilar fascia is attached.
4. To its lower end superior constrictor is attached.
5. *Pterygoid hamulus* – A hook shaped process at the lower end of the medial pterygoid plate. Tendon of tensor veli palatini glides around it. Gives attachment to **pterygomandibular raphe** and superior constrictor of muscle.

C. **Vaginal process** – Medial pterygoid plate is prolonged above as vaginal process below the body of sphenoid.

Sphenoidal process of the palatine bone forms palatovaginal canal with vaginal process. **Palatovaginal canal transmit pharyngeal branches of maxillary artery (3rd part) and pterygopalatine ganglion.**

With alae of the vomer form vomerovaginal canal with vaginal process. (Fig. 1.28)

Lateral pterygoid plate

a) **Lateral surface** – Origin of lower head of lateral pterygoid. It forms medial wall of infratemporal fossa.

b) **Medial surface** – origin of medial pterygoid.

c) **Anterior border** – forms posterior margin of pterygomaxillary fissure.

d) **Posterior margin** – occasionally presents pterygospinous process – for attachment of pterygospinous ligament.

(b) Greater wing of sphenoid (features)

A. ***Infratemporal surface***

a) *Anteriorly* – forms posterior margin of the inferior orbital fissure.

b) *Antero-lateral part* – forms the infratemporal crest.

c) *Postero laterally* – articulates with petrous part of temporal.

d) *Anterior & medially* – continuous with body and pterygoid process of sphenoid.

e) ***Spine*** – Junctional region between postero lateral and postero medial part. It is actually the posterior most part and very sharply pointed.

Attachment –

i) *Tip* – Spheno-mandibular ligament and derivative of Meckel's cartilage.

ii) Anterior aspect – Origin of posterior fibres of tensor veli palati.

– Attachment fo anterior ligament of malleus.

Relations –

i) *Laterally* – auriculotemporal nerve.

ii) *Medially* – chorda tympani nerve and auditory tube.

f) *Surface (Infratemporal)* – origin of upper head of lateral pterygoid and crossed by deep temporal and massetric nerves.

B. ***Foramina present in the greater wing***

a) ***Foramen ovale*** – situated lateral to scaphoid fossa – Transmits.

1. **Mandibular nerve**
2. **Accessory meningeal artery**
3. **Lesser petrosal nerve**
4. **Emissary vein connecting cavernous sinus with pterygoid venous plexus.**

b) ***Foramen spinosum*** – situated lateral to foramen ovale – Transmits

1. Middle meningeal artery (branch of first part of maxillary artery).
2. Its accompanying veins (venous sinus).
3. Meningeal branch (nervous spinosus) branch from trunk of mandibular nerve.

c) Occasionally **emissary sphenoidal foramen (foramen of vesalius)** – Situated between foramen ovale and scaphoid fossa. Transmitting an emissary vein connecting cavernous sinus with pterygoid venous plexus.

d) Sometimes **canaliculus innominatus** is situated between foramen ovale and foramen spinosum – when present, transmits lesser petrosal nerve.

e) ***Sulcus tubae*** – a groove between posteromedial margin of greater wing and petrous part of temporal – lodges cartilaginous part of pharyngo-tympanic tube.

(c) Inferior surface of petrous part of temporal bone (features)

a) ***Foramen lacerum*** – wide canal about 1 cm. near the apex of petrous part – which forms postero lateral boundary.

Formation

Medially – Basilar part of occipital and body of sphenoid.

Anteriorly – Root of pterygoid process and greater wing.

Postero laterally – Apex of petrous part of the temporal bone structures passing through:

1. Meningeal branch of ascending pharyngeal artery;
2. Emissary vein from cavernous sinus.

These structures pass through a cartilage covering the foramen.

b) *Rough anterior part* – origin of levator veli palati.

c) *Carotid canal* – near the apex and transmits

1. Internal carotid artery
2. Venous and sympathetic plexus around artery.

(d) Squamous part (mandibular fossa) of temporal bone [Features]

a) *Squamotympanic fissure* with projected tegmen tympani within it. Tegmen tympani divides the fissure into petro squamous and petrotympanic fissure.

Contents of petrotympanic fissure

a) anterior ligament of malleus.

b) anterior tympanic branch of maxillary artery.

c) chorda tympani nerve – in the anterior canaliculus situated at the medial end of the fissure.

Features

a) *Mandibular fossa* – situated in most lateral part of the floor of middle cranial fossa.

b) *Tubercle of root of zygoma* – for lateral ligament of temporo mandibular joint.

(e) Tympanic part of temporal bone (tympanic plate) [Features]

Situated in the angle between petrous and squamous parts.

a) It forms a sheath of styloid process.

b) Its upper curved part forms anterior, floor and part of posterior wall of the external accoustic meatus.

c) It forms non articular part of articular fossa containing a part of parotid gland.

III. POSTERIOR PART OF NORMA BASALIS (Part behind the anterior margin of foramen magnum).

1. **Median area** and **areas near the midline** – it presents from before backwards–
   a) *Foramen magnum,*
   b) *External occipital crest,*
   c) *External occipital protuberance,*
   d) *Area between superior and inferior nuchal line,*
   c) *Area below the inferior nuchal line.*
2. **Lateral areas on each side presents:**
   a) *Hypoglossal canal,*
   b) *Jugular foramen,*
   c) *Structures in the inferior surface of petrous part of temporal bone.*
      i) *Canaliculus for tympanic nerve*
      ii) *Jugular fossa*
      iii) *Mastoid canaliculus*
      iv) *Styloid process*
      v) *Stylomastoid foramen*
   d) *Mastoid notch.*

(1) Median area and **areas near the midline**

a) *FORAMEN MAGNUM* (Fig. 1.20)

Structures transmitting –

Alar ligament divides the foramen into smaller anterior part and larger posterior parts.

Structure passing through the anterior part

1. Apical ligament (with odontoid process);
2. Upper band of cruciate ligament;
3. Membrana tectoria.

Structure passing through the posterior part

1. Lower end of medulla oblongata with meninges.
2. Sometimes tonsils of the cerebellum.

In the subarachnoid space:

3. Spinal accessory nerve
4. Vertebral arteries (4th part)
5. Sympathetic plexus around the arteries
6. Posterior spinal arteries
7. Anterior spinal artery.

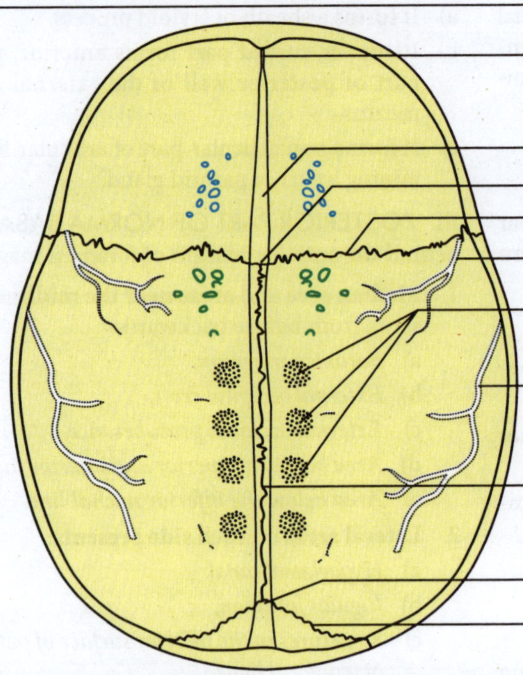

Fig. 1.12: Internal surface of the cranial vault (Calvaria)

[Attachments in the margins of the foramen:

Anterior margin – Anterior atlanto occipital membrane.

Posterior margin – Posterior atlanto occipital membrane.

Rough area: on the medial aspect of condyle – Alar ligaments.]

1\. b) EXTERNAL OCCIPITAL CREST – attachment of ligamentum nuchae.

1\. c) EXTERNAL OCCIPITAL PROTUBERANCE – origin of trapezius and beginning of ligamentum nuchae.

1\. d) AREA BETWEEN SUPERIOR AND INFERIOR NUCHAL LINES:

Insertion to:

a) Semispinalis capitis (medially)

b) Obliquus superior (laterally)

1\. e) AREA BELOW INFERIOR NUCHAL LINE:

Insertion to:

a) Rectus capitis posterior minor (medially)

b) Rectus capitis posterior major (laterally).

(2) Lateral area on each side

a) HYPOGLOSSAL CANAL:

Transmits –

1. Hypoglossal nerve;
2. Meningeal branch of ascending pharyngeal artery;
3. Emissary vein connecting basilar venous plexus; or connecting sigmoid sinus with internal jugular vein.
4. Meningeal branch of hypoglossal nerve.

b) JUGULAR FORAMEN (Fig. 20.21)

Transmits – Three compartments:

Through anterior –

1. Inferior petrosal sinus
2. Meningeal branch of ascending pharyngeal artery.

Through the middle – IXth, Xth & XIth cranial nerves.

Through the posterior – a) Sigmoid sinus continued as internal jugular vein; b) Meningeal branch of occipital artery.

c) STRUCTURES IN THE INFERIOR SURFACE OF PETROUS PART OF THE TEMPORAL BONE:

i) **Canaliculus for tympanic nerve** – It transmits tympanic branch of glossopharyngeal nerve.

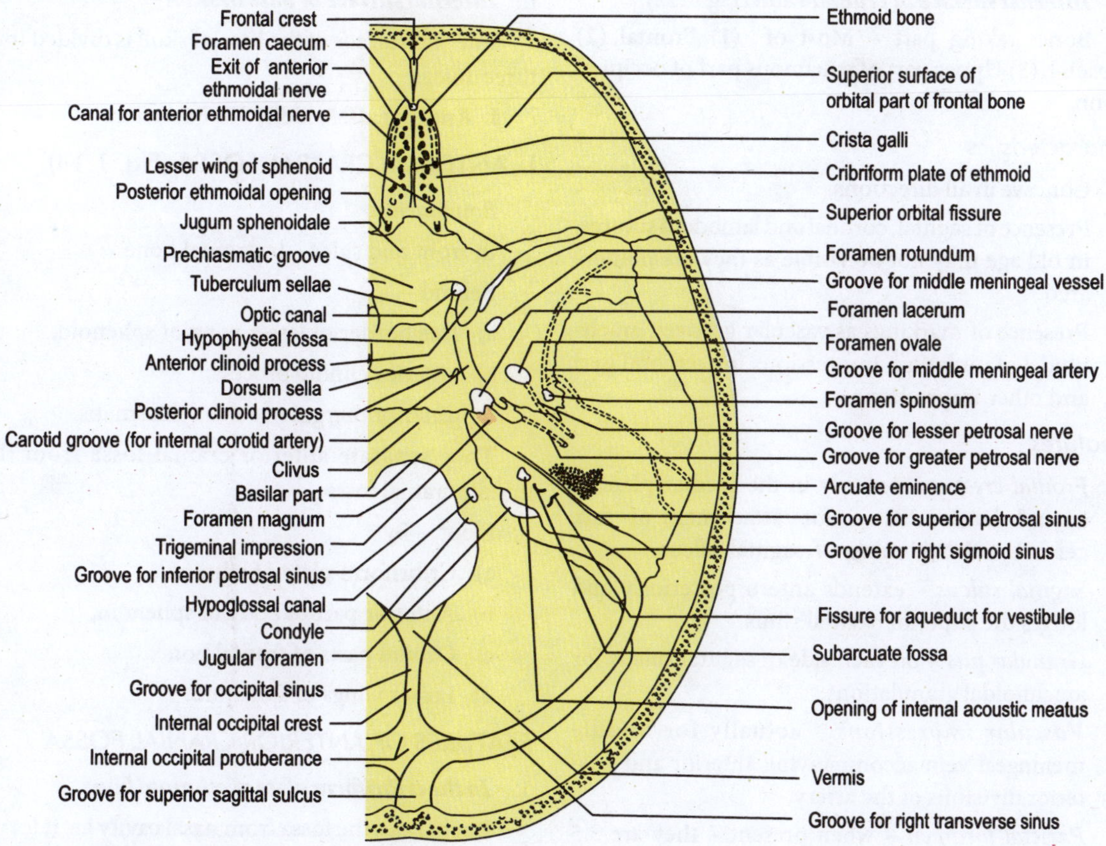

Fig. 1.13: Internal surface of the base of the skull

ii) **Jugular fossa** – It lodges superior jugular bulb of internal jugular vein.

iii) **Mastoid canaliculus** – It transmits auricular branch of vagus nerve.

iv) **Styloid process** – Refer page 7.

v) **Stylomastoid foramen** – It transmits facial nerve (exit) and stylomastoid branch of posterior auricular artery.

d) MASTOID NOTCH – Medial to mastoid process – **Origin of posterior belly of digastric** and medial to notch – a groove for occipital artery.

INTERIOR OF CRANIUM

The following characteristics should be kept in mind before study of the features of interior:

1. **Covering of bones:**
   a) Endosteum – Internal lining of the cranium (endosteal layer of dura).
   b) Pericranium – Outer lining of the cranium.

   Both are continuous with each other through foramen and sutures.
2. Bones are thinner in female than male.
3. Majority of the bones consist of :
   a) Outer compact (Table) and
   b) Inner compact (Table) and in between them
   c) Spongy bone filled with marrow substance known as diploe.

Interior of cranium is described under two parts:

I. **Internal surface of skull cap or cranial vault.** (Fig. 1.12)

II. **Internal surface of the base of skull.** (Fig. 1.13)

I. ***Internal surface of cranial vault*** (Fig. 1.12)

Bones taking part – Most of : (1) Frontal, (2) Parietal, (3) Upper part of squamous part of occipital bone.

Characteristics

1. Concave in all directions.
2. Presence of sagittal, coronal and lambdoid sutures, in old age may not be visible as they are obliterated.
3. Presence of markings as vascular grooves, arachnoidal granulation, impressions for cerebral gyri and other impressions.

Features

1. *Frontal crest* – anteriorly in the median plane – extend backwards – for attachment of falx cerebri and beginning of sagittal sulcus.
2. *Sagittal sulcus* – extends antero posteriorly and lodges the superior sagittal sinus.
3. *Granular pits* – on each side of sagittal sulcus for arachnoidal granulations.
4. *Vascular impressions* – actually for middle meningeal vein accompanying anterior and posterior divisions of the artery.
5. *Parietal foramen* – when present – they are 3.5 cms in front of lambdoid suture near the sagittal sulcus.
6. Impressions for cerebral gyri.
7. Sutures – (a) coronal, (b) sagittal, (c) lambdoid.

II. ***Internal surface of base of skull***

Internal surface of the base of skull is divided into three fossa:

I. Anterior, II. Middle, III. Posterior.

I. ANTERIOR CRANIAL FOSSA (Fig. 1.14)

Boundaries:

In front and sides – by frontal bone

Behind –

a) free border of lesser wing of sphenoid,
b) anterior clinoid process,
c) anterior margin of sulcus chiasmatis.

They separate anterior cranial fossa from the middle cranial fossa.

Floor – By

a) Cribriform plate of ethmoid,
b) Anterior part of body of sphenoid,
c) Orbital parts of frontal bone,
d) Lesser wings of sphenoid.

FEATURES OF ANTERIOR CRANIAL FOSSA

1. ***In the cribriform plate of ethmoid bone***

It separates the fossa from nasal cavity i.e. it forms the roof.

a) *Crista galli* – a crest like elevation for attachment of falx cerebri, and on each side of crista galli olfactory bulb is related.

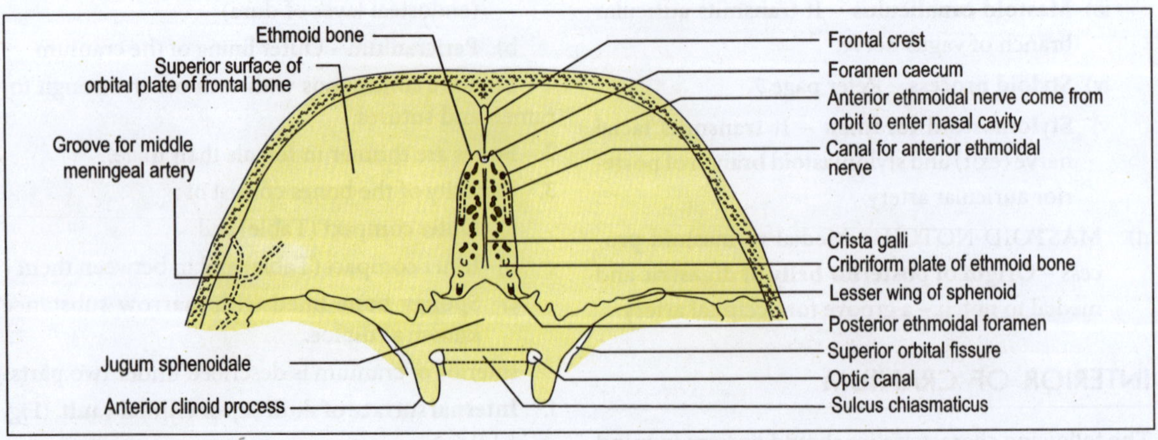

Fig. 1.14: Anterior cranial fossa

b) *Foramen caecum* – A small foramen in front of crista galli – for transmitting veins of the nose to superior sagittal sinus.

c) *Anterior ethmoidal canal* – behind and on each side of crista galli and transmit anterior ethmoidal nerve and vessels.

(Anterior ethmoidal nerve is a continuation of nasociliary nerve and posterior ethmoidal nerve is a branch of nasociliary, near the medial wall of orbit).

d) *Posterior ethmoidal foramen* – at the posterior-lateral part of the cribriform plate area – transmit posterior ethmoidal nerve and vessels.

e) *Numerous foramina in the cribriform plate* – for olfactory nerves (15 to 20 in number) terminating in olfactory bulb which also is situated on each side of crista galli.

2. ***Anterior part of body of sphenoid bone*:**

a) *Jugum sphenoidale* – It separates the fossa from sphenoidal air sinus. It lodges gyrus rectus and olfactory tract.

b) *Sulcus chiasmaticus* – lodges optic chiasma.

3. ***Orbital part of the frontal bone*:**

a) Impressions for cerebral gyri and supports inferior surface of frontal lobe.

b) It separates anterior cranial fossa from orbit and anterior ethmoidal sinuses.

c) Vascular impressions for meningeal vessels.

d) In front of cribriform plate – frontal crest.

4. ***Lesser wing of sphenoid bone*:**

a) *Posterior free border* – related with stem of lateral sulcus of brain.

b) *Anterior clinoid process* – prominent projection postero-medially – for attachment of free margin of tentorium cerebelli.

c) *Anterior* and *posterior roots* enclosing *optic canal* – transmitting optic nerve and ophthalmic artery.

d) It forms upper boundary of superior orbital fissure.

II. *MIDDLE CRANIAL FOSSA* (Fig. 1.15)

Boundaries:

In Front –

a) Posterior border of lesser wing,

b) Anterior clinoid process,

c) Anterior margin of sulcus chiasmaticus.

Behind –

a) Superior border of petrous temporal,

b) Dorsum sellae of sphenoid.

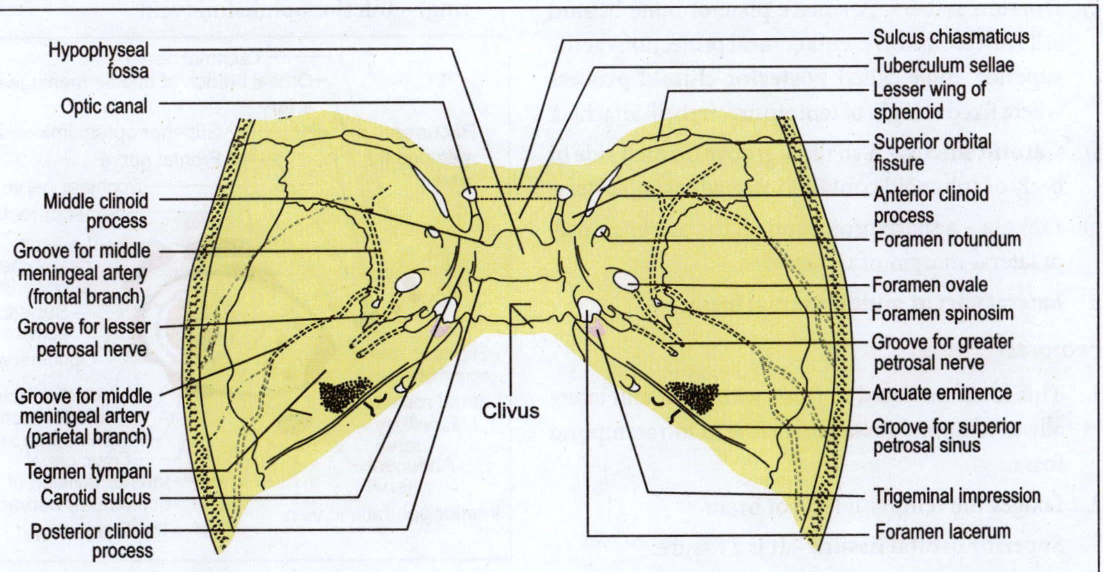

Fig. 1.15: Middle cranial fossa

On each side –

a) Greater wing of sphenoid,

b) Antero inferior angle of parietal,

c) Squamous part of temporal bone.

Bones taking part in the fossa or floor

1. Central part or median part by body of sphenoid.
2. Lateral part on each side:
   A. *Greater wing of sphenoid.*
   B. *Petrous part of temporal bone.*
   C. *Squamous part of temporal.*

1. **Central or median part**

Features

a) **Sulcus chiasmaticus** – It lodges optic chiasma. This sulcus leads to optic canal (which transmit optic nerve and ophthalmic artery) on each side.

b) **Tuberculum sellae** – It is an elevation behind sulcus chiasmaticus.

c) **Middle clinoid process** – Two projections from tuberculum sellae.

d) **Sella turcica** – A depressed area behind tuberculum sellae.

Hypophyseal fossa – Deepest part of sella turcica which lodges hypophysis cerebri.

e) **Dorsum sellae** – A square plate of bone behind sella turcica and presents conical projections at the superior angle called **posterior clinoid process** where fixed margin of tentorium cerebelli attached.

f) **Carotid sulcus** – A shallow groove on each side of body of sphenoid contains internal carotid artery.

g) **Lingula** – a sharp projection on the posterior part of lateral margin of the groove.

2. **Lateral part of middle cranial fossa**

Features

1. This fossa is related in front with orbit and laterally to temporal fossa and below to infratemporal fossa.
2. Lodges the temporal lobe of brain.
3. **Superior orbital fissure** – It is a fissure:
   i) Communication between anterior part of middle cranial fossa with the orbit.
   ii) Boundary – Above – Lesser wing
   Below – Greater wing
   Medially – Body of sphenoid
   iii) Medial part is wider than lateral
   iv) Long axis – directed upwards, laterally and forwards.

It is divided into three parts by common tendinous ring into (a) Middle part; (b) Lateral part; and (c) Medial part.

Structures transmitted through the fissure:

a) ***Middle part*** – (within common tendinous ring)

i) Superior and inferior divisions of oculomotor nerve.

ii) Nasociliary nerve in between divisions of oculomotor nerve.

iii) Abducent nerve – Lateral to inferior division of oculomotor nerve.

b) ***Lateral part*** – From medial to lateral (outside of the common tendinous ring)

i) Trochlear nerve (Fig. 1.16)

ii) Frontal nerve

iii) Lacrimal nerve.

Besides –

iv) Recurrent meningeal branch of lacrimal artery.

v) Orbital branch of middle meningeal artery

vi) Superior ophthalmic vein

c) ***Medial part*** (outside of the common tendinous ring) – Inferior ophthalmic vein

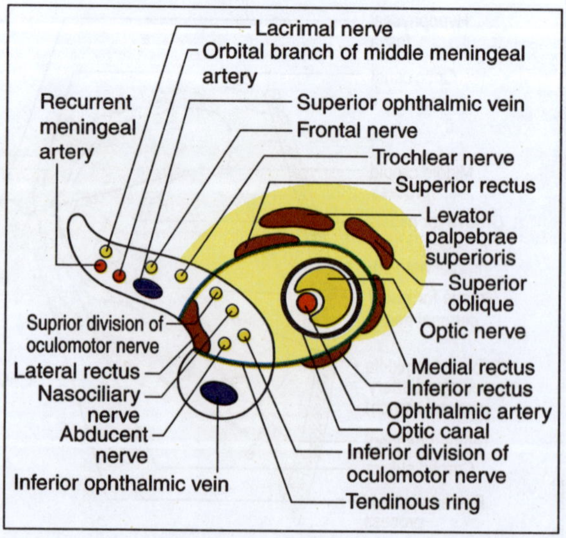

Fig. 1.16: Structures passing through superior orbital fissure & optic canal.

A. **GREATER WING OF SPHENOID**

Features:

1. **Foramen rotundum** – Situated below and medial to superior orbital fissure – transmits maxillary nerve to pterygopalatine fossa.
2. **Foramen ovale** – Refer page 12.
3. **Foramen spinosum** – situated postero-lateral to foramen ovale and in the spine of sphenoid bone.

   Refer page 12.
4. Grooves for middle meningeal vessels.

   Other Features:
5. **Foramen lacerum** – situated postero-medial to foramen ovale and at the posterior end of carotid sulcus – (Refer page 12)
6. **Emissary sphenoidal foramen** (Foramen of Vesalius) – Refer page 12.
7. **Canaliculus innominatus** – Refer page 12

B. **PETROUS PART OF TEMPORAL BONE**

Features:

1. **Trigeminal impression** – Situated near the apex of petrous part and behind foramen lacerum – lodges (a) *Trigeminal* (Gasserian) ganglion within dural cave (Meckel's cave). Between bone and ganglion (b) *Mandibular nerve* (Motor root), (c) *Greater petrosal nerve.*
2. Hiatus and groove for greater petrosal nerve.
3. Hiatus and groove for lesser petrosal nerve – Lateral to above hiatus.
4. **Arcuate eminence** – Lateral to above hiatuses – It is due to superior semi-circular canal.
5. **Tegmen tympani** – Thin plate of bone antero-lateral to arcuate eminence. It forms roof of following:

   (a) Tympanic antrum, (b) Tympanic cavity and (c) Canal for tensor tympani muscle.

   It divides squamotympanic fissure into petrosquamous and petrotympanic fissure.

   Tegmen tympani is a part of petrous temporal bone

   Petrotympanic fissure – refer page 13.
6. **Superior border of petrous part of temporal bone**

   a) groove – for superior petrosal sinus

   b) attachment of attached margin of the tentorium cerebelli

   c) crossing of branches of trigeminal nerve

C. **SQUAMOUS PART OF OCCIPITAL BONE**

Features:

a) Impressions of cerebral gyri of temporal lobe.

b) Grooves for middle meningeal vessels.

III. POSTERIOR CRANIAL FOSSA (Fig. 1.17)

Deepest of three cranial fossae.

Boundary:

In front –

a) superior border of petrous part of temporal.

b) posterior clinoid process and dorsum sellae of sphenoid.

Behind – Squamous part of occipital.

On each side –

a) Mastoid part of temporal.

b) Postero inferior angle of parietal.

Floor – Bones contributing to form the fossa.

I. In the central or median area – By

A) Clivus in front;

B) Squamous part of occipital.

II. In the lateral area (on each side)

A) Condylar part of occipital bone.

B) Posterior surface of petrous part of temporal.

C) Mastoid part of temporal bone.

D) Squamous part of occipital.

Contents of the fossa:

Parts of the hind brain which consists of (a) pons and (b) medulla, in front and (c) cerebellum – behind.

I. ***Central or median area***

Features

A. ***Clivus in front*** –

i) *Clivus* – a sloping surface formed by fused parts of (a) posterior part of body of sphenoid and (b) basilar part of occipital bone.

Relation:

ii) Basilar plexus of veins.

iii) Basilar artery (formed by the union of two vertebral arteries).

iv) Supports pons and medulla oblongata

Structures attached to lower part of clivus or area just in front of anterior margin of foramen magnum.

From front, backwards –

a) Membrana tectoria
b) Upper band of cruciate ligament
c) Apical ligament (remnant of notochord – other remnant is nucleus pulposus of intervertebral disc).
d) Anterior atlanto occipital membrane. (Fig. 1.19)

B. ***Squamous part of occipital bone***

1. *Internal occipital crest* – Extends from Internal occipital protuberance to margin of foramen magnum in the median plane – for attachment of (a) falx cerebelli containing (b)occipital sinus.
2. *Internal occipital protuberance* – A projection in the median plane just opposite to external occipital protuberance – related to confluence of sinuses.
3. *Transverse sulcus* – wide sulcus running laterally from the internal occipital protuberance to antero-inferior angle of parietal bone and continuous with sigmoid sulcus. It lodges *transverse sinus.* Attachment of attached margins of *tentorium cerebelli.* (Fig. 1.19)
4. *Vermian fossa* – It is a triangular depression in he midline in the squamous part of the occipital bone. Inferior vermis of cerebellum is related here.

II. **Lateral Area** (On each side of fossa)

A. ***Condylar part of occipital bone*** –

1. *Jugular tubercle* – groove for 9th, 10th and 11th cranial nerves.
2. *Hypoglossal canal* (Anterior condylar canal) – Situated below and behind the jugular tubercle. Transmits – Refer page 14.
3. *Condylar canal* (also called posterior condylar canal)

Transmits – emissary vein from sigmoid sinus.

B. ***Posterior surface of petrous part of temporal bone.*** It forms front and lateral part of posterior cranial fossa.

Features

1. *Jugular foramen* – formed by jugular notch of occipital bone below and behind and deep jugular notch of petrous part of temporal bone. Above and in front – structures passing through: Three compartments – refer page 14.
2. *Internal acoustic meatus* – Situated above the anterior part of jugular foramen. It is closed laterally by lamina cribrosa (a perforated lamina of bone) which separates the meatus from internal ear.

Transmits –

a) Motor and sensory roots of facial nerve,
b) Vestibulo cochlear nerve,
c) Internal accoustic (labyrinthine) branch of basilar artery with vein.

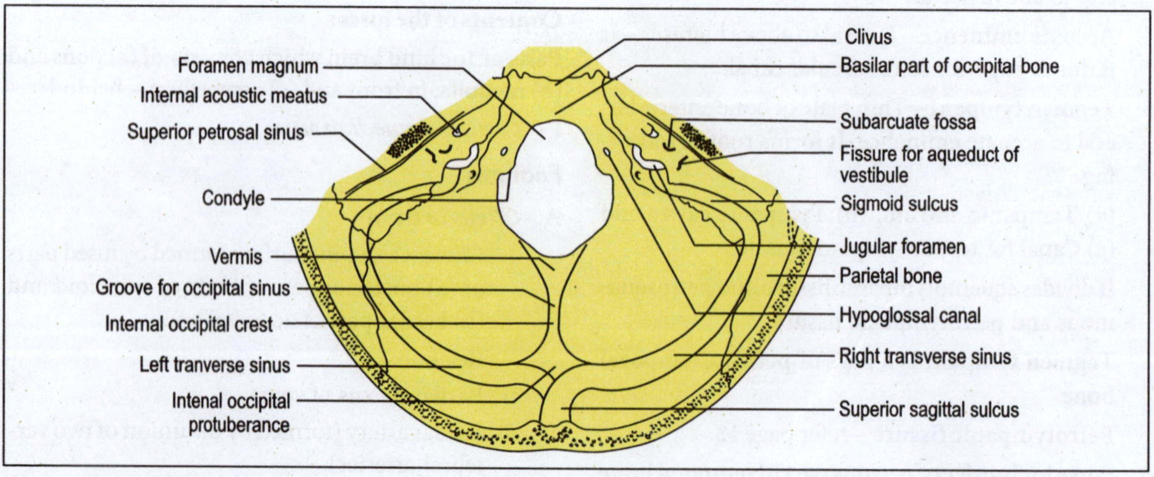

Fig. 1.17: Posterior cranial fossa

3. *Opening of aqueduct of vestibule* – a narrow slit behind the meatus – contains.
   a) saccus and ductus endolymphaticus,
   b) a small artery and vein,
4. *Subarcuate fossa* – It lies between aforesaid structures. It lodges process of dura mater.

C. ***Mastoid part of temporal bone*** – forming lateral wall of the fossa.

Features

1. *Sigmoid sulcus* – situated in front of this part of fossa. It is a downward continuation of transverse sulcus at the postero inferior (Mastoid) angle of parietal bone and ends at the jugular foramen.
   Lodges – *Sigmoid sinus* which is continued as *internal* jugular vein. *Related* – In front to *mastoid antrum.*
2. *Mastoid foramen* – Situated in front part of the sulcus near the posterior margin.
   Transmits –
   a) Emissary vein from the sigmoid sinus
   b) Meningeal branch of occipital artery

D. ***Squamous part of occipital bone*** –
1. Four fossae –
   Upper two – triangular – for occipital lobe
   Lower two – quadrangular – for cerebellum

Applied Aspects of Different Cranial Fossae

I. *Fracture of anterior cranial fossa* – may result in
   a) Black eye,
   b) Bleeding through nose,
   c) Discharge of cerebrospinal fluid through nose.

II. *Fracture of middle cranial fossa* – it may usually result in:
   a) Bleeding through ear,
   b) Discharge of C.S.F. through ear,
   c) When it involves sphenoid bone – there may be bleeding per nose or mouth,
   d) Injury to facial and vestibulo cochlear nerve if Internal accoustic meatus is involved,
   e) *Vertigo* may appear due to damage of semicircular canal.

Usual line of fracture in the Middle Cranial Fossa

Line from parietal eminence passing through parietal bone, squamous part of temporal, petrous part usually involving internal accoustic meatus.

III. *Fracture of posterior cranial fossa* – It usually forms a bruise over mastoid process spreading to sternocleidomastoid.

Factors usually preventing the fracture of skull

a) Elasticity and number of elastic arches in a single bone.
b) Shape – Round.
c) Covering muscles.

Sites and Reasons of fracture

a) It is the base of skull which is commonly fractured, because the base of skull is more fragile than the vault.
b) Inner table is more commonly injured – Why?

As the inner table is more brittle than the outer table so fracture or injury is more extensive than the outer table and usually limited to inner table.

Common sites of injury (fracture) of skull

a) In the vault – Parietal area.
b) In the base of skull – Middle cranial fossa – because of presence of so many foramina which weaken the bone.

Most common injury to facial bones

Nasal bone.

B. OCCIPITAL BONE

Anatomical Position

Bone should be held in such a manner so that:

1. Basilar part (quadrilateral plate of bone) should be directed forwards and upward; concavily of squamous part (backward and upward) forwards and convexity backwards.
2. Occipital condyles (oval articular processes) on each side of foramen magnum directed downwards.
3. Foramen magnum (large oval foramen) should be situated in front and lower part must be horizontal and parallel to the ground.

TABLE 1.4 : Different Parts of Occipital Bone

Parts of occipital bone

- Squamous (Behind and above foramen magnum)
- Basilar (Quadrilateral part in front of foramen magnum)
- Foramen magnum → Large oval foramen
- Two condylar parts → (Two lateral parts on each side of foramen magnum)

Squamous:

- Surfaces (Two)
- Angles (Three)
  - Superior forms lambda by two parietal bone and one occipital bone
  - Two lateral forms asterion between parietal and mastoid temporal bone
- Borders (Four)
  - Two lambdoid parietal bone articulate
  - Articulation between jugular process occipital bone and mastoid temporal bone

Surfaces:

External

a) External occipital protuberance
   An elevated prominence in the midway between superior angle and foramen magnum
   – Refer page 3

b) External occipital crest – It is a median crest extending from external occipital protuberance to margin of foramen magnum and ligamentum nuchae is attached

c) Highest nuchal lines – A faint line extend laterally from external occipital protuberance
   – Refer page 3

d) Superior nuchal lines – About 1cm below the above line, a prominent ridge extend laterally from external occipital protuberance
   – Refer page 3

e) Inferior nuchal lines – It runs laterally from midpoint of external occipital crest

f) Area between superior & inferior nuchal lines
   – Refer page 14

g) Area below inferior nuchal line (Fig. 1.18)
   – Refer page 14

Internal

a) Four fossae –
   1. Upper (two) – Triangular – for occipital lobes of cerebral hemisphere
   2. Lower (two) – Quadrangular – for cerebellar hemisphere

b) Internal occipital protuberance – A bony elevation close to the centre
   – Related to confluence of sinuses and posterior part of superior sagittal sinus

c) Internal occipital crest – A prominent ridge extends from internal occipital protuberance to the margin of foramen magnum
   – Attached: (a) Falx cerebelli containing occipital venous sinus

d) Vermian fossa – It is triangular depression in midline near foramen magnum and inferior vermis of cerebellum is related to this area

e) Transverse sulci – Margins of sulcus (extend laterally from internal occipital protuberance) gives attachment to attached margins of tentorium cerebelli containing transverse sinus

f) Sagittal sulcus – Margins of superior sagittal sulcus gives attachment to falx cerebri containing superior sagittal sinus (Fig. 1.19)

Confluence of sinus is formed by superior, occipital, right and left transverse and straight sinus. Right transverse sinus is usually the continuation of superior sagittal and left transverse is that of straight sinus. Confluence of sinus is located at the internal occipital protuberance.

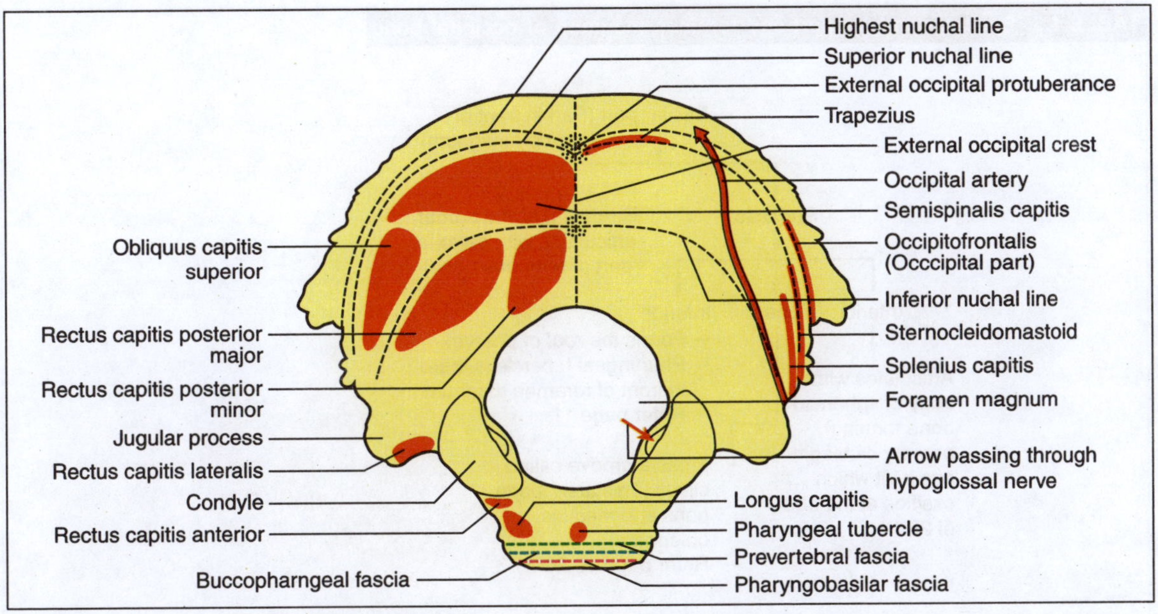

Fig. 1.18: External surface of the occipital bone

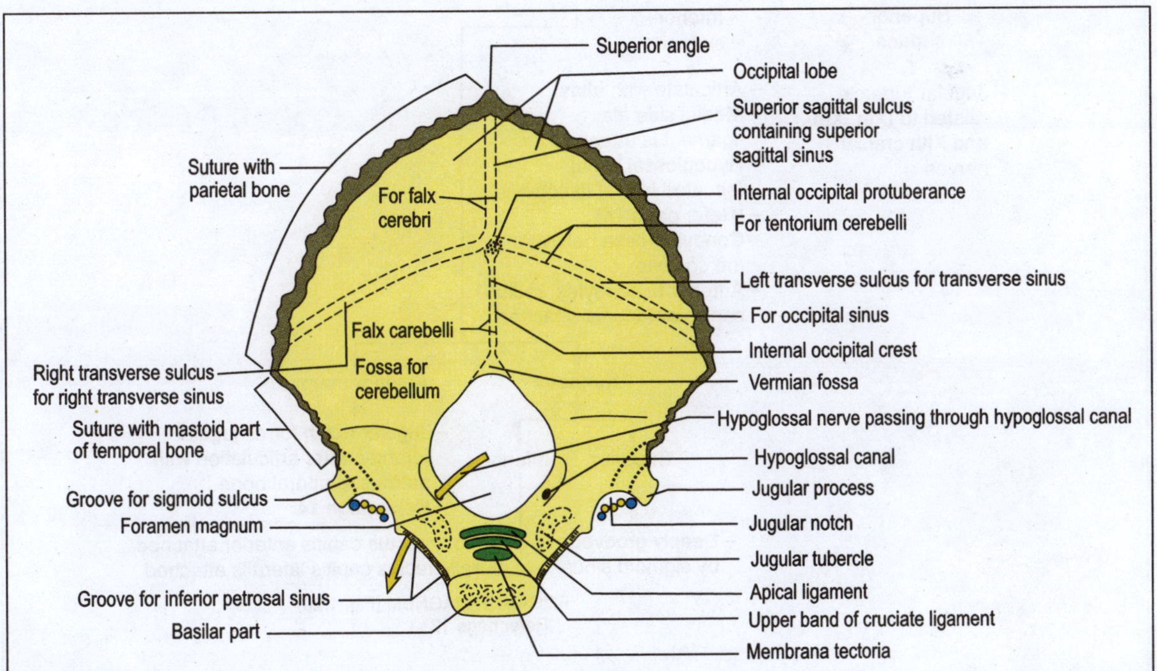

Fig. 1.19: Internal surface of the occipital bone

TABLE 1.5: Basilar, condylar part and foramen magnum of occipital bone

- **Basilar part (Part in front of foramen magnum)**
  - Surfaces
    - Anterior
      - Articulates with body of sphenoid bone forming primary cartilaginous joint which ossifies at the age of 25
    - Superior
      - It has a groove called clivus (This area lodge pons and medulla oblongata)
      - Refer page 19-20
    - Inferior
      - Forms the roof of pharynx
      - Pharyngeal tubercle is there in front of foramen magnum
      - Refer page 11
  - Borders (Lateral border articulates with petrous part of temporal bone)

- **Condylar part**
  - Medial part or occipital condyles
    - Superior surface
      - Jugular tubercle related to IXth, Xth and XIth cranial nerves
    - Inferior surface
      - Articulate with atlas
      - Medial side alar ligament is attached
      - Hypoglossal canal (situated lateral to condyle)
      - (Refer page 14)
      - Condylar fossa behind the condyle
      - Anterior to condyles, rectus capitis anterior is attached
  - Jugular process or lateral part
    - Surfaces
      - Superior
        - Deeply grooved by sigmoid sinus
      - Inferior
        - Anteriorly rectus capitis anterior attached
        - Laterally rectus capitis lateralis attached
    - Anterior margin
      - Jugular notch forms jugular foramen after articulation with petrous temporal bone
      - Refer page 14

FORAMEN MAGNUM (Fig. 1.20)
- Refer page 13

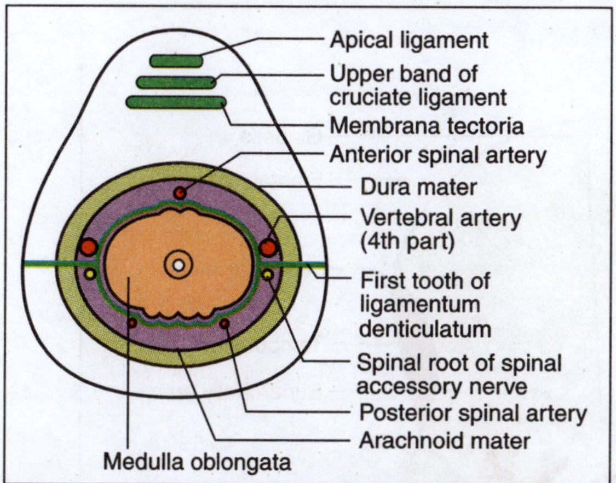

Fig. 1.20: Structures passing through foramen magnum

TABLE 1.6: Ossification of Occipital Bone

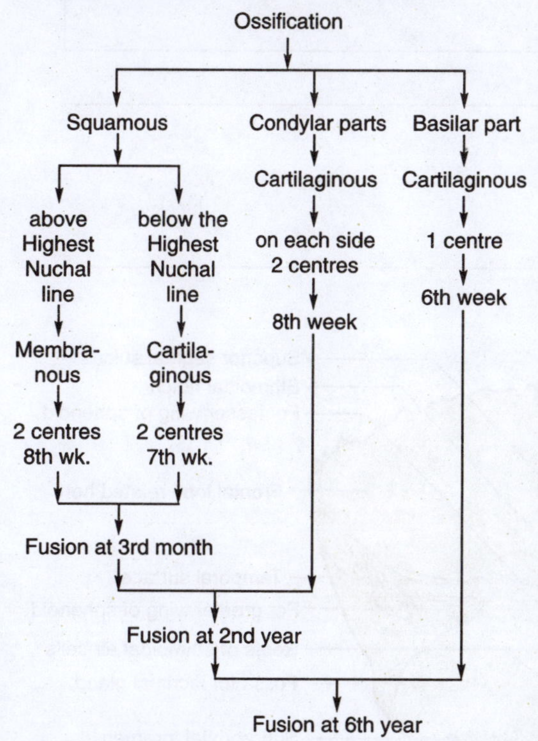

Important points

1. **Obstetrical hinge joint of budin** – At birth the *Junctional region between squamous* and condylar parts is cartilaginous and is known as *obstetrical hinge joint of Budin*. It plays an important role during the process of labour by moulding.

C. FRONTAL BONE

It forms forehead, roof of the orbit and a major part of anterior cranial fossa. It is cock-shell in shape.

Anatomical Position

It should be held in such a manner so that:

a) Squamous part is vertical and convex forwards.
b) Orbital plates will project backwards and downwards.
c) Nasal spine will be directed downwards and slightly forwards.

Three Parts:

(i) Squamous, (ii) Orbital, (iii) Nasal.

Squamous

Three surfaces:

(i) External, (ii) Internal, (iii) Temporal.

Borders – two:

(i) Upper (Parietal), (ii) Lower (Orbital).

I. **External surface** – Smooth and convex and presents the following features: (Fig. 1.21)
   1. Frontal eminence
   2. Superciliary arches
   3. Supra orbital margin
   4. Zygomatic process
   5. Metopic suture
   6. Temporal line

II. **Internal Surface** – It is concave. (Fig. 1.22)

III. **Temporal surface**

Ossification

1. Two primary centres appearing about 8th week of intrauterine life in the region of superciliary arch. It forms two halves of bone. It spreads upwards to form squamous part, backwards for orbital plate and downwards for nasal part.
2. 2 secondary centres may appear at the nasal spine. Two halves begin to fuse at the 2nd year from the upper part and usually completes by 8th year. There may be complete persistence of frontal suture. In 9% cases lower part of frontal suture may persist. (What is Wormian bone? A sutural bone and it may be found either in upper or lower part of frontal suture). It may be found in any suture of the skull).

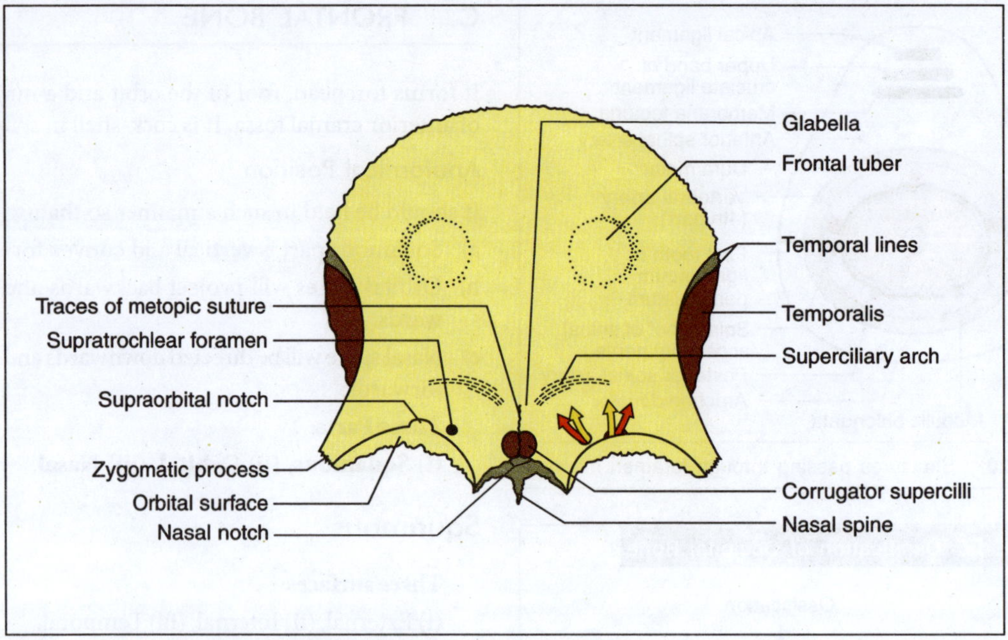

Fig. 1.21: External surface of the frontal bone

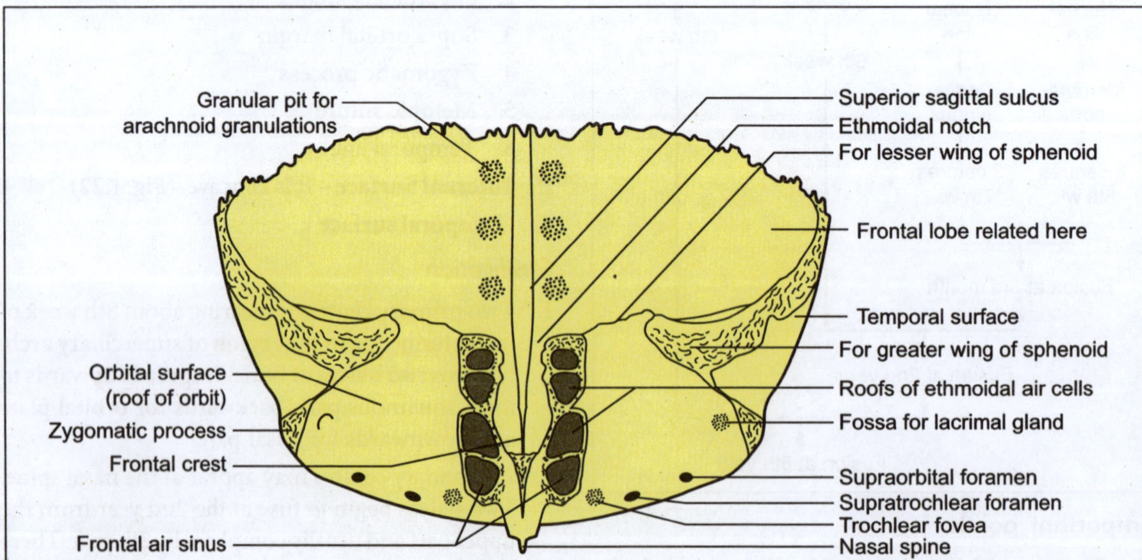

Fig. 1.22: Internal surface of the frontal bone

TABLE 1.7: Different Parts of Frontal Bone

Parts of frontal bone

- **Squamous**
  - Surfaces
    - Outer or External
      1. **Superciliary arches** Refer page 4
      2. **Glabella** Refer page 4
      3. **Supraorbital margin** Refer page 4
      4. **Supraorbital foramen** Refer page 4
      5. **Frontal eminence** Refer page 4
      6. **Supratrochlear notch** Refer page 4
      7. Metopic suture
         - Sometimes present
         - Its presence prove that frontal bone develop from two halves which unite later on
    - Internal or Cerebral
      1. **Superior sagittal sulcus**
         - Margin gives attachment to falx cerebri and lodges superior sagittal sinus
      2. **Frontal crest**
         - Gives attachment to falx cerebri
      3. **Foramen caecum**
         - Present in relation to frontal crest in articulated skull
         - Transmit an emissary vein to superior sagittal sinus
      4. **Granular pits**
         - Lodges arachnoid granulations
      5. Related to frontal lobe of cerebrum on each side of median plane
  - Borders
    - Articulate with parietal bone
- **Nasal part**
  - Nasal notch articulate with nasal bone, lacrimal bone and maxilla
  - Nasal spine articulate with perpendicular plate of ethmoid to form nasal septum
- **Zygomatic process (two)**
  - Articulate with zygomatic bone,
  - From posterior margin, temporal line starts and after proceeding superolaterally the line divides into superior & inferior temporal lines
- **Orbital plate**
  - Surface
    - Superior or Internal or Cerebral
      - Orbital surface of frontal lobe of cerebrum is related
    - Inferior or Orbital surface
      - Forms the roof of the orbital cavity and presents
        1. **Fossa for lacrimal gland** in the antero-lateral part
        2. **Trochlear fovea**: Pully for superior oblique muscle of eyeball is attached in this area which is present in the anteromedial part of this surface
  - Border
    - Articulate with greater wing of sphenoid
- **Ethmoidal notch**
  - To accommodate cribriform plate of ehtmoid Form anterior & posteiror ethmoidal canal for transmitting corresponding nerve & vessels
  - Frontal air sinus opens in the infundibulum of middle meatus of nasal cavity

D. PARIETAL BONE

Parietal bones are two in number and form major part of vault of skull and situated behind frontal, in front of occipital and above temporal bones. Each bone is quadrilateral in shape.

Anatomical position and side determination

Bone should be held in such a manner so that:

1. Convex and smooth (external) surface will be outwards and concave (internal) surface inwards.
2. Pointed angle (antero-inferior angle) and the inner surface of which presents grooves for anterior division of middle meningeal vessels will direct forwards and downwards.
3. Right angled angle is antero superior angle and the angle whose inner surface presents groove for sigmoid sinus is postero inferior angle and direct downwards and backwards.
4. Thick serrated straight border is the superior border and will look above and to the medium plane and arched border looks downwards and is the inferior border.
5. Convex external surface will direct to the side it belongs.

TABLE 1.8: Different parts of Parietal bone

Parietal bone (Quadrilateral bone)

Surfaces (Two)

External (outer)
- Convex
- Following features:
1. **Parietal tuberosity**– Most prominent part
2. **Superior & Inferior temporal lines** – Refer pages 2, 5 & 6
3. **Parietal foramen** – Sometimes near superior border & 2" in front of postero-superior angle and transmit a vein from superior sagittal sinus and a branch of occipital artery

Internal surface
- Concave & pitted; and presents:
1. **Sagittal sulcus** – Longitudinal groove along the superior sagittal border which lodges superior sagittal sinus
   - Lateral margin of the sulcus gives attachment to falx cerebri
2. **Groove for middle meningeal vessels** – Groove near the anteroinferior angle is formed by anterior division of middle meningeal
   - Grooves near the posteroinferior part is due to posterior division of middle meningeal artery
   - Grooves are usually formed by veins
3. **Granular pits** near the superior sagittal sulcus lodge arachnoid granulations
4. **Impression for cerebral gyri** – All the four lobes of cerebral hemisphere are related here; part of central sulcus & posterior ramus of lateral sulcus is related here
5. **Groove near posteroinferior angle**
   - Lodges sigmoid sinus

Borders (Four)

Superior or sagittal
Articulates with opposite parietal bone to form **sagittal suture**

Inferior or squamosal
Articulates with
a) Greater wing of sphenoid in front
b) Squamous temporal in the middle
c) Mastoid temporal posteriorly

Anterior or frontal
Articulate with frontal bone to form **coronal suture**

Posterior or lambdoid (occipital)
Articulate with occipital bone to form lambda

Angles (Four)

Antero superior (Frontal)
- Known as **bregma**
- Meeting point of sagittal suture & coronal suture

Antero inferior (Sphenoidal)
- Meeting point of four bones (**Pterion**):
  - Frontal bone
  - Temporal bone
  - Parietal bone
  - Greater wing four bone

Postero superior (Occipital)
- Meeting point of sagittal & lambdoid sutures
- Corresponds to **lambda**

Postero inferior (Mastoid)
- Articulates with occipital & mastoid temporal bone
- Known as **asterion**

Each parietal bone has two surfaces (external and internal) four borders (sagittal, squamosal, frontal and occipital) and four angles.

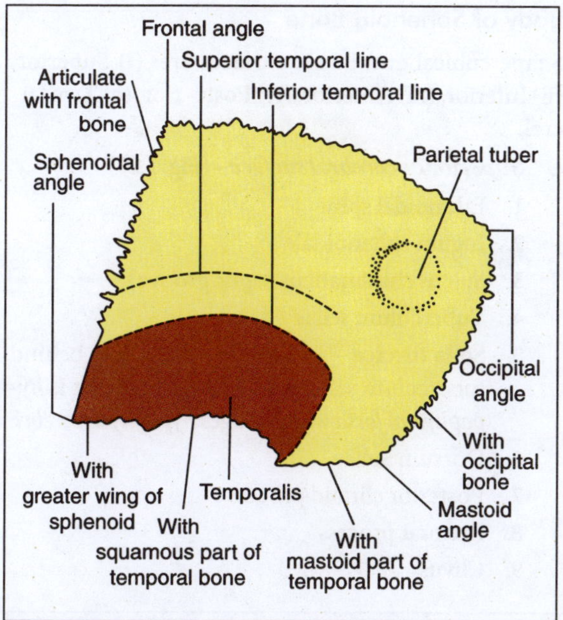

Fig. 1.23: External surface of the parietal bone (left)

I. **External Surface (Outer) (Fig. 1.23)**

Features

1. Convex and smooth.
2. Parietal eminence or tuber – It is the most prominent part of the surface.

[Importance – (a) Important bony land mark ; (b) Maximum transverse diameter of the skull when measured from one eminence to other ; (c) Centres of ossification start from this area and spread radially ; (d) Centre of printed and written words in angular gyrus (area 39) is located just deep to it.]

3. Temporal lines
4. Area above temporal lines
5. Area below the temporal lines
6. Parietal foramen (may be absent)

II. **Internal surface (Inner) (Fig. 1.24)**

Features

1. Granular foveolae (pits)
2. Grooves for middle meningeal artery

Angles

1. Anterosuperior (frontal)
2. Antero inferior (sphenoidal) angle
3. Postero-superior (occipital) angle
4. Postero inferior (mastoid) angle

Ossification

a) Membranous type.
b) Two centres one above the other appear at the parietal eminence (tuber) at the 7th week of intrauterine life.
c) Two centres fuse and proceed radially and the angles are last *parts to be ossified.*

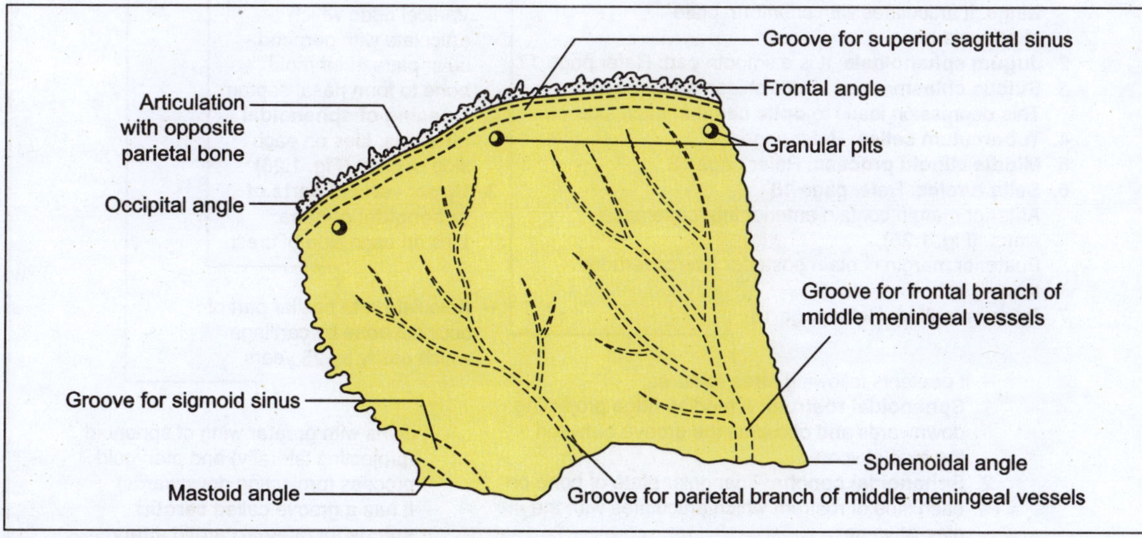

Fig. 1.24: Internal surface of the parietal bone (left)

E. SPHENOID BONE

It is situated in the base of the skull forming the middle cranial fossa and lies behind the frontal and in front of the temporal and basilar part of occipital bone. It is like a bat with outstretched wings.

Anatomical Position

Bone should be held in such a manner so that –

a) Pterygoid process is – vertically downwards.

b) Lesser wings in front and greater wings behind them.

c) Surface of body presenting opening of air sinus must be anterior and surface (usually cut) for basilar part of occipital bone behind.

d) Surface with sphenoidal crest inferiorly.

Body of Sphenoid Bone

Shape cubical and its six surfaces are: (i) Superior, (ii) Inferior, (iii) Anterior, (iv) Poste- rior, (v) Two lateral.

I. ***Superior or cerebral surface*** – (Fig. 1.25)

1. Ethmoidal spine
2. Jugum sphenoidale
3. Sulcus chiasmaticus (optic groove)
4. Tuberculum sellae
5. **Sella turcica** – A deep depressed area behind tuberculum sellae and deepest part of it is *hypophyseal fossa* which lodges *hypophysis cerebri.*
6. Dorsum sellae
7. Posterior clinoid process
8. Petrosal process
9. Clivus

TABLE 1.9: Different parts of Sphenoid

Parts of sphenoid bone

- Surfaces of body
- Greater wings
- Lesser wings
- Pterygoid processes

Surfaces of body:

Superior

On cerebral surface:
From front backwards the following features:

1. **Ethmoidal spine:** A triangular projection between two lesser wings. It articulates with cribriform plate of ethmoid bone
2. **Jugum sphenoidale**: It is a smooth part. Refer page 17
3. **Sulcus chiasmaticus**: Optic chiasma relates here. This depression leads to **optic canal** in each side
4. **Tuberculum sellae**: Refer page 18
5. **Middle clinoid process**: Refer page 18
6. **Sella turcica**: Refer page 18
   Anterior margin contain anterior intercavernous sinus. (Fig. 1.25)
   Posterior margin contain posterior intercavernous sinus
7. **Dorsum sellae**: Refer page 18

Inferior

– It presents following three features:

1. **Sphenoidal rostrum:** A median ridge projecting downwards and occupies the groove between the alae of vomer
2. **Sphenoidal concha**: Triangular plate of bone on each side of rostrum which articulates with the alae of vomer
3. **Vaginal process**: (Refer page 12)

Anterior

It presents following features

1. **Sphenoidal crest:** Vertical ridge which articulate with perpendicular plate of ethmoid bone to form nasal septum
2. **Opening of sphenoidal air sinus**: Lies on each side of crest (Fig. 1.26)
3. **Upper vertical parts of sphenoidal concha:** Lies on each side of crest

Posterior

– Articulate with basilar part of occipital bone by cartilage which ossify by 25 years

Lateral

– Joins with greater wing of sphenoid (projecting laterally) and pterygoid process (projecting downwards)
– It has a groove called **carotid sulcus** for internal carotid artery

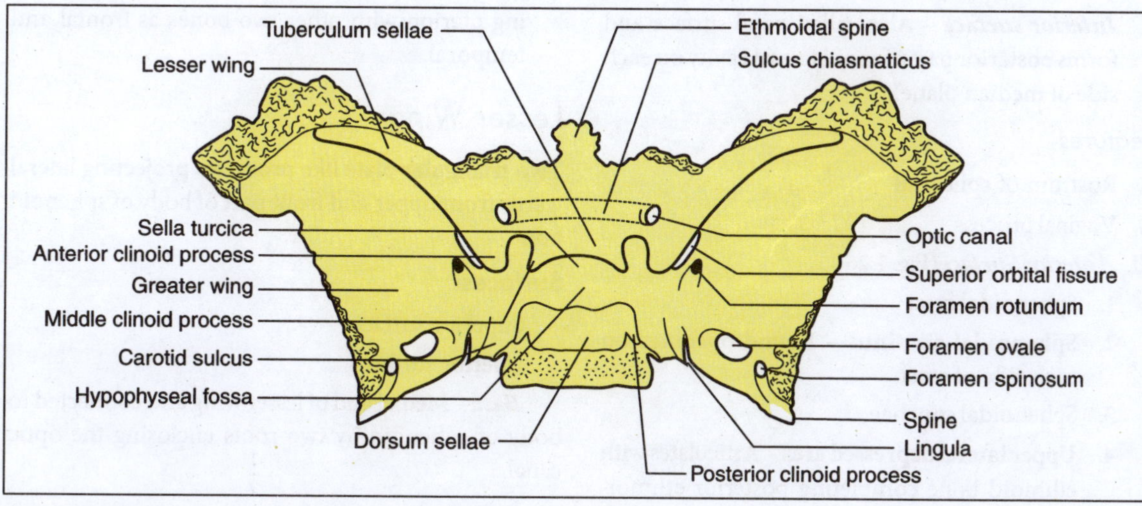

Fig. 1.25: Superior aspect of sphenoid bone

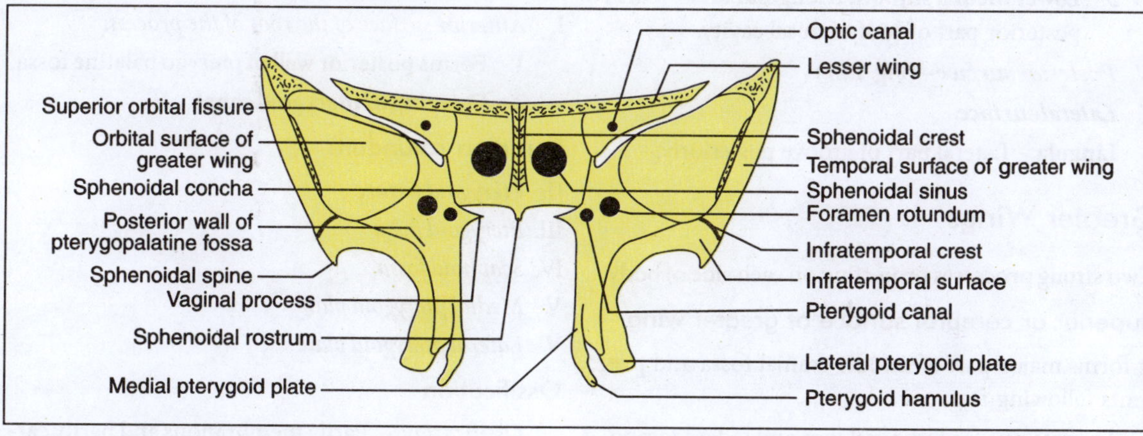

Fig. 1.26: Anterior aspect of sphenoid bone

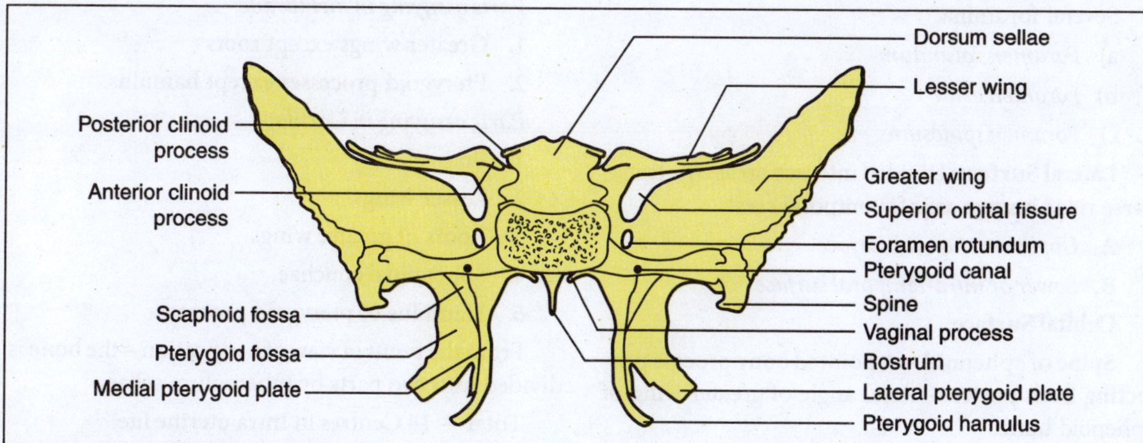

Fig. 1.27: Posterior aspect of sphenoid bone

II. ***Inferior surface*** – Also called nasal surface and forms posterior part of roof of nasal cavity on each side of median plane.

Features

1. Rostrum of sphenoid
2. Vaginal process

III. ***Anterior Surface*** (Fig. 1.26)
   1. Sphenoidal crest
   2. **Sphenoidal air sinus** – Round openings on each side of crest.
   3. Sphenoidal conchae
   4. **Upper lateral depressed area** – Articulates with ethmoid bone completing posterior ethmoidal air sinus.
   5. **Lower medial smooth triangular area** – Form posterior part of roof of nosal cavity.

IV. ***Posterior surface*** – (Fig. 1.27)

V. ***Lateral surface***:

Lingula – Lateral part of groove posteriorly.

Greater Wings

Two strong processes projecting on each side of body.

Superior or cerebral surface of greater wing

It forms major part of middle cranial fossa and presents following features:

1. Impressions for temporal gyri and lodges temporal lobe.
2. Several foramina
   a) *Foramen rotundum*
   b) *Foramen ovale*
   c) *Foramen spinosum*

Lateral Surface: Divided into two areas by a transverse ridge known as infratemporal crest.

A. *Upper or temporal surface*

B. *Lower or infra-temporal surface*

Orbital Surface:

Spine of sphenoid – A pointed bony process projecting from postero-lateral angle of greater wing of sphenoid bone.

1. **Tip or parietal border** – articulates with antero-inferior (sphenoidal) angle of parietal bone forming pterion with other two bones as frontal and temporal.

Lesser Wings

Two triangular plate like processes projecting lateral wards from upper and front part of body of sphenoid bone.

Surfaces

Superior surface

Inferior surface

Base – Medial end of lesser wing and connected to body of sphenoid by two roots enclosing the optic canal.

Pterygoid processes

I. *Anterior surface of the root of the process:*
   1. Forms posterior wall of pterygo palatine fossa.
   2. **Opening of pterygoid canal**

Foramen rotundum

II. *Pterygoid fissure*

III. *Pterygoid fossa*

IV. *Scaphoid fossa*

V. *Medial pterygoid plate*

VI. *Lateral pterygoid plate*

Ossification

Ossification – Partly membranous and partly cartilaginous.

Parts ossifying in membrane –

1. Greater wings except roots
2. Pterygoid processes except hamulus.

Parts ossifying in Cartilage –

1. Body.
2. Lesser wings.
3. Roots of greater wings.
4. Sphenoidal conchae.
5. Hamulus of pterygoid process.

From the point of view of ossification – the bone is divided into two parts by tuberculum sellae.

Total — 14 Centres in Intra uterine life.

1. Pre-sphenoidal part — 6 centres
2. Post-sphenoidal part — 8 centres.

TABLE 1.10: Features of Greater Wing, Lesser wing & Pterygoid process

Greater Wing (Lateral processes extending from each side of body)

- **Surfaces**
  - Superior or cerebral
    - Forms the part of middle cranial impressions for temporal gyri – presence of
      - a) **Foramen rotundum** give exit to maxillary nerve
      - b) **Foramen ovale** situated postero lateral to foramen rotundum. (Refer page 12)
      - c) **Foramen spinosum** (Fig. 1.25) lateral to foramen ovale. (Refer page 12)
  - Lateral
    - Infratemporal crest divides lateral surface into:
      - Upper or temporal surface
        - Forms the part of temporal fossa
        - Gives origin to temporalis muscle (Fig. 1.26)
      - Lower or infratemporal surface
        - Forms the part of infratemporal fossa, & in its lateral part infratemporal crest is present
        - Gives origin to upper head to lateral pterygoid muscle
  - Orbital surface
    - Smooth, quadrilateral forms postero-lateral wall of orbital cavity
- **Spines** (Refer page 12)
- **Borders**
  - Posterior
    - Medial half forming anterior boundary of foramen lacerum
    - Lateral half articulates with petrous part of temporal
      - At the site of articulation, two bones forms sulcus inferiorly, **sulcus tubae**, which lodges auditory tube (cartilaginous part)
  - Squamosal or lateral border
    - Articulates with squamous part of temporal bone
      - Anterior end of this border articulates with anteroinferior angle of parietal bone to form **pterion**

Lesser wings (Triangular piece of the bone attached with anterior half of body of sphenoid by two roots which encloses optic canal)

- **Surfaces**
  - Superior or Cerebral
    - Continuous with superior surface of body (Jugum sphenoidale) forms a part of anterior cranial fossa lodge frontal lobe
  - Inferior or Orbital
    - Forming upper boundary of superior orbital fissure. It also form the posterior half of roof of orbit
- **Borders**
  - Anterior
    - Articulates with posterior border of orbital surface of frontal bone
  - Posterior
    - Non articulated medial end forms **anterior clinoid process** to which free margin of the tentorium cerebelli is attached; it lodges sphenoparietal sinus

Pterygoid process

- Refer page 11

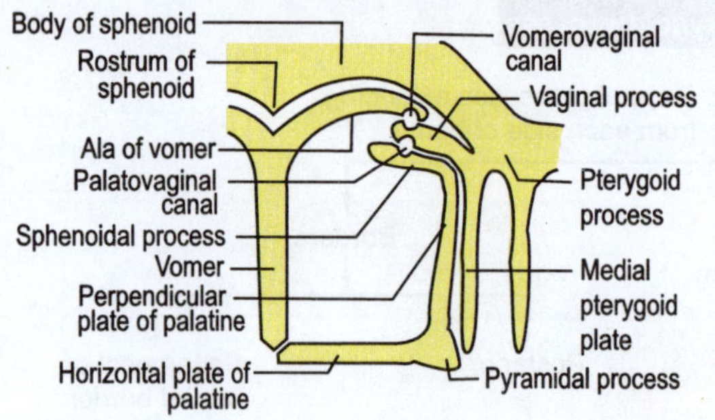

Fig. 1.28: Relations between sphenoid, vomer & palatine bone

1. Pre-sphenoidal part

   ↓

   Part in front of tuberculum sellae and consists of:

   a) Part of body in front of tuberculum Sellae — 2 centres

   b) Lesser wings — 2 centres

   c) Sphenoidal conchae — 2 centres.

2. Post-sphenoidal part

   ↓

   Part behind tuberculum sellae — 8 centres

   4th month → Post sphenoidal part of body — as Sellae turcica and Dorsum Sellae — 2 centres.

   8th week → Greater wing — 2 centres and lateral pterygoid plate.

   8 – 10th week → Medial pterygoid plate — 2 centres.

   4th month → Lingula — 2 centres.

Fusion or Union

6th month before birth: Union between Lateral and Medial Pterygoid plate.

8th month before birth: Union between Pre and Post Sphenoidal parts of body.

Just after birth: The bone consists of three parts – (i) Body with lesser wings and (ii) and (iii) on each side greater wing with Pterygoid processes.

Union of these three parts

Union between body and greater wings takes place in the first year. *Body of sphenoid unites with Basilar part of occipital bone at the age of 25th year forming primary Cartilaginous Joint.*

F. TEMPORAL BONE

These bones form side and base of skull.

Different Parts

It consist of following parts (morphologically):

1. *Squamous part* – for protection of cerebrum.
2. *Petro-mastoid part* – to preserve orientation of membranous labyrinth.
3. *Tympanic part* – forms external accoustic meatus in man for conduction of sound waves to tympanic membrane.
4. *Styloid process* – derived from skeletal element of second branchial arch (Reichert's cartilage).

Anatomical position and side determination

Bone should be held in such a manner so that –

1. Squamous part is directed upwards and in front.
2. Mastoid part behind and process directed downwards.
3. Zygomatic process arising from outer surface will be directed forwards.
4. Petrous part will be fused with squamous part at its base and its apex will be directed forwards and medially.
5. External acoustic meatus is directed laterally and will direct to the side it belongs.

Outer or temporal surface of squamous part (Fig. 1.29)

1. It forms greater part of temporal fossa.
2. *Groove* for middle temporal artery (branch of superficial temporal artery).
3. *Supramastoid crest* – A curved ridge in the posterior part which runs upwards and backwards – for attachment of *temporal fascia* and limits the origin of temporalis muscle.

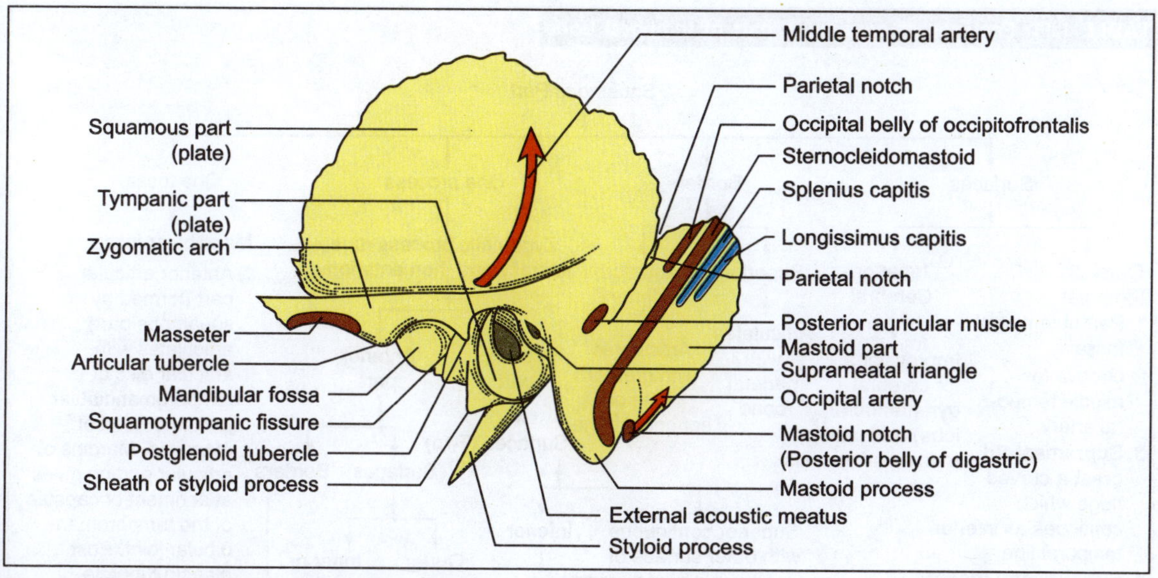

Fig. 1.29: External surface of temporal bone (left)

Inner or cerebral surface of squamous part (Fig. 1.30)

1. Concave and *impressions for cerebral* gyri of temporal lobe.
2. Grooves for middle meningeal vessels.

Borders

Superior border – Articulates with inferior border of parietal bone.

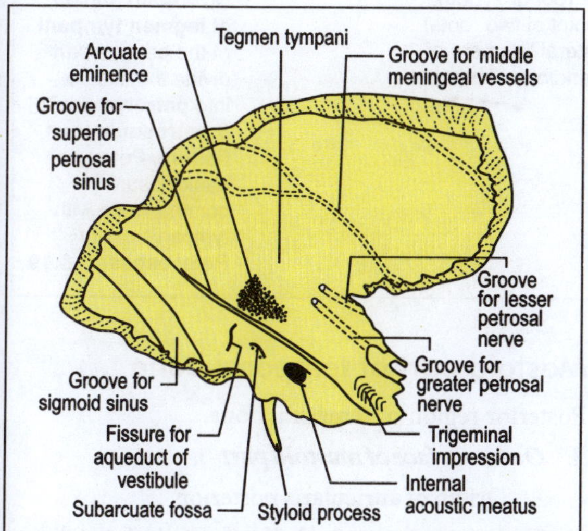

Fig. 1.30: Internal surface (medial view) of temporal bone

Antero inferior border – Articulates with greater wing of sphenoid bone.

Zygomatic process of temporal bone – It projects from lower part of outer surface. It has two parts:

I. *Posterior Part* (it has two surfaces)

A. **Superior** – Concave and continuous with outer surface of squamous part.

B. **Inferior** – Consists of two roots and tubercle of root of zygoma –

a) *Anterior root* – it forms *articular tubercle* or *eminence* in front of mandibular fossa.

b) *Posterior root.*

c) *Tubercle of root of zygoma.*

II. *Anterior part of zygomatic process:*

As the anterior part is twisted it presents two borders: (a) Upper, (b) Lower. Two surfaces: (i) Lateral and (ii) Medial and one anterior end.

Anterior rough end – Articulates with temporal process of zygomatic bone to form zygomatic arch.

Upper border – for temporal fascia

Lower border – origin of few fibres of masseter

Medial surface – origin of masseter

Lateral surface – subcutaneous.

TABLE 1.11: Features of squamous part of temporal bone

Squamous Part

- **Surfaces**
  - Outer or Temporal
    1. Part of temporal fossa
    2. Groove for middle temporal artery
    3. **Supramastoid crest** a curved ridge which continues as inferior temporal line
    4. **Suprameatal triangle** triangular area between anterior end of supramastoid crest and postero superior part of external acoustic meatus.
       - Important landmark for tympanic antrum (lies depth of 1.25 cm)
       - Refer page 6 (Fig. 1.29)
  - Inner or Cerebral
    - Impressions for cerebral gyri (temporal lobe) and middle meningeal vessels
- **Borders**
  - Superior
    - Articulates with parietal bone
  - Anterior inferior
    - Articulates with greater wing of sphenoid bone
- **One process**
  - Zygomatic process runs laterally and then anteriorly
    - Posterior part
      - Surfaces (Two)
        - Superior continuous with outer surface of squamous part
        - Inferior
          - Two roots
            - Anterior
              - Forms anterior boundary of mandibular fossa & is called articular tubercle
            - Posterior begins above the external acoustic meatus continuous with supramastoid crest
          - Tubercle or root or zygoma (meeting point of two roots) attaches lateral ligament of temporomandibular ligament
    - Anterior part
      - Surfaces
        - Ourter – subcutaneous
        - Inner or medial attaches masseter
      - Borders
        - Superior – Attaches temporal fascia
        - Inferior – Attaches masseter
- **One fossa**
  - Mandibular fossa
    - a) Anterior articular part (formed by squamous part) articulates with articular disc of temporomandibular joint and head of mandible. Margins of articular portion gives attachment of capsule of the temporomandibular joint. Post glenoid tubercle separates the articular part from nonarticular part (Figs. 1.31 & 1.33)
    - b) Posterior or nonarticular formed by the tympanic part of temporal bone & lodges part of parotid gland
    - **Squamotympanic fissure**:
      - It is situated in the mandibular fossa between articular & nonarticular parts
      - Downward portion of **tegmen tympani** of the petrous part divide the fissure into **petrotympanic** & **petrosquamous fissure**. Petrotympanic fissure communicate with tympanic cavity
      - Refer pages 13 & 19

Mandibular Fossa

Situated behind the articular tubercle or eminence.

FEATURES: consists of two parts: (Fig. 1.24c)

I. *Anterior articular part*

II. *Non-Articular Part* – (Fig. 1.31)

Squamotympanic fissure can be seen.

Mastoid part of temporal bone

Posterior region of temporal bone.

I. ***Outer surface of mastoid part***

1. Origin of auricularis posterior
2. Origin of occipital belly of occipitofrontalis
3. *Mastoid foramen* – May or may not be present.

TABLE 1.12: Features of Mastoid, Tympanic part and Styloid process of temporal bone

- **Mastoid part** (Posterior region of temporal bone)
  - Surfaces
    - Outer → Origin of auricularis posterior & occipital belly of occipitofrontalis muscle
    - Inner → Sigmoid sinus is present here
  - Border
    - Posterior → Articulate with occipital bone
  - Mastoid air cells → Extend in different parts of temporal bone
  - Mastoid process
    - Surfaces
      - Lateral → Gives insertion of sternocleidomastoid, splenius capitis & longissimus capitis
      - Medial → Deep groove is known as **mastoid notch** which gives origin of posterior belly of digastric muscle
  - Mastoid antrum → Refer page 6

- **Tympanic part** (Curved plate of bone between squamous & mastoid part)
  - Surfaces
    - Anterior
      - Concave
      - Forms non-articular part of mandibular fossa & lodges parotid gland
    - Posterior
      - Forms floor & anterior wall of external auditory meatus
      - At the medial end presents tympanic sulcus for tympanic membrane
  - Borders
    - Lateral → Margin of external acoustic meatus for attachment of cartilaginous part
    - Superior → Forms the posterior boundary of petrotympanic fissure
    - Inferior → Extend from carotid canal to enclose (as sheath of styloid process) styloid process

- **Styloid process**
  - Parts
    - Base is enclosed by tympanic part
    - Distal free part
  - Attachments
    - Refer page 7

If present transmits – (a) an emissary vein connecting sigmoid sinus with posterior auricular vein, (b) a small branch of occipital artery.

II. ***Cerebral or inner***

a) Sigmoid sulcus – For sigmoid sinus

b) *Mastoid foramen* – May be present in the floor.

III. *Posterior* – Articulates with inferior border of squamous part of occipital bone from lateral angle to jugular process.

Mastoid air cells and tympanic (mastoid antrum)

I. *Mastoid air cells*

II. *Tympanic* (mastoid antrum)

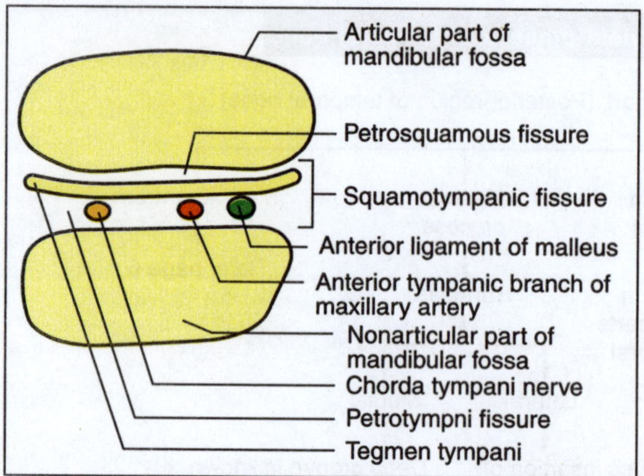

Fig. 1.31: Petrotympanic & petrosquamous fissure

Petrous Part

It is the triangular pyramid shaped part of bone and at the base of skull is wedged between greater wing of sphenoid and occipital bone.

Surfaces of Petrous Part

A. **Anterior Surface:**

1. Trigeminal impression
2. Arcuate eminence
3. Tegmen tympani
4. Hiatus and groove for greater petrosal nerve – (Fig. 1.32)
5. Hiatus and groove for lesser petrosal nerve

B. **Posterior Surface:**

1. Opening of internal acoustic meatus
2. Opening of aqueduct of the vestibule
3. Subarcuate fossa
4. Internal acoustic meatus

A short canal about 1 cm. length and of 3 to 5 mm. diameter.

A perforated plate of bone is present at the bottom or lateral end of the canal. This plate forms the medial wall of the internal ear. This plate is divided into two areas:

I. *Upper area*:

1. *Anterior part* – Opening for beginning of facial canal for facial nerve.
2. *Posterior or superior vestibular area* – Numerous small foramina for nerves to ampullae of superior and lateral semicircular ducts and utricle.

II. *Lower area*:

1. *Anterior part or cochlear area* – It corresponds to base of Cochlea. It consists of (a) Central canal – for nerves to apex of cochlea, (b) A

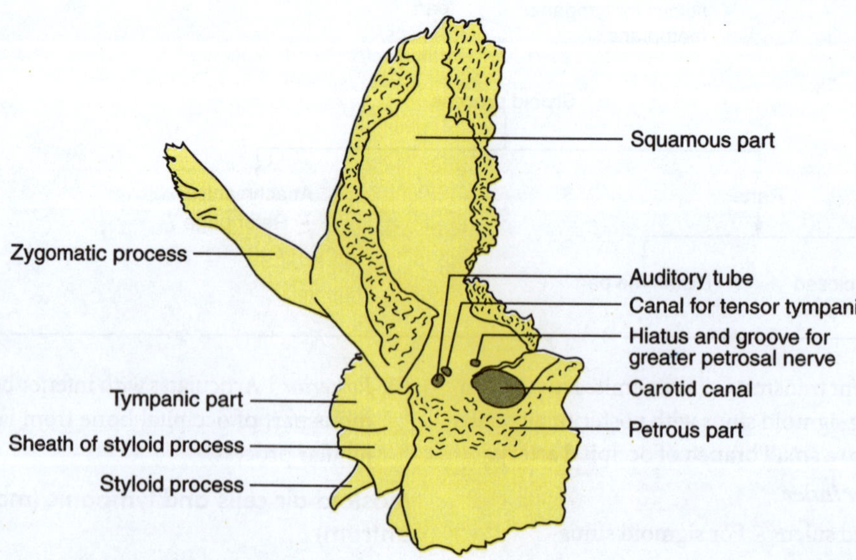

Fig. 1.32: Right temporal bone from the front

TABLE 1.13: Different parts of Petrous part of temporal bone

Petrous part (Triangular pyramid shaped part of bone lie between greater wing of sphenoid and occipital bone)

- **Base**
  - Fused with
    - a) Squamous part by petrosquamosal suture
    - b) Mastoid Part
- **Apex**
  - Projects forwards medially and slightly upwards and forms posterolateral boundary of foramen lacerum and opening of carotid canal; articulates with petrosal process of sphenoid
- **Surfaces**
  - **Anterior**
    - It forms the posterior part of middle cranial fossa
    - – Presents the following features:
      1. **Trigeminal impression**: Close to apex of petrous tempora bone
         – It lodges trigeminal ganglion
      2. **Arcuate eminence**: Behind the trigeminal impression, there is an elevated area, the arcuate eminence (due to superior semicircular canal)
      3. **Tegmen tympani**: It is thin plate of bone, & it is part of petrous temporal bone. Rest refer to page 19
      4. Presents two foramina with grooves (lateral & medial);
         – Lateral foramen transmit lesser petrosal nerve
         – Medial foramen transmit greater petrosal nerve (Fig. 1.30)
  - **Posterior**
    - Three important features
      1. **Internal acoustic meatus**: Refer page 20
      2. **Aqueduct of vestibule**: It lodges ductus endolymphaticus
      3. **Subarcuate fossa**: It lodges a process of dura mater
  - **Inferior**
    - Important features:
      1. Origin of levator veli palatini near the apex
      2. **Carotid canal**: Transmit internal carotid artery with sympathetic plexus
      3. **Tympanic canaliculus**: Transmit tympanic branch of glossopharyngeal nerve in between carotid canal and jugular fossa
      4. **Triangular depression**: It lodges inferior ganglion of glossopharyngeal nerve
      5. **Jugular fossa**: It lodges superior bulb of internal jugular vein
      6. **Mastoid canaliculus**: It transmit auricular branch of vagus
      7. **Jugular surface**: Quadrilateral surface articulate with jugular process of occipital bone
      8. **Styloid process** (Refer page 7)
      9. **Stylomastoid foramen**: It transmits facial nerve and stylomastoid artery of posterior auricular artery
- **Borders**
  - **Anterior**
    - – Articulate with sphenoid bone
    - – At the site of articulation, **sulcus tubae** is present at the base of skull which lodges auditory tube (cartilaginous part)
  - **Superior**
    - – Lodges superior petrosal sinus
  - **Posterior**
    - – Articulates with occipital bone & forms jugular foramen

spiral tract surrounding the central canal with foramen and known as *tractus spiralis foraminosus* – for nerves to rest of cochlea.

2. Posterior part or *inferior vestibular area* for which presents foramen for nerves to saccule.
3. *Foramen singulare* – In the posterior most part for nerves to ampulla of posterior semicircular duct.

C. **Inferior Surface**: It is rough, irregular and more or less triangular in shape. (Fig. 1.33, Fig. 1.34)

1. Quadrilateral rough area
2. Lower opening of carotid canal
3. Jugular fossa
4. Triangular notch
5. Cochlear canaliculus
6. Tympanic canaliculus
7. Mastoid canaliculus
8. Jugular surface

D. **Borders of petrous part**

I. ***Superior***

II. ***Posterior border***

III. ***Anterior border***

IV. ***Tympanic part***

V. ***Styloid process***

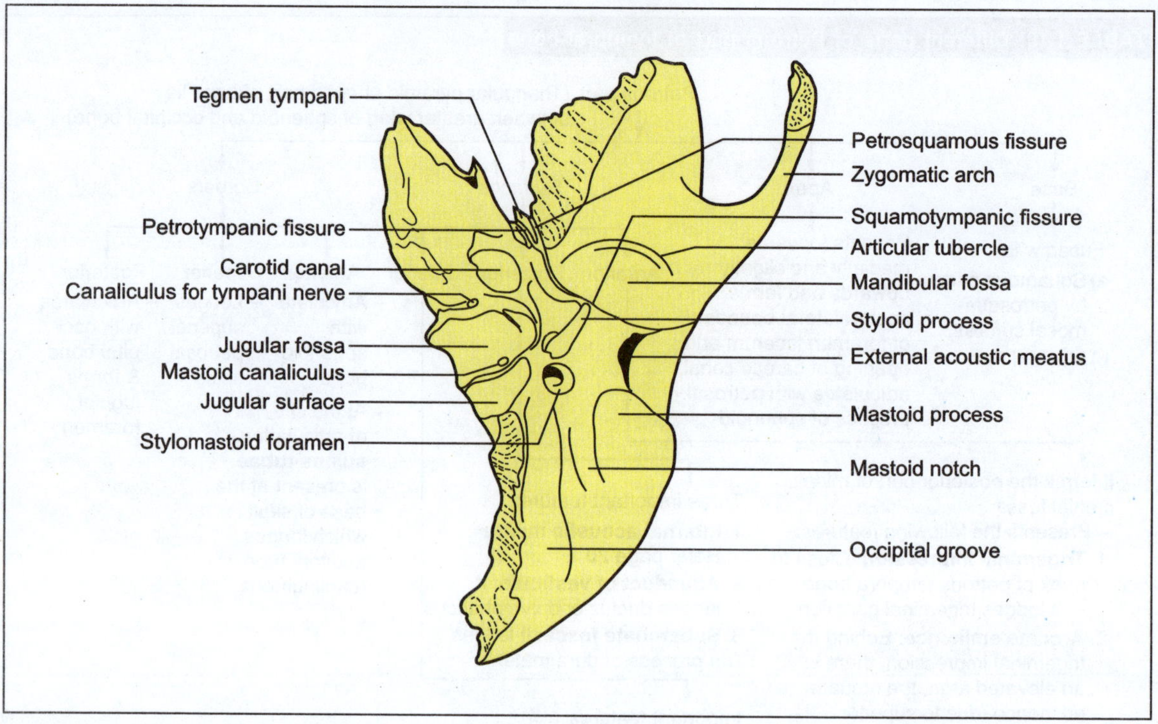

Fig. 1.33: Inferior surface of the left temporal bone

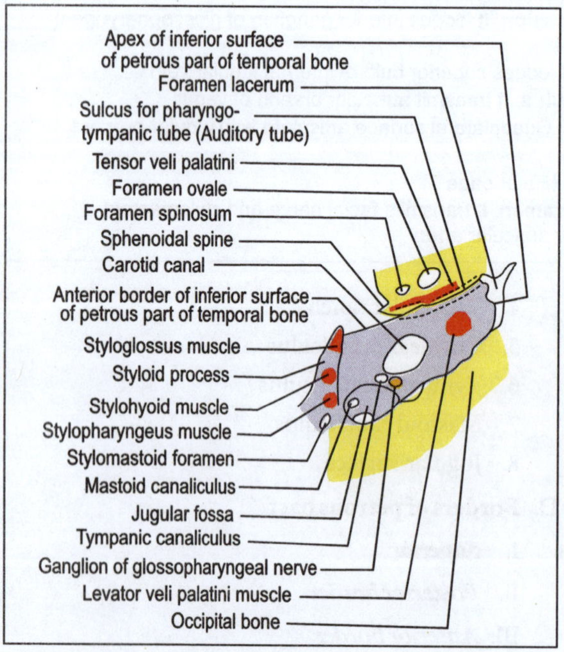

Fig. 1.34: Inferior surface of petrous part of left temporal bone & adjacent part of sphenoid

Relations:

1. *Facial nerve* when within parotid gland crosses the base laterally.
2. *Internal Jugular vein* medially but separated by stylopharyngeus.
3. *External carotid artery* – Crosses the tip when it lies within parotid gland.
4. *Parotid gland* – Covers it laterally.
5. *Stylomastoid Foramen* – It is the lower end of facial canal and situated between styloid process and mastoid process.

Transmits:

a) Exit of facial nerve.

b) Entrance of stylomastoid branch of posterior auricular artery.

TABLE 1.14: Ossifications of Temporal bone and Fusion of Component

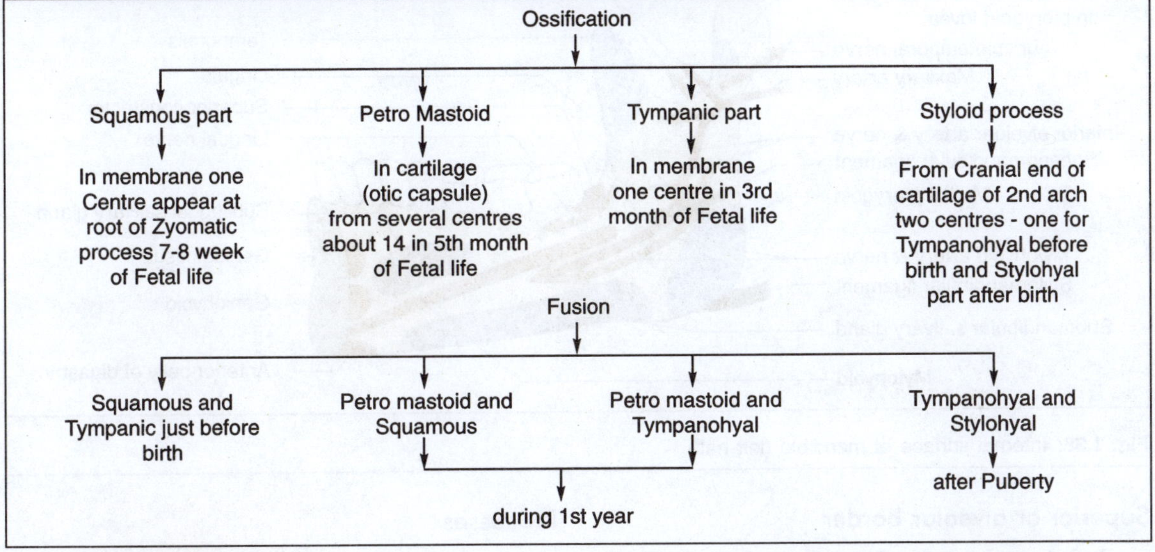

G. MANDIBLE

1. Largest and strongest bone of the face consists of :
   a) Body which is horse-shoe shaped.
   b) Two Rami projecting upwards (quadrila-teral in shape).

Body of Mandible

External or Outer Surface (Fig. 1.35)

FEATURES:

1. **Symphysis menti**

Internal or Inner Surface (Fig. 1.36)

FEATURES:

1. Mylohyoid line
2. Mylohyoid groove
3. Genial tubercles
4. Area behind the 3rd molar tooth
5. Origin of superior constrictor
6. Relation of lingual nerve

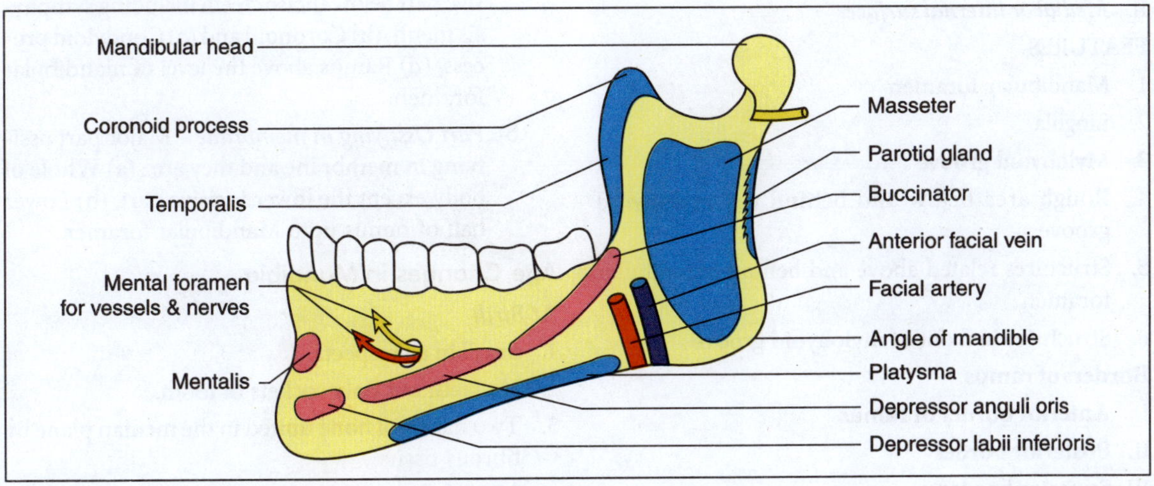

Fig. 1.35: Features of external surface of mandible (left half)

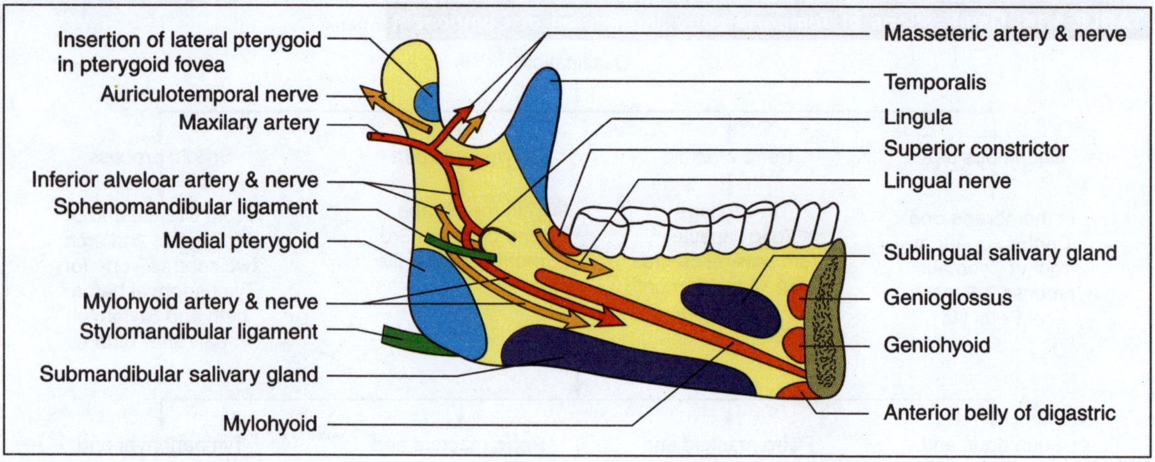

Fig. 1.36: Internal surface of mandible (left half)

Superior or alveolar border

Inferior or lower border – It forms the base of mandible.

FEATURES

1. **Digastric fossa**
2. **Attachment of investing layer of deep cervical fascia**
3. **Platysma**

Ramus of mandible

I. *External or lateral surface*
   1. *Upper and posterior smooth part*
   2. *Major rough area or part*

II. *Medial or internal surface*

FEATURES

1. Mandibular foramen
2. Lingula
3. Mylohyoid groove
4. Rough area below and behind the mylohyoid groove
5. Structures related above and behind mandibular foramen
6. Structures in front of mylohyoid groove

Borders of ramus:

I. **Anterior border of ramus**
II. **Posterior border**
III. **Superior border**
IV. **Inferior border**

Processes

I. ***Condyloid*** – Strong upward projection from postero-superior part of ramus.

Ossification

1. It is the second bone to ossify in the body (first is the clavicle).
2. It is partly membranous and partly cartilaginous in ossification and the centre in each half of mandible appears in 6th week of fetal life.
3. Centre appears at the anterior end of Meckel's cartilage (cartilage skeletal element of first branchial arch).
4. a) *Part Ossifying in Cartilage* – They are : (a) Incisive part below Incisor teeth including symphysis menti, (b) Coronoid and (c) Condyloid process, (d) Ramus above the level of mandibular foramen.

   b) *Part Ossifying in membrane* – Major part ossifying in membrane and they are : (a) Whole of body except the lower incisive part, (b) Lower half of ramus upto Mandibular foramen.

Age Changes in Mandible

At Birth

1. Small in all respects.
2. No teeth but only sockets of tooth.
3. Two halves of bone united in the median plane by fibrous tissue.
4. Mental foramen – just opposite first deciduous molar tooth at the lower border.

TABLE 1.15: Features of body of the Mandible

- Mandible
  - Body
    - Surfaces
      - External or outer surface
        - Features:
          1. **Symphysis menti**: Faint midline ridge indicate line of fusion of two halves
          2. **Mental protuberance**: Triangular elevation formed by bifurcation lower end of symphysis
          3. **Mental tubercle**: Small tubercles at the infero-lateral angles of mental protuberance
          4. **Mental foramen**: Situated between first & second premolars. Give exist to mental nerve & vessel
          5. **Mental fossa**: On each side of median ridge. Gives origin to mentalis muscle
          6. **Oblique line**: It is the continuation of anterior border of coronoid process up to mental tubercle. Gives origin to buccinator, depressor anguli oris and depressor labii inferioris
          7. **Junction of body & ramus**: Related to facial artery & anterior facial vein
      - Internal or inner
        - Features:
          1. **Mylohyoid line**: An oblique line running downwards & forwards from the third molar (behind) tooth to symphysis menti. Mylohyoid muscle is attached.
          2. **Sublingual fossa**: Above the mylohyoid line there is a depression which lodge sublingual gland
          3. **Submandibular fossa**: Below the mylohyoid line there is a depression for submandibular gland
          4. **Lingual nerve**: It is related on inner side of body to medial side of the root of the 3rd molar tooth
          5. **Mylohyoid groove**: It lies below mylohyoid line. Lodges mylohyoid nerve and vessel
          6. Area below third molar tooth (above mylohyoid line).
             - Gives origin to superior constrictor of pharynx and attachment to pterygomandibular raphe
          7. **Genial tubercles**: Upper & inferior tubercles on either side
             a) **Upper genial tubercles** (two): Gives origin to genioglossus muscle
             b) **Lower genial tubercles** (two): Gives origin to geniohyoid muscle
    - Borders
      - Superior or alveolar
        - It passes socket for teeth
      - Inferior or base
        - It is continuous with lower border of ramus. On each side of midline in the internal or inner surface, there is digastric fossa which gives origin to anterior belly of digastric muscle
        - Attachment of investing layer of deep cervical fascia through out the border
        - Platysma is attached on the external surface near inferior border
  - Ramus
    - Table 1.16

5. Mandibular canal nearer to lower border.
6. Angle – obtuse about 140".
7. Coronoid process higher than condyloid processes.

After first year and in Children

1. Grows in length behind mental foramen.
2. Mandibular canal – little higher.
3. Union of two halves or bone (after 1st year).
4. Coronoid and condyloid process are more or less at the same level.
5. Ramus grows in height.

In Adults

1. Angle – reduces to 110" – 120" (Roughly at right angle).
2. Mental foramen – midway between upper and lower borders.
3. Alveolar parts are well-developed and teeth are erupted.
4. Mandibular canal runs parallel with mylohyoid line.
5. Ramus becomes almost vertical.
6. Condyloid process is at higher level than coronoid process.

TABLE 1.16: Features of Ramus of the Mandible

Ramus of the mandible

- **Surfaces**
  - **Internal or medial**
    1. **Mandibular foramen**: It is located a little above the centre of the ramus. It leads to mandibular canal. Transmits – inferior alveolar nerve & artery
    2. **Lingula**: A bony projection at medial margin of the mandibular foramen.
       - Attaches sphenomandibular ligament
    3. **Mylohyoid groove**: Lodges mylohyoid nerve & vessel
    4. **Rough area**: This area lies posteroinferiorly & gives attachment to medial pterygoid muscles
  - **External or lateral**
    1. **Posterosuperiorly**: Related to parotid gland
    2. **Major rough area**: This area lies posteroinferiorly & gives attachment to masseter muscle
- **Borders**
  - **Anterior border**: Thin & sharp – insertion of temporalis muscle
  - **Posterior border**
    - Thick
    - Related to parotid gland
  - **Superior border**
    - Concave
    - Forms **mandibular notch**
    - Mandibular notch transmits masseteric vessels & nerves
  - **Inferior border**
    - This border is continuous with inferior border of body
    - Platysma attached on the external surface near the inferior border
    - Attachment of investing layer of deep cervical fascia. At the angle of mandible the investing layer proceeds upwards & attached to styloid process to form stylomandibular ligament
- **Processes**
  - **Head & neck**
    1. **Head:** Upper expanded thick end covered with fibrocartilage & form temporomandibular joint with articular fossa of temporal bone
    2. **Neck:**
       a) **Pterygoid fovea**: A depression on anterior surface
          – Gives attachment to lateral pterygoid muscle
       b) Medially related to auriculotemporal nerve above and maxillary artery below
       c) Laterally: Its **lateral aspect** gives attachment to the **temporomandibular ligament**
  - **Coronoid process**
    - Projection from anterosuperior part of ramus, in front of mandibular notch. At the apex, lateral aspect and margins temporalis muscle is inserted

In Old Age

1. Falling of teeth with absorption of alveolar border.
2. Mental foramen and mandibular canal are close to alveolar process.
3. Ramus – oblique; angle becomes again obtuse, about 140".
4. Bending backwards of condyloid process.

Growth of Mandible

1. Lengthwise growth takes place at the posterior border.
2. Growth in width and between two angles takes place at the lateral slope of the posterior border.
3. Growth in thickness takes place at the external surfaces.
4. Growth in height is due to growth in alveolar process.

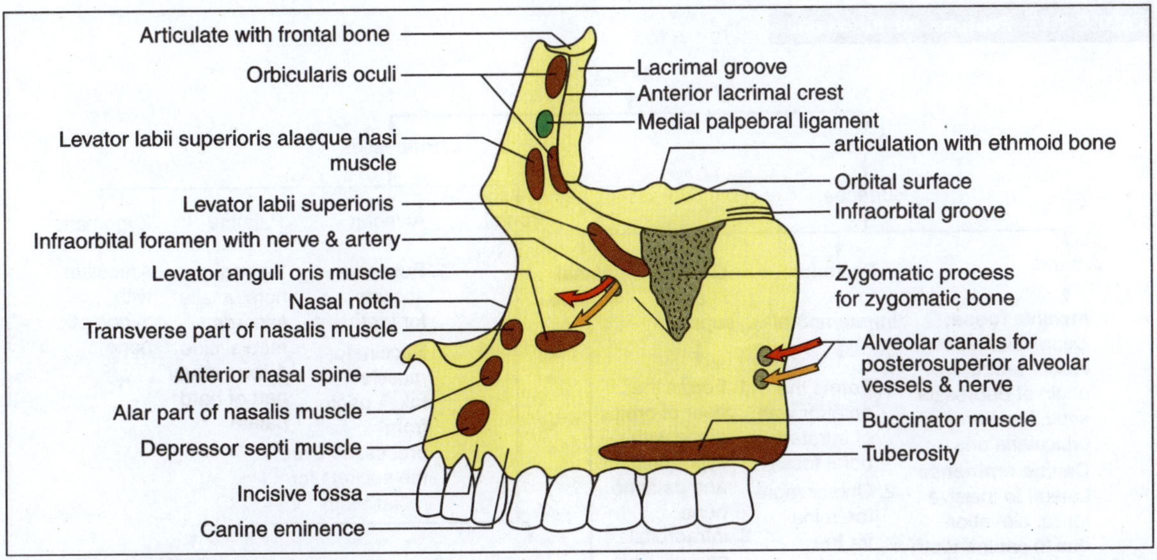

Fig. 1.37: Lateral surface of left maxilla

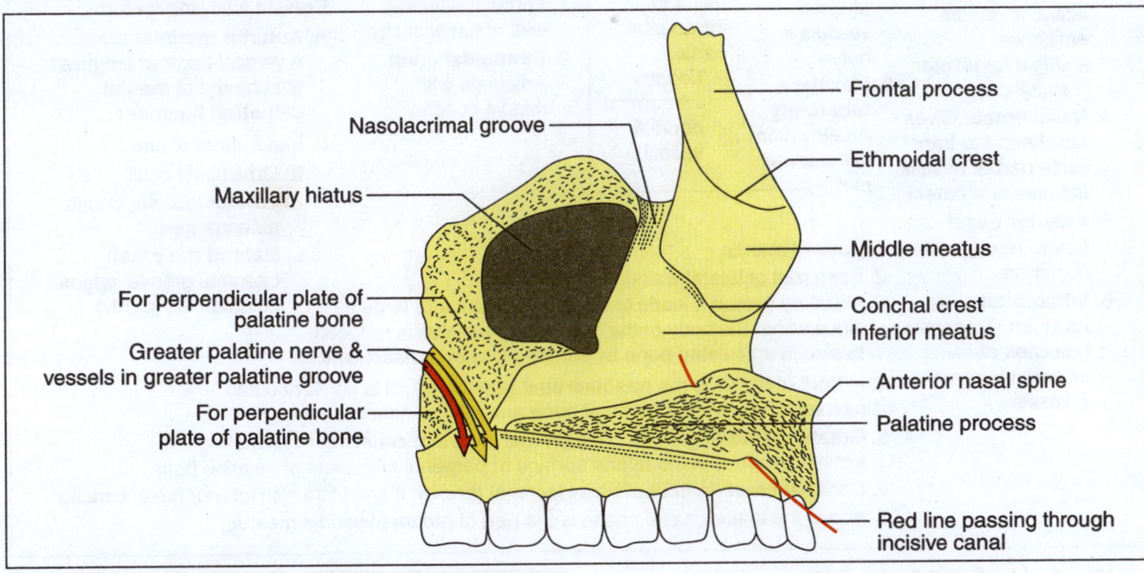

Fig. 1.38: Medial aspect of left maxilla

5. Shape of the mandible is maintained by remodelling work by alternate osteoblastic (bone formation) and osteoclastic (resorption of bone) at the opposite borders and surfaces.

H. MAXILLA

It is the largest bone of the face except mandible. It takes part in the formation of the upper jaw, face, nose, orbit, nasal cavity, infratemporal and Pterygo palatine fossa.

Anatomical position and side determination

It should be held in such a manner:

1. Concave nasal notch in front and medially.
2. Longest process (frontal) directed upwards.
3. Convex surface – posteriorly.
4. Large and irregular opening maxillary hiatus medially.

TABLE 1.17: Features of the Maxilla

Maxilla

- **Body**
  - Surfaces
    - **Anterior**
      1. **Incisive fossa**: Depression above incisor teeth, origin of depressor septi, few fibres of orbicularis oris
      2. **Canine eminence**: Lateral to incisive fossa, elevation due to canine tooth
      3. **Canine fossa**: Larger depression lateral to canine eminence
         – Origin for levator anguli oris
      4. **Nasal notch**: Gives attachment to transverse part of nesalis (compressor nares)
      5. **Anterior nasal spine**: A projection in midline
      6. **Infraorbital foramen**: Transmits branches of infraorbital nerve & vessel
    - **Posterior or Infratemporal**
      1. Forms the anterior wall of Infratemporal fossa
      2. One or more foramina for the postero-superior alveolar vessels & nerve
      3. **Maxillary tuberosity**: An elevation in the lower part
    - **Orbital or superior**
      1. Forms the floor of orbit along with zygomatic and palatine bone
      2. Infraorbital groove: This groove leads to infraorbital canal.
         – Lodges infraorbital nerve & vessel
    - **Nasal surface**
      1. Base of maxilla
      2. Form part of lateral wall of nasal cavity
      3. Maxillary hiatus: It leads to maxillary air sinus (a large air sinus within the body of the maxilla). The hiatus is reduced to size in articulated bone by ethmoid & inferior nasal concha
      4. In front of hiatus is the **nasolacrimal groove** which is converted into nasolacrimal canal by lacrimal bone and inferior nasal concha
      5. **Greater palatine groove**: This groove turns into canal after articulating with similar groove with the lateral surface of perpendicular plate of palatine bone
      6. **Conchal crest**: In front of nasal lacrimal groove. It articulate with inferior nasal concha
      7. Above the inferior nasal cocha is the part of atrium of middle meatus
- **Processes**
  - **Frontal**
    - Surfaces
      - **Medial**
        1. Forms the lateral wall of nasal cavity
        2. **Ethmoidal crest**: Articulate with middle concha
      - **Lateral**
        Present following features:
        A. **Anterior lacrimal crest**: A vertical ridge which gives attachment of **medial palpebral ligament**
        B. Part in front of crest:
           a) Orbicularis oculi
           b) Levator labii superioris alaeque nasi
           c) **Behind the crest**: Lacrimal groove lodges lacrimal sac (partly)
  - **Alveolar**
    1. Posseses sockets for teeth
    2. Buccinator muscle takes origin from processes over the sockets for molar teeth
  - **Palatine**
    - Extend horizontally towards medial side & form major part of hard palate
  - **Zygomatic**
    - Articulate with zygomatic bone

5. Alveolar border with sockets for tooth downwards and its convexity outwards.
6. Rough triangular area (Zygomatic process) laterally.
7. Zygomatic process directs to the side it belongs or Maxillary Hiatus belongs to the opposite side it belongs.

Different Parts of Bone

1. Body.
2. Processes: (i) Frontal, (ii) Zygomatic, (iii) Alveolar, (iv) Palatine.

TABLE 1.18: Ossification of the Maxilla

Ossification—(Membranous)

- One for maxilla proper 6th week of intrauterine life above the canine fossa
  - Forms main mass with processes
- Two for pre-maxila
  - 1st or main 7th week of intrauterine life above the Incisive fossa
  - Second
    - Anterior margin of nasal septum

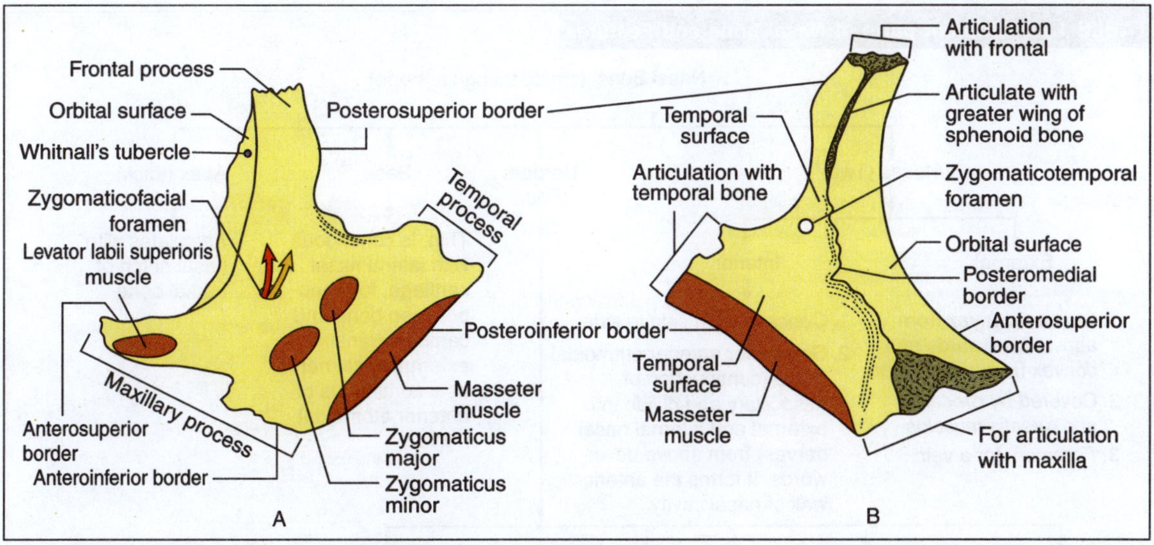

Fig. 1.39: Left zygomatic bone; A – Lateral aspect; B – Medial aspect

I. ZYGOMATIC BONES

Two in number and forms infero-lateral part of orbital opening.

Anatomical position and side determination

It should be held in such a manner so that (a) non-articular border (Postero-superior) resembling letter 'F' will be directed upwards and backwards, (b) Frontal process will look upwards, (c) The convex (lateral) surface will direct to the side it belongs

Surfaces of zygomatic – Three:

I. *Lateral or malar surface* — Convex and directed laterally and forwards.

TABLE 1.19: Features of different part of Zygomatic bone

Zygomatic bone (It forms the prominence of the cheek)

- **Body** → Surfaces (Three)
  - Lateral or malar → Convex → Features:
    1. **Zygomaticofacial foramen**: Transmit zygomaticofacial nerve and vessels
    2. Elevation below the foramen: Origin of zygomaticus major and minor muscle
    3. Near the posteroinferior margin: Origin of masseter
    4. Near the infraorbital margin: Origin of levator labii superioris
  - Medial or temporal → Concave → Features:
    1. Zygomaticotemporal foramen: Transmit zygomaticotemporal nerve and vessels
    2. It forms part of temporal fossa
  - Orbital → Forms lateral wall and floor of orbit → Features:
    1. Zygomatico-orbital foramen
    2. Whitnall's tubercle: 1cm below the frontozygomatic suture
       Attachment: 1. Lateral palpebral ligament
       2. Lateral check ligament
- **Processes** (Two)
  - Frontal → Articulate with a) Zygomatic process of frontal bone above
  - Temporal → Articulate with zygomatic process of temporal bone forming zygomatic arch

TABLE 1.20: Different parts of Nasal bone and Features

Nasal Bone (small, triangular bone)

- Surfaces (Two)
  - External
    1. Concavoconvex from above downwards and convex from side to side
    2. Covered by p*rocerus* and n*asalis muscles*
    3. *Foramen*–for a vein
  - Interior
    1. Concave from side to side
    2. Groove for anterior ethmoidal nerve (continuation of nasociliary and divide into external and internal nasal nerves) from above downwords. It forms the anterior wall of nasal cavity
- Borders (Four)
  - Superior: Articulates with nasal part of frontal bone
  - Inferior: Continuous with lateral nasal cartilage of nose
  - Lateral: Articulates with frontal process of maxilla
  - Medial:
    1. Articulates with opposite bone forming nasal crest
    2. Nasal crest articulates from above downwards
       a) Nasal spine of frontal
       b) Perpendicular plate of ethmoid
       c) Cartilage of nasal septum
- Base: Thin, is continuous with lateral nasal cartilage, foramen between bone and cartilage transmits external nasal nerve as a continuous of anterior ethmoidal nerve
- Apex (thick): Articulates with nasal notch of frontal bone

J. NASAL BONE (Fig. 1.40)

Two small oblong bones forming bridge of nose

Side determination and anatomical position

1. Shortest and thickest border upwards.

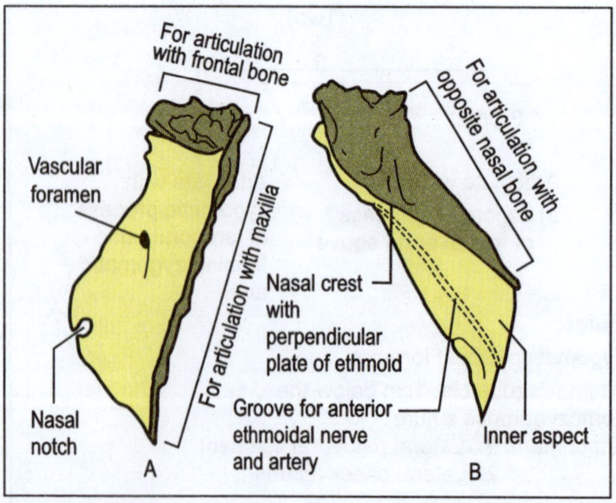

Fig. 1.40: Nasal bone; A – External aspect; B – Internal aspect

2. Thick border – medially and projecting.
3. Part from upper end look backwards.
4. Concavo-convex surface laterally and will direct to the side it belongs.

OSSIFICATION:

From *one centre in 3rd month of intrauterine life and membranous in type.*

K. ETHMOID BONE

Situated below the ethmoidal notch of frontal and in front part of base of Cranium. Exceedingly light and fragile. It forms roof, lateral wall, septum of the nose, medial wall of orbit and front part of anterior cranial fossa.

Anatomical Position

Should be held in such a manner so that:

1. Cribriform plate should be horizontally placed and looks upwards and crista galli must be in front.
2. Perpendicular plate will be in between two lateral masses & direct vertically downwards.

TABLE 1.21: Features of different part of Ethmoid

Ethmoid (Unpaired bone that located between two orbits, forms roof, lateral & medial wall [nasal septum] of nasal cavity as well as medial wall of orbit)

Horizontal cribriform plate
- Median part of upper surface of bone
- It fills the ethmoidal notch between the orbital plates of the frontal bone
- It separates the roof of the nasal cavity & anterior cranial fossa

Features:
1. Crista galli: Triangular process which gives attachment to falx cerebri. In front of it foramen caecum can be seen in articulated skull
2. Lateral to crista galli
   - Related to olfactory bulb
   - Contains several foramina for passages of olfactory nerve

Perpendicular plate

Projects downwards in the midline from lower surface of cribirform plate. It forms upper part of nasal septum

Labyrinths

Composed of large number of air cells grouped into anterior, middle & posterior ethmoidal air sinuses

Surfaces:

Medial

Forms lateral wall of nasal cavity

Features:
1. **Middle nasal concha**
2. **Bulla ethmoidalis**: Refer nasal cavity
3. **Hiatus semilunaris**: Refer nasal cavity
4. **Superior concha**: Refer nasal cavity
5. **Infundibulum**: Refer nasal cavity
6. **Sphenoethmoidal recess**: Refer nasal cavity

Lateral

Bony plate called orbital plate which forms medial wall of the orbit

Anterior
- It is having anterior ethmoidal air sinus
- **Uncinate process**: A hook like process projects downwards & backward helps to reduce opening of the maxillary air sinus

Posterior
- It is having posterior ethmoidal air sinus

Superior
- It is having anerior and posterior ethmoidal canal for transmitting correspon-ding nerve and vessels

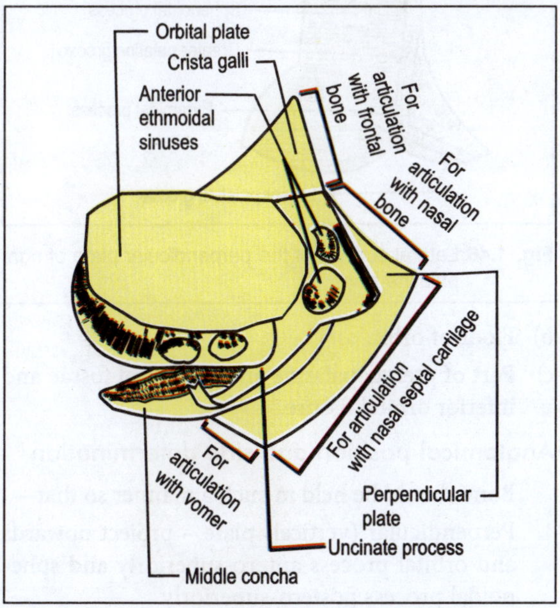

Fig. 1.41: Lateral view of the ethmoid bone

3. Orbital plate of the labyrinth (lateral surface) will look lateralwards. (Fig. 1.41)

OSSIFICATION – In cartilage

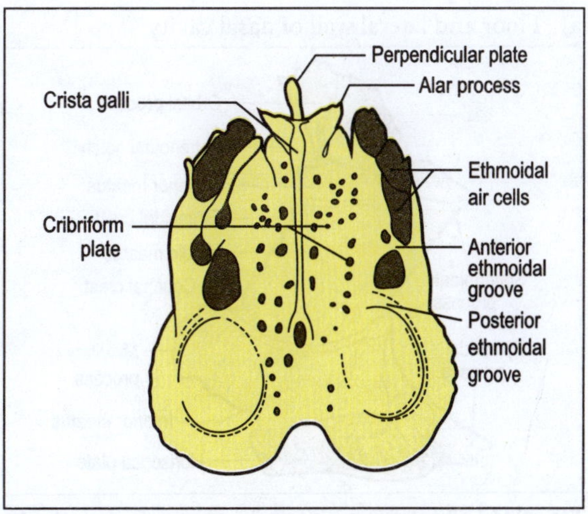

Fig. 1.42: Superior aspect of ethmoid bone

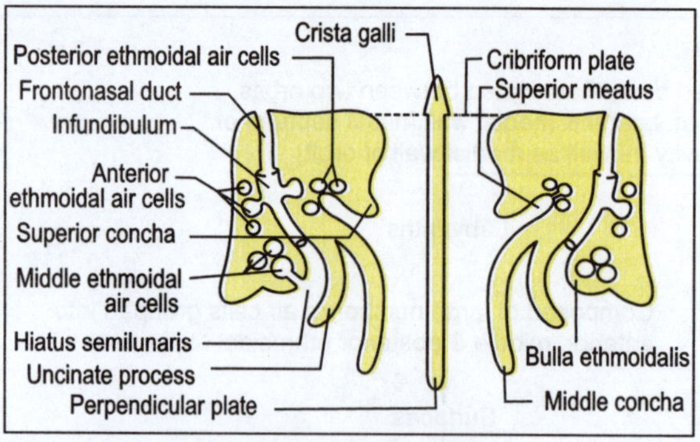

Fig. 1.43: Coronal section of ethmoid bone

TABLE 1.22: Ossification of Ethmoid

Ossification by 3 centres

- **Two** → One in each *labyrinth* 4th or 5th *month of life* also forming ethmoidal concha and a portion of cribriform plate
- **One** → For *perpendicular plate in* 1st *year after birth* and also forms crista galli and remaining part of cribriform plate

↓

Fusion at the *end of* 2nd *year*

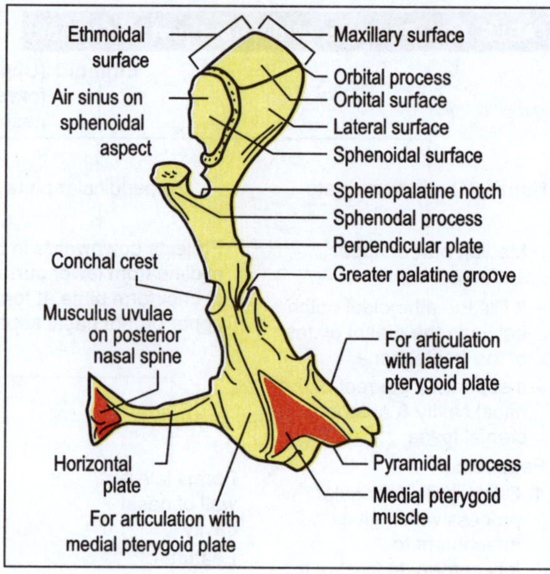

Fig. 1.45: Palatine bone posterior aspect (right side)

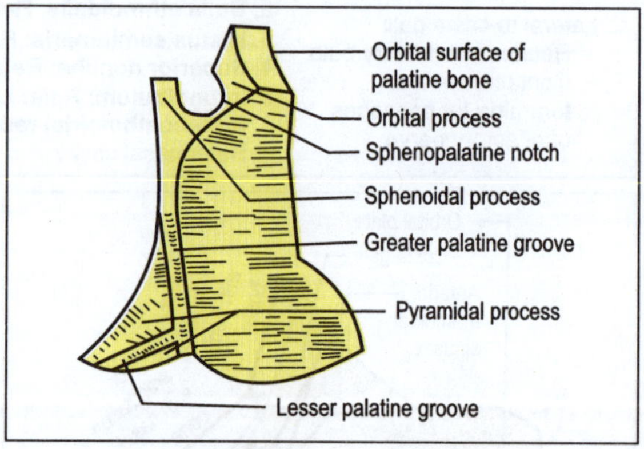

Fig. 1.46: Lateral surface of the perpendicular plate of right palatine bone

L. PALATINE BONE

Two 'L'-shaped bones situated in the posterior part of nasal-cavity and between pterygoid processes of sphenoid bone and maxillae.

It takes part in the formation of –

a) Floor and lateral wall of nasal cavity –

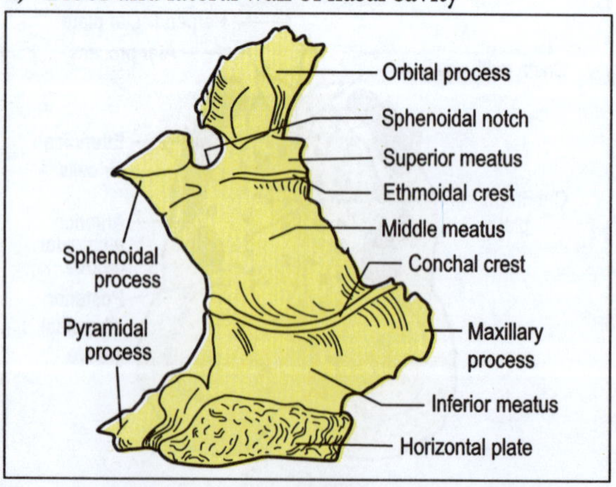

Fig. 1.44: Left palatine bone (medial aspect of perpendicular plate)

b) Floor of orbit.

c) Part of pterygopalatine and pterygoid fossae and inferior orbital fissure.

Anatomical position and side determination

Bone should be held in such a manner so that—

1. Perpendicular (vertical) plate – project upwards and orbital process antero-superiorly and sphenoidal process postero-superiorly.
2. Pyramidal process – projecting backwards downwards laterally from the junction of vertical and horizontal plates.
3. Medial surface of vertical plates show two ridges (crests) and three areas.

TABLE 1.23: Features of Palatine bone

Palatine bone (Each resembles a letter L in its horizontal and perpendicular plate) (Located in between maxilla & pterygoid process of sphenoid and forms one-fourth of hard palate)

- Horizontal plate (forms posterior one-fourth of hard palate)
  - Project medially & unites with its conterpart of opposite bone
    - Surfaces
      - Superior or nasal surface
        - Forms the floor of nasal cavity
        - Forms **nasal crest** in the midline
        - Nasal crest forms the part of nasal septum
      - Inferior or oral surface
        - Forms posterior 1/4 of the hard palate
        - **Palatine crest** – Refer page 10
- Perpendicular plate
  - Surfaces
    - Medial
      - **Conchal crest** give attachment to inferior concha & space below it inferior meatus
      - **Ethmoidal crest** give attachment to middle nasal concha & space below it middle meatus
    - Lateral
      - Present **greater palatine groove**
  - Borders
    - Its upper border present:
      - a) **Orbital process**
      - b) **Sphenoidal process**:
      - This processes enclose sphenopalatine notch which is converted into foramen
- Three processes
  - Orbital
    - Form floor of orbit
  - Sphenoidal
    - It articulate with vaginal process of medial pterygoid plate to form palato-vaginal canal
  - Pyramidal
    - It project from the junction of horizontal plate and perpendicular plate
    - **Lesser palatine groove** can be seen in this process

4. Pyramidal process will direct to side it belongs.
5. Horizontal plate – Anteriorly rough and articular – Medial border of this plate will direct to the opposite side to which it belongs.

OSSIFICATION:

In membrane from one centre appearing at the 8th week in the Intra uterine life in the perpendicular plate.

M. INFERIOR NASAL CONCHA

These are two curved laminae of bones – one on each side situated in the lower part of lateral wall of nasal cavity.

Anatomical position and side determination

Bone should be held in such a manner so that –

1. Tapering end posteriorly.
2. Border carrying processes upwards – in front – Lacrimal and behind ethmoidal.
3. Concave Surface – Lateral wards and determine the side it belongs.

Inferior Nasal Concha

OSSIFICATION:

In cartilage – one centre appearing 5th month of Intra uterine life.

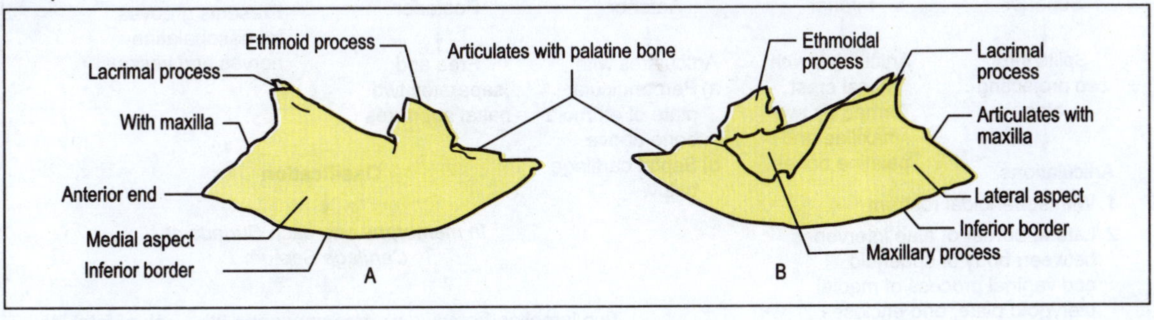

Fig. 1.47: Right inferior nasal concha; A – Medial aspect; B – Lateral aspect

TABLE 1.24: Features of different parts of Inferior Nasal Concha

Inferior nasal concha (a pair of curved bony plate)

- Surfaces (Two)
  - Medial → Convex and grooves for vessels are present
  - Lateral → Concave and forms medial wall of Inferior meatus
- Borders (Two)
  - Superior
    - Anterior end → Articulates with conchal crest of maxilla
    - Posterior end → Articulates with conchal crest of palatine bone
    - Intermediate → Three Process
      - Lacrimal → Articulates with descending process of lacrimal bone forming nasolacrimal canal
      - Ethmoidal → Articulates with uncinate process of ethmoid bone
      - Maxillary → Aarticulate with maxilla
  - Inferior → Non-articular and more or less rounded

N. VOMER

Thin flat and more or less quadrilateral bone and forms postero inferior part of nasal septum.

Anatomical Position – To be held in such a manner so that

a) The border which splits into two alae must be above and behind.

b) Free and non-articulating border behind i.e. posterior.

TABLE 1.25: Features of Vomer and Ossification

Vomer (quadrilateral, unpaired bone, forms posteroinferior part of nasal septum)

- Borders
  - Superior → Splits into two projecting alae → Articulations
    1. With sphenoidal rostrum
    2. Lateral border of alae intervenes between body of sphenoid and vaginal process of medial pterygoid plate, and encloses vomerovaginal canal
  - Inferior → Articulates with nasal crest formed by two maxillae and palatine bones
  - Anterior → Articulates with
    - a) Perpendicular plate of ethmoid bone above
    - b) Septal cartilage below
  - Posterior → Free and separates two nasal apertures
- Surfaces
  - Two lateral surfaces
  - Presents grooves for nasopalatine nerves and vessels

Ossification

→ *In membrane* one each *Surface of Cartilage Septum*

→ Two lamellae from two centres appearing 8th week of fetal life. 12th week two centres fuse below the cartilage

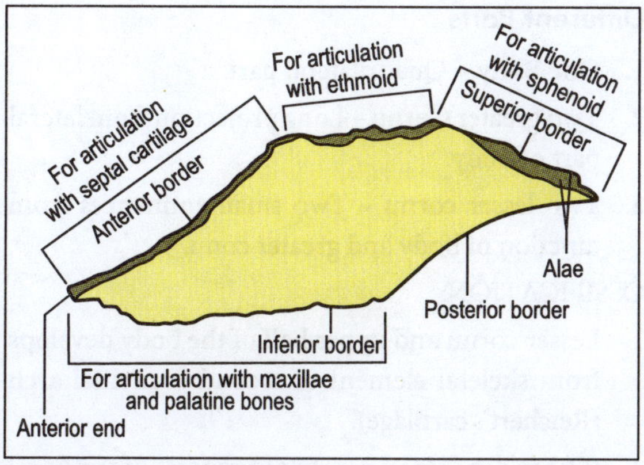

Fig. 1.48: Vomer

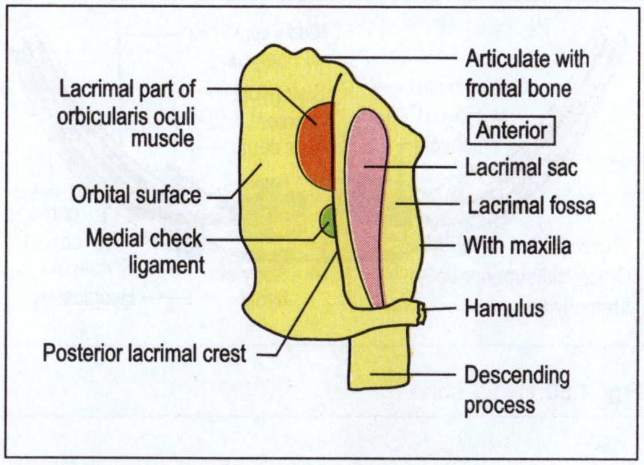

Fig. 1.49: Right lacrimal bone (lateral aspect)

O. LACRIMAL BONES

Most fragile and smallest of the cranial bones – Two in number and take part in the formation of medial wall of orbit.

Anatomical position and side determination

Bone should be held in such a manner that –

1. Groove-bearing surface looks laterally and the groove should be in front of the ridge;
2. Pointed process would direct downwards (uncinate);
3. A process (Lacrimal hamulus) should direct forwards and medially from the lower part of the ridge. This hamulus or process will direct to the side it belongs.

Lesser Lacrimal Bone – When hamulus exists as a separate bone – it is known as Lesser Lacrimal bone.

Ossification – In membrane – one centre appearing at 12th week of intra uterine life.

TABLE 1.26: Different parts of Lacrimal bone

Lacrimal bone

- Surfaces (Two)
  - Lateral (orbital) (Lateral surface is divided into anterior part & posterior part by posterior lacrimal crest)
    - Anterior part
      1. This groove area form lacrimal fossa for lodging lacrimal sac
      2. Descending process: Nasolacrimal duct lodges here.
    - Posterior lacrimal crest (In the middle)
      1. Attachment of lacrimal fascia, lacrimal part of orbicularis oculi & medial cheek ligament
      2. Hamulus: Here upper opening of nasolacrimal duct is present
    - Posterior part
      - Forms a part of medial wall of orbit
  - Medial or Nasal
    - Contribute partly to middle meatus
- Borders
  - Anterior → Articulates with maxilla
  - Posterior → Articulates with ethmoid
  - Superior → Articulates with frontal bone
  - Inferior → Articulates with maxilla

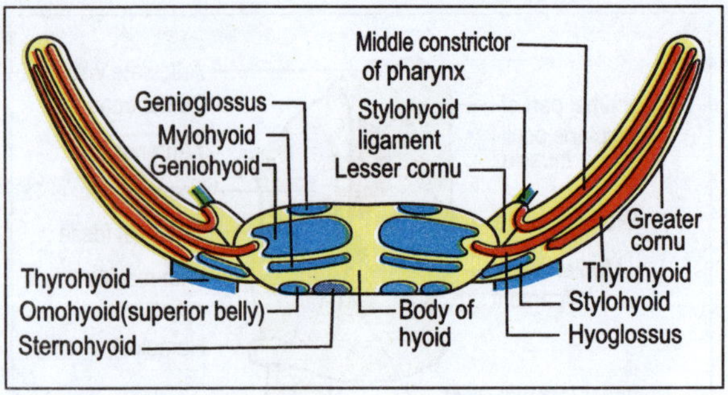

Fig. 1.50: Hyoid bone

P. HYOID BONE

'U'-shaped bone.

Anatomical Position

1. Convex and rough surface of body in front,
2. Concave and smooth surface looks behind and downwards.
3. Convex surface also presents –
   a) Transverse line and
   b) Vertical ridge looks forwards and upward.

Different Parts

1. One Body – Quadrilateral part.
2. Two greater Cornu – Long projection from lateral part of body.
3. Two lesser cornu – Two small eminences from junction of body and greater conu.

OSSIFICATION:

1. Lesser cornu and upper half of the body develops from skeletal element of second branchial arch (Reichert's cartilage).

   (Other derivatives are styloid process of temporal bone, stylohyoid ligament, stapes).
2. Greater cornu and lower half of the body develops from 3rd branchial arch.

   Ossification from six centres —

1. Two for body – Appearance of centre before or just after birth.
2. One for each greater cornu centre appears at the end of fetal life.
3. One for each lesser cornu centre appears at puberty.

TABLE 1.27: Features of different parts of Hyoid bone

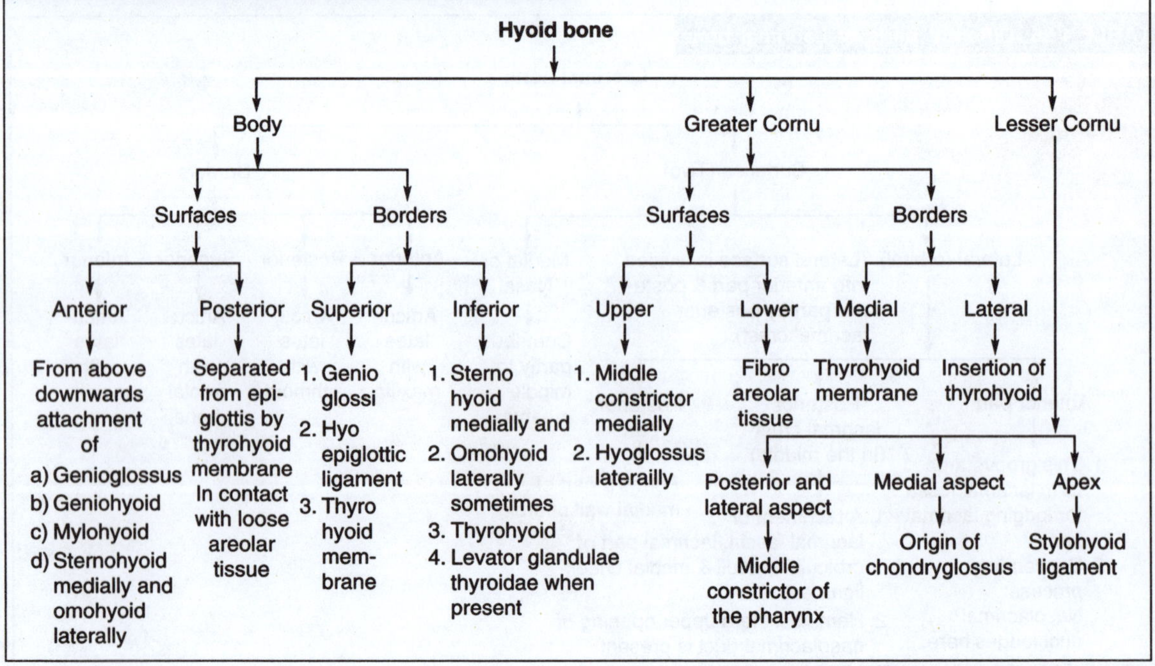

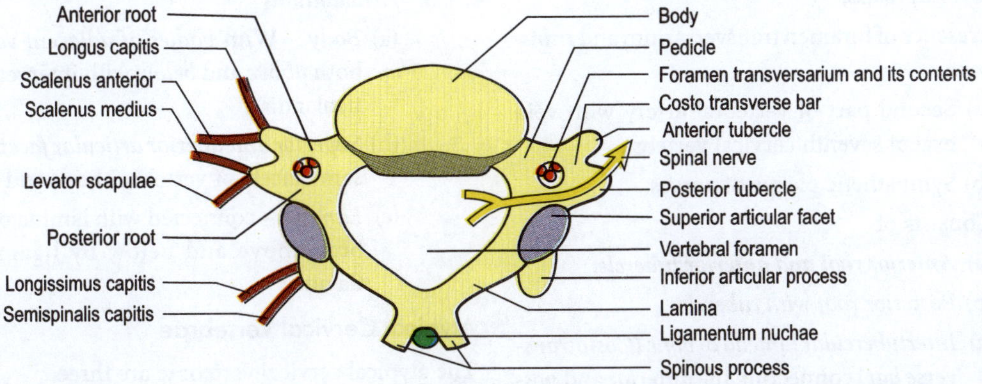

Fig. 1.51: Typical cervical vertebrae

Q. CERVICAL VERTEBRAE

1. *Seven* in number.
2. Identified by presence of *foramen transversarium* – a foramen in each of Transverse process.
3. (a) **Atypical** – First, second and seventh have got special features for identification so they are *atypical.*

   (b) **Typical** – The rest of the cervical vertebrae cannot be identified as to which number they belong. So they are *typical.*

Typical Cervical Vertebrae

Anatomical Position – Bone should be held in such a manner so that (a) Body should be directed forward and spinous process backwards. (b) Concave surface of body upwards and convex surface downwards. (c) Thin margin of the lamina upwards and medially.

FEATURES:

I. **Body**:

1. It is small and side to side broad.
2. Four Surfaces:

   (a) *Upper surface* – Concave and related to intervertebral disc.

   (b) *Lower surface* – Convex from side to side and related to intervertebral disc.

   (c) *Anterior surface* – Convex and attachment of *anterior longitudinal ligament*

   (d) *Posterior surface* – Flat and presents two or three openings for basivertebral veins, and is covered by *posterior longitudinal ligament* (extends from back of body of axis to sacral canal. It continues above as *membrana tectoria*).

II. **Vertebral Foramen** – Larger and triangular.

III. **Vertebral Arch**:

1. *Pedicle*: Arises from posterolateral part of body, and *directed laterally* and *backwards*.

   Superior and inferior vertebral notches are of equal size.

   Gap between pedicle is known as intervertebral foramen.

2. *Laminae*: Pedicles continue medially as laminae towards spine.

   Upper borders and lower part of anterior surface for *ligamentum flavum* from lamina of one vertebra to other.

IV. **Processes**:

A. *Superior and inferior articular processes*:

1. Form articular pillar at the junctional region of pedicles and laminae.
2. *Superior articular facets* – articulate with inferior articular facet of vertebra above and *inferior articular facet* with superior articular facet of vertebra below.

B. *Spinous process*:

1. Short and bifid.
2. Attachment:

   (a) Ligamentum nuchae – in the tip (extends from external occipital crest above to spine of seventh cervical vertebra below).

   (b) Deep muscles of back.

C. *Transverse process*:

1. Presence of foramen transversarium and *transmits*
   (a) Second part of vertebral artery with vein except seventh cervical vertebra.
   (b) Sympathetic plexus of nerves.
2. Consists of
   (a) *Anterior root and anterior tubercle.*
   (b) *Posterior root with tubercle.*
   (c) *Intertubercular lamella of bone (Costotransverse bar)* connecting the *anterior* and *posterior roots.*

Thus transverse process consists of two parts:

(i) *Costal element* – It consists of anterior root with tubercle, intertubercular lamella and poste-rior root.

(ii) *True transverse process* – Only the *posterior root*

3. *Carotid tubercle* – enlarged anterior tubercle of sixth cervical vertebra and related to common carotid artery and it can be compressed against it.
4. *Attachment*
   (a) *Anterior tubercle* – *origin of scalenus* anterior.
   (b) *Posterior tubercle* – origin of levator scapulae and scalenus medius.
5. *Articulations*
   (a) *Body* – With *bodies of adjacent vertebrae* both *above* and *below* with intervening articular disc.
   (b) *Superior and inferior articular facets* – with same facets of vertebra above and below.
   (c) *Lamina* – connected with lamina of vertebrae above and below by ligamentum flavum.

Atypical Cervical Vertebrae

The atypical cervical vertebrae are three:

1. Atlas or first cervical vertebra
2. Axis or second cervical vertebra
3. Seventh cervical vertebra.

Atlas

It is the first cervical vertebra and popularly called atlas.

It is so called atlas because atlas is a greek mythological giant who supports this globe or world. The first cervical vertebra supports the 'globe' of head and so is called *atlas*.

Identification

1. A ring of bone and has no body. Body has become fused with body of second cervical vertebra (Axis) to form dens (odontoid process).
2. Spinous process is absent and represented by a tubercle (**Posterior tubercle**). If there would have

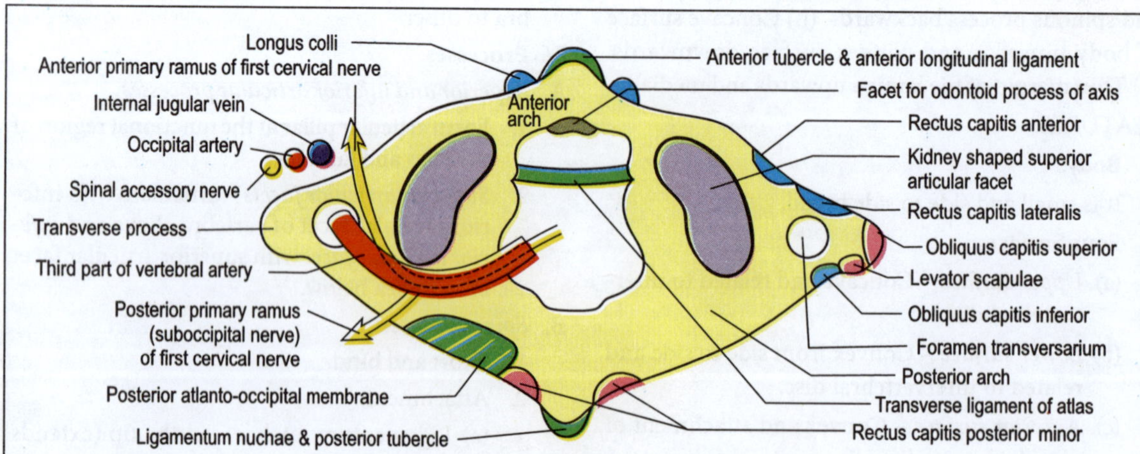

Fig. 1.52: Superior aspect of atlas

TABLE 1.28: Atlas

Atlas

- **Anterior arch**
  - Anterior surface → Centrally for anterior longitudinal ligament and on each side for origin of longus colli & rectus capitis anterior
  - – Upper margin for anterior atlanto-occipital membrane
    – Lower margin for anterior longitudinal ligament
  - Posterior surface → Facet for articulation with odontoid process of axis
- **Transverse process**
  - – Origin for obliquus capitis superior, rectus capitis lateralis and levator scapulae
  - – Insertion of obliquus capitis inferior
  - – Foramen transverium transmits vertebral artery, vein & sympathetic plexus
  - – Structure in front of tip of transverse process:
    - Internal jugular vein
    - Spinal accessory nerve
    - Occipital artery
- **Lateral mass**
  - Superior articular facet → Kidney shaped and for articulation with condyles of occipital
  - Inferior articular facet for → Articulation with superior facet of axis
  - Medial tubercle → For attachment of transverse ligament of atlas
- **Posterior arch**
  - Upper Surface →
    a) In front groove for third part of vertebral artery and sub-occipital nerve deep to it
    b) Behind for posterior atlanto occipital membrane
  - Posterior Tubercle → For ligamentum nuchae and rectus capitis posterior minor on each side
  - Inferior surface → Ligamentum flavum

been a spinous process – then it would hinder the movement of extension of head.

3. Transverse process is unusually long. The width between the tips is maximum except in case of seventh cervical vertebra. It provides good amount of leverage for rotatory movement of head.

Anatomical Position – The bone should be held in such a manner so that

1. Shorter arch in front and longer arch behind.
2. Kidney-shaped concave facets should direct upwards and circular flat facet will direct downwards.
3. Groove in the posterior arch will direct upwards.

Different Parts

1. Two arches – Anterior and Posterior
2. Two lateral masses
3. Two Transverse Processes.

II. **Posterior Arch**:

1. Longer than the anterior arch.

Articulations:

1. With *odontoid process of Axis forming Synovial joint (Pivot type).*
2. *Superior articular facet* with condyles of occipital bone forming two Atlanto occipital joints (for *nodding and lateral flexion of head. Synovial and Condyloid type*).
3. *Atlanto occipital membranes and ligamentum flavum* connect Atlas with occipital and Axis respectively forming fibrous type of Joints.

Second Cervical Vertebra or Axis

It is called axis due to presence of odontoid process or dens around which head with atlas rotates.

FEATURES FOR IDENTIFICATION:

1. Presence of *dens* or *odontoid process* – a tooth-like process projecting from upper part of body.
2. Spinous process – large and bifid.
3. Very much ragged lateral mass.
4. Inferior vertebral notches are very deep.

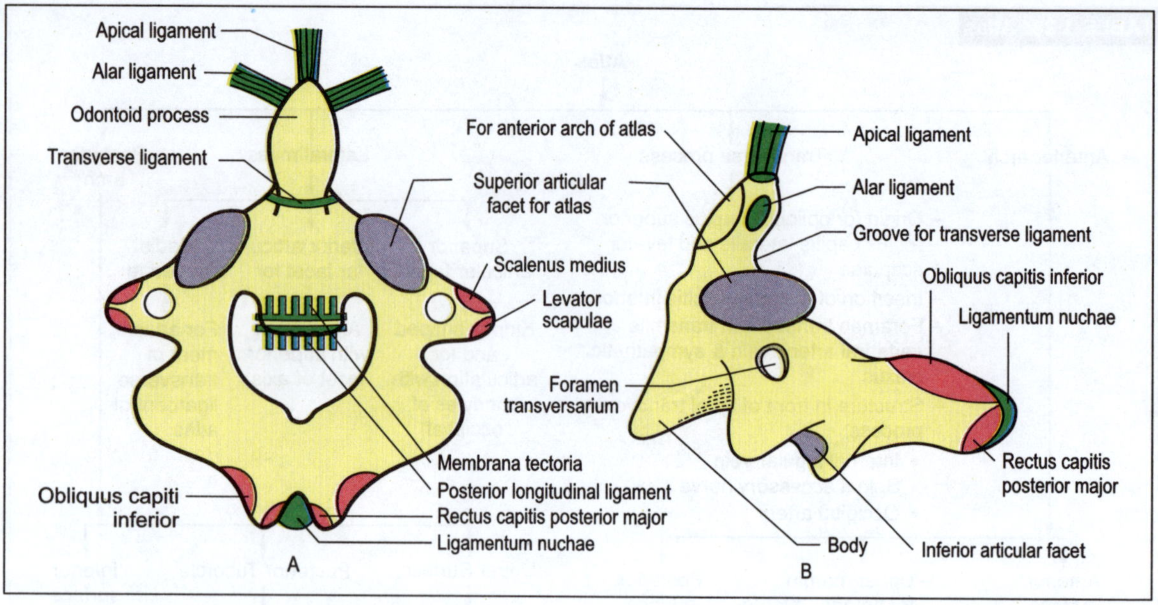

Fig. 1.53: Superior and lateral view of axis

Anatomical Position – It should be held in such a manner that

1. Body will be in front
2. Odontoid process upwards
3. Spinous process behind.

SEVENTH CERVICAL VERTEBRA OR VERTEBRA PROMINENS

It is called vertebra prominens due to its prominence of spinous process.

CHARACTERISTICS FOR IDENTIFICATION:

1. Spinous process is *long* and *horizontal* and not bifid like other cervical but ends in Knob like enlargement.
2. Foramen Transversarium is small.
3. Transverse process is large specially the posterior part.

Anatomical Position – Bone should be held in such a manner that

1. Body should be directed in front.
2. Spinous process will be directed behind and in the median plane.
3. Upper border of Lamina will be more in front than the lower border.

FEATURES:

I. **Body**:

A. *In Front* – Anterior Longitudinal ligament and Longus colli.

B. *Behind* – Posterior Longitudinal ligament.

II. **Spinous Process**:

A. *In the Tubercle*:

1. Lower end of Ligamentum nuchae.
2. Origin of Trapezius, Rhomboideus minor and other deep muscles of back.

III. **Transverse Process**:

A. *Prominent posterior tubercle* for

1. Scalenus minimus
2. Apex of Supra pleural membrane (Sibson's fascia).
   (It extends to inner border of First rib. It is a dome-shaped fascia covering cervical pleura. It represents degenerated scalenae muscles and endothoracic fascia.)

B. *Lower border* – for origin of first pair of Levatores costarum.

C. *Foramen Transversarium* – Very small and transmits only vertebral veins and sympathetic plexus and not vertebral artery.

D. *Anterior Part* – Short and slender and costal element may form a *cervical rib*.

TABLE 1.29: Features of Atlas

Axis

- Odontoid process (Represents the body of atlas)
  - Tip → Apical ligament → Represents the remnants of notochord
  - One each side → Alar ligaments
  - Anterior facets for anterior arch of atlas
  - Posterior groove for transverse ligament of atlas
- Body (surfaces)
  - Anterior → 1. Anterior longitudinal ligament 2. Longus colli
  - Posterior → Posterior longitudinal ligament (upper part) which is continuous with membrana tectoria
  - Inferior surface → Articulate with body of third cervical vertebra
- Pedicle
  - Superior vertebral notches → Shallow
  - Inferior notches → Deep
- Laminae → Thick and massive for ligamentum flavum
- Articular process
  - Superior → Articulate with inferior facet of atlas
  - Inferior → Articulate with superior facet of 3rd cervical vertebra
- Spinous process → Bifid and large gap →
  1. On each side for origin of obliquus capitis inferior and rectus capitis posterior major
  2. In the gap for ligamentum nuchae and deep muscles of back
- Transverse process
  A tubercle for origin of
  1. Scalenus medium; 2. Levator scapulae
  3. Splenius cervicis

  Foramen transversarium:
  Transmits: a) Vertebral artery, (2nd part)
  b) Vertebral vein; c) Sympathetic plexus

(When cervical rib present – it may extend up to first rib. It may be wholly bony or fibrous or partly bony. So, if bony will be visualised by X'ray, otherwise not visible. It may or may not produce symptom. If it compresses subclavian artery and Lower Trunk of Brachial Plexus – then *pain* along *medial border of forearm* and cause *aneurysm* of the artery which may be potential source of embolus to the hand and may cause gangrene).

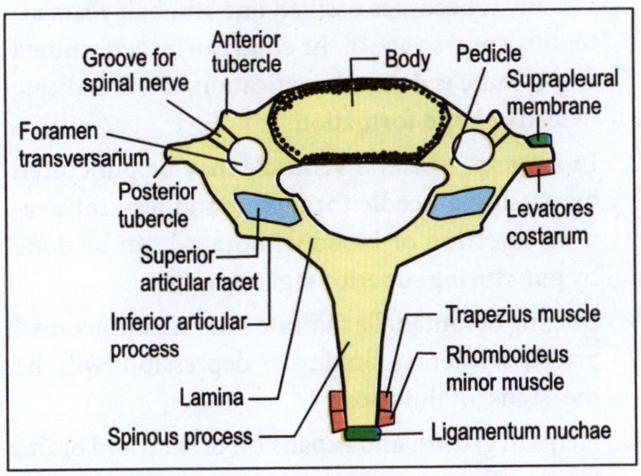

Fig. 1.54: Postero-superior aspect of Seventh Cervical Vertebra

NEONATAL SKULL

Features of neonatal skull

1. **Fontanelles** – Six unossified areas on fontanelles are found in the vault of newborn.

   Unpaired anterior & posterior fontanelles lies in the midline.

   The fontanellies helps during delivery without pressure on brain.

Anterior fontanellae & its importance

a) It is the largest & diamond shaped.

b) It is situated at the site of future bregma.

c) It is bounded by two halves of frontal bone in front and two parietal bone behind.

d) Measurements: Length – 4cm
Breadth – 2.5cm

e) below the fontanelle, superior sagittal sinus lies.

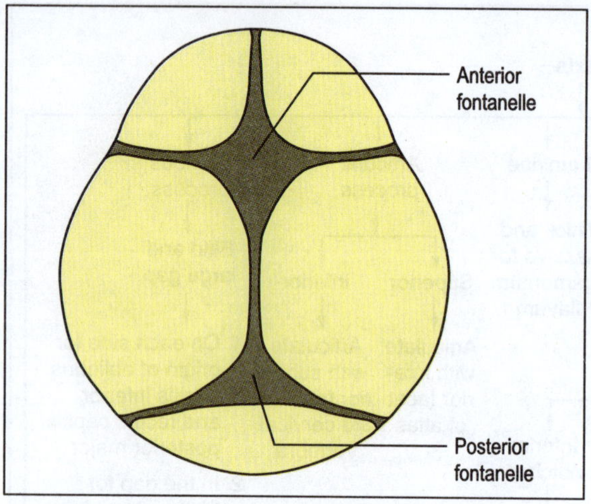

Fig. 1.55: Anterior and posterior fontanelle

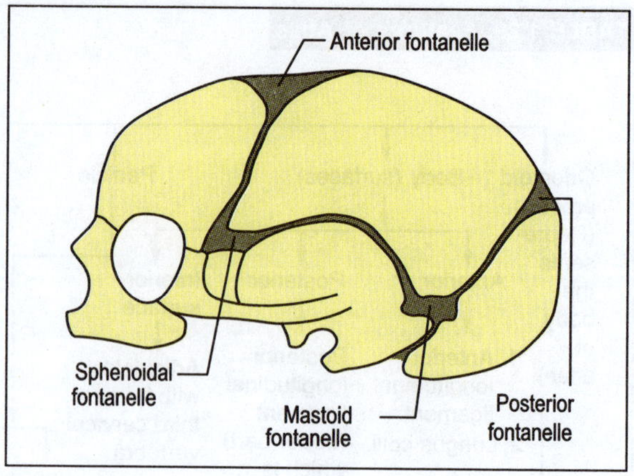

Fig. 1.56: Sphenoidal, mastoid, anterior and posterior fontanelle.

f) It usually closes by 18 months or 2 yrs.

g) Pulsation can be seen.

Clinical importance of anterior fontanelle

a) Delay in closing in Vit. D deficiency.

b) Abnormal bulging occur in increase in intracranial tension.

c) Depressed in dehydration.

d) Withdrawal of blood or intravenous transfusion of fluid or drugs with the help of superior sagittal sinus.

Posterior fontanellae is situated at the site of future lambda.

Sphenoidal fontanellaes are closed during third month.

Mastoid fontanellaes closes at the 2nd of first year.

2. **Mastoid process** – Mastoid process is absent at birth, appear in second year. Stylomastoid foramen is exposed at birth.

   Mastoid antrum lies 2mm deep to suprameatal triangle. Every year, there is an increase of 1mm in thickness until it reaches 12 to 15mm in adult.

3. **Small skull** – The facial skeleton of the newborn is very small, which is due to small size of mandible and maxilla, small size of maxillary air sinus, and nasal cavities, and non-eruption of teeth.

   The angle of mandible is about 140° at birth. The two halves of mandible unites & form symphysis menti by one year.

4. **Paranasal air sinus**:

   a) Maxillary air sinus is small at birth & development complete by 15-20 yrs.

   b) Frontal air sinus – absent at birth
   – grows by 15-20 yrs.

Bony part of external auditory meatus is yet to develop at birth. The tympanic membrane is close to surface in new born.

Growth of facial skeleton is related to eruption of teeth, growth of orbits, nasal cavities along with paranasal air sinuses.

Importance of fontanelles

Its importances are:

1. Usually it becomes ossified one and half years after birth and so age of the child can be determined and if there is delayed ossification, it will indicate defective bone formation.
2. In surgery – Lateral ventricle may be punctured by passing a needle through it and also intravenous injection or blood withdrawal can be done by puncturing superior sagittal sinus.
3. Bulging of fontanelle indicate increase intracranial pressure whereas sinking or depression will be the signs of fluid-loss.
4. Helps in growth and expansion of skull and brain.
5. During labour (delivery of a baby), the position of baby may be known by feeling the fontanelle through a vaginal examination.

chapter 2

THE SCALP, THE TEMPLE AND THE FACE

AT A GLANCE

- *Scalp—Layers; Arterial supply; Venous drainage; Nerve supply; Lymphatic drainage; Applied anatomy*
- *Temple—Boundary; Contents*
- *Face—Muscles of facial expression; Arterial supply; Venous drainage; Lymphatic drainage; Nerve supply; Applied anatomy; Development with anomalies*
- *Eyelids—Features; Structure; Blood supply; Nerve supply; Applied anatomy*
- *Conjunctiva—Different parts; Fornices, conjunctival sac; Bulbar & palpebral conjunctiva; Blood & nerve supply*
- *Lacrimal apparatus—Lacrimal gland (Different parts, Accessory lacrimal glands, Ducts of lacrimal gland, Structure of lacrimal gland, Functions of tears, Nerve supply); Conjunctival sac; Lacrimal puncta and canaliculi; Lacrimal sac; Nasolacrimal duct*

THE SCALP

Layers

The scalp consists of **five layers:** (Fig. 2.1)

(a) **Skin** – Thick very hairy with numerous sebaceous & sweat gland.

(b) **Connective tissue** – Network of fibro-fatty tissue with blood vessels & nerve. It connects the skin and aponeurotic layer, lobules of fat. The wall of vessels are adherent to the fibrous network.

(c) **Aponeurosis** of occipitofrontalis muscle. The aponeurosis (epicranial) or galea aponeurotica is attached:

1. Anteriorly – No bony attachment
2. Posteriorly – External occipital protuberance & highest nuchal line
3. Laterally – Zygomatic arch after an attachment to superior temporal line

OCCIPITOFRONTALIS MUSCLE –

Occipital bellies

– Two bellies, separated by a gap. (Fig. 2.2)

Origin – From lateral two-third of the superior nuchal line

Insertion – Aponeurosis.

Nerve supply – Posterior auricular nerve of the facial nerve.

Frontal bellies

– Both bellies are close to the midline. Frontal fibers continuous with procerus, corrugator supercilli and orbicularis oculi.

Origin – From skin of the forehead near the root of nose

Insertion – Aponeurosis.

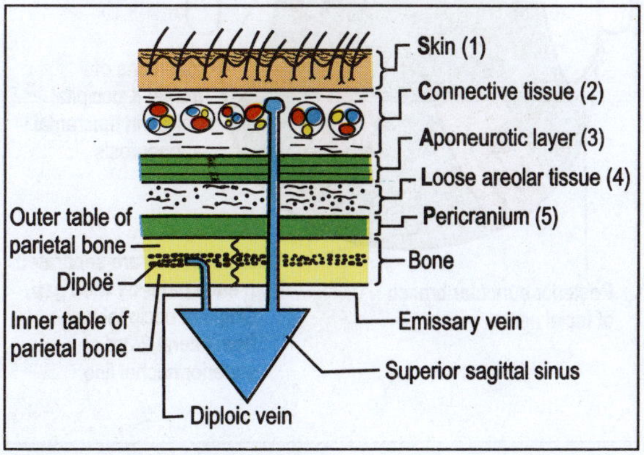

Fig. 2.1: Layers (1 to 5) of the scalp

Nerve supply – Temporal branch of the facial nerve.

Action: 1. Alternate contraction of two bellies move the scalp forward & backward.

2. Frontal fibers elevate the eyebrow during the expressions of surprise.

3. Frontal bellies also form transverse wrinkles.

(d) **Loose areolar tissue** – forms a potential space below aponeurosis. Traversed by emissary vein. This layer extends into eyelids. Emissary vein passes through this layer.

Extend – anteriorly up to the eyelids.

Posteriorly – highest nuchal line

Laterally – Superior temporal line.

(e) **Pericranium** – loosely attached to the skull bone, formed by periosteum

– firmly attached to the sutures.

Arterial supply: Arteries supplying the scalp mentioned in the Table 2.1

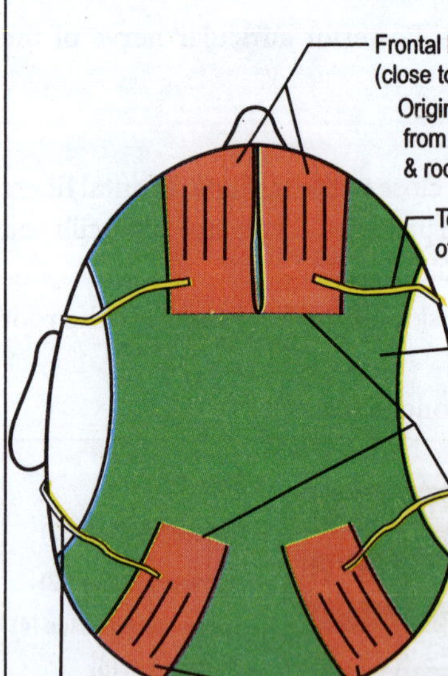

Fig. 2.2: Occipitofrontalis muscle

TABLE 2.1: Arteries supplying the scalp

In front of auricle	Behind the auricle
1. **Supratrochlear artery**, a branch of ophthalmic artery which is a branch of internal carotid artery	1. **Posterior auricular artery**, a branch of external carotid artery
2. **Supraorbital artery**, a branch of ophthalmic artery	2. **Occipital artery**, a branch of external carotid artery
3. **Superficial temporal artery** one of the terminal branch of external carotid artery	

Venous drainage – All the veins accompany the arteries

(a) **Supratrochlear vein + Supraorbital vein**

↓

Angular vein (at the medial angle of eye)

↓

Facial vein

(b) **Superficial temporal vein + maxillary vein**

↓

Retromandibular vein

(c) **Posterior division of retromandibular vein + Posterior auricular vein**

↓

External jugular vein → Subclavian vein

(d) **Anterior division of retromandibular vein + Facial vein**

↓

Common facial vein → Internal jugular vein

(e) **Occipital veins** → Suboccipital venous plexus

(f) **Emissary veins** – It connects the extracranial veins with the intracranial venous sinuses.

Usually two sets – Parietal and mastoid

1. **Parietal emissary veins**

↓ passes through the parietal foramen to communicate with the superior sagittal sinus

2. **Mastoid emissary vein**

↓ passes through the mastoid foramen to communicate with the sigmoid sinus

Nerve supply of scalp

Nerves supplying the scalp mentioned in the Table 2.2.

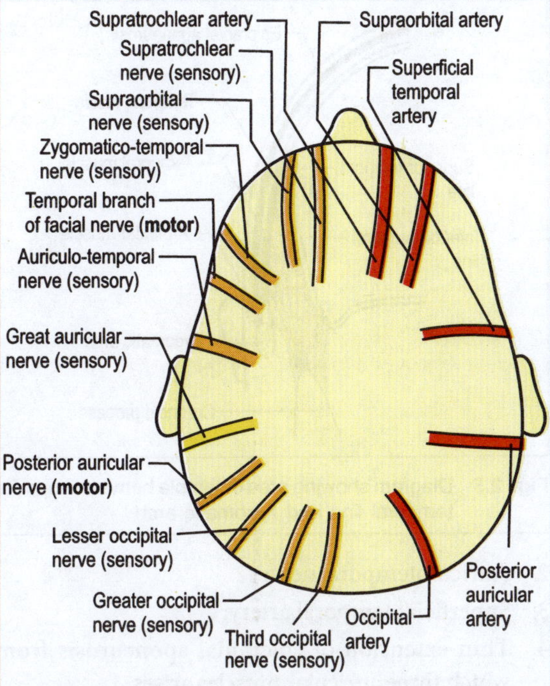

Fig. 2.3: Arterial and nerve supply of the scalp

TABLE 2.2: Nerves of the scalp

In front of auricle	Behind the auricle
Sensory nerves:	***Sensory nevers:***
1. *Supratrochlear branch* of frontal nerve (which is a branch of ophthalmic division of trigeminal nerve)	1. *Great auricular nerve* from ventral rami of $C_{2,3}$ cervical plexus
2. *Supraorbital nerve*, a branch of frontal nerve (which is a branch of ophthalmic division of trigeminal nerve)	2. *Lesser occipital nerve* (C_2) from ventral ramus of 2nd cervical nerve (sensory)
3. *Zygomatico-temporal nerve*, a branch of zygomatic nerve (which is a branch of maxillary division of trigeminal nerve)	3. *Greater occipital nerve* (C_2) from dorsal ramus of 2nd cervical nerve (sensory)
4. *Auriculo-temporal nerve*, a branch of posterior division of mandibular nerve (which is a branch of trigeminal nerve)	4. *Third occipital nerve* (C_3) from dorsal ramus of 3rd cervical nerve (sensory)
Motor nerve:	***Motor nerve:***
1. *Temporal branch of facial nerve*	1. *Posterior auricular nerve*, a branch of facial nerve

Nerves behind the auricle (form before backwards)

1. Great auricular nerve ($C_{2,3}$) – Sensory.
2. Post auricular branch of facial nerve – Motor
3. Lesser occipital nerve (C_2) – Sensory.
4. Greater occipital nerve (C_2) – Sensory.
5. Third occipital nerve (C_2) – Sensory.

Lymphatic drainage of scalp

1. Anterior part of scalp → Preauricular lymph nodes (superficial or parotid lymph nodes).
2. Posterior part of scalp → Postauricular lymph nodes or mastoid lymph nodes.

APPLIED ANATOMY OF SCALP (FIVE DIFFERENT LAYERS)

1. **Dangerous area of scalp** – Blood & pus move freely in the layer of loose areolar tissue. Infection may travel readily through the emissary vein into the intracranial venous sinuses. So, this layer is known as dangerous area of the scalp.
2. **Black eye** – Blood (following head injury) collect in the 4th layer. Blood cannot travel posteriorly & laterally because of the attachments of galea aponeurotica. The blood flows anteriorly because the galea aponeurotica has no bony attachment anteriorly. So blood collect around the upper eyelid, after few hours causing black discoloration of the skin around eye. This condition is known as **black eye** (Fig. 2.4).

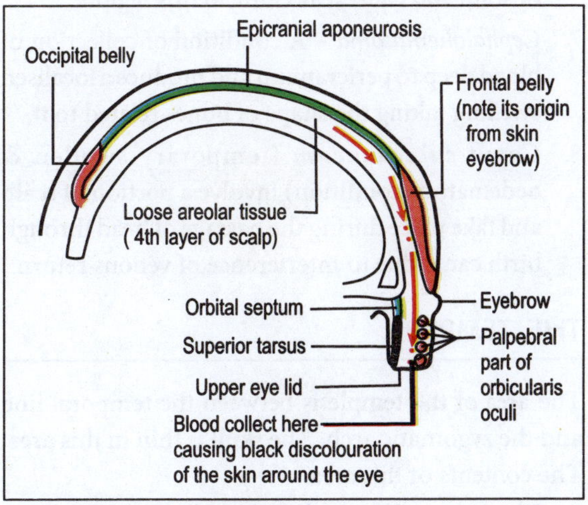

Fig. 2.4: Migration of blood in the 4th layer of scalp

3. Scalp is common site for formation *sebaceous cysts* because skin is provided with numerous sebaceous glands.
4. Scalp injury even minor *cause profuse bleeding.* It occurs because the walls of the blood vessels are firmly attached with the fibrous network of the dense connective tissue layer and so when the vessels are torn the *wall cannot retract* and *cause profuse bleeding.* Pressure against the bone can stop bleeding.

   There may be *pain due to rich sensory supply of the scalp.*

   Due to *rich arterial supply scalp wound heals well* and even when a large area of the scalp is avulsed, if it is replaced and stitched, it will heal quickly.
5. Wounds of scalp usually do not gap unless the epicranial aponeurosis is cut transversely.
6. *Safety-valve haematoma of the scalp* – In children, when fracture of vault of the skull (with torn dura mater) occurs, the blood from intracranial haemorrhage passes to the loose areolar tissue zone and the signs of cerebral compression do not develop till the fourth layer (loose areolar tissue) is filled with blood; this is *safety valve haematoma of the scalp.*

   Traumatic cephalohydrocele is a condition in children when cerebrospinal fluid (due to fracture of vault and tearing of meninges) pass to fourth layer of scalp and cause a swelling in this region.
7. *Cephalohematoma* – A condition of collection of blood deep to pericranium and produce a localised swelling taking the shape of bones related to it.
8. *Caput succedaneum* (temporary swollen & oedematous condition) involve a portion of scalp and take place during the passage of head through birth canal due to interference of venous return.

THE TEMPLE

The area of the temple is between the temporal line and the zygomatic arch. The skull is thin in this area. The contents of this area:

1. The temporalis muscle (covered by **temporal fascia**);

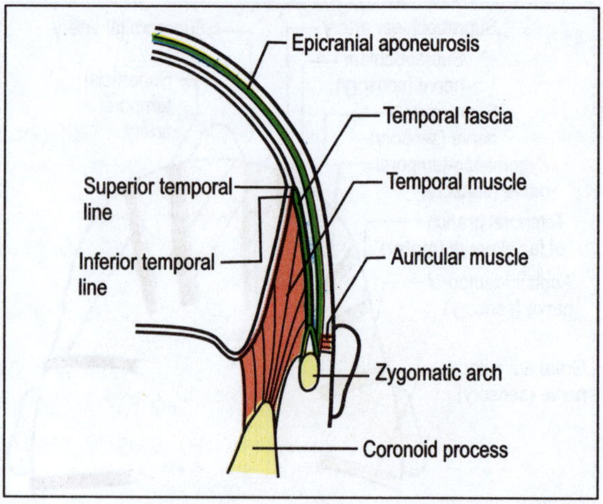

Fig. 2.5: Diagram showing area of temple between superior temporal line and zygomatic arch

2. Auriculotemporal nerve;
3. Superficial temporal artery;
4. Thin extension of epicranial aponeurosis from which three auricular muscles arises.

THE FACE

The skin of the face is highly vascular with numerous sebaceous glands. Superficial fascia contain facial muscles, vessels and nerves; provide attachment to facial muscles.

Muscles of the face

A. **Characteristics** –

   1. Muscles of the face are inserted to the skin of the face.
   2. These are muscles of the facial expression.
   3. *Morphologically* – represent *remnants of panniculus carnosus.*
   4. *Developmentally they are mesodermal and derived from myotome of second branchial arch* and so *supplied by the facial nerve.*
   5. They are grouped according to their position and around the different orifices of the face.
   6. *Functionally* the muscles are

      a) *regulators of the openings of mouth, eye, nose and early sphincters and dilators [Sphincters are circular and dilators are radiating fibres]*

b) *control facial expressions.*

[**Cleavage lines of skin**: These lines coincide with natural wrinkle lines of face. These lines are prominent in old age. It is important to know about these lines to avoid big scars.]

Facial muscles are arranged in groups around eye, nose, mouth and ears. (Figs. 2.6 and 2.7)

Deep fascia is absent in front of masseter, and over the masseter and parotid region, it is present as parotido-masseteric fascia.

Skin is lax in greater part of skin of face; skin is firmly adherent to cartilage of auricle and nose.

A. Muscles around the eye:

(a) Orbicularis oculi : Described in the Table 2.3

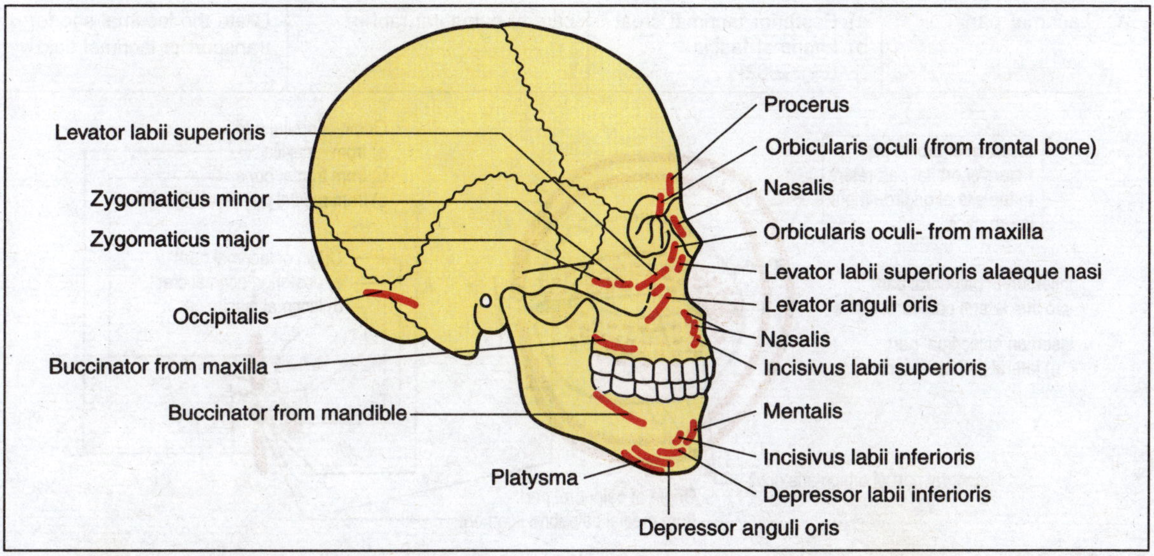

Fig. 2.6: Bony attachments of muscles of face

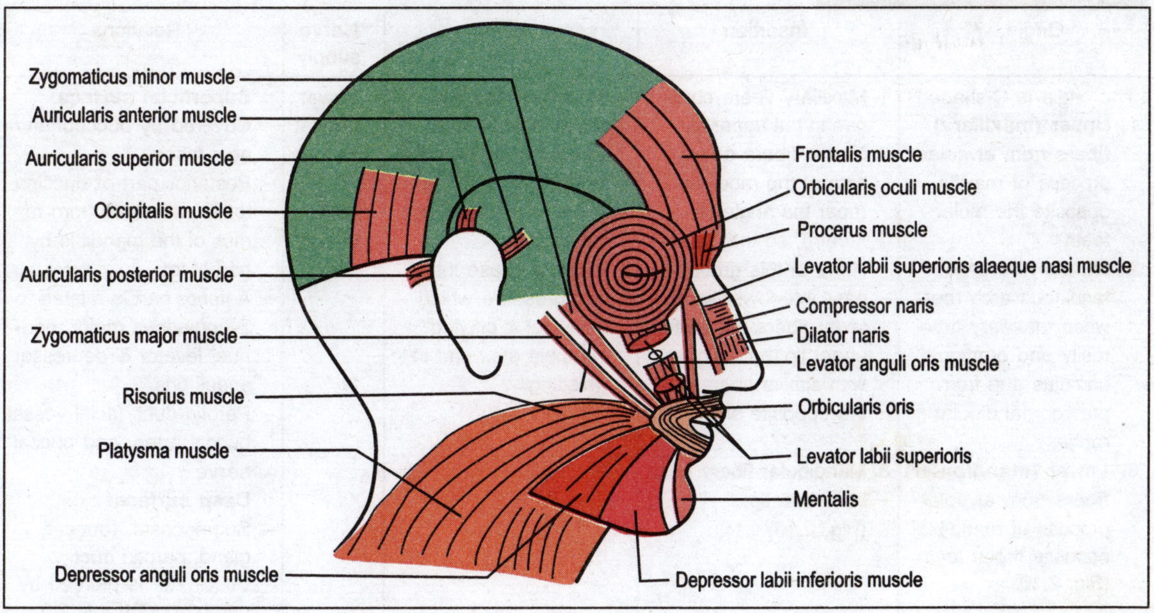

Fig. 2.7: Muscles of facial expression

TABLE 2.3: Muscle of face

Name of the muscle	Origin	Insertion	Action
1. Orbicularis oculi: three parts: (Fig. 2.8)			
A. Orbital part	a) Medial palpebral ligament b) Adjoining bones (frontal and maxilla bone)	Return to the site of the origin without interruption	Protect from the intense light and injury
B. Palpebral part	Medial palpebral ligament	Lateral palpebral raphe	Closes the eye gently in sleep
C. Lacrimal part	a) Posterior lacrimal crest b) Lacrimal fascia (Fig. 2.32)	Lateral palpebral raphe	Dilate the lacrimal sac for transport of lacrimal fluid

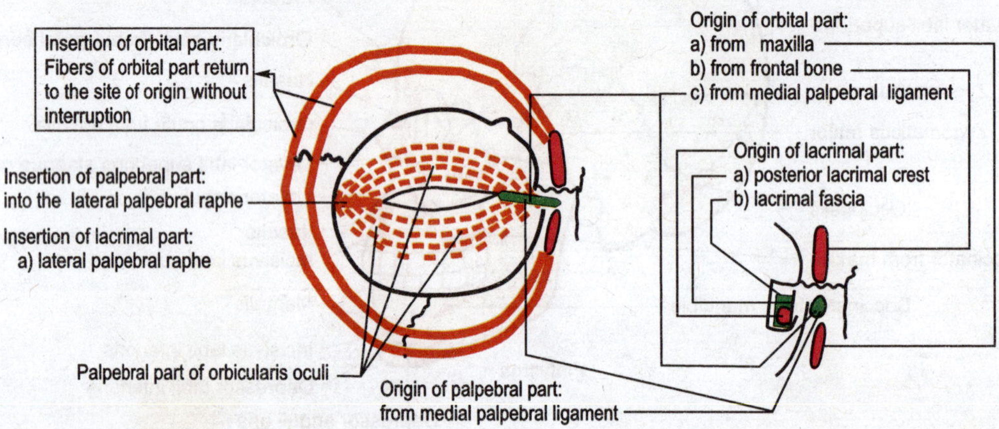

Fig. 2.8: Origin and insertions of orbital, palpebral and lacrimal part of orbicularis oculi

TABLE 2.4: Buccinator muscle

Origin	Insertion	Action	Nerve supply	Relations
The origin is C-shaped 1. **Upper (maxillary) fibers** from alveolar process of maxilla opposite the molar teeth 2. **Middle fibers** from tendinous arch (between maxillary tuberosity and pterygoid hamulus and from pterygomandibular raphe 3. **Lower (mandibular) fibers** from alveolar process of mandible opposite molar teeth (Fig. 2.10)	1. Maxillary fibers continue in the upper lip 2. Middle fibers decussate at the modiolus (near the angle of mouth), so that upper fibers of this group pass into lower lip and lower fibers pass into upper lip to continue with similar fibers of the opposite side. 3. Mandibular fibers pass into lower lip. (Fig. 2.10)	1. It compresses the cheek against gum and teeth. It prevents food from collecting in the vestibule during mastication 2. It can increase intra-oral pressure which is helpful in playing trumpets etc., and in whistling	1. Lower buccal branch of facial nerve	**Superficial surface**: – Covered by buccopharyngeal fascia – Posterior part of buccinator is separated from ramus of the mandible by pad of fat – Anterior part is related to zygomaticus major, risorius, levator & depressor anguli oris – Parotid duct, facial vessel, buccal artery and buccal nerve **Deep surface**: – Submucosal, (buccal) gland, parotid duct Buccinator is pierced by parotid duct (Figs. 2.9, 2.10, 2.11)

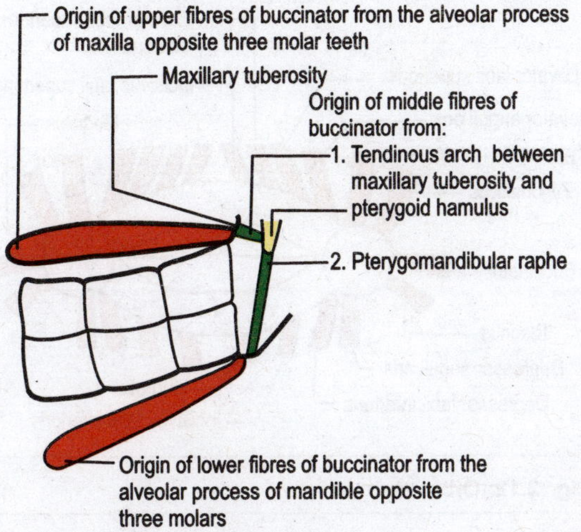

Fig. 2.9: Origin of buccinator

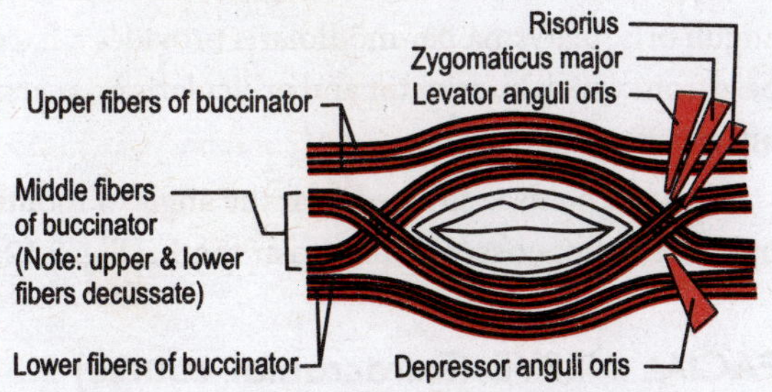

Fig. 2.10: Superficial relations of buccinator and showing the arrangement of fibers of buccinator

TABLE 2.5: Facial expressions and muscles

Facial expression	Muscles
1. Smiling and laughing	1. Zygomaticus major
2. Sadness	2. Levator labii superioris, levator anguli oris and depressor anguli oris
3. Frowing	3. Corrugator supercilli and procerus
4. Anger	4. Dilator nares and depressor septi
5. Surprise	5. Frontalis
6. Doubt	6. Mentalis
7. Irony	7. Depressor labii inferioris
8. Grinning	8. Risorius
9. Contempt or disdain	9. Zygomaticus minor

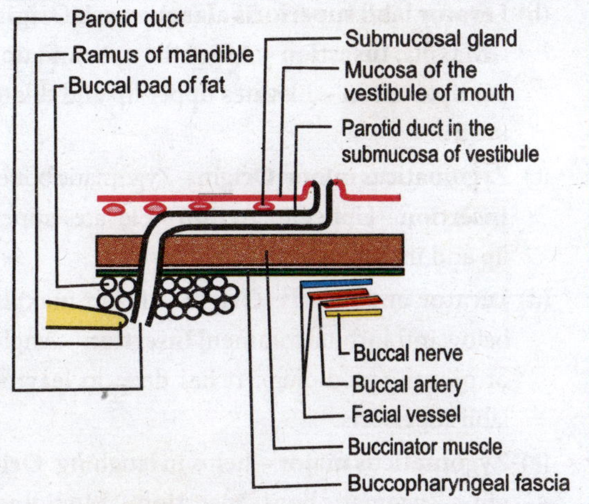

Fig. 2.11: Relations of buccinator muscle

(b) **Corrugator supercilli**

Origin – Frontal bone; Insertion: Skin of eyebrow; Action: Protects eye from bright sunlight & vertical wrinkles in frowning.

(c) **Occipito frontalis** – Described in scalp.

(d) **Levator palpebrae superioris** – Mentioned in orbit.

B. **Muscles around nose:**

(a) **Procerus: Origin**: Fascia covering nasal bone; Insertion: Skin between eyebrows; Action: It produces transverse wrinkles across bridge of nose in frowning.

(b) **Nasalis**: It consists of transverse & alar part. **Transverse part or compressor naris: Origin** – Maxilla; Insertion – continuous with the muscle of opposite side;

Alar part or **dilator naris**: **Origin** – Maxilla; **Insertion** – ala of the nose; **Action**: 1. Transverse part compresses the nasal apertures; 2. Alar part dilates the nasal apertures.

(c) **Depressor septi**: **Origin** – Incisive fossa of maxilla; **Insertion** – mobile part of nasal septum; **Action** – Dilatation of nasal aperture in anger.

C. **Muscles around the mouth:**

(a) **Levator labii superioris: Origin** – above the infraorbital foramen; Insertion – Upper lip; Action – Elevates upper lip.

(b) **Levator labii superioris alaeque nasi: Origin** – Maxilla; **Insertion** – Ala of the nose and upper lip; **Action** – Elevates upper lip and dilate nostril.

(c) **Zygomaticus minor: Origin** – Zygomatic bone; **Insertion** – Upper lip; **Action** – Elevates upper lip and increases naso-labial furrow.

(d) **Levator anguli oris**: **Origin** – From maxilla below infraorbital foramen; **Insertion** – Angle of mouth (modiolus). It lies deep to leavtor labii superioris.

(e) **Zygomaticus major** – helps in laughing: **Origin** – Zygomatic bone; **Insertion** – Modiolus.

(f) **Depressor labii inferioris: Origin** – From oblique line of the mandible; **Insertion** – Lower up.

(g) **Depressor anguli oris: Origin** – From oblique line of the mandible; **Insertion** – Modiolus.

(h) **Mentalis: Origin** – From incisive fossa of the mandible; **Insertion** – Skin of lower up.

(i) **Risorius: Origin** – From posterior fibers of platysma; **Insertion** – Modiolus.

(j) **Buccinator** – Described in the Table 2.4.

(k) **Orbicularis oris** – It is a complex muscle surrounds oral orifice. It comprises both (a) Extrinsic and (b) Intrinsic parts.

Extrinsic part: Following muscles converge around the mouth: a) risorius, b) zygomaticus major & minor, c) levator anguli oris, d) levator labii superioris, e) levator labii superioris alaeque nasi, f) depressor anguli oris, g) depressior labii inferioris, h) mentalis.

Intrinsic part: They lie in between outer skin and mucous membrane of the lips.

Action – The actions of the muscles – pursing, twisting etc.

The modiolus and its role in movement

The shape and dimensions of the modiolus are variable according to individuals, age, sexual and ethnic variation.

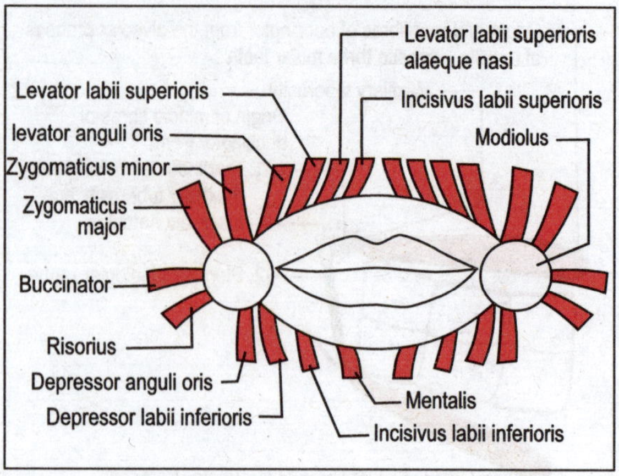

Fig. 2.12: Orbicularis oris

Zygomatic major, levator anguli oris, depressor anguli oris, platysma par modiolaris provides a fixed base from which buccinator and orbicularis oris carry out specific action.

The modiolus is situated near the angle of mouth opposite to upper second premolar tooth. (Fig. 2.12)

FACIAL NERVE (Extracranial course) (Fig. 2.13)

a) After emerging from stylomastoid foramen, the facial nerve lies superficial to styloid process.

b) Thereafter, the nerve enters the parotid gland & divide into two trunks – temporo-facial & cervico-facial trunks.

c) Temporo-facial trunk divides into temporal & zygomatic branch within the parotid gland.

d) Cervico-facial trunk divides into buccal, marginal mandibular and cervical branches inside the parotid gland. Buccal branch divides into upper and lower buccal branch.

e) All the branches emerges from the parotid gland. Branching pattern is known as pes anserinus, as the branches look like goose's foot. The branches and distributions of facial nerve have been mentioned in Table 2.6.

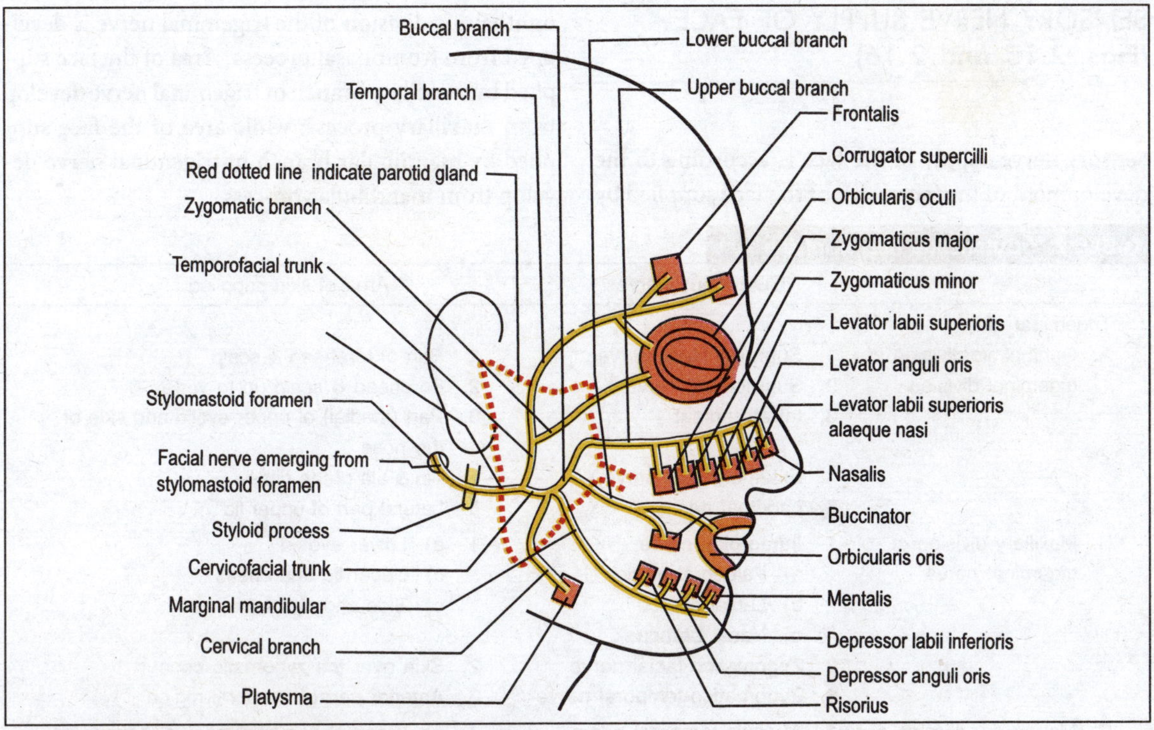

Fig. 2.13: Motor supply of muscles of facial expression

TABLE 2.6: Showing branches & distribution of facial nerve

Branches	Muscles supplying
1. Temporal	1. Auricularis anterior, auricularis superior, frontalis, corrugator supercilli, orbicularis oculi
2. Zygomatic	2. Lower part of orbicularis oculi
3. Buccal: i) Upper buccal	3. i) Upper buccal – runs above the parotid duct & supply zygomaticus major, zygomaticus minor, levator labii superioris, levator anguli oris, levator labii superioris alaeque nasi, nasalis.
ii) Lower buccal	ii) Lower buccal passes below the parotid duct & supplies buccinator, orbicularis oris.
4. Marginal mandibular	4. Risorius, depressor anguli oris, depressor labii inferioris, mentalis.
5. Cervical branch	5. Platysma

Bell's palsy – It is lower motor paralysis of facial muscles due to involvement of the facial nerve (injury or infection) below the stylomastoid foramen. (Fig. 2.14)

Following manifestations can be observed on the affected side of paralysis:

1. Face becomes asymmetrical due to action of muscles of the normal side.
2. Transverse wrinkles of the forehead disappear–due to involvement of frontal belly of occipital frontalis muscle.
3. Palpebral fissure becomes wider as orbicularis oculi (which is paralysed) cannot close the eye.
4. Tears flow down the cheek (epiphora), due to paralysis of orbicularis oculi. There may be corneal ulcers, which may lead to blindness.
5. Disappearance of nasolabial fold.
6. Angle of mouth becomes motionless (during smiling)–due to paralysis of zygomaticus major.
7. Food accumulates in the vestibule of the mouth due paralysis of buccinator.
8. Saliva flow down (dribbling) from the angle of the mouth.
9. The patient cannot move the lip in the affected side, causing disturbance of labial speech.

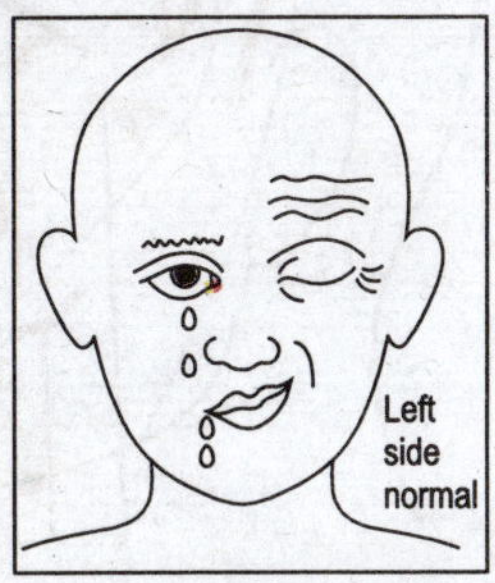

Fig. 2.14: Bell's palsy of right side

SENSORY NERVE SUPPLY OF FACE (Figs. 2.15 and 2.16)

Sensory nerve supply of the face is according to the development of the face. Area of the face supplied by ophthalmic division of the trigeminal nerve is developed from frontonasal process. Area of the face supplied by maxillary branch of trigeminal nerve develop from maxillary process; while area of the face supplied by mandibular branch of trigeminal nerve develop from mandibular process.

TABLE 2.7: Cutaneous nerves of the face

	Cutaneous nerves	Area of skin supplied
1. Trigeminal nerve		
A. Ophthalmic division of trigeminal division	1. Supratrochlear nerve	1. Part of forehead & scalp
	2. Supraorbital nerve	2. Forehead & scalp up to vertex
	3. Infratrochlear	3. Part (medial) of upper eyelid and side of the nose
	4. External nasal nerve	4. Tip & ala of the nose
	5. Lacrimal nerve	5. Lateral part of upper lid
B. Maxillary division of trigeminal nerve	1. Infraorbital nerve	
	a) Palpebral branch	1. a) Lower eye lid
	b) Labial branch	b) Upper lip and cheek
	c) Nasal branch	c) Side and ala of the nose
	2. Zygomatico-facial nerve	2. Skin over the zygomatic bone
	3. Zygomatico-temporal nerve	3. Anterior part of temporal region
C. Mandibular division of trigeminal nerve	1. Auriculo-temporal nerve	
	a) Auricular branch	1. a) External acoustic meatus, tympanic membrane and pinna of the ear
	b) Temporal branch	b) Part of temporal region
	2. Buccal	2. Cheek
	3. Mental nerve	3. Lower lip (part)
2. From cervical plexus	1. Great auricular nerve	1. The angle of the mandible

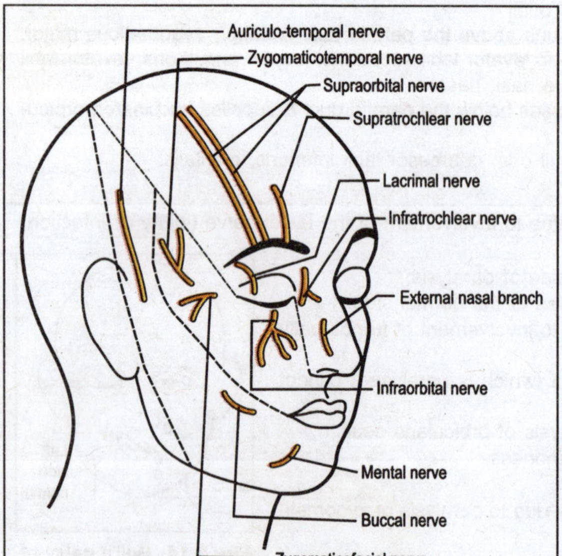

Fig. 2.15: Sensory nerves of the face

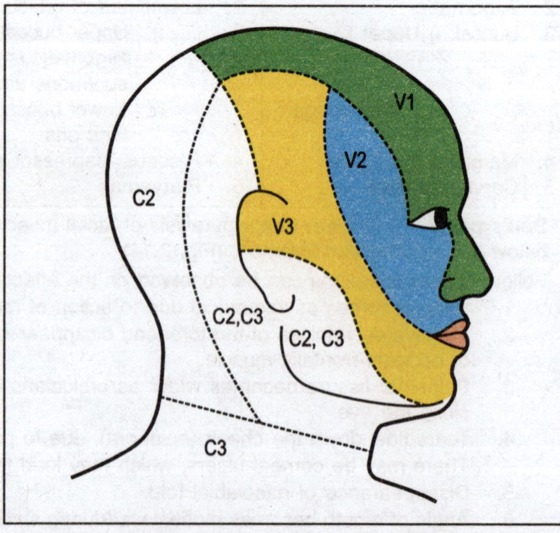

Fig. 2.16: Sensory nerve supply of head: V_1 – Ophthalmic division of trigeminal nerve; V_2 – Maxillary division of trigeminal nerve; V_3 – Mandibular division of trigeminal nerve

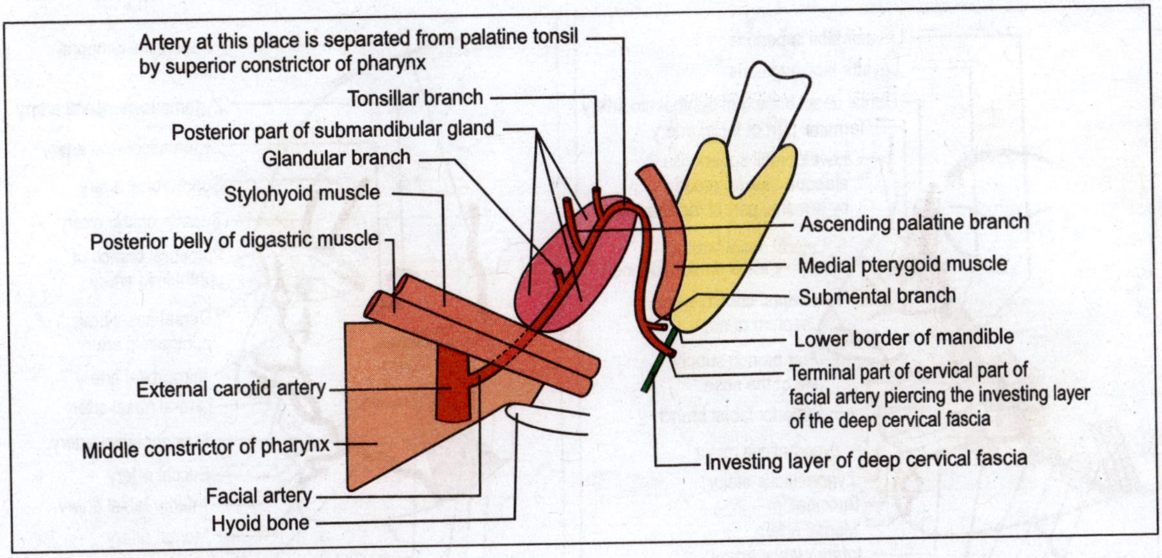

Fig. 2.17: Cervical part of facial artery

ARTERIES OF FACE

Arteries of the face are as follows: (a) Facial artery, (b) Transverse facial artery, and (c) Arteries that accompany the cutaneous nerves.

A. **Facial artery** – It has two parts: (a) Cervical part; (b) Facial part.

Origin – It takes origin from external carotid artery above the tip of greater cornu of hyoid bone.

Termination – It terminates at medial angle of eye after anastomosing with dorsal nasal branch of ophthalmic artery.

(a) Cervical part – From its origin the artery runs upwards & forwards deep to posterior belly of digastric and stylohyoid muscles, ascend in a groove at the posterior end of submandibular gland and presents a loop with a convexity upward. From the loop the artery descends between the medial pterygoid and lateral surface of submandibular gland. At the lower border of mandible the artery pierces the investing layer of deep cervical fascia to enter the face at the anteroinferior angle of the masseter. (Fig. 2.17)

The branches of the cervical part are:

1. Glandular (to submandibular gland)
2. Tonsillar (to palatine tonsil)
3. Ascending palatine branch supplies soft palate, tonsil, wall of pharynx & auditory tube.
4. Submental artery supply mylohyoid & adjoining structures.

(b) Facial part: The artery ascends tortuously. The artery lies on the mandible, buccinator & levator anguli oris. The artery covered by platysma, risorius, zygomaticus major, zygomaticus minor and levator labii superioris. The artery lies 1.25cm lateral to angle of mouth. The artery pierces levator labii superioris alaeque nasi and anastomoses with dorsal nasal branch of ophthalmic artery at the medial angle of eye. (Fig. 2.18)

The branches of the facial artery in the face are:

1. **Inferior labial artery**: It supplies the lower lip.
2. **Superior labial artery**: It supplies the upper lip & gives branches: (a) Alar branch – supplies ala of nose; (b) Septal branch – supplies mobile part of nasal septum.
3. **Lateral nasal branch**: It supply the ala and dorsum of the nose.

B. **Transverse facial artery**: The artery is a branch of superficial temporal artery. It supplies parotid gland. Refer page 142.

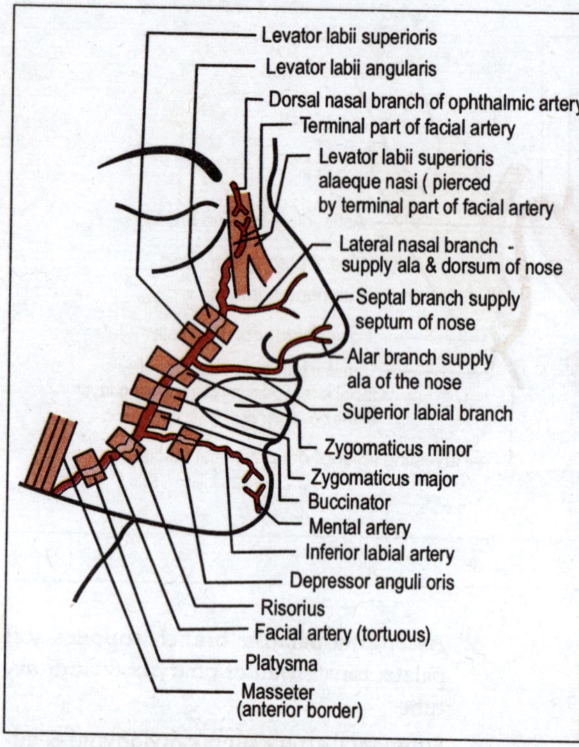

Fig. 2.18: Relation of facial part of facial artery

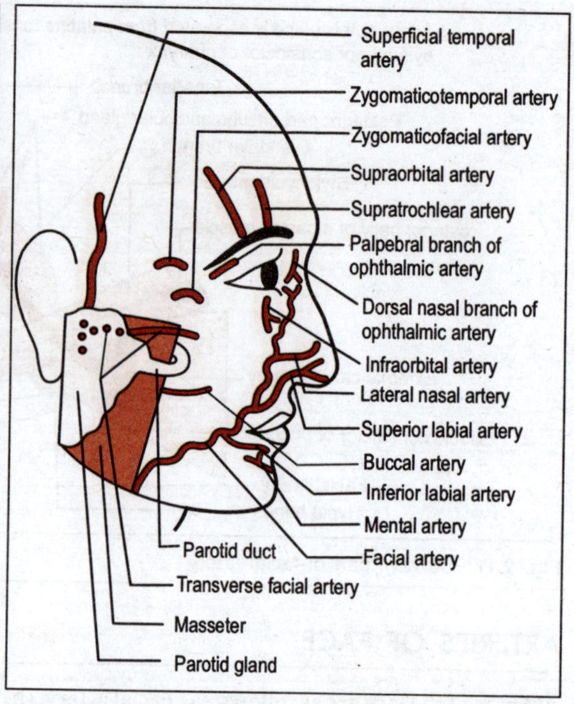

Fig. 2.19: Arteries of face

C. Arteries that accompany the cutaneous nerves: Refer Fig. 2.19.

VENOUS DRAINAGE OF THE FACE (Fig. 2.20)

1\.

Supratrochlear vein + Supraorbital vein	Superficial temporal vein + Maxillary vein
↓	↓
Angular vein (at medial angle of eye)	Retromandibular vein (with in parotid gland)
↓	↓
Facial vein + Anterior division or retro-mandibular vein	Posterior division of retro-mandibular vein + Posterior auricular vein
↓	↓
Common facial vein	External jugular vein
↓	↓
Internal jugular vein	Subclavian vein

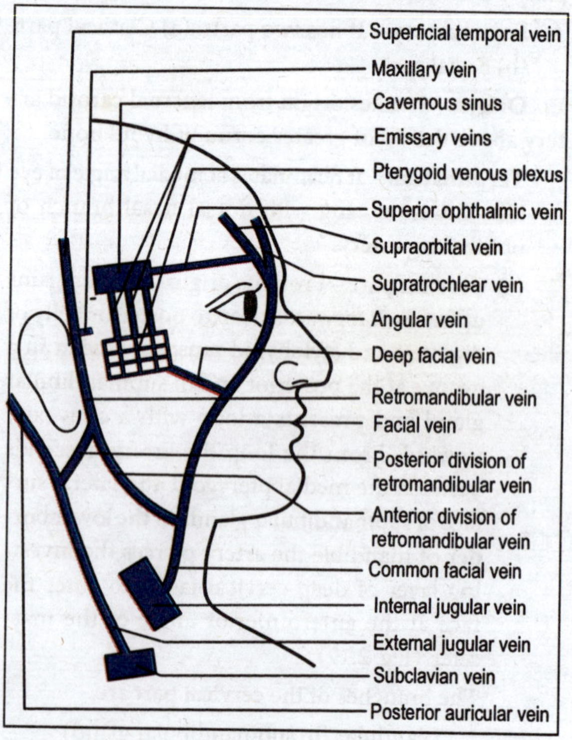

Fig. 2.20: Venous drainage of face

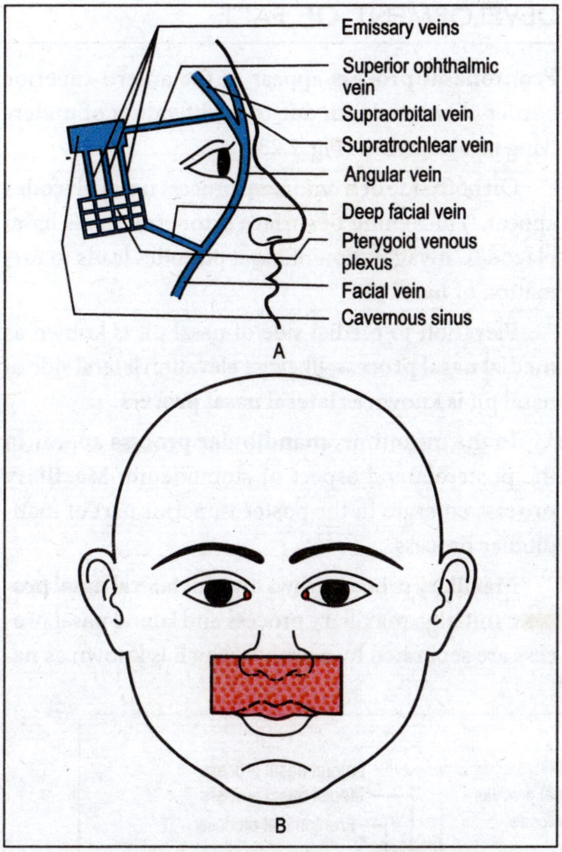

Fig. 2.21: (A) Connections of cavernous sinus to show the spread of infection from dangerous area of face; (B) Dangerous area of the face

2. **Supraorbital vein** is connected with **cavernous sinus** through **superior ophthalmic vein.** Facial vein is connected with pterygoid venous plexus through deep facial vein. Pterygoid venous plexus communicates with cavernous sinus through emissary veins.

DANGEROUS AREA OF THE FACE (Fig. 2.21)

The lower part of the nose and the upper lip is known as dangerous area of face. Infections from this area can spread to the cavernous sinus and can cause thrombosis of the cavernous sinus due to communications between supraorbital vein and facial vein with cavernous sinus through superior ophthalmic vein. Facial vein is connected with cavernous sinus through deep facial vein; pterygoid venous plexus and emissary veins. Infection usually spread in a retrograde direction.

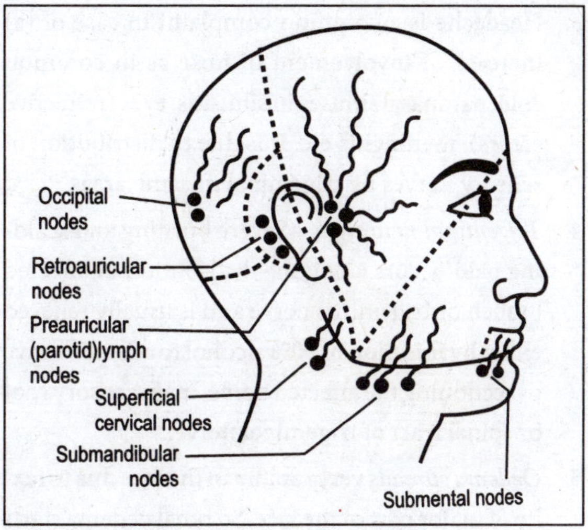

Fig. 2.22: Lymphatic drainage of face

LYMPHATIC DRAINAGE OF THE FACE (Fig. 2.22)

Lymphatics of the face are drained from three areas.

I. *Upper* – It includes greater part of forehead, temple, lateral halves of eyelids and conjunctiva and cheek and parotid area and drains into *preauricular* or *superficial parotid lymph nodes.*

II. *Middle* – It includes central part of forehead frontal sinuses, medial halves of eyelids, conjunctiva, nose with maxillary sinuses, upper lip, lateral part of lower lip, medial part of cheek and greater part of lower jaw and drains into *submandibular lymph nodes.*

III. *Lower area* – It includes lower part of chin, central part of lower lip and drains into *Submental lymph nodes.*

APPLIED ANATOMY

1. *Presence of Acne glands* in the face. Skin of face is rich in sebaceous glands and when they are inflamed there will be retention of secretion and form Acne. These glands are under influence of sex hormones.
2. *Injury in face* heals quickly due to high vascularity. Cut injury in the face bleeds profusely.

3. Headache is a common complaint in case of (a) increase of involvement of nose as in common cold, paranasal sinuses in sinusitis, eyes (refractive errors), meningitis etc. It is due to distribution of sensory nerves by trigeminal in same areas.
4. *Trigeminal neuralgia* – Severe burning and scalding paid occurs along the distribution of affected branch or trigeminal nerve and is usually relieved either by injection of 90% alcohol to affected nerve or sectioning the affected nerve, main sensory root or spinal tract of trigeminal nerve.
5. *Oedema spreads* very rapidly in the face due to laxity of major part of the face. So renal oedema starts first in eyelid.
6. Inflammatory conditions in nose and ear are very painful because the skin is fixed to underlying cartilages.

DEVELOPMENT OF FACE

Frontonasal process appear at the antero-superior border of stomodeum due to proliferation of underlying mesenchyme. (Fig. 2.23)

On both side of frontonasal process **nasal placodes** appear. Thickening of surface ectoderm forms nasal placodes. Invagination of nasal placodes leads to formation of **nasal pit**.

Elevation to medial side of nasal pit is known as **medial nasal process**, likewise elevation lateral side of nasal pit is known as **lateral nasal process.**

In the meantime, **mandibular process** appear in the posterolateral aspect of stomodeum. **Maxillary process** emerges in the posterosuperior part of mandibular process.

Maxillary process grows towards **lateral nasal process**. Initially, maxillary process and lateral nasal process are separated by a groove which is known as **na-**

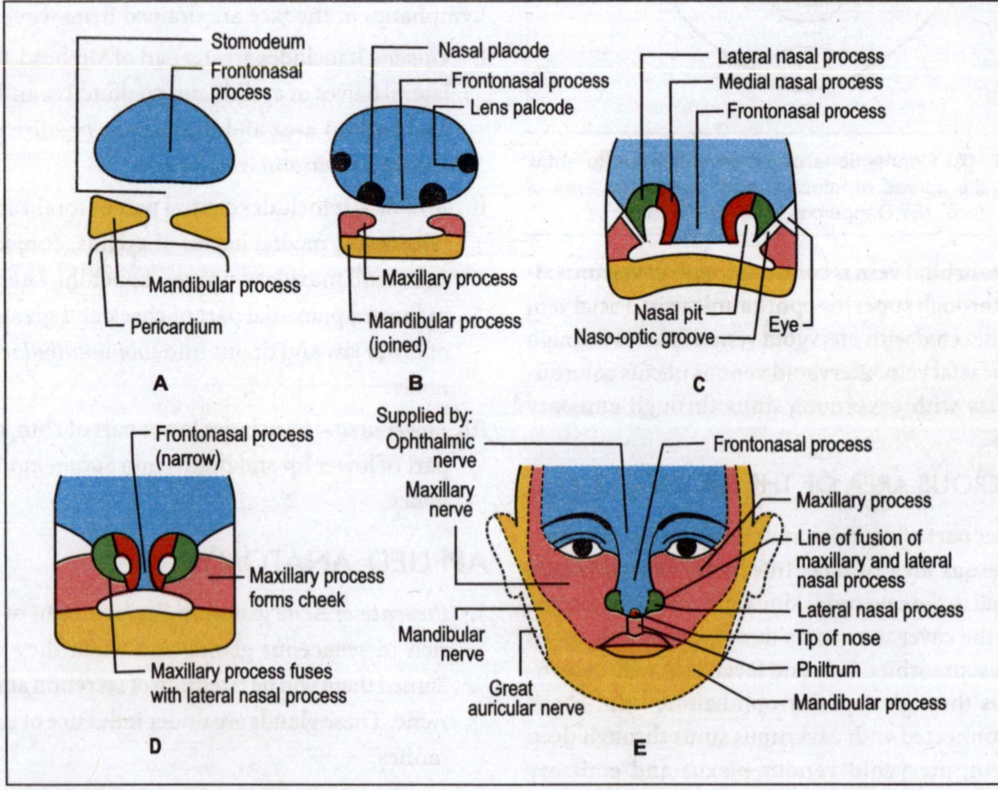

Fig. 2.23: Development of face (A to E)

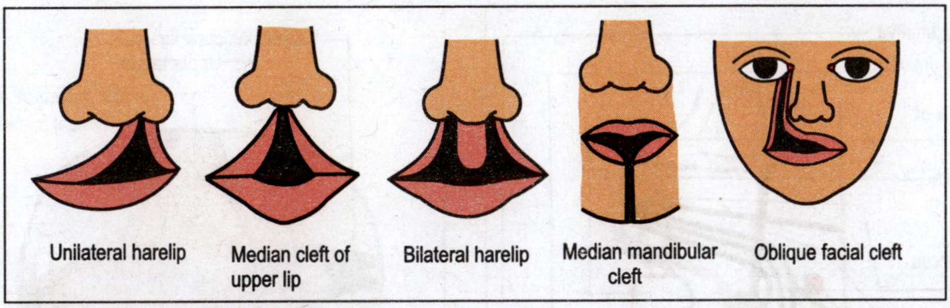

Fig. 2.24: Developmental anomalies of face

solacrimal groove. Nasolacrimal groove helps in the formation of **nasolacrimal duct**.

Maxillary process joins with the lateral nasal process and medial nasal process forming **anterior nasal nares**. Maxillary process joins with opposite side maxillary process forming upper lip & check.

Frontonasal process contribute for the formation of forehead, bridge of nose, medial and lateral nasal prominences.

Maxillary process helps in the formation of cheek and upper lip.

Medial nasal process contributes for the formation of crest and tip of the nose.

Lateral nasal process forms alae of the nose.

Mandibular process helps in the formation of lower lip and mandible.

Congenital anomalies of the face (Fig. 2.24)

1. Hare lip – It occurs usually in the upper lip due to nonfusion of maxillary process with medial nasal process of one side (unilateral) or both side (bilateral).

   Median cleft lip is due to incomplete fusion of medial nasal process in the midline.
2. Oblique facial clefts occur due to nonfusion of maxillary process with lateral nasal process. In this case, nasolacrimal duct cannot be formed.
3. Macrostomia (wide mouth) forms due to inadequate fusion of maxillary and mandibular process.

   Microstomia (small mouth) occur due to more fusion.
4. In hypertelorism, eyes are widely separated.
5. Median mandibular cleft – It is due to incomplete fusion of mandibular process.

EYELIDS (Fig. 2.25)

These are two movable curtains – upper and lower situated infront of eyeball.

Function

1. Protection of eye from injury, foreign body and bright light.
2. Keep the cornea moist and clean.

   Upper eyelid: The upper eyelid is more movable and larger than the lower eyelid.

Features

1. **Palpebral fissure** – Margins of eyelids are separated by palpebral fissure. Margin of upper eyelid partially covers the cornea. Margin of lower eyelid lies usually at the lower limit of cornea. So sclera can be seen at the side of cornea.

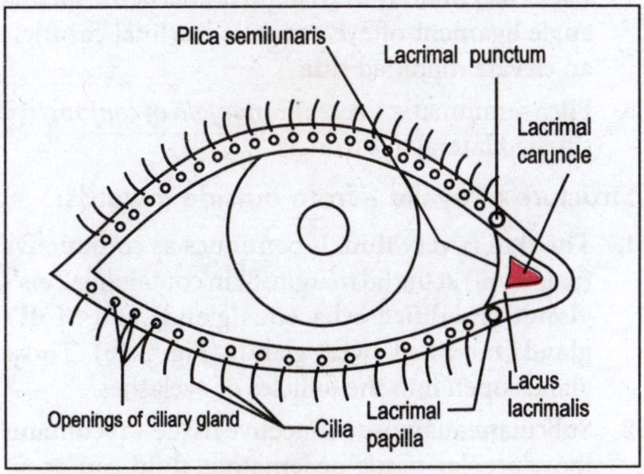

Fig. 2.25: Structures of the eyelids and medial angle between the eyelids

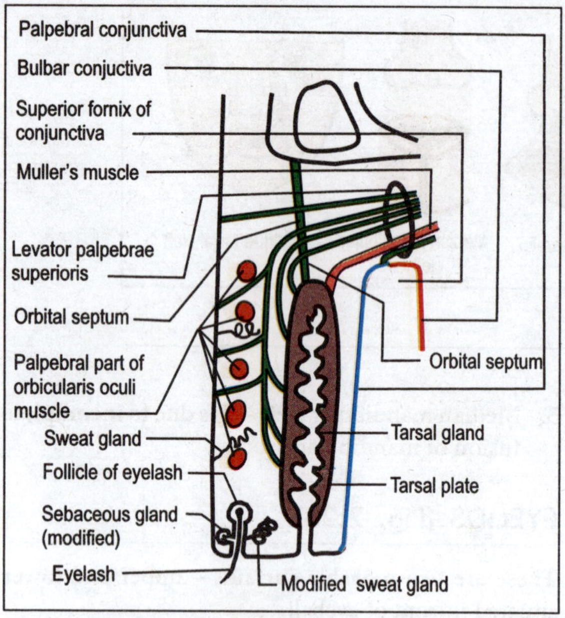

Fig. 2.26: Structure of upper eyelid

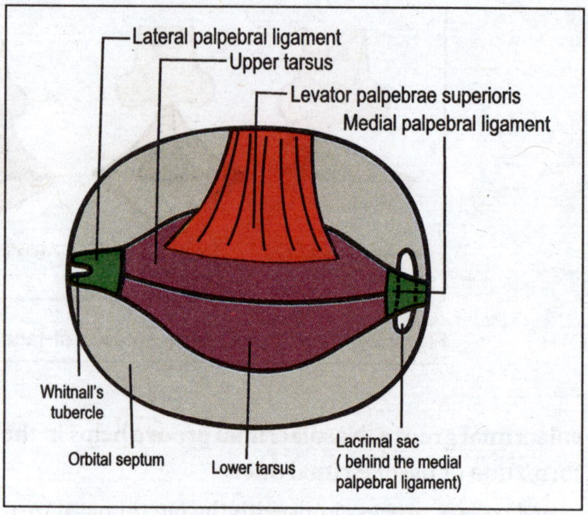

Fig. 2.27: Tarsal plates & orbital septum

2. **Canthi or lateral angles** – Angles at the meeting of two eyelids at the two ends of fissure form **medial** and **lateral canthus**.
3. Lid margin –
   a) Lateral five-sixth has outer rounded lip and sharp inner lip. Outer lip presents eye lashes or cilia with sebaceous and sweat glands (ciliary glands). Inner lip presents openings of tarsal glands.
   b) Medial one sixth has no eye lashes but present lacrimal canaliculi.
4. **Lacus lacrimalis** – A triangular area at the medial angle ligament of eye contains lacrimal caruncle an elevate modified **skin**.
5. Plica semilunaris – A *semilunar fold of conjunctiva* situated lateral to caruncle.

Structure of eyelid – from outside inwards:

1. The skin is very thin. It continues as conjunctiva (palpebral) at the lid margin. Skin containing **Zeis's glands** (modified sebaceous gland) and **Moll's gland** (modified sweat gland) (Fig. 2.26). Those glands open into the follicles of eyelashes.
2. Subcutaneous loose connective tissue – It contains loose areolar tissue oedematous fluid can accumulate in this layer.
3. Fibres of orbicularis oculi – The palpebral fibres of orbicularis oculi lie parallel with the palpebral fissure. A layer of loose areolar tissue (deep to muscle fibres) is continuous with scalp's subaponeurotic layer so that blood or pus at this layer can pass down from the scalp into upper eyelid.
4. a) ***Palpebral fascia*** – It forms orbital septum which lines the margin of orbit.
   b) ***Tarsal plate*** – Condensed and thickened palpebral fascia forms tarsal plate. They are connected medially with medial palpebral ligament and laterally with lateral palpebral ligaments. Upper tarsal plates are reinforced by tendinous slips from levator palpebrae superioris. (Fig. 2.27)
   c) ***Tarsal glands (Meibomian glands)*** – They are *sebaceous glands* in the posterior aspect of tarsal plates and their ducts open behind cilia.
   d) The ciliary glands are present close (behind) to the root of eyelashes, so that their duct also open on the lid margin close to the eyelashes.

Conjunctiva – At the posterior surface of eye

Blood supply

Arterial supply –

Superior and inferior palpebral branches of ophthalmic artery supplies eyelids.

Lateral palpebral branch of lacrimal artery. They form an arterial arch in each lid.

Venous drainage: Drain into ophthalmic and facial veins.

Nerve supply

Upper eyelid is supplied by supratrochlear and supraorbital branches of ophthalmic division of trigeminal nerve.

Lower eyelid is supplied by infraorbital nerve (Maxillary nerve).

Lymphatic drainage

Medial half drains to submandibular nodes. Lateral half to preauricular lymph nodes.

Applied anatomy

1. Foreign body is usually lodged in a groove 2mm from the margin of the lid.
2. Stye is inflammation of Zeis's gland. Chalazion is inflammation of tarsal or Meibomian glands and blepharitis is swelling of lid margin in inflammation.
3. For jaundice, bulbar conjunctiva is examined and for anaemia, conjunctivitis, palpebral conjunctiva is seen.

CONJUNCTIVA

It is transparent, moist membrane covering the front of cornea, sclera and inner surface of eyelid.

Different parts – Two:

1. Bulbar or ocular – Part lining the eyeball.
2. Palpebral – Part lining the eyelid.

Fornices – The line of junction between bulbar and palpebral parts are known as fornices. They are two in number.

a) Superior – At the upper eyelid
b) Inferior – At the lower eyelid.

Conjunctival sac – It is the potential space between the palpebral and bulbar conjunctiva. It contain fluid mainly from lacrimal gland watery and also mucous from conjunctiva and oily from tarsal glands. (Fig. 2.28)

Bulbar conjunctiva – Characteristic features:

a) Transparent
b) Loosely attached to sclera for the movement of eyeball
c) Adherent at the sclerocorneal junction with cornea and continuous with corneal epithelium

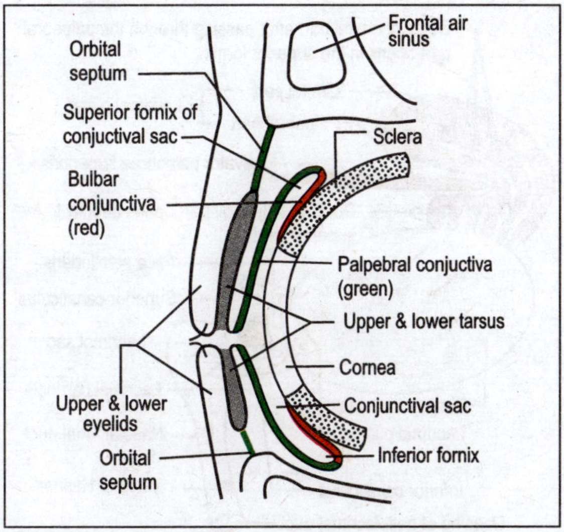

Fig. 2.28: Conjunctival sac

d) It is *trilaminar* – Superficial columnar, middle polygonal and deeper flattened cell layer.

Palpebral conjunctiva – characteristic features

a) Very much vascular.
b) Adherent with tarsal plates.
c) Continuous with skin at the margin of lid and lacrimal ducts at upper fornix.
d) *Structurally* – at the *margin* lined by *stratified squamous epithelium*, on the *posterior surface* of eyelid *bilaminar* superficial columnar and deep flattened cell layer. At the *fornices trilaminar* like bulbar conjunctiva.

Blood supply –

a) Bulbar conjunctiva – Bulbar conjunctiva is supplied by anterior and posterior conjunctival arteries. Anterior artery is from *marginal arterial arcade* and posterior artery is from anterior ciliary arteries.
b) Palpebral conjunctiva – Arterial supply to palpebral conjunctiva is from marginal *arterial arcades* in eyelids formed by branches of ophthalmic and lacrimal arteries.

Nerve supply –

a) Bulbar conjunctiva and upper palpebral conjunctiva – Both are supplied by ophthalmic division of trigeminal nerve.
b) Lower palpebral conjunctiva is supplied by maxillary division of trigeminal nerve.

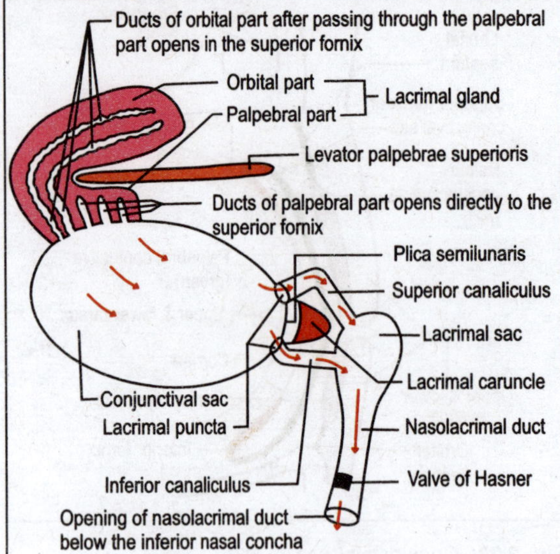

Fig. 2.29: Lacrimal apparatus. Red arrows indicate the pathway of lacrimal fluid secreted by lacrimal gland

LACRIMAL APPARATUS (Fig. 2.29)

Lacrimal apparatus consist of following parts: (1) Lacrimal gland & its duct; (2) Conjunctival sac; (3) Lacrimal puncta and lacrimal canaliculi; (4) Lacrimal sac; (5) Nasolacrimal duct.

1. Lacrimal gland

It is a serous gland.

Situation – Antero-lateral part of roof of orbital cavity.

Parts – It is divided into two parts by levator palpebrae superioris:

(a) **Orbital part** – This part is larger and is lodged in the lacrimal fossa which is in the anterolateral part of the roof of orbit. This part lie behind the orbital septum and inferiorly the orbital part rest on aponeurosis of the levator palpebrae superioris.

(b) **Palpebral part** – Smaller. One-third of the size of orbital part. The palpebral part lies below the levator palpebrae superioris and behind the lateral part of upper eyelid. The palpebral part reaches near the superior fornix of the conjunctival sac.

Two parts are continuous with each other.

Ducts of both parts of the gland open in the superolateral part of fornix.

Ducts of orbital part (4 or 5) passes through palpebral part to open into fornix. Ducts of palpebral part are 6-8, directly open into the superior fornix.

Removal of palpebral part is functionally more or less equal to total removal of the gland because the ducts of orbital part passes through the palpebral part.

Arterial supply of the gland

Lacrimal branch of ophthalmic artery.

Nerve supply of the gland

The gland is supplied by lacrimal nerve which has both sensory and parasympathetic component, along with sympathetic part (Flow chart 2.1).

Flowchart 2.1: Parasympathetic & sympathetic pathways for lacrimal gland

Parasympathetic or secretomotor pathway:

Lacrimatory nucleus (origin of preganglionic fibres) of pons
↓
Nervus intermedius of facial nerve
↓
Geniculate ganglion
↓
Greater petrosal nerve + Deep petrosal nerve
↓
Nerve to pterygoid canal
↓
Relay in pterygopalatine ganglion & postganglionic fibers

Sympathetic pathway:

Postganglionic fibres arises from superior cervical ganglion of sympathetic chain
↓
Plexus around internal carotid artery
↓
Deep petrosal nerve + Greater petrosal nerve
↓
Nerve to pterygoid canal
↓
Passes through pterygopalatine ganglion without relaying

Both pathways:
↓
Joins with maxillary nerve
↓
Zygomatic branch of maxillary nerve
↓
Zygomaticotemporal branch of zygomatic nerve
↓
Lacrimal nerve
↓
Lacrimal gland

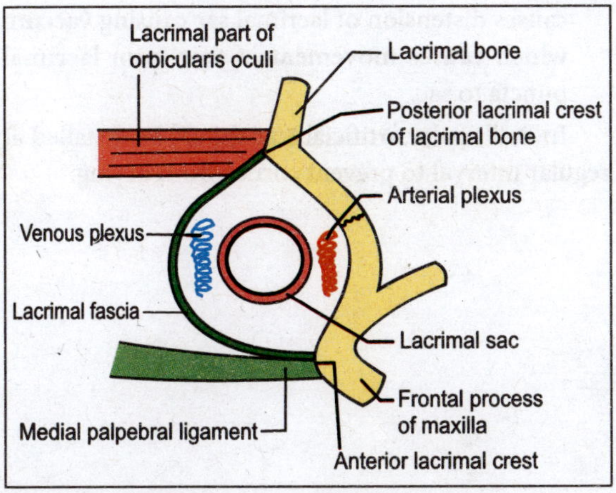

Fig. 2.30: Relations of the lacrimal sac

Lacrimal fluid secreted by the lacrimal gland passes in conjunctival sac.

2. Conjunctival sac

The potential space between palpebral conjunctiva & bulbar conjunctiva is known as conjunctival sac.

Palpebral conjunctiva is continues with bulbar conjunctiva at fornix. Bulbar conjunctiva continues as anterior epithelium on cornea.

The lines of reflection between palpebral and bulbar conjunctiva (behind the upper & lower eyelid) form superior and inferior fornices. (Figs. 2.28 & 2.29).

3. Lacrimal puncta and canaliculi

The lacrimal fluid reach the lacrimal puncta which are situated at the medial angle of palpebral fissure. Lacrimal puncta is a small opening in lacrimal papilla. Lacrimal papilla is a conical elevation. Lacrimal puncta continues as canaliculi. Canaliculi is 10mm long. Each canaliculi open into lacrimal sac. **Superior canaliculus** runs upwards and then bend downwards to open in lacrimal sac. **Inferior canaliculus** almost proceed horizontally to open in lacrimal sac.

At the bending each canaliculus presents small dilatation called **ampulla**. Canaliculi are lined by stratified squamous epithelium and elastic fibres in the walls.

4. Lacrimal sac

It is about 14mm long and 5mm wide. It continues as nasolacrimal duct. Lacrimal sac lies in lacrimal fossa formed by lacrimal bone posteriorly and frontal process of maxilla anteriorly. It is having fundus, body and neck. The lacrimal fascia encloses lacrimal sac. (Fig. 2.30)

Relations:

Anteriorly – Medial palpebral ligament.

Posteriorly – Lacrimal part of orbicularis oculi.

Laterally – Lacrimal fascia, plexus of veins.

Medially – Lacrimal fossa, arterial pelxus.

5. Nasolacrimal duct

It is about 18mm long. It opens at inferior meatus in nasal cavity. It lies in the bony canal fromed by lacrimal bone, maxilla and inferior nasal concha. At the site of termination, **Hasner's valve** is present. The valve is produced by mucosal fold.

APPLIED ANATOMY

Dacryocystitis is an inflammatory condition of the sac causing overflowing of tear (Epiphora).

Accessory lacrimal gland – Small glands found in or near the fornices and more in the upper eyelid than in lower lid. [So *when lacrimal gland is removed* – the *conjunctiva does not become dried due to presence of accessory glands.*]

Epiphora: Tears flow down the cheek may be due to obstruction of lacrimal fluid pathway.

TEARS

Secretion of lacrimal gland when overflowed forms tear.

FUNCTIONS OF TEARS (secretion of lacrimal gland)

a) Keeps the cornea moist and transparent.

b) Provides nutrition to cornea.

c) Kills bacteria.

d) Emotional expression is the shedding of tears.

FACTORS FOR MOVEMENT OF TEAR TO LACRIMAL SAC

1. Blinking of eyelids, tear reaches lacrimal puncta.
2. The contraction of lacrimal part of orbicularis oculi causes distension of lacrimal sac causing vaccum which causes movement of tear from lacrimal puncta to sac.

In Bell's palsy artificial tear should be installed at regular interval to prevent cornea from drying.

chapter 3

The Side of the Neck

AT A GLANCE

- *Superficial fascia*
- *Deep cervical fascia—Investing layer; Pretrocheal layer; Prevertebral layer; Carotid sheath; Buccopharyngeal layer; Fascial spaces – Retropharyngeal space, Lateral pharyngeal space*
- *Posterior triangle—Boundary; Contents*
- *External jugular vein*
- *Sternocleidomastoid*

FASCIA OF NECK

In the head and neck region two kinds of fascia are usually found—superficial and deep. Of these deep cervical fascia is very important to study.

SUPERFICIAL FASCIA

Characteristics:

a) A thin fascia covering platysma muscle of neck and not clearly demonstrable.

b) May present some amount of fat, specially in female.

c) Not a membrane like other superficial fascia but consists of loose connective issue between skin and platysma.

Superficial veins of neck lie between the platysma and investing layer of deep fascia, injury of neck bleed profusely, due to retraction of the divided platysma keep the veins (injured) open (unable to collapse) due to the attachment to the underlying fascia. After the division of deep fascia veins retract.

DEEP CERVICAL FASCIA

Before considering the fascia, one fundamental principle must be borne in mind. Secondary mesoderm forms loose areolar tissue which are found in between the organs of head and neck region. This is like cotton. When cotton is spanned it gives rise to sheet of cloth. So a single fascia takes different names in different regions and is continuous with each other—other directly or indirectly-through loose areolar tissue. This is same in every region of the body regarding fascia.

The deep cervical fascia is also known as fascia colli and it lies deep to platysma in the interval between muscles, vessels and organs of cervical region. It gives different laminae by condensation and thickening.

The deep fascia of the neck forms the following layers:

1. Investing layer;
2. Pretracheal layer;
3. Prevertebral layer;
4. Buccopharyngeal fascia;
5. Pharyngobasilar fascia;
6. Carotid sheath.

1. INVESTING LAYER

It is the superficial lamina of the deep cervical fascia and disposed in a cylindrical manner; it lies just deep to platysma.

The layer forms roof of the posterior & anterior triangle.

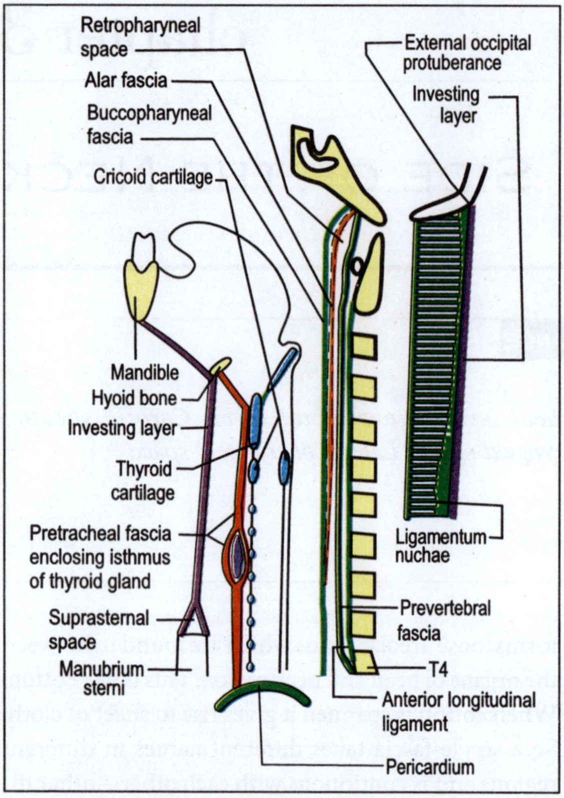

Fig. 3.1: Vertical disposition of deep cervical fascia

Attachments:

Superiorly—(from behind forward)

a) External occipital protuberance; (Fig. 3.1)

b) Superior nuchal line;

c) Mastoid process;

d) Lower border (base) of the mandible.

Inferiorly—(from behind forward)

a) Ligamentum nuchae at seventh cervical spine;

b) Spine of scapula;

c) Acromium process of capula

d) Superior surface of clavicle; and

e) Manubrium sterni. (Jugular notch)

Posteriorly—

a) Ligamentum nuchae.

Anteriorly—

a) Symphysis menti

b) Hyoid bone;

c) It continues to the opposite side as same fascia.

The investing layer presents following features:

a) Encloses two muscles: trapezius and sternocleidomastoid. (Fig. 3.2)

b) Forms roof of two triangles—anterior triangle and posterior triangle.

c) Encloses two glands: parotid gland & submandibular gland.

d) Forms two pulleys or fascial slings:

1. For inferior belly of omohyoid
2. For intermediate tendon of diagastric.

e) Thickened twice to form

1. Parotido-masseteric fascia – Superficial, strong layer attached to lower border of zygomatic arch, covers the superficial surface of the parotid gland.
2. Stylomandibular ligament deep layer – attached to styloid process (strong) [& lower border of lympanic plate (weak)] and angle of the mandible. Stylomandibular ligament separate parotid gland from submandibular gland.

f) Helps to form

1. Pretracheal layer
2. Prevertebral layer
3. Carotid sheath.

Vertical tracing of the investing layer (from below upwards)

Investing layer of lower part encloses two spaces:

1. **Suprasternal space**: Above the suprasternal notch it splits into two layers (attached to antrior & posterior borders of suprasternal notch). It contains:
   a) Sternal head of sternocleidomastoid muscle.
   b) Interclavicular ligament.
   c) Jugular venous arch
   d) Sometimes lymph nodes. (Fig. 3.3)
2. **Supraclavicular space**: It lies above the middle third of the clavicle. It splits into two layers which attached to anterior & posterior borders of clavicle. It contains:
   a) External jugular vein;
   b) Supraclavicular nerves; (Fig. 3.4)

Further vertical tracing –

A. At the lower part of submandibular gland, it splits

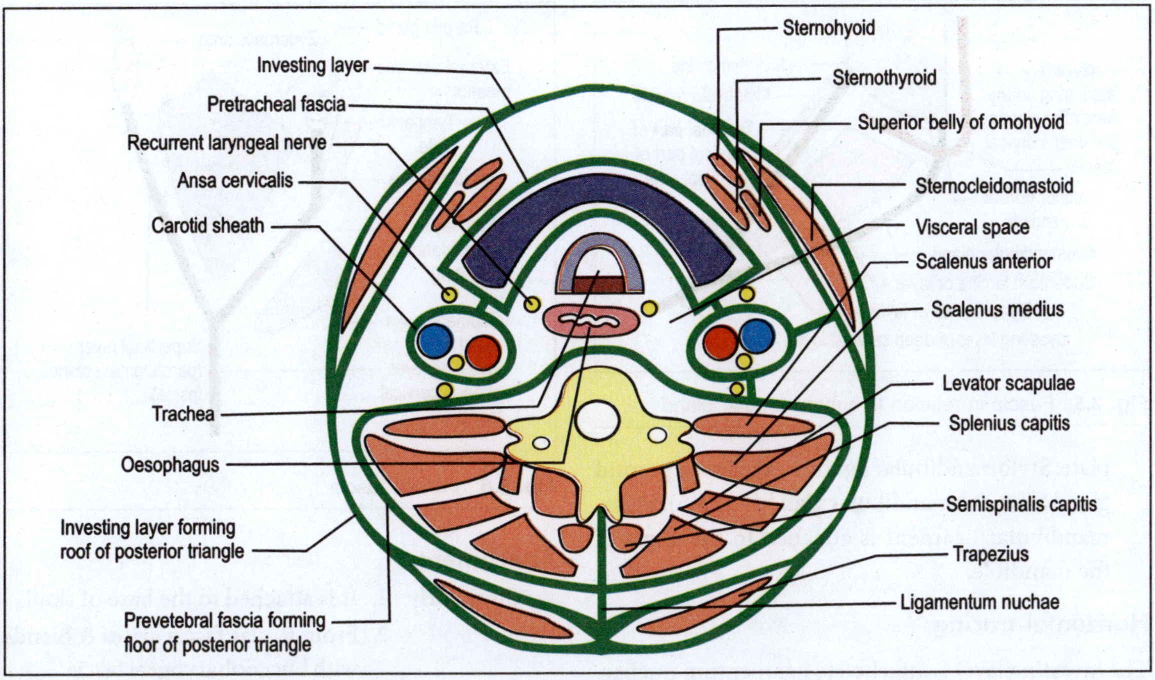

Fig. 3.2: Horizontal disposition of deep cervical fascia

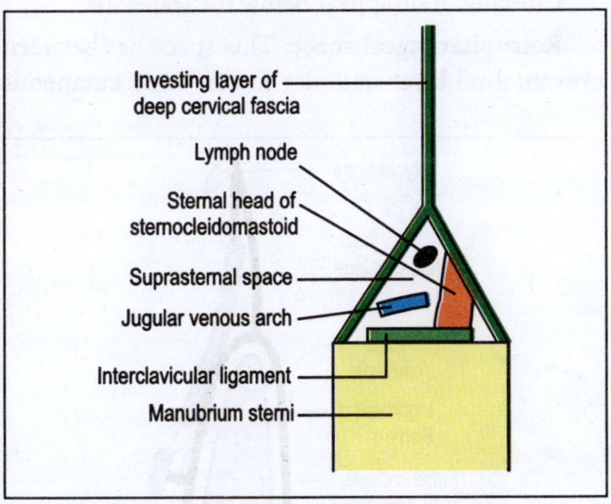

Fig. 3.3: Suprasternal space

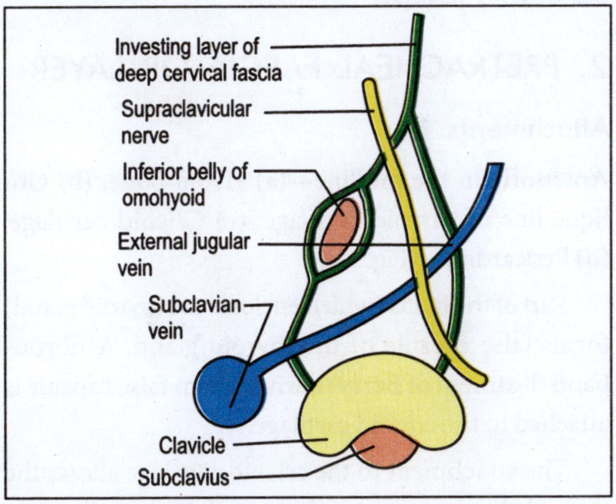

Fig. 3.4: Supraclavicular space

into two layers and encloses superficial part of submandibular salivary gland. The superficial layer is attached to lower border of body of mandible after covering inferior surface of submandibular gland & submandibular lymph nodes. The deep layer after covering the medial surface of submandibular gland attached to mylohyoid line. (Fig. 3.5)

B. *In the parotid region*: At the lower part of parotid gland, the investing layer splits to enclose parotid gland. The superficial layer passes superficial to parotid gland as parotido-masseteric fascia and is attached to zygomatic arch. The deep layer passes deep to parotid gland and is attached to styloid process (stylomandibular ligament) and tympanic

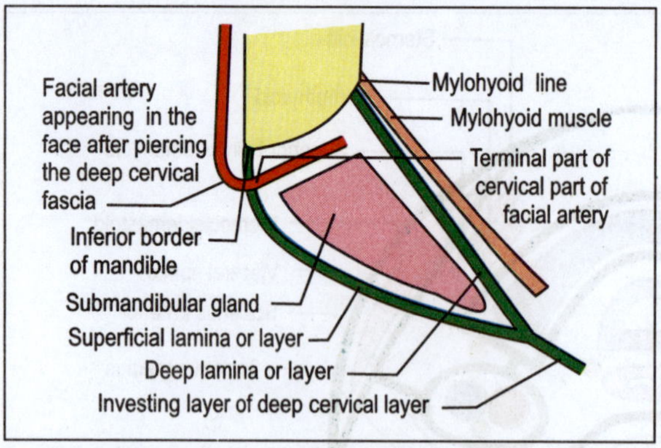

Fig. 3.5: Fascia in relation to submandibular gland

plate. Stylomandibular ligament separates parotid gland from submandibular gland (Fig. 3.6). Stylomandibular ligament is attached to the angle of the mandible.

Horizontal tracing

The investing layer is attached to ligamentum nuchae. It encloses the trapezius & sternocleidomastoid muscles. It forms the roof of the posterior triangle & the anterior triangle.

2. PRETRACHEAL FASCIA OR LAYER

Attachments:

Anteriorly in the midline—(a) Hyoid bone; (b) Oblique line of thyroid cartilage; (c) Cricoid cartilage; (d) Pericardium. (Fig. 3.7)

Part of the fascia (which encloses the thyroid gland) forms false capsule of the thyroid gland. A fibrous band (ligament of Berry) derived from false capsule is attached to the cricoid cartilage.

The attachment to the cricoid cartilage allows the thyroid gland to move up & down during swallowing. Part of layer in the posterior surface of thyroid gland ill-defined which allows the gland to enlarge posteriorly causing dysphagia compressing oesophagus.

3. PREVERTEBRAL LAYER OR FASCIA

It lies anterior to the prevertebral muscles. The part of the fascia in the posterior triangle forms floor of the triangle.

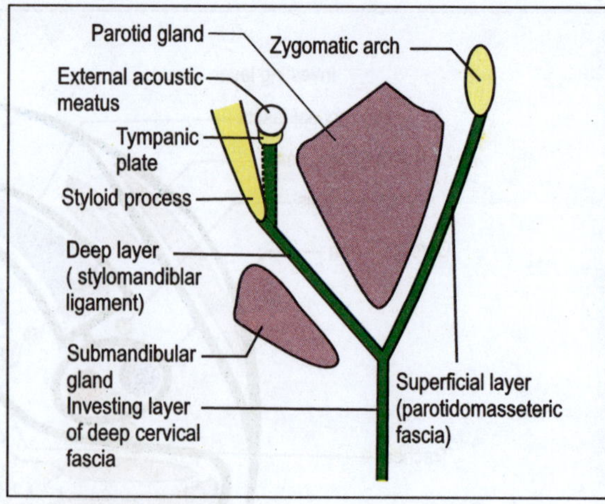

Fig. 3.6: Parotid fascia

Attachments:

Superiorly: 1. It is attached to the base of skull.
2. From it, alar fascia arises & blends with buccopharyngeal fascia.

Inferiorly: Lower border of body of the fourth thoracic vertebra.

Laterally: It disappear below the trapezius.

Retropharyngeal space: This space lies between preventebral layer and alar fascia. Four cutaneous

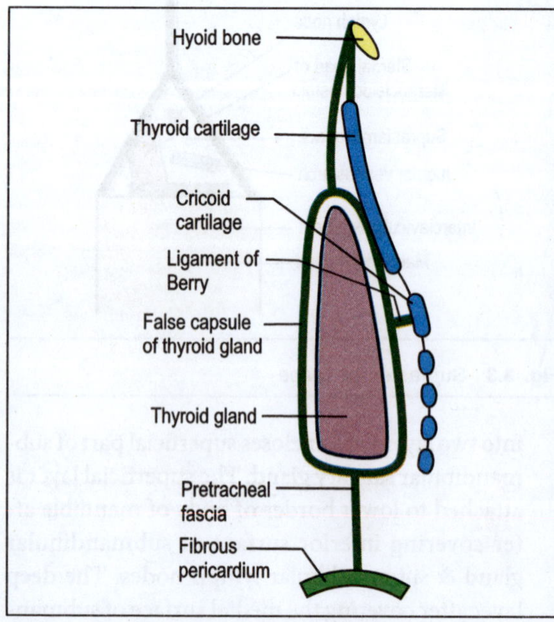

Fig. 3.7: Vertical disposition of pretracheal fascia

branches of cervical plexus pierces the prevertebral fascia. Cervical plexus and brachial plexus lies behind the fascia.

Inferolaterally, prevertebral layer continue as axillary sheath which extends into axilla. Axillary sheath encloses axillary artery, axillary vein and branchial plexus.

4. BUCCOPHARYNGEAL FASCIA

It covers externally the constrictor muscles of pharynx. Superiorly, the fascia is attached to the base of the skull. It extends on the buccinator muscle.

5. PHARYNGOBASILAR FASCIA

Submucous layer of upper part of pharynx thickened to form pharyngo-basilar fascia. Pharyngobasilar fascia closes the sinus of morgagni (space between upper border of superior constrictor of pharynx and base of the skull).

6. CAROTID SHEATH

Carotid sheath (tubular condensation of deep cervical fascia) encloses internal jugular vein, common carotid artery, internal carotid artery and vagus nerve. It extends from base of the skull to the arch of aorta. Sheath is thick over artery and thin over vein. Sheath joins with tunica adventitia of arch of aorta.

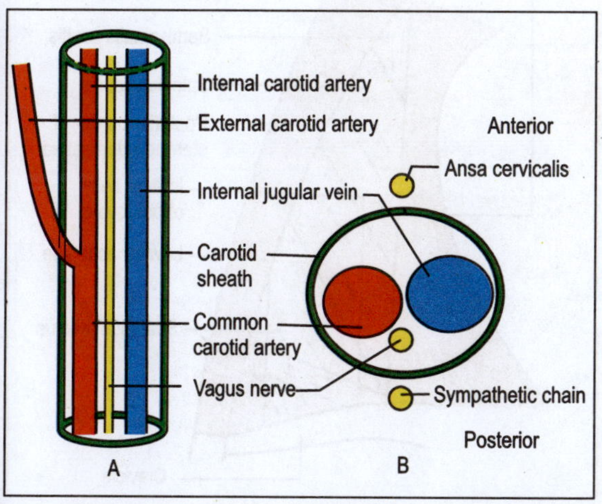

Fig. 3.8: Carotid sheath: A. Vertical view; B. Sectional view

Pretracheal fascia along with investing layer, forms the anterior wall of the sheath. Prevertebral layer forms the posterior wall of carotid sheath.

Ansa cervicalis lies on the anterior wall.

Sympathetic chain lies in between the carotid sheath and the prevertebral layer.

Carotid sheath lies behind the sternocleidomastoid muscle (Fig. 3.8).

RETROPHARYNGEAL SPACE

It is an inverted pyramidal shaped potential fascial space situated behind the pharynx and oesophagus.

Extent: It extends from base of skull above and is continuous with superior mediastinum of thorax below. (Fig. 3.9)

Boundaries:

In front – Buccopharyngeal fascia.

Behind – Prevertebral fascia.

On each side: Carotid sheath.

Division: Divided into right and left parts by alar fascia which is a midline fascial septum extending between buccopharyngeal fascia in front and prevertebral fascia behind.

Contents:

1. Loose areolar tissue.
2. Few retropharyngeal lymph nodes with lymph vessels.
3. Plexus of nerves and vessels.

APPLIED ANATOMY

Retropharyngeal abscess is collection of pus in the retropharyngeal space which may extend downwards into the superior mediastinum or may extend later-

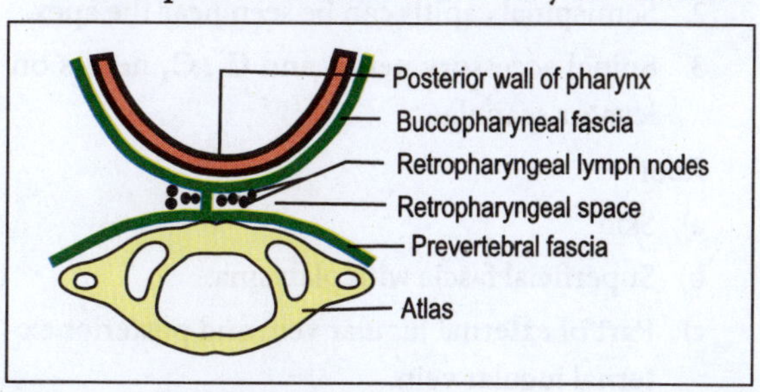

Fig. 3.9: Retropharyngeal space

ally and pass behind the carotid sheath or along buccopharyngeal fascia in the face. This abscess in acute retropharyngeal abscess. Sometimes pus may be collected on one side causing one side (paramedian) swelling.

Chronic retropharyngeal abscess: It is collection of pus behind prevertebral fascia in the mid line and in front of vertebral column due to caries spine. It does not occur in true retropharyngeal space. These two types of retropharyngeal abscesses are distinguished by inspecting bulging in the posterior pharyngeal wall.

Pus due to tuberculosis of the vertebrae behind the prevertebral layer may appear in the axilla after passing through the axillary sheath.

Retropharyngeal lymph nodes involvement produces unilateral paramedian bulge in the posterior pharyngeal wall due to adhesion of buccopharyngeal fascia to the prevertebral fascia in the median plane.

POSTERIOR TRIANGLE

Boundaries: (Fig. 3.10)

Anterior: Posterior border of sternocleidomastoid.

Posterior: Anterior border of trapezius.

Base: Middle third of clavicle (superior aspect).

Apex: Junctional part of sternocleidomastoid & trapezius.

Floor:

1. Prevertebral layer of deep fascia covering following muscles:
   a) Splenius capitis.
   b) Levator scapulae
   c) Scalenus medius (Fig. 3.11)
2. Semispinal capitis can be seen near the apex.
3. Spinal accessory nerve, and C_3, C_4 nerves on levator scapulae.

Roof:

a) Skin

b) Superficial fascia with platysma.

c) Part of external jugular vein and posterior external jugular vein.

d) Parts of supraclavicular nerve, lesser occipital nerve and great auricular never. Sometimes, transverse cervical nerve.

e) Investing layer between sternocleidomastoid & trapezius muscles.

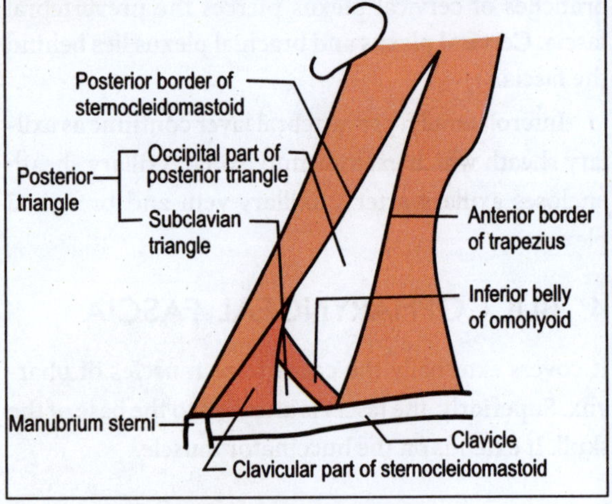

Fig. 3.10: Boundaries of posterior triangle

Divisions of posterior triangle:

The triangle is subdivided by inferior belly of omohyoid into two triangles:

a) Occipital triangle: Larger, upper part.

b) Subclavian triangle: Smaller, lower part.

The contents of posterior triangle mentioned in the Table 3.1.

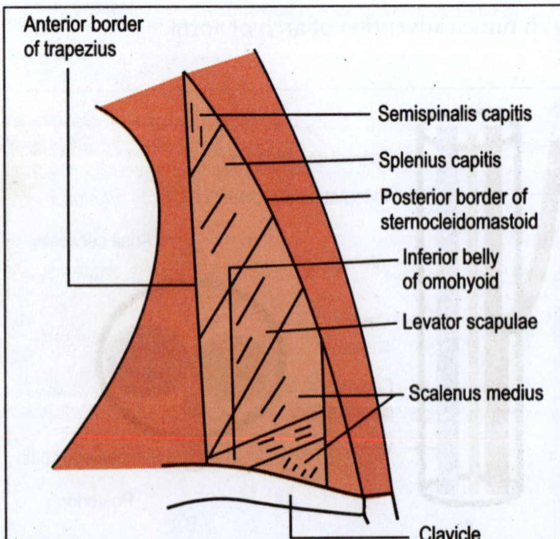

Fig. 3.11: Boundaries & floor of posterior triangle

TABLE 3.1: Contents of posterior triangle (Fig. 3.12)

	Occipital triangle	Subclavian triangle or supraclavicular triangle
1. Nerves	1. Spinal accessory nerve accompanied by two proprioceptive branches to trapezius (C_3, C_4) 2. Branches of cervical plexus— (a) Cutaneous branches— i) Lesser occipital nerve (C_2) ii) Great auricular nerve (C_2, C_3) iii) Transverse cutaneous branch (C_2, C_3) iv) Supraclavicular nerve (C_3, C_4) (b) Muscular branches— i) Two branches to levator scapulae (C_3, C_4) 3. Parts of brachial plexus— (a) Roots of brachial plexus (C_5, C_6) (b) Dorsal scapular nerve	1. Three trunks of brachial plexus. 2. Long thoracic nerve (C_5, C_6, C_7) 3. Suprascapular nerve (C_5, C_6) 4. Nerve to subclavius (C_5, C_6)
2. Vessels	1. Transverse cervical artery & vein 2. Occipital artery	1. Third part of subclavian artery 2. Part of subclavian vein 3. Transverse cervical artery 4. Terminal part of external jugular vein 5. Suprascapular artery & vein
3. Lymph nodes	1. Along the spinal accessory nerve; & Occipital nodes	1. Supraclavicular lymph nodes

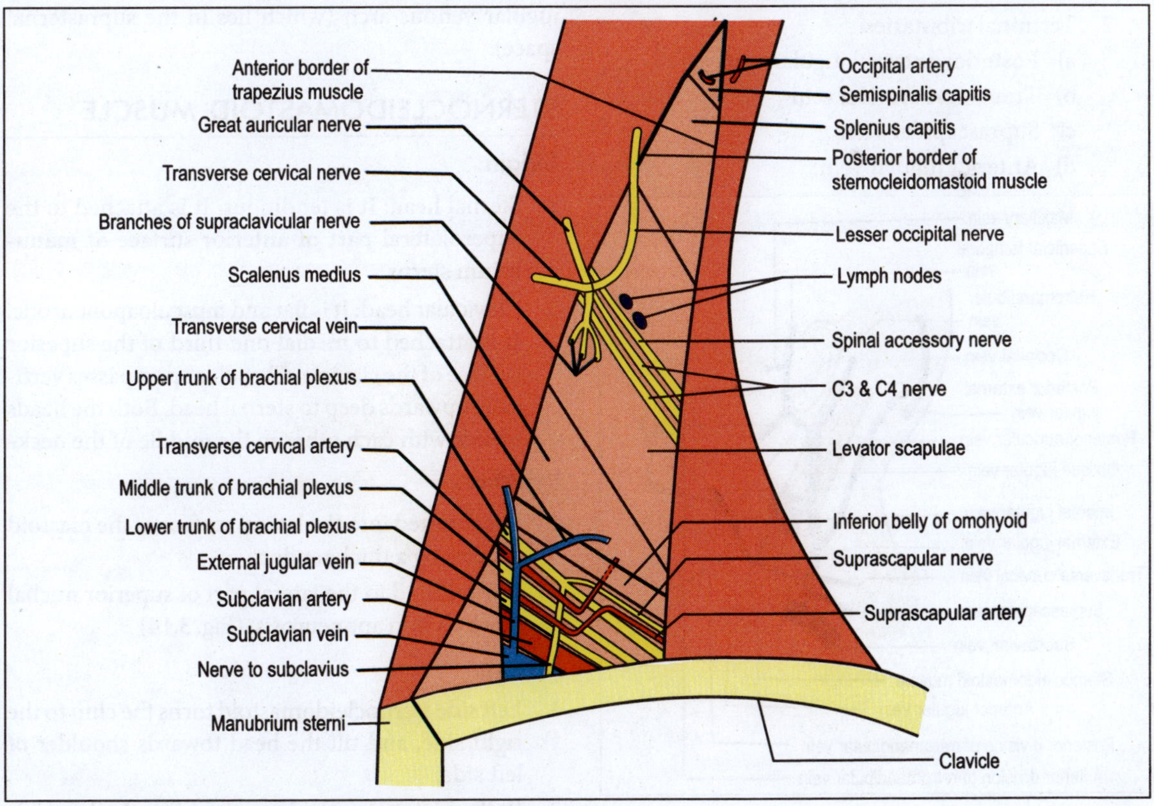

Fig. 3.12: Boundaries, floor and contents of posterior triangle

APPLIED ANATOMY

During operations for removal of lymph nodes or doing biopsy of lymph nodes spinal accessory nerve may be injured in this region as it lies superficial to prevertebral fascia and intimately related to lymph nodes, other nerves escape being deep to prevertebral fascia.

EXTERNAL JUGULAR VEIN

Formation & course: It is formed by the union of posterior auricular vein with the posterior division of the retromandibular vein. It begins near the apex of the parotid gland. It runs obliquely downwards on the sternocleidomastoid muscle. It lies under the platysma. It pierces the investing layer of deep cervical fascia and appears the subclavian or supraclavicular triangle.

Termination: It ends in the subclavian vein. (Fig. 3.13)

Tributaries:

1. Formative tributaries: Posterior auricular vein and anterior division of retromandibular vein.
2. Terminal tributaries:
   a) Posterior external jugular vein.
   b) Transverse cervical vein
   c) Suprascapular vein.
   d) Anterior jugular vein.
   e) Oblique jugular vein: It communicate external jugular vein with internal jugular vein.

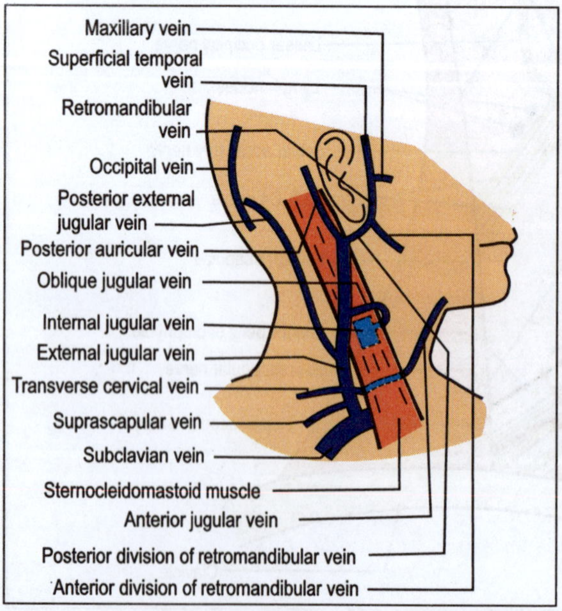

Fig. 3.13: Course & tributaries of external jugular vein

APPLIED ANATOMY

1. The walls of external jugular vein is adherent to the deep fascia of the neck through which it passes. If the vessel is cut in this region, air embolism occur. To avoid such condition, pressure (finger) should be applied immediately.
2. The external jugular vein is used to know about venous pressure.
3. Engorgement of the vein occur in patients with right heart failure.

ANTERIOR JUGULAR VEIN

It is formed in the submental triangle. It descends in the superficial fascia & enters the suprasternal space at about 2.5cm above the suprasternal notch. Then the vein runs sharply laterally below the sternocleidomastoid muscle to terminate in the external jugular vein. Anterior jugular veins of both side are joined by jugular venous arch (which lies in the suprasternal space).

STERNOCLEIDOMASTOID MUSCLE

Origin:

1. Sternal head: It is tendinous. It is attached to the superolateral part of anterior surface of manubrium sterni.
2. Clavicular head: It is flat and musculoaponeurotic. It is attached to medial one-third of the superior surface of the clavicle. Clavicular part passes vertically upwards deep to sternal head. Both the heads blends with each other in the middle of the neck.

Insertion:

1. It is inserted into the lateral surface of the mastoid process by a thick tendon.
2. It is inserted to the lateral part of superior nuchal line by a thin aponeurosis. (Fig. 3.14)

Action:

1. Left side sternocleidomastoid turns the chin to the right side, and tilt the head towards shoulder of left side.
2. Both sides sternocleidomastoid flex the head towards manubrium sterni.

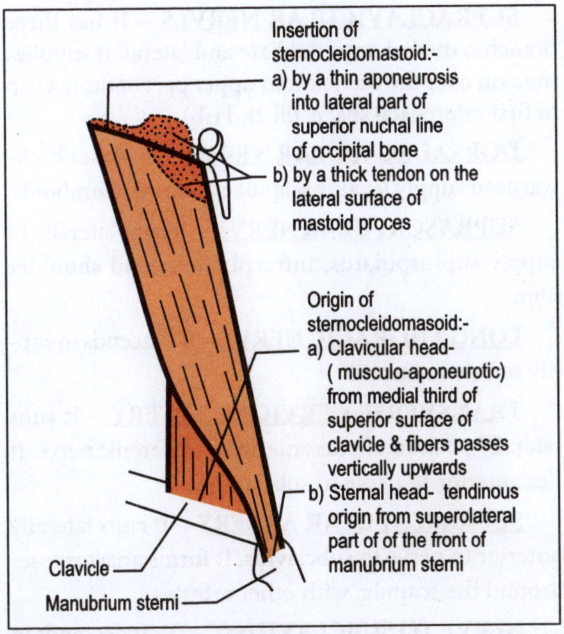

Fig. 3.14: Sternocleidomastoid muscle

3. Both sides sternocleidomastoids are used in forced inspirations.

Relations:

Superficial: (a) Platysma; (b) External jugular vein with superficial lymph nodes; (c) Great auricular nerve; (d) Transverse cutaneous nerve; (e) Medial supraclavicular nerve; (f) Parotid gland; (g) Occipital nerve. (Fig. 3.15)

Deep:

1. ***Muscles***: (a) Sternohyoid; (b) Sternothyroid; (c) Omohyoid; (d) Scalenus anterior; (e) Scalenus medius; (f) Levator scapulae; (g) Splenius capitis; (h) Posterior belly of digastric; (i) Rectus capitis lateralis;
2. ***Blood vessels***: (a) Common carotid artery; (b) Internal carotid artery; (c) Sternocleidomastoid branches of occipital & superior thyroid arteries; (d) Subclavian artery; (e) Suprascapular artery; (f) Transverse cervical artery; (g) Internal jugular vein; (h) Anterior jugular vein; (i) Common facial vein; (j) Lingual vein.
3. ***Nerves***: (a) Vagus nerve; (b) Spinal accessory nerve; (c) Cervical plexus; (d) Phrenic nerve; (e) Ansa cervicalis. (Fig. 3.16)

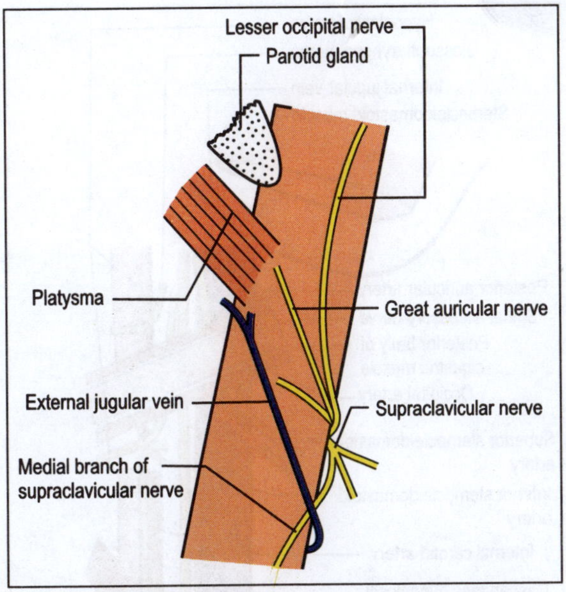

Fig. 3.15: Superficial relations of sternocleidomastoid

Nerve supply:

1. Motor part: By spinal accessory nerve.
2. Sensory part: Proprioceptive through ventral rami of C_2 and C_3.

Blood supply:

Arterial supply: Branches from superior thyroid artery, posterior auricular artery, suprascapular artery, & occipital artery.

Veins: Suprascapular vein drains to external jugular vein. Superior thyroid vein drains to internal jugular vein. Occipital vein to the suboccipital venous plexus.

APPLIED ANATOMY

1. Wry neck – Deformity of neck due to which head is bent on one side & chin point opposite side due to spasm of sternocleidomastoid.
2. Spasmodic **torticollis** – Due to repeated painful contraction of trapezius and sternocleidomastoid muscles of one side.

LESSER OCCIPITAL NERVE

It ascends at the posterior border of sternocleidomastoid. It supplies cranial surface of auricle and the skin over the mastoid process (Fig. 3.17).

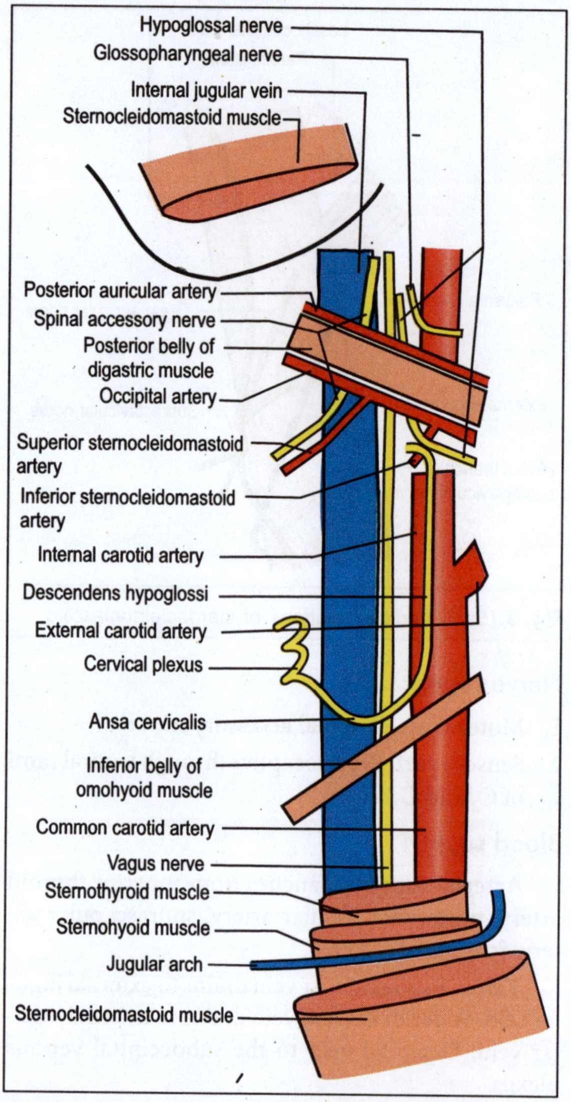

Fig. 3.16: Deep relations of sternocleidomastoid

GREAT AURICULAR NERVE – It ascends round the posterior border of sternocleidomastoid and divides into anterior & posterior branch. Anterior branch supplies skin of the lower 1/3rd of lateral surface of the auricle and its connection with auriculotemporal nerve involves for manifestation in Frey's syndrome; it also supply skin over the angle of mandible. Posterior division supply skin to the medial surface of the auricle.

TRANSVERSE NERVE OF NECK – It lies superficial to sternocleidomastoid to supply of skin over the front of neck.

SUPRACLAVICULAR NERVES – It has three branches medial, intermediate and lateral. It supplies the skin over the clavicle and upper part of thorax (up to first intercostal space, till 2nd rib).

DORSAL SCAPULAR NERVE – It passes backwards to supply levator scapulae and two rhomboids.

SUPRASCAPULAR NERVE – It runs laterally to supply supraspinatus, infraspinatous and shoulder joint.

LONG THORACIC NERVE – It descends to supply serratus anterior.

TRANSVERSE CERVICAL ARTERY – It runs laterally on the scalenus anterior and phrenic nerve. It lies anterior to nerve to subclavius.

SUPRASCAPULAR ARTERY – It runs laterally anterior to nerve to subclavius. It forms anastomoses around the scapula, with other arteries.

NERVE TO SUBCLAVIUS ($C_{5,6}$) – It descends in front of brachial plexus and subclavian vessels. The nerve descends posterior to the transverse cervical artery, suprascapular artery, omohyoid and clavicle, to reach the deep surface of subclavius.

Nerve to subclavius gives a branch called accessory phrenic nerve (33%) which passes below the subclavian vein to join the phrenic nerve. (Fig. 3.12)

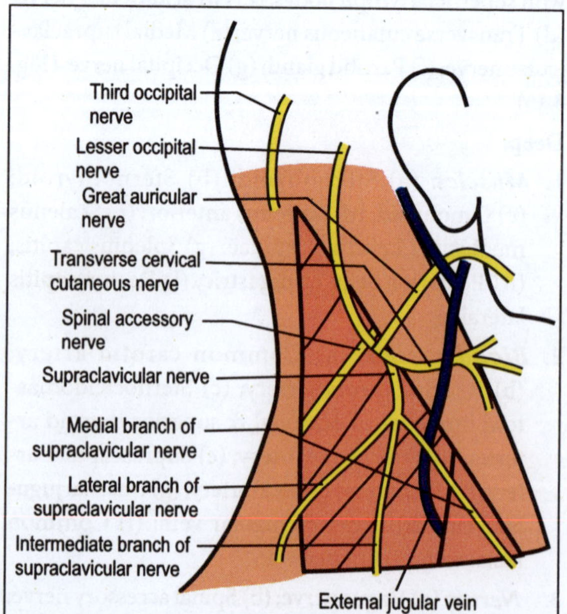

Fig. 3.17: Superficial nerves of the neck

chapter 4

BACK OF THE NECK

AT A GLANCE

- *Upper & lower limit of neck*
- *Muscles of back of neck—First layer – Trapezius, latissimus dorsi; Second layer – Levator scapulae, rhomboids, two serratus posterior and splenius capitis with cervicis; Third layer – Erector spinae, semispinalis capitis & longissimus capitis; Suboccipital triangle – Boundary, Conents.*
- *First cervical nerve, Greater occipital nerve, Occipital artery*

Upper limit of the back of neck is the external occipital protuberance and superior nuchal line; while lower limit is the seventh cervical spine and horizontal lines on either side up to acromial process of scapula.

The suboccipital triangle, lies below the three layers of muscles of the back of the neck.

First layer of muscles of the back of neck are trapezius & latissimus dorsi.

Second layer muscles are levator scapulae, the rhomboids, two serratus posterior and splenius.

Deep layer of muscles are splenius capitis, longissimus capitis and semispinalis capitis in the neck.

Below the semispinalis capitis, suboccipital triangle can be seen.

TRAPEZIUS

It is a paired muscle and actually belongs to scapular muscles and connect upper limb with vertebral column.

It forms roof of suboccipital triangle and its lateral margin forms the posterior border of the posterior triangle.

Origin: Mentioned in the Fig. 4.1.

Insertion: Mentioned in the Fig. 4.1.

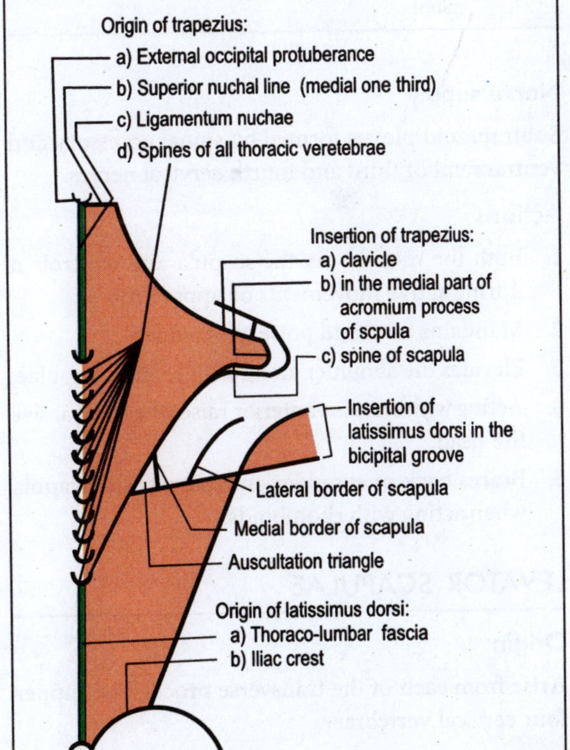

Fig. 4.1: Trapezius & latissimus dorsi

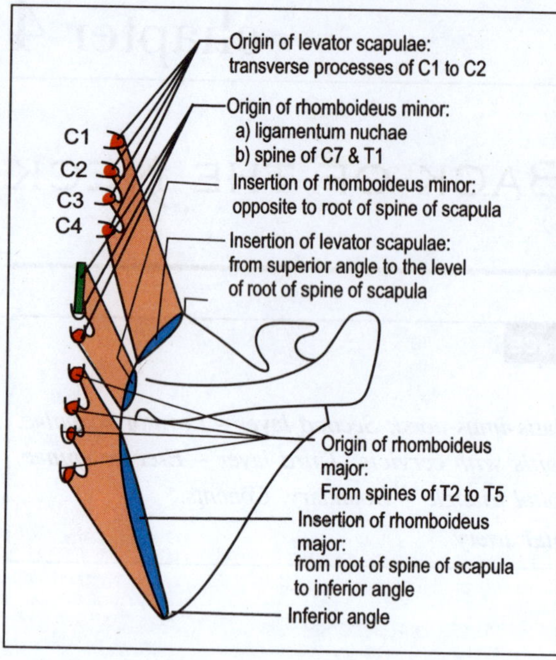

Fig. 4.2: Levator scapula and rhomboideus major and minor

Nerve supply

Subtrapezoid plexus formed by spinal accessory and ventral rami of third and fourth cervical nerves.

Actions

1. Both the muscles fix the scapula and controls it during active movements of upper limb.
2. Maintains level and poise of shoulder.
3. Elevates the shoulder along with levator scapulae.
4. Acting with serratus anterior raises the hand above the head.
5. Braces back of shoulder and retracts the scapula when acting with rhomboids.

LEVATOR SCAPULAE

Origin

Arise from each of the transverse processes of upper four cervical vertebrae.

Insertion

Medial border of scapula from superior angle up to root spine.

Nerve supply

1. Ventral rami of C_3 and C_4
2. Dorsal scapular nerve (C_5)

Action

Elevate the scapula.

POSTERIOR SERRATE MUSCLES

a) **Serratus posterior superior:**

Origin: Spines of seventh cervical and upper two or three thoracic vertebrae.

Insertion: Second to fifth ribs.

b) **Serratus posterior inferior:**

Origin: Lumbar fascia

Spines of lower two thoracic vertebrae.

Insertion: Last four ribs.

Nerve supply:

1. Second to fourth intercostal nerves.
2. Lower intercostal & subcostal nerves.

Action: Both are inspiratory muscles.

Superior elevates ribs.

Inferior by holding the ribs down against the pull of the diaphragm.

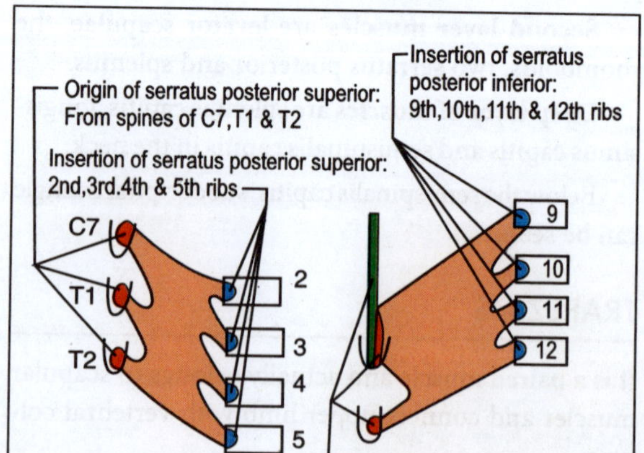

Fig. 4.3: Serratus posterior superior & inferior

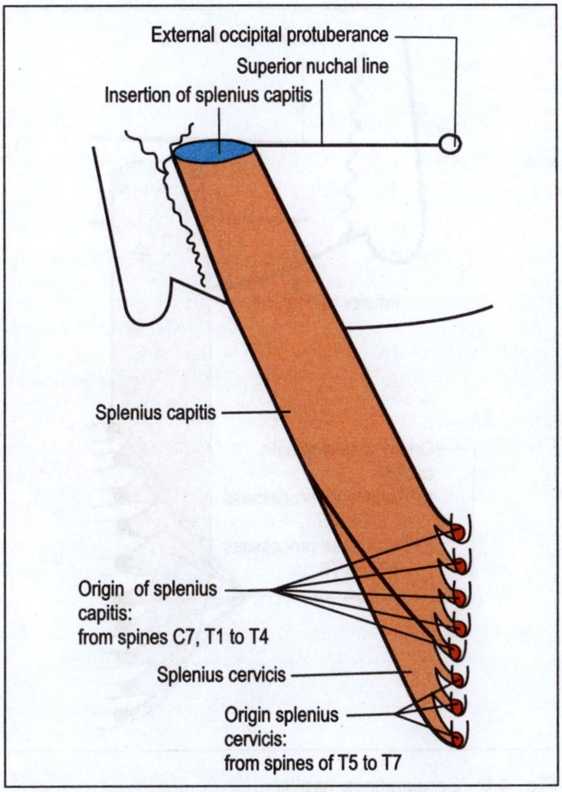

Fig. 4.4: Splenius capitis

SPLENIUS CAPITIS

Origin

Form ligamentum nuchae, spine of seventh cervical vertebra, spines of upper three or four thoracic vertebrae. (Fig. 4.4)

Insertion

To the mastoid process of temporal and below lateral third of superior nuchal line of occipital bone.

Nerve supply

Lateral branches of the dorsal rami of middle cervical nerves.

Splenius cervicis can be seen in between C_2 to C_6 vertebrae.

Nerve supply

Lateral branches of the dorsal rami of middle cervical nerves.

Action of Splenii

a) Draws the head directly backwards when muscles of both sides act together.

b) Draws the head to one side and slightly rotate when act separately. So they act as synergist with opposite sternocleidomastoid.

ERECTOR SPINAE (SACROSPINALIS)

Thick muscle extending from lumbar to thoracic and cervical regions in a groove on each side of vertebral column.

Nerve supply

All the above muscles are supplied by dorsal rami of lower cervical, thoracic and lumbar nerves.

Action

Extensors and lateral flexors of vertebral column.

LONGISSIMUS

1. **Longissimus thoracis:**
   a) Fused with iliocostalis
   b) Posterior surfaces of transverse and accessory processes of lumbar vertebrae
   c) Middle layer of thoracolumbar fascia.

   In the thoracic region – attached
   a) To tip transverse processes of all the thoracic vertebrae
   b) To part between tubercles and angles of nine to ten ribs.

2. **Longissimus cervicis:**
   a) Situated medial to thoracis

3. **Longissimus capitis**: Situated between longissimus cervicis and semispinalis capitis. (Fig. 4.5)

   Origin: From transverse processes of upper four of five thoracic vertebrae and articular processes of lower three of four cervical vertebrae.

   Insertion: To posterior margin of the mastoid process.

   Nerve supply of longissimus: Dorsal rami of lower cervical, thoracic and lumbar nerves.

   Actions:

   a) Longissimus thoracis and vervicis bend the vertebral column backwards and laterally.

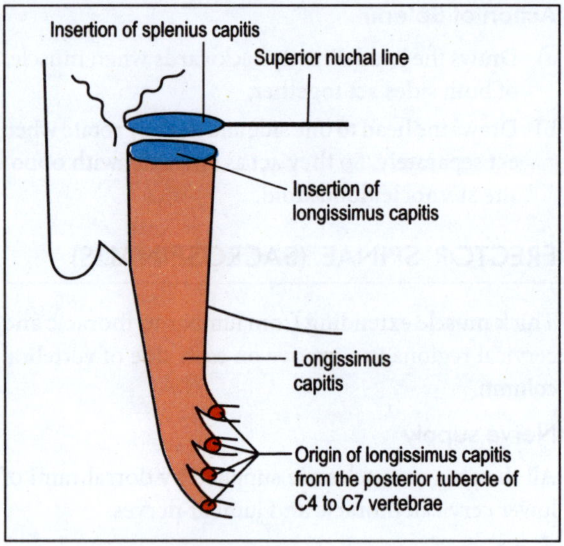

Fig. 4.5: Longissimus capitis

b) Longissimus capitis extends the head and turns the face towards the same side.

SPINALIS

1. **Spinalis thoracis**: It is medial continuation of erector spinae and situated medial to longissimus thoracis.
2. **Spinalis cervicis**: An inconstant muscle.
3. **Spinalis capitis**: More or less blended with semispinalis capitis.

Nerve supply: Spinalis are supplied by dorsal rami of lower cervical and thoracic spinal nerves.

Actions: Extensors of vertebral column.

TRANSVERSOSPINALIS

Consists of

1. Semispinalis thoracis, cervicis and capitis.
2. Multifidus.
3. Rotatores thoracis, cervicis and lumborum.

All these muscles arise from transverse processes and pass obliquely upwards and medially to be inserted into the spines of the vertebrae.

Semispinalis thoracis: It is present in between sixth to tenth thoracic vertebrae.

Semispinalis cervicis is present in the upper five or six thoracic vertebrae.

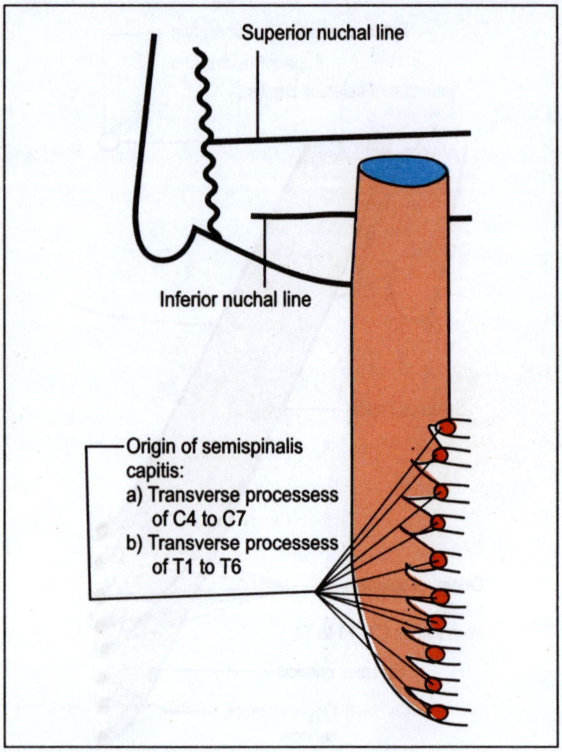

Fig. 4.6: Semispinalis capitis

Semispinalis capitis

Situated at the back of the neck and forms roof of suboccipital triangle. (Fig. 4.6)

Origin: From

a) Tips of transverse processes of upper six or seven thoracic and seventh cervical vertebrae.

b) Articular processes of fourth to sixth cervical vertebrae and sometimes spines of seventh cervical or first thoracic vertebrae.

Insertion: To the medial part of area between superior and inferior nuchal lines of occipital bone.

Nerve supply: By dorsal rami of cervical and thoracic spinal nerves.

Actions:

a) Semispinalis thoracis and cervicis: Extensor of cervical and thoracic part of vertebral column.

b) Semispinalis capitis: Extensor of the head and turns the head slightly to the opposite side.

MULTIFIDUS

Small fleshy muscles occupying the spaces on each side of spines from sacrum below to axis above.

ROTATORES (CERVICIS, THORACIS AND LUMBORUM)

Best developed in thoracic region and situated deep to multifidus.

Rotatores thoracis:

Action:

a) Mainly as postural muscle
b) Controlling the movements of small individual joints during motion of vertebral column as a whole.

SUBOCCIPITAL REGION

The region is in between inferior nuchal line & spine of axis vertebra.

Suboccipital muscles

The muscles of the suboccipital triangle are:

1. Rectus capitis posterior major
2. Rectus capitis posterior minor
3. Obliquus capitis superior
4. Obliquus capitis inferior

Suboccipital triangles

These are paired triangular spaces situated in the deeper aspect on the back of neck and on each side of midline.

Boundary

1. **Above and medially**: Rectus capitis posterior major and supplemented by minor.
2. **Above and laterally**: Obliquus capitis superior.
3. **Below**: Obliquus capitis inferior.
4. **Roof**: Covered by dense fibrous tissue which is covered by
   a) *Medially*: Semispinalis capitis.
   b) *Laterally*: Longissimus capitis and occasionally splenius capitis.

In the roof two important structures are found:

a) *Occipital artery*: Lies in the superolateral part.
b) *Greater occipital nerve* lies in the inferomedial part and finally it winds the lower border of obliquus capitis inferior and runs upwards and medially.

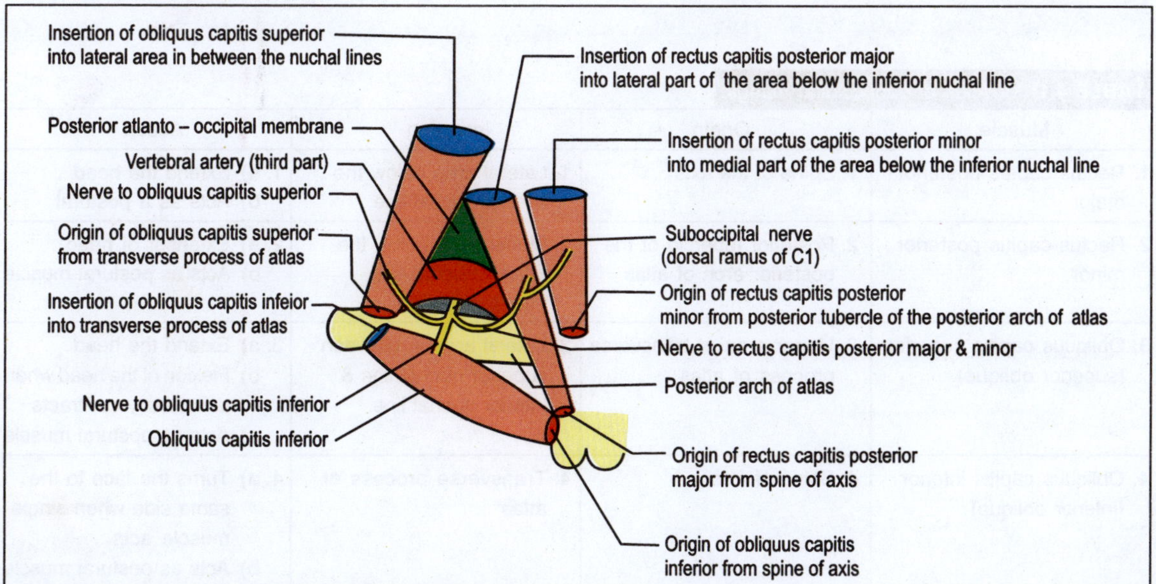

Fig. 4.7: Suboccipital triangle (boundaries & contents)

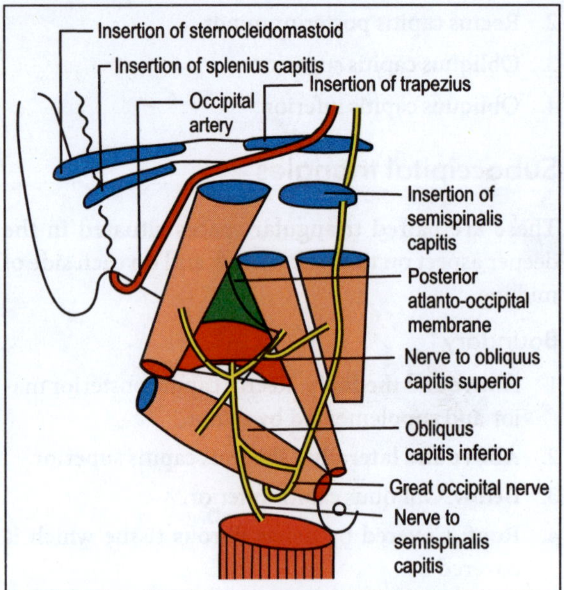

Fig. 4.8: Structures around suboccipital triangle

This nerve is a guide to expose the triangle.

- Trapezius with investing layer of deep cervical fascia and skin lies superficially.

Floor:

a) Posterior arch of atlas and

b) Posterior atlanto-occipital membrane.

Contents:

1. Third part of vertebral artery.
2. Suboccipital nerve (dorsal ramus of first cervical nerve) and nerve lies deep to artery and on the posterior arch.
3. Suboccipital plexus of veins.

The muscles of the suboccipital triangle are described in the Table 4.1.

APPLIED ANATOMY

1. **Cisternal puncture**: This region is important to surgeon for *cisternal puncture* for collection of C.S.F. from cisterna magna and site of puncture is just above spine of axis and the needle should be directed upward and forward direction (in direction parallel to an imaginary line extending from nasion to external acoustic meatus). The needle pierces the atlanto occipital membrane at a dept of about 4 to 5cm after that needle's resistance is lost. Too much insertion of needle will cause injury to medulla oblongata, which will be fatal.
2. In case of meningitis, tetanus, retraction of head due to spasm or cervical spondylitis – this region is important for both physician as well as surgeon.

TABLE 4.1: Muscles of suboccipital triangle

Muscle	Origin	Insertion	Action
1. Rectus capitis posterior major	1. Spine of the axis	1. Lateral area below the inferior nuchal line	1. a) Extend the head b) Acts as a postural
2. Rectus capitis posterior minor	2. Posterior tubercle of the posterior arch of atlas	2. Medial area below the inferior nuchal line near the midline	2. a) Extensor of head b) Acts as postural muscle
3. Obliquus capitis superior (superior oblique)	3. Upper area of transverse process of atlas	3. Lateral area in between superior nuchal line & inferior nuchal line	3. a) Extend the head b) Flexion of the head when unilaterally contracts c) Acts as postural muscle
4. Obliquus capitis inferior (inferior oblique)	4. Spine of axis	4. Transverse process of atlas	4. a) Turns the face to the same side when single muscle acts b) Acts as postural muscle

All the muscles are supplied by dorsal ramus of C_1.

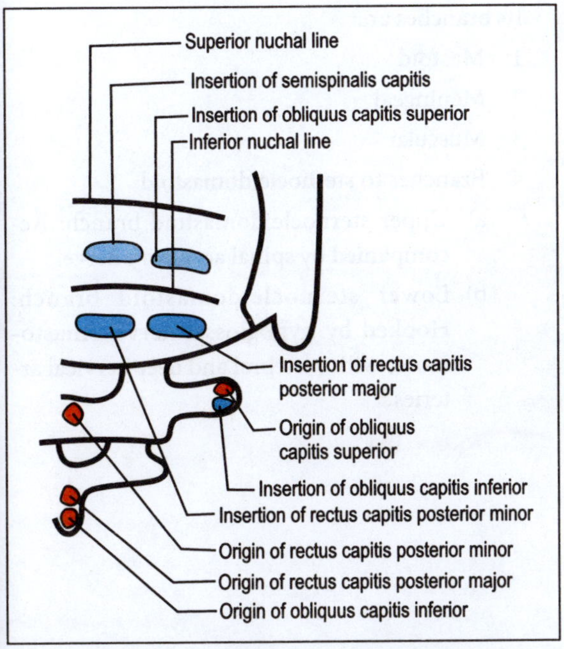

Fig. 4.9: Muscles in relations to suboccipital triangle

VERTEBRAL ARTERY

It is the first branch of subclavian artery. This artery mainly supplies the central nervous system. The artery is having four parts. Third part of this artery lies in the suboccipital triangle. This artery appear in the suboccipital triangle after passing through foramen transversarium of the atlas and lies on the posterior arch of atlas, then leaves the triangle below the posterior atlanto- occipital membrane. In between the artery and posterior arch of atlas first cervical nerve lies.

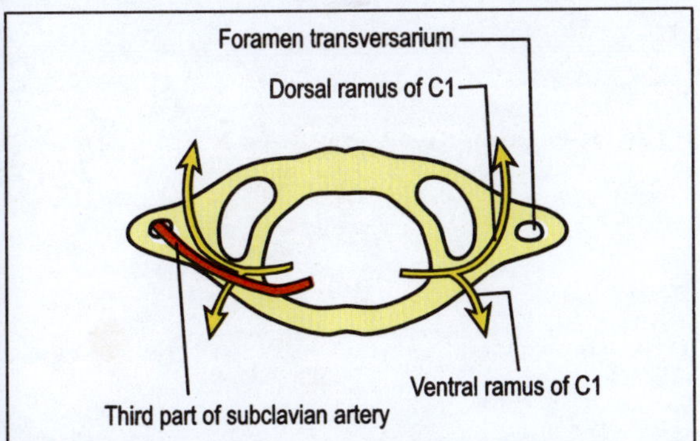

Fig. 4.10: Relations of superior aspect of atlas

FIRST CERVICAL NERVE (C_1)

This nerve is called suboccipital nerve. This nerve passes behind the lateral mass of atlas, and divides into dorsal and ventral rami.

The dorsal ramus runs backward between the third part of the vertebral artery and posterior arch of atlas. It supplies five muscles. Before supplying the muscles the nerve divides into five muscular branches. The branches are for rectus capitis posterior major, rectus capitis posterior minor, superior oblique, inferior oblique and semispinalis capitis. The nerve to inferior oblique joins with greater occipital nerve (which is derived from dorsal ramus of C_2). This nerve do not supply the skin. The ventral rami after passing in between rectus capitis lateralis and rectus capitis anterior joins with hypoglossal nerve. The ventral rami supply two muscles namely rectus capitis lateralis and rectus capitis anterior. Here the nerve joins with the hypoglossal nerve supplies thyrohyoid and geniohyoid muscles.

SUBOCCIPITAL PLEXUS OF VEINS

It can be seen within and around the suboccipital triangle. It drains blood from muscles, occipital veins, internal vertebral venous plexus, emissary veins. It drains into vertebral veins.

GREATER OCCIPITAL NERVE (C_2)

It is the thickest cutaneous of the body. It is a medial branch of dorsal ramus of second cervical nerve. It runs upward and medially after going around the lower border of inferior oblique muscle. It pierces the semispinalis capitis and trapezius after crossing the suboccipital triangle. It reaches up to vertex. It supplies posterior part of scalp up to vertex.

THIRD OCCIPITAL NERVE

It is the medial branch of the dorsal ramus of C_3 nerve. After piercing the semispinalis capitis and trapezius, it runs medial to greater occipital nerve. It supplies the skin of the back of the neck up to the external occipital protuberance.

OCCIPITAL ARTERY

It arises from the external carotid artery, almost opposite to the origin of facial artery. It runs (along the lower border posterior belly of digastric) upwards backwards. It crosses the splenius capitis, longissimus capitis, and semispinalis capitis and finally pierces the trapezius and lie near the greater occipital nerve.

Its branches are:

1. Mastoid
2. Meningeal
3. Muscular
4. Branches to sternocleidomastoid:
   a) Upper sternocleidomastoid branch: Accompanied by spinal accessory nerve.
   b) Lower sternocleidomastoid branch: Hooked by hypoglossal nerve. Anastomoses with vertebral and deep cervical arteries.

chapter 5

Anterior Triangle of the Neck

AT A GLANCE

- *Anterior median line of nec and structures in the line*
- *Platysma*
- *Anterior triangle*
- *Subdivisions of anterior triangle—(Submental triangle; Diagastric trialge; Carotid triangle; Muscular triangle)–Boundaries & content.*
- *Ansa cervicalis*

STRUCTURES IN THE ANTERIOR MEDIAN REGION OF THE NECK

The anterior median line extends from the symphysis menti to the suprasternal notch.

Structures at the anterior median line of neck are as follows:

1. **Median fibrous raphe** extending from symphysis menti to hyoid bone.
2. Hyoid bone lies opposite to C_3 vertebra. The regions above and below the hyoid are called suprahyoid and infrahyoid regions.
3. Thyrohyoid membrane: It is pierced by internal laryngeal nerve and superior laryngeal vessels. The membrane is attached to the upper border of hyoid bone and separated from the membrane by subhyoid bursa.
4. Angle of thyroid cartilage: Thyroid cartilage lies opposite of C_4 and C_5 vertebrae. Angle of thyroid cartilage is formed by the fusion of anterior border of two thyroid laminae. Angle of thyroid cartilage is acute in male and becomes prominent. So, angle of thyroid cartilage in male is known as laryngeal prominence which is known as Adam's apple (Fig. 5.1).
5. Median cricothyroid ligament (conus elasticus) and a pair of cricothyroid muscles.
6. Cricoid cartilage: It is an unpaired cartilage and lies opposite to C_6 vertebra. The lower border of cri-

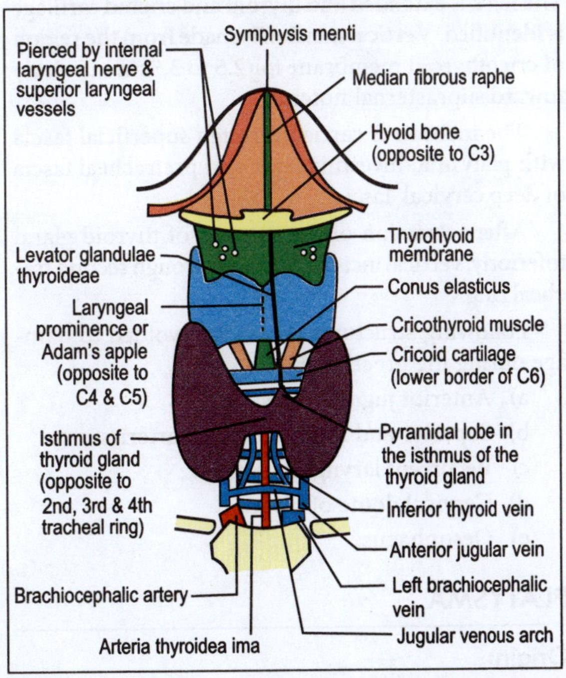

Fig. 5.1: Structures in anterior median region of the neck

coid cartilage corresponds to lower border of C_6 vertebra.

7. Isthmus of thyroid gland lies opposite 2nd, 3rd and 4th tracheal ring. Sometimes pyramidal lobe extends upwards from left side of the upper border of isthmus of the thyroid gland. Sometimes, pyramidal lobe is connected with hyoid bone through levator glandulae thyroideae (fibromuscular band).
8. Around the upper border of isthmus of thyroid gland anastomoses between both sides superior thyroid arteries.
9. At the lower border of isthmus inferior thyroid veins, sometimes arteria thyroidea ima can be seen.
10. Jugular venous arch is present above the suprasternal notch. Brachiocephalic artery can be seen in the right side of the median line.
11. Occasionally left brachiocephalic vein can be seen above the suprasternal notch.

Clinical note:

Tracheostomy is a life saving surgical procedure which is done to make an opening in trachea to place endotracheal tube.

Steps in tracheostomy

The neck is extended and thyroid and cricoid cartilage is identified. Vertical incision is made from the region of cricothyroid membrane for 2.5 to 3.5cm inferiorly toward suprasternal notch.

The incision is carried through superficial fascia with platysma, investing layer and pretracheal fascia of deep cervical fascia.

After retraction of the isthmus of thyroid gland inferiorly, vertical incision is made through second tracheal ring.

Following structures should be avoided to damage during the procedure:

a) Anterior jugular veins
b) Superior and inferior thyroid arteries
c) Recurrent laryngeal nerve
d) Cervical dome of pleura
e) Oesophagus.

PLATYSMA

Origin:

It takes origin from skin and deep fascia covering the anterior part of deltoid and pectoralis major up to the level of second rib.

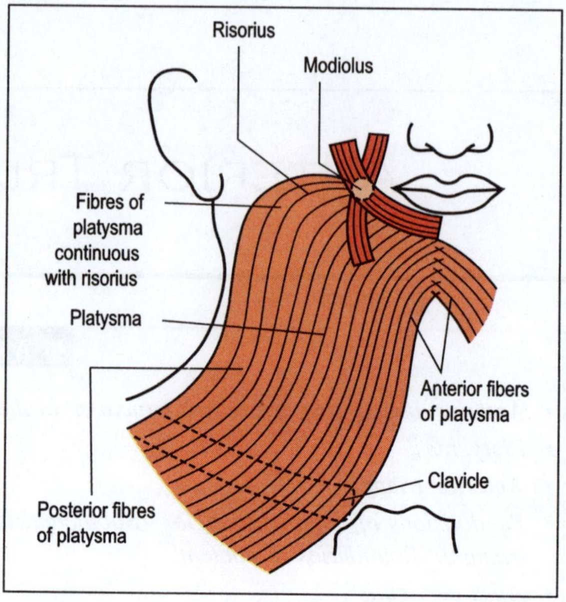

Fig. 5.2: Platysma

Insertion:

The fibres of the muscle passes upward and forward superficial to sternocleidomastoid and clavicle. It forms the roof of the posterior triangle & upper part of anterior triangle. It is inserted into:

a) Posterior & middle fibers are inserted to lower border of body of the mandible.
b) Some posterior fibers crosses the angle of mandible to be inserted to the angle of mouth (modiolus) through risorius.
c) Anterior fibres decussate (Fig. 5.2), in the midline.

Nerve supply

Cervical branch of facial nerve.

Action

a) Contraction of the whole muscle produces oblique wrinkles of the neck.
b) Anterior fibers depresses the mandible.
c) Posterior fibers draw the angle of mouth in surprise.

Clinical note:

In lacerations and surgical incisions in the neck,

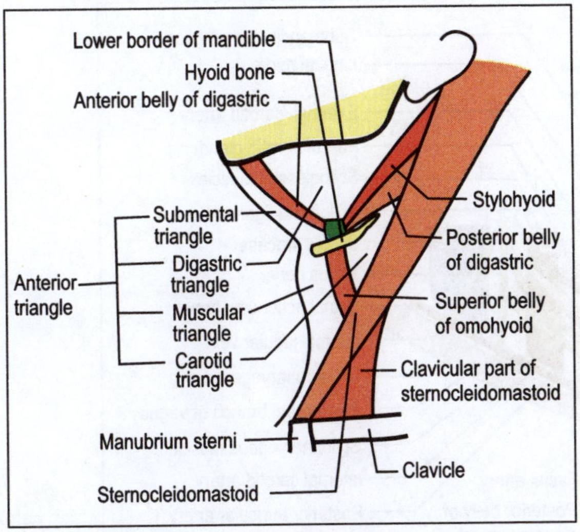

Fig. 5.3: Boundaries and subdivisions of antrior triangle

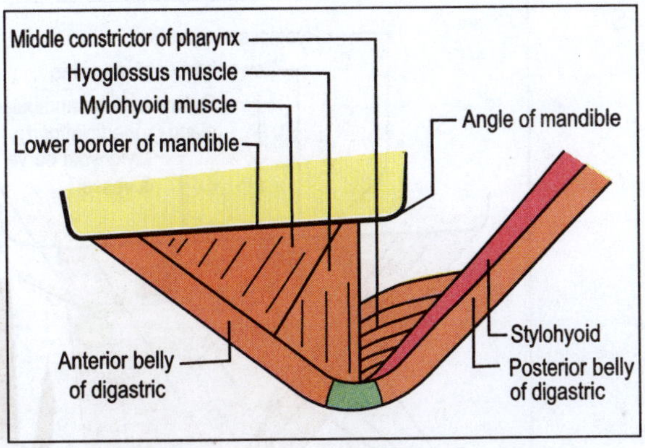

Fig. 5.4: Boundaries & floor of digastric triangle

platysma should be sutured carefully, otherwise broad scars will be produced due to contractions of platysma.

Due to damage of cervical branch of facial nerve may distort the shape of mouth.

ANTERIOR TRIANGLE OF THE NECK

Boundaries:

Medially: Anterior median line (Fig. 5.3).

Superiorly: Lower border of mandible and a line joining angle of mandible up to mastoid process.

Laterally: Anterior border of sternocleidomastoid.

Roof: Investing layer of deep cervical fascia.

Subdivision:

Anterior triangle is subdivided by posterior belly of digastric and superior belly of omohyoid into:

a) Digastric triangle
b) Carotid triangle
c) Submental triangle
d) Muscular triangle

Digastric triangle

Boundaries (Fig. 5.4)

Superiorly: Lower border or base of the mandible and a line (imaginary) joining the angle of the mandible to the mastoid process.

Anterior inferiorly: Anterior belly of digastric.

Postero inferiorly: Posterior belly of digastric and stylohyoid.

Roof: Skin, superficial fascia with platysma, cervical branch of facial nerve & part of investing layer of deep cervical fascia.

Floor: Mylohyoid, hyoglossus and middle constrictor of pharynx (small part) form floor.

Contents (Fig. 5.5)

1. Structures on mylohyoid: Mylohyoid nerve & vessels, part of the submandibular salivary gland.
2. Structures on the hyoglossus muscles (above downwards) are:
   a) Lingual nerve;
   b) Submandibular ganglion;
   c) Hypoglossal nerve with venae comitantes.
3. Structures in the posterior part of triangle:
   a) Styloglossus;
   b) Stylopharyngeus with glossopharyngeal nerve;
   c) Pharyngeal branch of vagus nerve;
   d) External carotid artery;
   e) Internal carotid artery;
   f) Vagus nerve;
   g) Internal jugular vein;
   h) Facial artery.
   i) Spinal accessory nerve.
   j) Hypoglossal nerve.

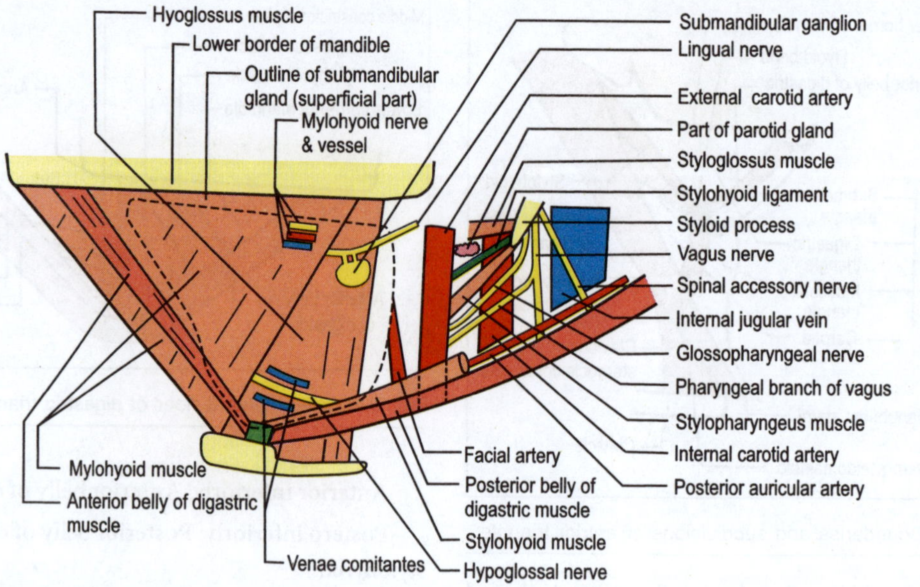

Fig. 5.5: Contents of digastric triangle

Carotid triangle

Boundaries (Fig. 5.6)

Anterosuperiorly: Stylohyoid and posterior belly of digastric muscle.

Anteroinferiorly: Superior belly of omohyoid.

Posteriorly: Anterior border of sternocleidomastoid muscle.

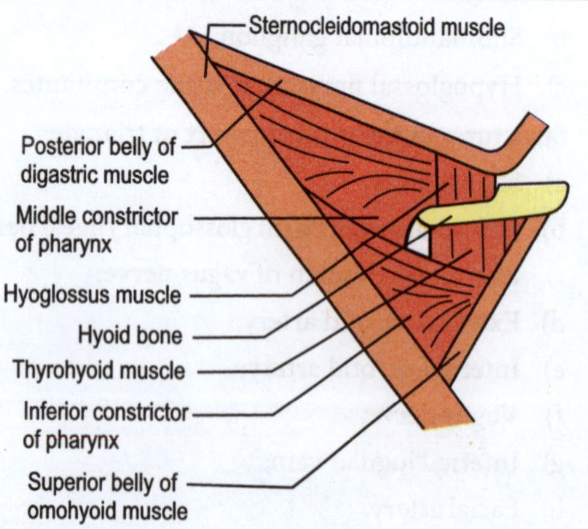

Fig. 5.6: Boundaries & floor of carotid triangle

Roof: Skin, superficial fascia with platysma.

Deep cervical fascia (investing layer), cervical branch of facial nerve, and transverse cervical nerve.

Floor: Thyrohyoid muscle, hyoglossus muscle, middle and inferior constrictor of pharynx.

Contents of carotid triangle (Fig. 5.7)

Nerves

a) Superior laryngeal nerve (a branch of vagus nerve) divides into external and internal laryngeal nerve;
b) Vagus nerve;
c) Spinal accessory nerve;
d) Hypoglossal nerve;
e) Part of ansa cervicalis;
f) Sympathetic chain.

Arteries

a) Common carotid artery;
b) Internal carotid artery;
c) External carotid artery;
d) Carotid sinus & carotid body;

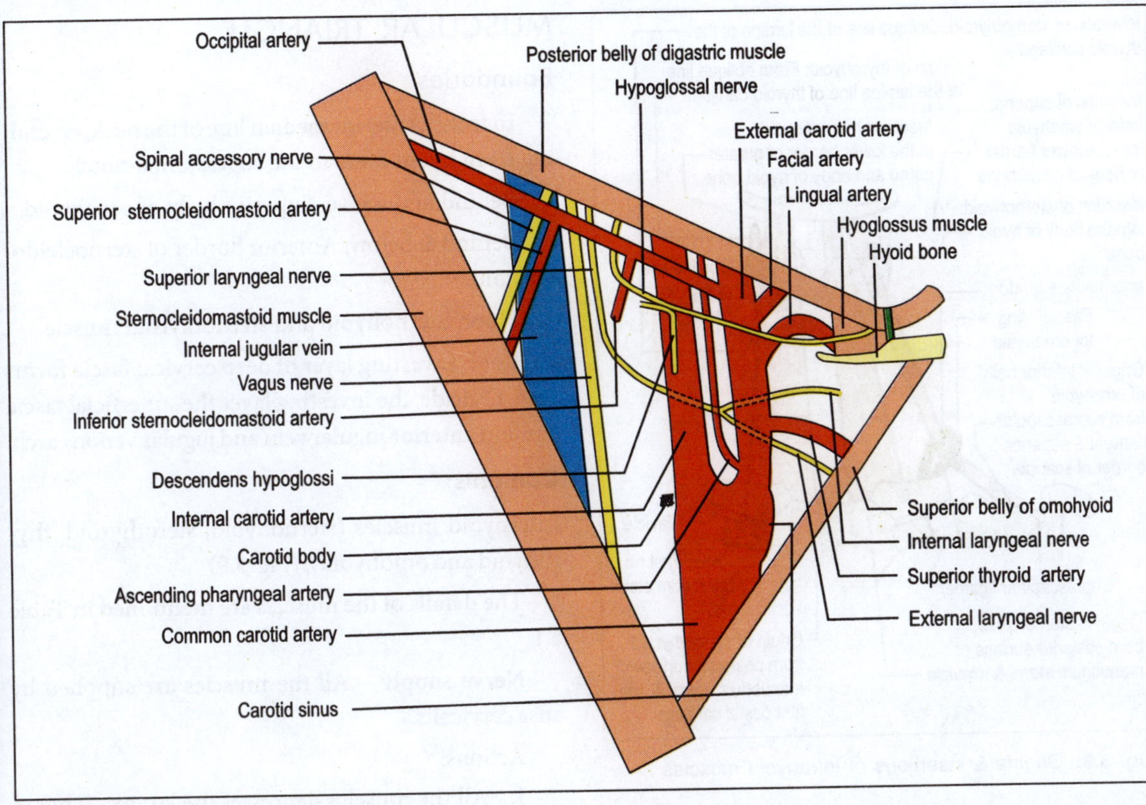

Fig. 5.7: Contents of carotid triangle

e) Branches of external carotid artery:
1. Ascending pharyngeal artery;
2. Superior thyroid artery;
3. Lingual artery;
4. Facial artery;
5. Occipital artery with its superior & inferior sternocleidomastoid branch.

Veins:
a) Internal jugular vein;
b) Common facial vein;
c) Lingual vein.

Lymph nodes: Deep cervical lymph nodes.

SUBMENTAL TRIANGLE (Fig. 5.8)

Boundaries:

Base: Body of the hyoid bone.

Apex: Symphysis menti (lower border)

Sides: Anterior belly of digastric muscles of both sides.

Floor: Mylohyoid.

Roof: Investing layer of deep cervical fascia.

Contents:

a) Submental lymph nodes;

b) Part of anterior jugular vein.

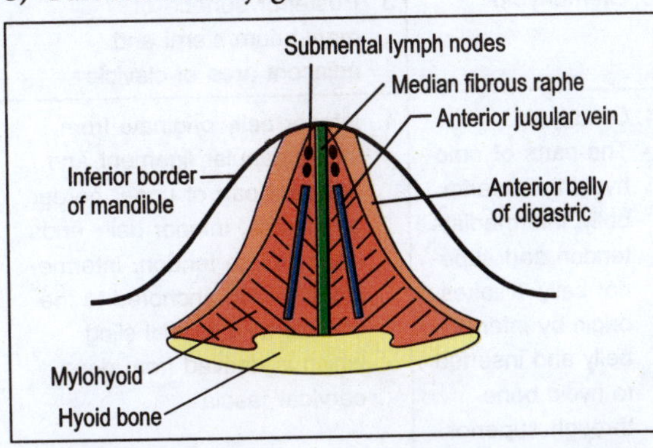

Fig. 5.8: Boundaries & content of the submental triangle

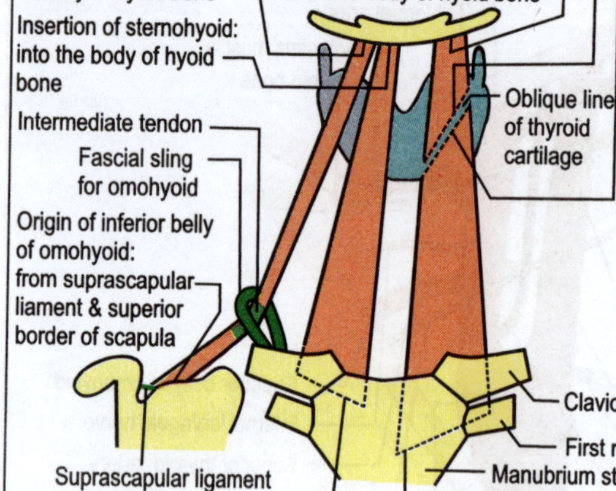

Fig. 5.9: Origins & insertions of infrahyoid muscles

MUSCULAR TRIANGLE

Boundaries

In front: Anterior median line of the neck, extending from hyoid bone to the suprasternal notch.

Behind and above: Superior belly of omohyoid.

Behind & below: Anterior border of sternocleidomastoid.

Floor: Sternohyoid and sternothyroid muscle.

Roof: Investing layer of deep cervical fascia forms roof. Outside the investing layer the superficial fascia contain anterior jugular vein and jugular venous arch.

Contents:

Infrahyoid muscles (sternohyoid, sterothyroid, thyrohyoid and omohyoid). (Fig. 5.9)

The details of the muscles are mentioned in Table 5.1.

Nerve supply – All the muscles are supplied by ansa cervicalis.

Actions:

1. All the muscles depresses the larynx, & hyoid bone.

TABLE 5.1: Infrahyoid muscles

Muscle	Origin	Insertion	Actions
1. Sternothyroid	1. Posterior surface of manubrium sterni and adjacent area of first costal cartilage	1. Oblique line of the lamina of thyroid cartilage	Depreses the larynx after its elevation in deglutition
2. Thyrohyoid	2. Oblique line of the lamina of thyroid cartilage	2. Lower border of body and greater cornu of hyoid bone	a) Depresses the hyoid bone b) Elevates the larynx when hyoid bone is fixed
3. Sternohyoid	3. Posterior surface of manubrium sterni and adjacent area of clavicle	3. Medial part of lower border of hyoid bone	Depresses the hyoid bone after its elevation during swallowing
4. Omohyoid: The parts of omohyoid are inferior belly, intermediate tendon and superior belly. It takes origin by inferior belly and inserted to hyoid bone through superior belly	4. Inferior belly originate from suprascapular ligament and adjacent part of upper border of scapula. Inferior belly ends intermediate tendon. Intermediate tendon anchored to the clavicle by a fascial sling which is derived from deep cervical fascia	4. Lower border of hyoid (lateral to sternohyoid) through superior belly	Depresses the hyoid bone after its elevation during swallowing

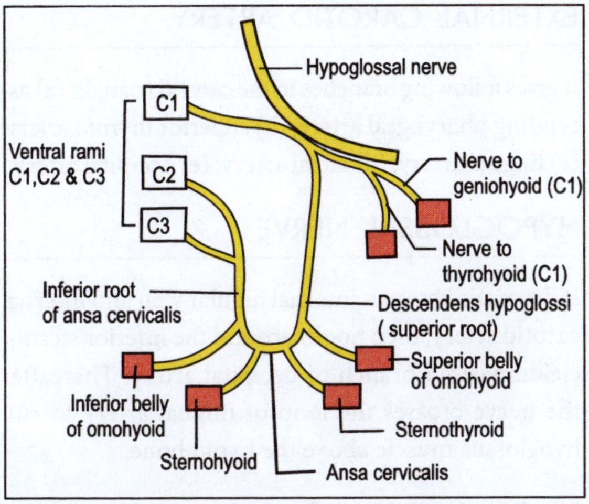

Fig. 5.10: Ansa cervicalis

2. Infrahyoid muscles stabilises the hyoid bone during depression of mandible.

SUPRAHYOID MUSCLES

The muscles are digastric muscles, stylohyoid, mylohyoid and geniohyoid.

DIGASTRIC MUSCLE

It consists of following parts: (a) Anterior belly; (b) Posterior belly; and (c) Intermediate tendon.

a) Anterior belly

Origin: It arises from digastric fossa of the mandible.

Insertion: Intermediate tendon.

b) Posterior belly:

Origin: Mastoid notch.

Insertion: Intermediate tendon.

c) Intermediate tendon: It is kept in position by facial sling of deep fascia which anchors the tendon to the hyoid bone.

Stylohyoid muscle bifurcate on both side of tendon before insertion to hyoid bone.

ANSA CERVICALIS (Fig. 5.10)

It lies in the anterior wall of the carotid sheath. It has two root:

1. **Superior root**: Nerve fibres of ventral ramus of C_1 (first cervical nerve) join with hypoglossal nerve.

   Some nerve fibres supply thyrohyoid and geniohyoid muscles.

   Other nerve fibres forms superior root (descendens hypoglossi) which descends from hypoglossal nerve on the internal and common carotid artery.

2. **Inferior root**: Nerve fibres of ventral rami of second and third cervical nerves curve round the internal jugular vein and passing anteroinferiorly to join the superior root (on the common carotid artery) to form a loop called ansa cervicalis.

Distribution

The ansa cervicalis supplies remaining infrahyoid muscles (sternohyoid, sternothyroid and omohyoid).

SUPERIOR LARYNGEAL NERVE

It is a branch of vagus nerve. It runs on deep plane & divides into external and internal laryngeal nerves in between external and internal carotid arteries.

Internal laryngeal nerve (sensory) pierces the thyrohyoid membrane to supply laryngeal mucosa.

External laryngeal nerve (motor) accompany the superior thyroid artery to supply the cricothyroid and inferior constrictor of pharynx.

PHARYNGEAL BRANCH OF VAGUS (motor)

It runs inferiorly on the middle constrictor of pharynx to form pharyngeal plexus. Pharyngeal branch (sensory) of glossopharyngeal nerve and pharyngeal branch (vasomotor) of superior cervical sympathetic ganglion also contribute to form pharyngeal plexus.

COMMON CAROTID ARTERY

The right common carotid artery arises from branchiocephalic artery behind the right sternoclavicular joint. The left common carotid artery arises form the arch of aorta in the superior mediastinum. It divides into internal and external carotid artery at the level of upper border of the thyroid cartilage.

Carotid sinus: Terminal part of common carotid artery or the beginning of internal carotid artery shows dilatation, called the carotid sinus. Tunica adventitia is relatively thick which contain branches from glossopharyngeal nerve. It act as a baroreceptor. Tunica media is thinner.

Carotid body: The carotid body is a small structure which lies posteriorly at the site of bifurcation of common carotid artery. The carotid body is supplied by glossopharyngeal nerve. It is a chemoreceptor. It is sensitive to excess carbon dioxide and low oxygen tension.

EXTERNAL CAROTID ARTERY

It gives following branches in the carotid triangle: (a) ascending pharyngeal artery; (b) superior thyroid artery; (c) lingual artery; (d) facial artery; (e) occipital artery.

HYPOGLOSSAL NERVE

It descends between internal jugular vein and internal carotid artery, then hooks around the inferior sternocleidomastoid branch of occipital artery. Thereafter the nerve crosses the loop of lingual artery to run hyoglossus muscle above the hyoid bone.

LINGUAL VEIN, COMMON FACIAL VEIN AND SUPERIOR THYROID VEIN

All the veins end in the internal jugular vein.

chapter 6

THE CRANIAL CAVITY

AT A GLANCE

- *Meninges of cranial cavity*
- *Folds of dura mater*
- *Blood supply dura mater*
- *Nerve supply of dura mater*
- *Falx cerebri, Falx cerebelli, Tentorium cerebelli, Diaphragma sellae*
- *Features of intracranial venous sinus—*
- *Superior sagittal sinus*
- *Inferior sagittal sinus*
- *Straight sinus*
- *Occipital sinus*
- *Transverse sinus*
- *Petrosquemous sinus*
- *Sigmoid sinus*
- *Cavernous sinus, Intercavernous sinus*
- *Superior petrosal sinus*
- *Inferior pertrosal sinus*
- *Hypophysis cerebri*
- *Trigeminal ganglion*
- *Middle meningeal artery*

INTRODUCTION

The cranial cavity contains brain. The brain is covered by three meninges: dura, arachnoid and pia mater. (Figs. 6.1, 6.2, 6.3 and 6.4).

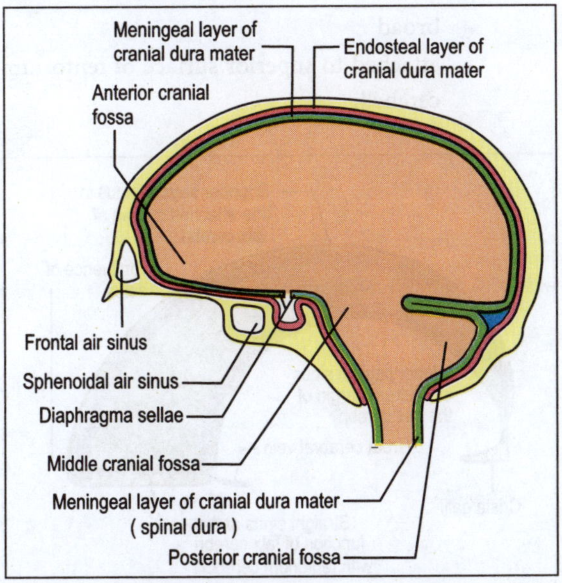

Fig. 6.1: Sagittal section showing showing anterior, middle & posterior cranial fossa

CRANIAL DURA

- It consists of
  a) outer endosteal layer
  b) inner meningeal layer.
- Outer endosteal layer serves as a periosteum or endocranium. Cranial dura present no extradural space. It is continuous with sclera of orbit.

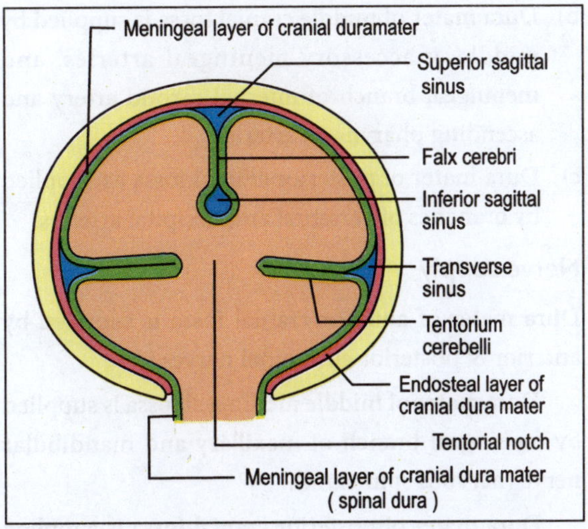

Fig. 6.2: Coronal section of the cranial cavity

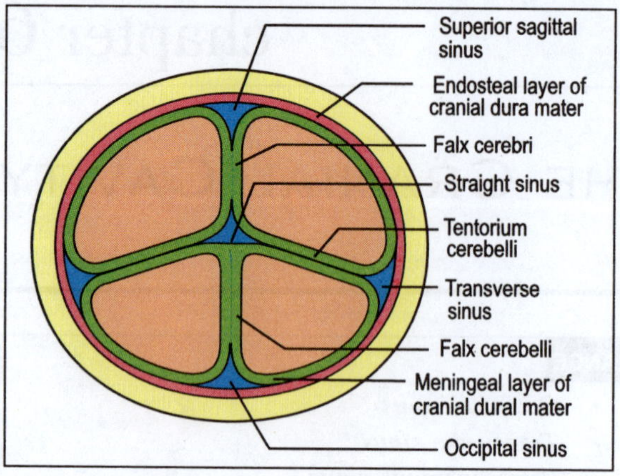

Fig. 6.3: Coronal section of the posterior part of the cranial cavity

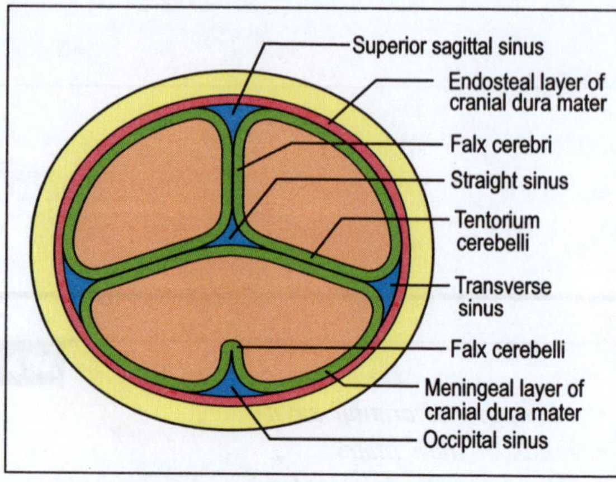

Fig. 6.4: Coronal section of the anterior part of the posterior cranial fossa

- Inner meningeal layer projects inwards to form four folds.
  a) Falx cerebri
  b) Tentorium cerebelli
  c) Falx cerebelli
  d) Diaphragma sellae

Blood supply of dura mater

a) Dura mater of anterior cranial fossa is supplied by meningeal branch of ophthalmic, anterior and posterior ethmoidal arteries, and branch from middle meningeal artery.

b) Dura mater of middle cranial fossa is supplied by middle & accessory meningeal arteries, and meningeal branch of internal carotid artery and ascending pharyngeal arteries.

c) Dura mater of posterior cranial fossa as supplied by branches of vertebral and occipital arteries.

Nerve supply

Dura mater of anterior cranial fossa is supplied by anterior & posterior ethmoidal nerves.

Dura mater of middle meningeal fossa is supplied by meningeal branch of maxillary and mandibular nerve (nervous spinosum).

Dura mater of posterior cranial fossa is supplied by meningeal branches of vagus & hypoglossal nerve.

FALX CEREBRI (Fig. 6.5)

1. It is large sickle shaped fold of dura mater occupying the median longitudinal fissure (between two cerebral hemisphere).
2. To ends:
   a) anterior end:
   - narrow
   - attached to crista galli

   b) posterior end
   - broad
   - attached to superior surface of tentorium cerebelli.

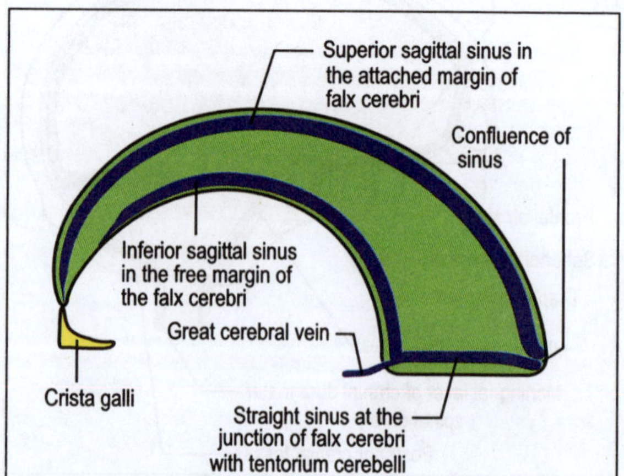

Fig. 6.5: Falx cerebri

3. Margins
   a) Upper margin
      – convex
      – attached to lips of sagittal sulcus of skull vault.
   b) lower margin
      – Concave
      – Free, lie above corpus callosum
4. Venous sinuses encloses in falx cerebri
   – Superior sagittal sinus is present in the upper margin
   – Inferior sagittal sinus is present along the inferior margin
   – Straight sinus is present along the line of attachment of falx cerebri & tentorium cerebelli.

TENTORIUM CEREBELLI (Fig. 6.6)

- Tentorium cerebelli is tent-shaped fold of dura mater, forming the roof of posterior cranial fossa
- It separate the occipital lobe of cerebrum from cerebellum.
- It divides the posterior part of cranial cavity into supratentorial and infratentorial compartment.
- Infratentorial compartment is known as posterior cranial fossa, & contain lower part of midbrain & hind brain.

Margins

a) Free margin
   – Anterior margin is 'U' shaped & free.
   – Ends of the 'U' are attached anteriorly to anterior clinoid process.
   – Inner free margin encloses tentorial notch which is related to midbrain.

b) Outer attached margin
   – Convex
   – Attached to (before backwards):
     1. Posterior clinoid process
     2. Superior border of petrous temporal bone (containing superior petrosal sinus)
     3. Lips of transverse sulcus in parietal bone (posterio-inferior angle) and occipital bone containing transverse sinus.

Free & attached margins cross each other near apex of petrous temporal bone. There is a triangular area which is related to cavernous sinus and pierced by oculomotor nerve.

Surfaces:

Superior surface
   – Convex
   – In the midline falx cerebri is attached (straight sinus is present along the line of attachment).
   – Related to occipital lobes of cerebrum.

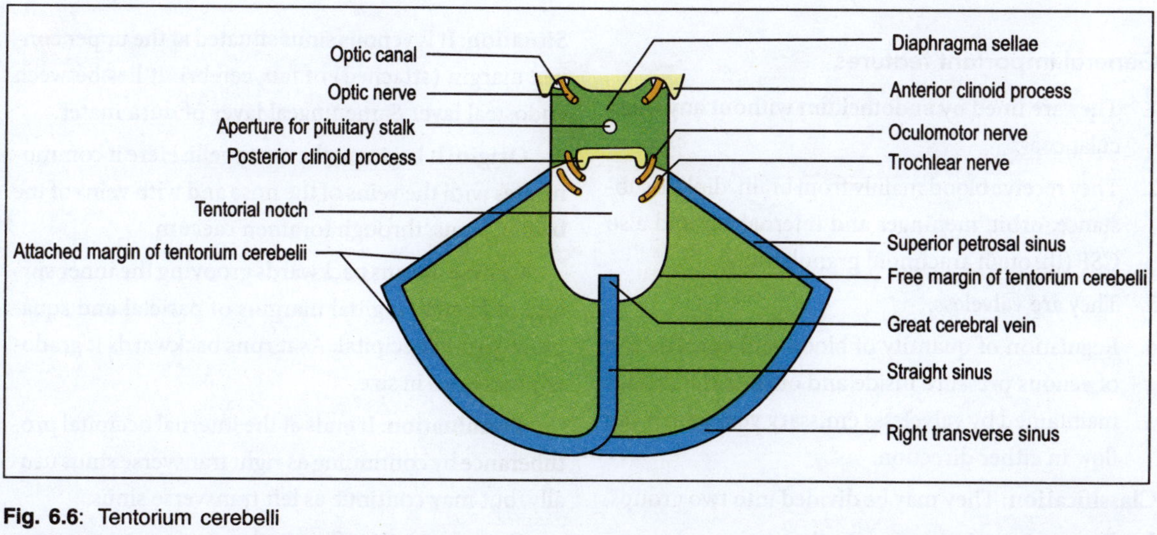

Fig. 6.6: Tentorium cerebelli

Inferior surface

- Concave
- Related to cerebellum
- Falx cerebelli is attached.

FALX CEREBELLI

- Small sickle shaped fold of dura mater
- Project in the cerebellar notch.
- Base of sickle is attached to posterior part of inferior surface (in the midline) of tentorium cerebelli.
- Its posterior margin is attached to internal occipital protuberance along the internal occipital crest up to margin of foramen magnum. Posterior margin is convex. Anterior margin is concave and free.

DIAPHRAGMA SELLAE

- Small circular horizontal fold of dura mater which form roof of hypophyseal fossa.
  Anteriorly: attached to tuberculum sellae
  Posteriorly: attached to dorsum sellae
  Each side: continuous with dura mater of the middle cranial fossa.

  It has a central aperture through which stalk of hypophysis cerebri passes.

INTRACRANIAL VENOUS SINUSES (OF DURA MATER)

General important features

1. They are lined by endothelium without any muscular coat.
2. They receive blood mainly from brain, diploic substance, orbit, meninges and internal ear and also CSF (through arachnoid granulations).
3. They are valveless.
4. Regulation of quantity of blood and equalisation of venous pressure inside and outside the skull is maintained by valvelesss emissary vein which can flow in either direction.

Classification: They may be divided into two groups.

I. **Posterosuperior group**: In the upper and posterior part of cranial cavity. They may again be paired and unpaired.

A. **Unpaired**
1. Superior sagittal sinus
2. Inferior sagittal sinus
3. Straight sinus
4. Occipital sinus

B. **Paired**
1. Transverse sinus
2. Sigmoid sinus
3. Petrosquamous sinus

II. **Anteroinferior group** in the base of skull.

A. **Unpaired**
1. Anterior intercavernous
2. Posterior intercavernous
3. Basilar

B. **Paired**
1. Cavernous sinus
2. Superior petrosal sinus
3. Inferior petrosal sinus
4. Sphenoparietal sinus
5. Middle meningeal sinus.

SUPERIOR SAGITTAL SINUS (Fig. 6.7)

Situation: It is venous sinus situated at the upper convex margin (attached) of falx cerebri. It lies between endosteal layer & meningeal layer of dura mater.

Origin: It begins at the crista galli. Here it communicates with the veins of the nose and with veins of the frontal sinus, through foramen caecum.

Course: It runs backwards grooving the inner surface of frontal, sagittal margins of parietal and squamous part of occipital. As it runs backwards it gradually increases in size.

Termination: It ends at the internal occipital protuberance by continuing as right transverse sinus usually, but may continue as left transverse sinus.

On cross section: Triangular.

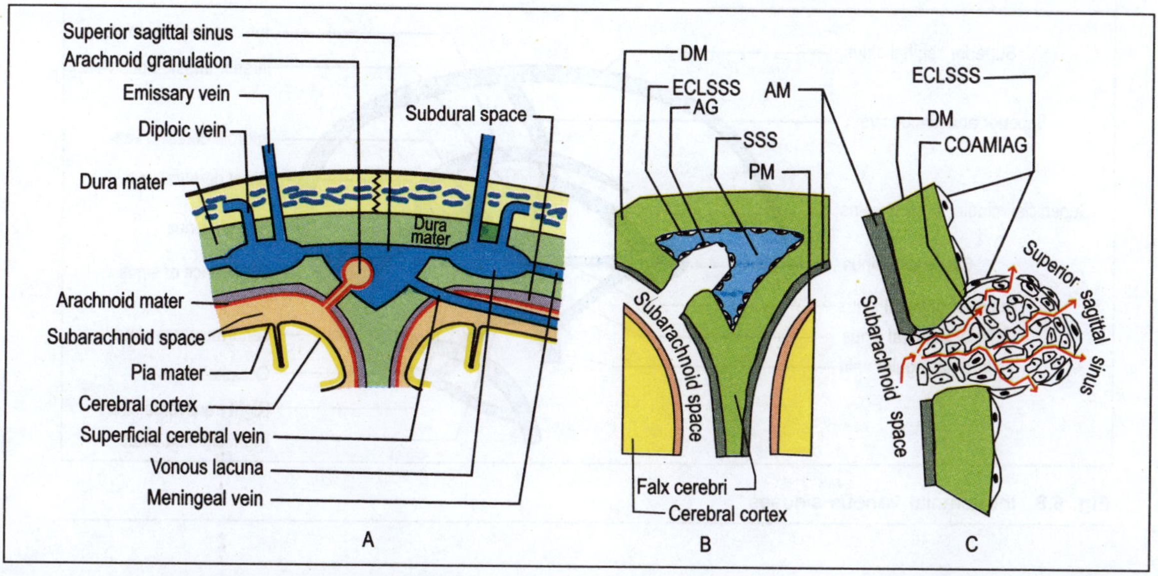

Fig. 6.7: **(A)** A coronal section through superior sagittal sinus; **(B)** Coronal section showing arachnoid granulation—DM: Dura mater; AG: Arachnoid granulation; SSS: Superior sagittal sinus; AM: Arachnoid mater; PM: Pia mater; ECLSSS: Endothelial cells lining superior sagittal sinus; **(C)** Magnified arachnoid granulation; COAMIAG: Cells of arachnoid mater in arachnoid granulation; Red lines indicate pathway of CSF from subarachnoid space to superior sagittal sinus

Features of interior of the sinus

1. Opening of superior cerebral veins.
2. Projections of arachnoidal granulations (for absorption of CSF).
3. Numerous fibrous stands at the inferior angle.
4. Opening of venous lacunae which are usually three on each side.

   [Diploic and meningeal veins open in the lacunae].

Tributaries:

1. Veins from nose & frontal air sinus.
2. Superior cerebral vein: 8-12 in numbers from cerebral hemisphere.
3. Parietal emissary vein.
4. Venous lacunae – three on each side draining diploe and meningeal veins.
5. Communicate with cavernous sinus by superior anastomatic vein and superficial middle cerebral vein. (Fig. 6.8)

Applied anatomy: Infection from nose, scalp and diploe may cause thrombosis of superior sagittal sinus. This results in increased intracranial tension due to defective absorption of CSF. It may also give rise to paraplegia (due to involvement of paracentral lobule of both side); delirium and convulsion by congestion of superior cerebral veins.

Inferior sagittal sinus (Fig. 6.8)

It is a venous sinus situated in the posterior two thirds of lower free margin of falx cerebri. It ends by uniting with great cerebral vein and forming straight sinus (great cerebral vein is formed by the union of two internal cerebral veins and receives two basal veins at the terminal part).

It receives

a) some veins of falx cerebri

b) few veins from medial surfaces of cerebrum.

STRAIGHT SINUS

It is a venous sinus situated at the junction of falx cerebri and tentorium cerebelli.

Formation: Formed by the union of inferior sagit-

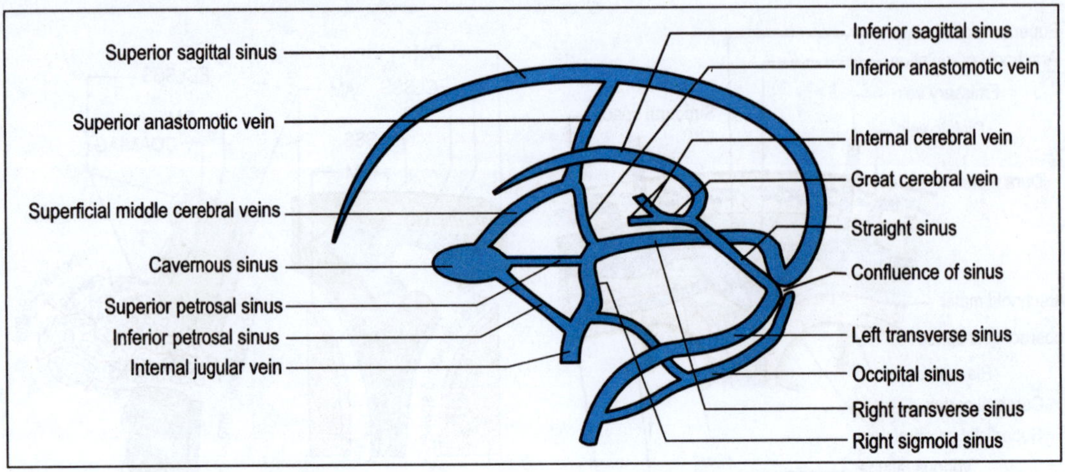

Fig. 6.8: Intracranial venous sinuses

tal sinus and great cerebral vein. It is also said to be continuation of inferior sagittal sinus.

Course: It runs backward and downwards and ends by continuing as left transverse sinus. It also communicates with confluence of sinus.

Tributaries:

1. Inferior sagittal sinus
2. Great cerebral vein
3. Few superior cerebellar veins.

[Great cerebral vein is formed by the union of two internal cerebral veins and basal veins from each side at its termination in straight sinus. It is guardes by a valve at its formation and the valve is formed by arachnoidal granulation tissue containing sinusoidal plexus of blood vessels. This valve forms a ball valve mechanism for regulation of formation of CSF in the lateral ventricles].

OCCIPITAL SINUS

1. The smallest venous sinus situated along the attached margin (along the internal occipital crest) of falx cerebelli.
2. It begins from the margin of foramen magnum as some small venous channels.
3. It ends in confluence of sinus.
4. It communicates with sigmoid sinus and internal vertebral plexus.

TRANSVERSE SINUSES

These are large paired sinuses – right and left usually.

Features:

1. Situation: It lies in the attached margin of tentorium cerebelli a first at the squamous part of occipital and then at mastoid (postero-inferior) angle of parietal bone.
2. Beginning: At the internal occipital protuberance, the superior sagittal sinus continues as right transverse sinus & straight sinus continues as left transverse sinus.
3. Course: It runs laterally and forwards to the posterolateral part of petrous part of temporal bone and forms a gentle curve convex upwards and ends at the mastoid angle.
4. Size and shape on cross section: Right is larger than the left and it is triangular on cross section.
5. End: At the mastoid angle it ends by continuing as sigmoid sinus.
6. Tributaries
   a) Superior petrosal sinus at the termination
   b) Inferior cerebral veins

c) Posteior temporal diploic vein
d) Inferior anastomotic vein connecting transverse sinus with superifical middle cerebral vein.
e) Inferior cerebeller veins
f) Petrosquamous sinus.

PETROSQUAMOUS SINUS

It is small venous sinus and situated in the groove at the junction of squamous and petrous part of temporal bone.

In front it communicates with retromandibular vein and ends in transverse sinus.

SIGMOID SINUSES

There are paired venous sinuses situated one on each side in 'S' shaped groove on the mastoid part of temporal and jugular process of occipital bone.

Features:

1. Beginning: It is the direct continuation of transverse sinus at the mastoid angle of parietal bone.
2. Course: Each sinus courses downwards and medially in a curved manner in a deep groove on the mastoid part of temporal bone and then crosses the jugular process of occipital bone and finally turns forward to the posterior compartment of jugular foramen.
3. End: It ends in the posterior compartment of jugular foramen by forming superior bulb and continues as internal jugular vein.
4. Important relation: In front a thin plate of bone separates its upper part from mastoid antrum and air cells.
5. Tributaries
   a) Communication with veins of pericranium by mastoid emissary vein and
   b) Communication with suboccipital venous plexus by condylar emissary veins.
   c) Labyrinthine veins.
   d) Cerebellar veins.

Applied: Infected thrombosis of sinus may occur from infection of tympanic cavity and tympanic (mastoid) antrum as they are closely related.

CAVERNOUS SINUSES (Fig. 6.9)

Situation: These are large paired venous sinuses situated in the middle cranial fossa and one on each side of body of sphenoid bone.

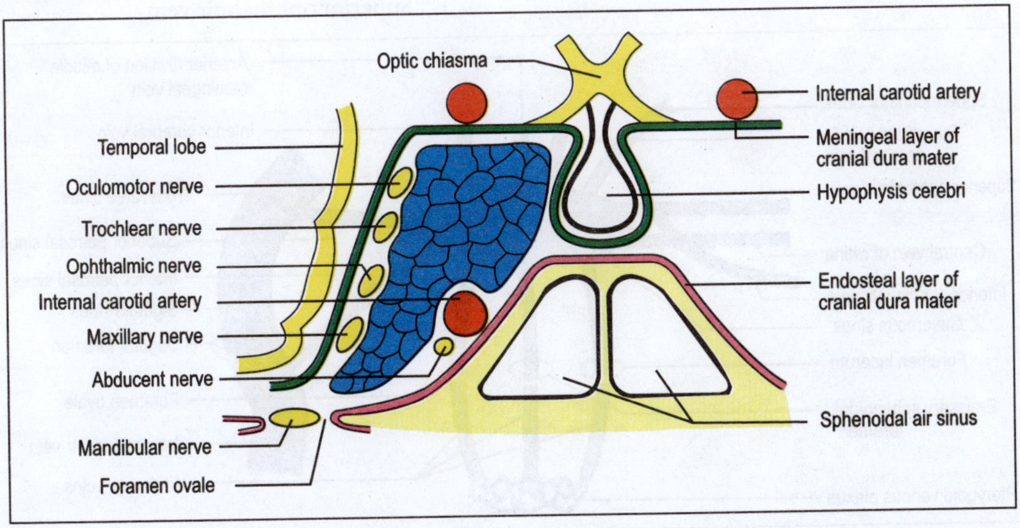

Fig. 6.9: Cavernous sinus

Its interior is divided into numerous small spaces or caverns by trabaculae. So it is called cavernous sinus.

Formation: It is the sapce between endosteal and meningeal layers of dura mater

Roof and lateral wall: is formed by meningeal layer

Floor and medial wall: is formed by endosteal layer.

Extention: Anteriorly: Up to medial end of superior orbital fissure.

Posteriorly: Apex of the petrous part of temporal bone.

Dimensions: Lengthh: 2cm; width: 1cm.

Relations (External): Medially

a) Sphenoidal air sinus

b) Hypophysis cerebri (pituitary gland)

Laterally

a) Uncus of temporal lobe

b) Cavum trigeminale with trigeminal ganglion

In front

a) Medial end of the superior orbital fissure

b) Apex of the orbit

Behind

a) Apex of petrous part of temporal bone.

b) Crus cerebri of midbrain.

Above

a) Optic tract

b) Optic chiasma

c) Internal carotid artery.

d) Anterior perforated substance

Below

a) Foramen lacerum

b) Junction between body and greater wing of scapula.

Content: True content is blood. Other structures which pass through it are separated by layer of endothelium.

Structures passing through the sinus

1. Internal carotid artery with sympathetic and venous plexus around it.
2. Abducent nerve lying below and lateral to internal carotid artery.

Structures in the lateral wall of the sinus

From above downwards

a) Oculomotor nerve

b) Trochlear nerve

c) Ophthalmic nerve

d) Maxillary neerve

Tributaries (Figs. 6.10, and 6.11)

I. **From orbit**

1. Superior ophthalmic vein

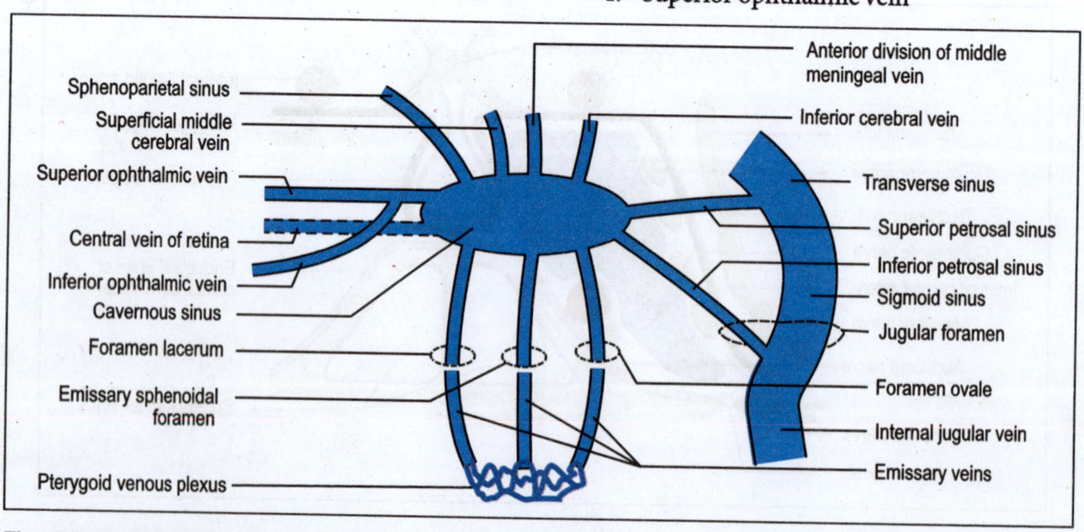

Fig. 6.10: Tributaries of cavernous sinus

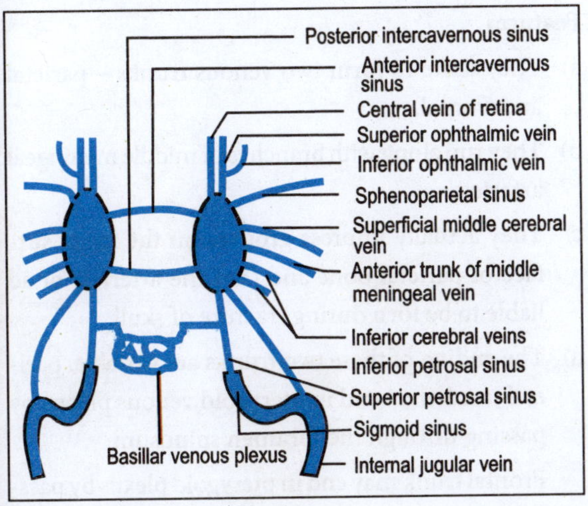

Fig. 6.11: Tributaries of cavernous sinus (superior view)

2. Inferior ophthalmic vein
3. Central vein of retina

II. **From brain**
4. Superficial middle cerebral veins
5. Some inferior cerebral veins

III. **Meningeal**
6. Sphenoparietal sinus
7. Anterior trunk of middle meningeal vein

Communications

1. With transverse sinus by superior petrosal sinus.
2. With internal jugular vein by inferior petrosal sinus.
3. With pterygoid venous plexus by emissary veins through foramen lacerum, foramen ovale, foramen spinosum, emissary sphenoidal foramen (foramen vesalius).
4. With facial vein by:
   a) Superior ophthalmic vein and angular vein.
   b) Emissary vein, pterygoid venous plexus and deep facial vein.
5. With superior sagittal sinus by superior anastomotic and superficial middle cerebral veins.
6. With opposite cavernous sinus by anterior and posterior intercavernous sinuses.

All these communications are valveless and blood can flow in either direction.

Factors helping blood flow in the sinus

1. Transmitted pulsation of internal carotid artery.
2. Gravity.
3. Change of position of head.

APPLIED ANATOMY

1. Arterio-venous aneurysm may occur by repturing of internal carotid artery into the cavernous sinus as a result of head injuries and give symptoms like:
   a) Loud systolic murmur is heard over the eye
   b) Unilateral pulsatile exophthalmos with oedema of eyelids, conjunctivitis.

   Treatment is ligation of internal carotid artery but may cause hemiplegia.
2. Thrombosis of cavernous sinus resulting in meningitis may occur due to septic infections in the dangerous area of face, scalp, nose and paranasal air sinuses. It may give rise to severe pain in the eye, forehead, ophthalmoplegia, oedema of eyelids and exophthalmos. Third, fourth and sixth cranial nerves may be involved.

Development: It is developed from primary head veins which are persistent intracranial part of anterior cardinal veins.

INTERCAVERNOUS SINUSES

These are two **anterior** and **posterior.**

Features:

1. They connect the two cavernous sinuses across the median plane.
2. They are situated at the anterior and posterior attached margins of diaphragma sellae.
3. They, along with two cavernous sinuses, form a venous circle (circular veins).
4. Small irregular venous sinuses below hypophysis cerebri drain into intercavernous sinuses.

BASILAR VENOUS SINUSES OR PLEXUS

It consists of a number of intercommunicating venous channels situated between the layers of duramater over the clivus of the skull.

It connects two inferior petrosal sinuses and communicates with internal vertebral venous plexus.

SUPERIOR PETROSAL SINUSES

They are paired small venous channels draining blood of cavernous sinus into transverse sinus – so it is a connection between cavernous and transverse sinuses.

Course: Each sinus starts from posterosuperior part of cavernous sinus and runs backwards and laterally along the attached margin of tentorium cerebelli and crosses the trigeminal nerve. Then it lies at the superior border of petrous part of temporal bone. Ultimately it ends by joining with the transverse sinus at the point where it is continued as sigmoid sinus.

Tributaries

1. Some cerebellar veins
2. Inferior cerebral vein
3. Veins from tympanic cavity

INFERIOR PETROSAL SINUSES

They are small paired venous channels draining blood of cavernous sinuses with corresponding internal jugular veins.

Course: It arises from postero-inferior part of the cavernous sinus and runs backwards in the groove between the petrous part of temporal and basilar part of occipital bone. Then it passes through the anterior compartment of jugular foramen and finally end in superior bulb of internal jugular vein and forms its first tributary.

Tributaries

1. Labyrinthine veins from cochlea canaliculus.
2. Veins from aqueduct of cochlea
3. Vein from medulla oblongata, pons, inferior surface of cerebellum.

MIDDLE MENINGEAL SINUS

These are venous channels communicating cavernous sinus with superior sagittal sinus above through venous lacunae.

Features

a) They unite to form two venous trunks – parietal and frontal.
b) They run along with branches of middle meningeal arteries.
c) They actually impress grooves on the inner surface of parietal bone and (not the arteries) or so liable to be torn during fracture of skull.
d) The ending of these two trunks are variable. parietal trunk may end in pterygoid venous plexus by passing through the foramen spinosum.

Frontal trunk may end in pterygoid plexus by passing through foramen ovale or may end in spheno-parietal or cavernous sinus.

Tributaries

1. Meningeal veins
2. Some inferior verebral veins
3. Diploic veins
4. Superficial middle cerebral veins.

The last two are communications.

HYPOPHYSIS CEREBRI OR PITUITARY GLAND

It is a small neuro-glandular endocrine gland (also known as **leader of endocrine orchestra** because it controls so many endocrine glands by so many hormones secreted by it but it is *under control of hypothalamus*). (Fig. 6.12)

Situation: The gland lies in the hypophyseal fossa or pituitary fossa of **sella turcica** of body of sphenoid bone. Suspended from floor of third ventricle by infundibulum (stalk) and is roofed by diaphragma sellae (dural process).

Shape: Ovoid.

Measurements

a) Length – (antero-posterior): 8mm
b) Breadth – (transverse): 12mm
c) Weight: 500mg

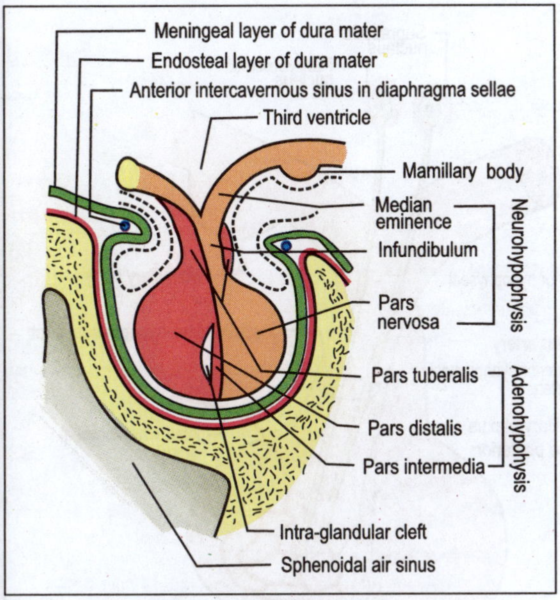

Fig. 6.12: Parts of pituitary gland

Different parts: It consists of two parts:

I. Anterior lobe or adenohypophysis

II. Posterior lobe or neurohypophysis

Subdivisions

I. **Adenohypophysis**: Three parts:

1. Pars anterior: Larger part in front of intraglandular cleft (which is present in the adenohypophysis)
2. Pars intermedia: Small part behind the cleft (this part is rudimentary and represents lumen of Rathke's pouch)
3. Pars tuberalis: An upward extension from the pars anterior along the infundibular stem.

II. **Neurohypophysis or Posterior lobe**

Three parts:

1. Pars nervosa: Smaller part situated in the concavity of large anterior lobe.
2. Infundibulum: It is the connection of posterior lobe with hypothalamus.
3. Median eminence of tuber cinereum is continuous with infundibulum.

Relations

I. Above: Diaphragma sellae separating
   a) Optic chiasma
   b) Anterior communicating artery
   c) Floor of third ventricle

II. Below: Sphenoidal air sinus separated by plate of bone (forming hypophyseal fossa).

III. In front and behind: Anterior and posterior intercavernous sinuses respectively.

IV. On each side: Cavernous sinus and its contained structures:

1. Internal carotid artery with sympathetic plexus.
2. Adbucent nerve
3. Nerves in the lateral wall – from above downwards:
   a) Oculomotor nerve
   b) Trochlear nerve
   c) Ophthalmic nerve
   d) Maxillary nerve

Arterial supply: Arteries supplying the hypophysis cerebri are: (Fig. 6.13)

1. Superior and
2. Inferior hypophyseal branches of internal carotid artery.

Mode of supply

1. **Superior hypophyseal artery** after entering into infundibulum forms primary capillary plexus in the vicinity of median eminence and infundibulum. Primary capillary plexus in the upper part of infundibulum receives releasing and inhibitory factors from the axon teminals of neurons of hypothalamus.

Hypothalamohypophyseal portal system: The **hypothalamohypophyseal portal veins** (long & short portal vessels) begin in the primary capillary plexus at the infundibulum and ends in the secondary capillary plexus around the cells of the adenohypophysis. The portal vessels (hypothalamo-

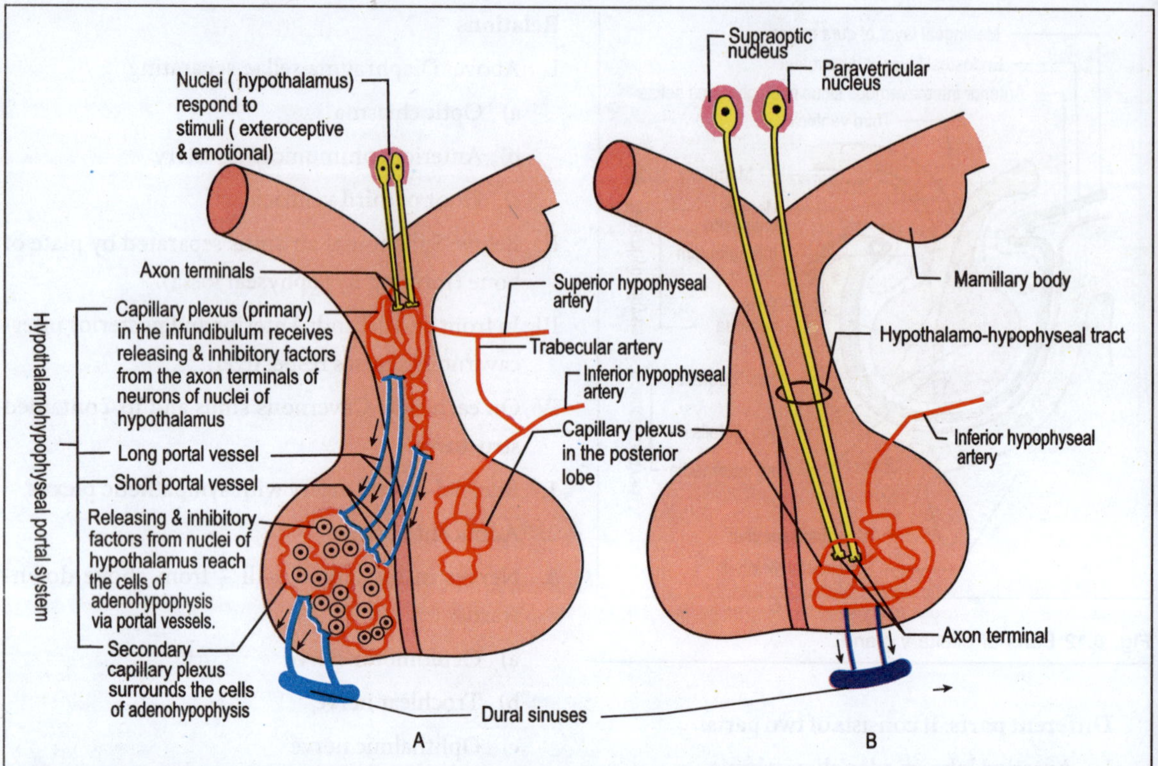

Fig. 6.13: Blood supply of pituitary gland; A – Hypothalamohypophyseal portal system; B – Hypothalamohypophyseal tract

hypophyseal portal system) are of great functional importance because they carry releasing & inhibitory factors from the axon terminals of neurons of hypothalamus. The releasing & inhibitory factors regulate the activities of the cells of the adenohypophysis. (Fig. 6.13)

2. **Inferior hypophyseal artery** forms a capillary plexus around the neurohypophysis and supply it. This plexus drains directly into cavernous and intercavernous sinus.

Hypothalamohypophyseal tract: This tract consist of unmyelinated nerve fibres (about 1,00,000) which are derived from supraoptic and paraventricular nuclei of hypothalamus. The fibres of the tract passes through infundibular stem. Supraoptic nucleus secretor vasopressin or antidiuretic (ADH), and paraventricular nucleus secretes oxytocin. These hormones are transported by nerve fibres of the tract and stored in the nerve terminals (Herring bodies) which are present near the capillary plexus of posterior lobe.

Oxytocin stimulates myoepithelial cells of alveoli of mammary gland.

Vasopressin or antidiuretic hormone increases water absorption at distal convoluted tubules of nephron of kidney.

Venous drainage

Short veins emerge from the gland to nearby dural venous sinuses (mainly cavernous sinus). Hormones released from pituitary gland to reach the target cells of the different endocrine glands.

MICROSCOPIC FEATURES OF PITUITARY GLAND

I. **Adenohypophysis**: Consists of

a) Irregular groups of cells with
b) Reticular fibres and
c) Sinusoids and capillaries

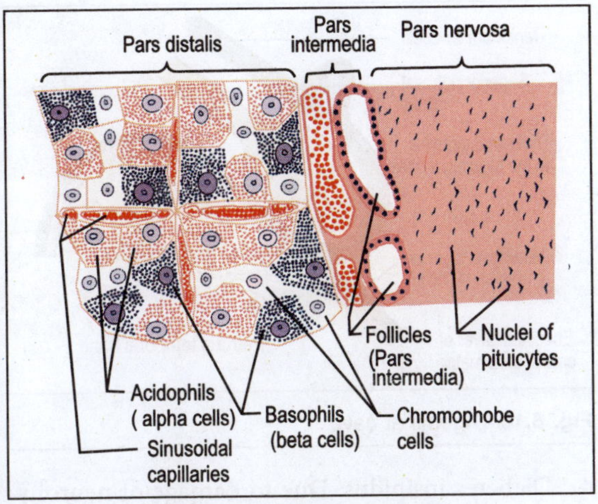

Fig. 6.14: Microscopic features of pituitary gland

Cells: Using routine staining procedures cells of adenohypophysis can be divided into two types:

1. **Chromophobe cells** 50% (agranular cytoplasm): They are nonsecretory or perhaps the precursors of chromophil cells.
2. **Chromophilic cells** (granular cytoplasm): Depending upon the staining of the cytoplasmic granules the cells are:
   a) **Acidophilic or alpha cells** 40%. They stain with eosin (acid stain). These are two types:
      1. **Somatotrophs** secrete growth hormone (STH, GH)
      2. **Mammotrophs** secrete prolactin.
   b) **Basophilic or beta cells**: 10%. They stain with basic stain like haematoxylene and these are of three types:
      1. **Thyrotrophs** secretes thyroid stimulating hormone (TSH)
      2. **Gonadotrophs** secrete follicle stimulating hormone (FSH), leutining hormone (LH), or interstitial cell stimulating hormone (ICSH).
      3. **Corticotrophs** secrete adrenocorticotropic hormone (ACTH).

II. **Pars intermedia** (Intermediate lobe) consists of basophil cells and chromophobe cells. It secretes melanocyte stimulating hormone (MSH).

III. **Neurohypophysis** (posterior lobe): Consists of
   a) Nonmyelinated nerve fibres (from hypothalamus)
   b) Capillary plexus
   c) Pituicytes: Specialised neuroglial cells.
   d) **Herring bodies**: Knob-like terminals of nerve fibres. (Fig. 6.14)

Hormones secreted are:

1. **Vasopressin** (ADH) – acts on renal tubules producing more urine.
2. **Oxytocin** – acting on uterus for contraction and also mammary smooth muscles.

These hormones are not actually synthesised by neurohypophysis (posterior lobe) but synthesised by hypothalamus and transported by hypothalamo-hypophyseal tract (carrier) to neurohypophysis.

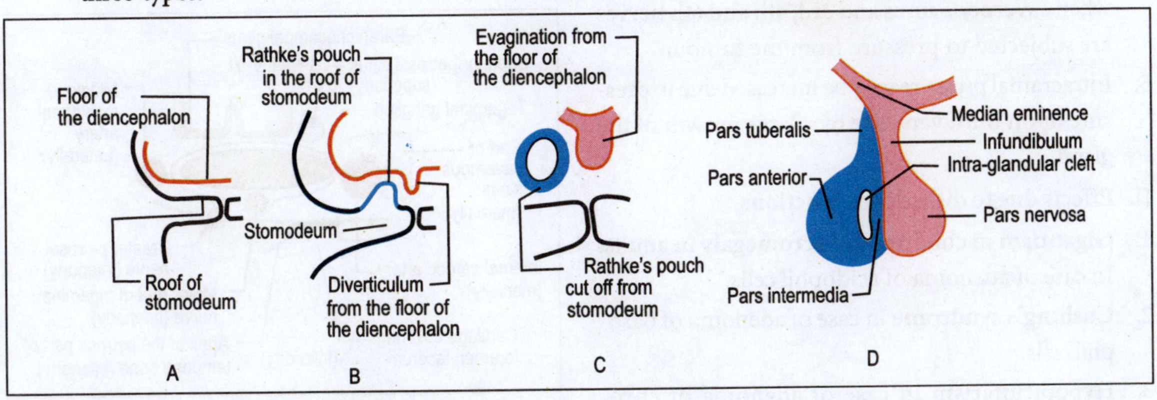

Fig. 6.15: Development of pituitary gland

DEVELOPMENT OF PITUITARY GLAND

Hypophysis cerebri is ectodermal in development. (Fig. 6.15)

Adenohypophysis is developed from surface ectoderm and from the **'Rathke's pouch'** which is an outgrowth from the roof of the stomodeum. Rathke's pouch get detached from the roof of the stomodeum & proceeds towards outgrowth from the floor of diencephalon.

Neurohypophysis is developed from an outgrowth downwards from floor of diencephalon.

Distal end of the Rathke's pouch persist as intraglandular cleft (Fig. 6.15).

APPLIED ANATOMY:

When a tumour in hypophysis cerebri occur – It will produce:

I. Effects due to pressure;
II. Effects due to disorders of function.

I. Effects due to pressure

1. Enlargement of sella turcica which may cause headache if duramater is stretched or nasal discharge when sphenoidal air sinus is involved.
2. Often **bitemporal hemianopia** is usual effect due to involvement of optic chiasma when the growth expands upwards.
3. Hypothalamus may be involved and may cause obesity of **Frohlich's syndrome.**
4. Exophthalmos and ophthalmoplegia may result when cavernous sinus and 3rd, 4th and 6th nerves are subjected to pressure from the tumour.
5. Intracranial pressure may be increased due to pressure upon third ventricle by a large growth of the gland.

II. Effects due to disorder of functions

1. **Gigantism** in children and **acromegaly** in adults: In case of adenoma of acidophil cells.
2. **Cushing's syndrome** in case of adenoma of basophil cells.
3. Hypopituitarism in case of adenoma of chromophobe cells.

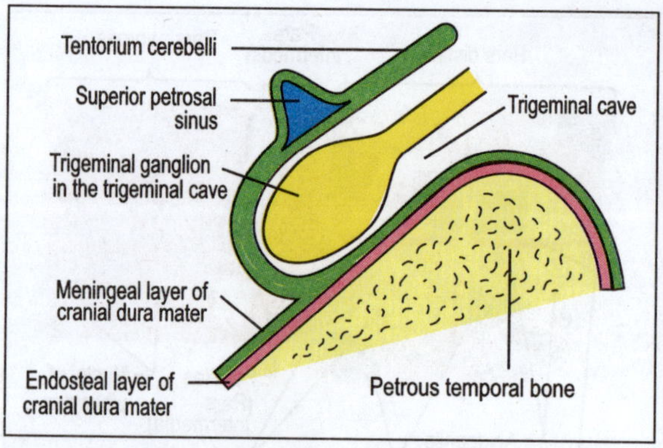

Fig. 6.16: Trigeminal cave

4. Diabetes insipidus: Due to damage of neurohypophysis (actual lesion is in hypothalamus).

Pituitary gland can be removed in pituitary adenoma through trans- nasal approach (Nasal cavity → rostrum → sphenoidal air sinus → pituitary gland).

TRIGEMINAL GANGLION

Also known as semilunar or gasserian ganglion. It is a sensory ganglion of fifth nerve which corresponds to posterior root ganglions of a spinal nerve.

Situation: It is situated over an impression at the apex of the anterior surface of petrous part of temporal bone within trigeminal or meckel's cave which is a special space of a duramater. (Fig. 6.16)

Shape: Semilunar with convexity directed antero laterally (three divisions emerge) and concavity posteriorly (attachment of sensory root).

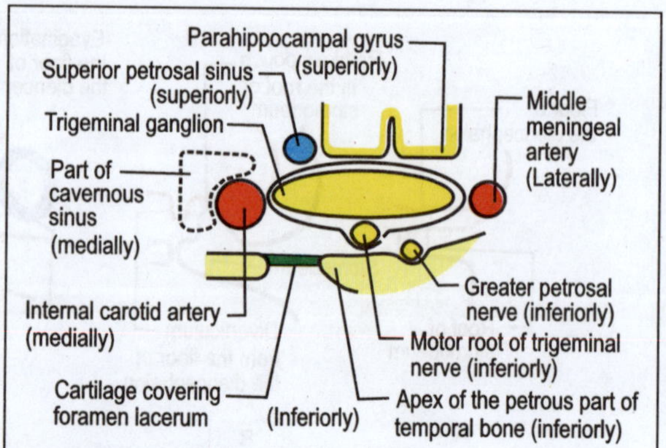

Fig. 6.17: Relations of trigeminal ganglion

Relations:

Superior surface: Parahippocampal gyrus of temporal lobe. Free margin of tentorium cerebelli and superior pertrosal sinus.

Inferior surface related to:

a) Bed to the ganglion (hollow) or impression on the apex of petrous part of temporal bone and cartilage covering foramen lacerum. (Fig. 6.17)

b) Motor root of 5th nerve.

c) Greater petrosal nerve.

Medially: Part of cavernous sinus and internal carotid artery.

Laterally: Middle meningeal artery.

Borders:

Posterosuperior border: It is concave and gives off sensory root.

Anteroinferior border: Convex – emergence of three divisions:

a) Ophthalmic division

b) Maxillary division

c) Mandibular division

Roots and their fate: Both the roots (motor and sensory) run side by side up to pons – sensory – larger, motor – smaller.

I. **Sensory root**: Central processes of the ganglion cells form the sensory root. It enters into the pons to end in different nuclei. The peripheral processes of ganglion cells (pseudounipolar neurons) form ophthalmic, maxillary and mandibular division of trigeminal nerve.

II. **Motor root**: It is a smaller than sensory root. It arises from motor neucleus and emerge from the pons. It passes deep to ganglion and joins the mandibular nerve below the foramen ovale to form the trunk of mandibular nerve.

Arterial supply– branches of:

a) Internal carotid artery; b) Middle meningeal artery, c) Accessory meningeal artery.

Nerve supply: Meningeal branch (nervous spinosus) of mandibular trunk. It supplies perimysium only.

Development: From neural crest epithelium.

APPLIED ANATOMY

Trigeminal neuralgia (intractable facial pain) may be due to acute glaucoma, frontal sinusitis, dental caries of upper jaw, malignant growth in maxillary sinus, dental carries of lower jaw, ulcer or cancer tongue. Treatment usually adopted – first by medicines to relieve pain but if it fails:

a) Injection of alcohol in the trigeminal ganglion by 10cm long lumbar puncture needle through foramen ovale. Thermocoagulation of the ganglion also gives very good result.

b) If ophthalmic neuralgia occurs, section of spinal tract at the lower part of medulla or below it.

c) If ophthalmic nerve is not involved, section of the inferolateral part of sensory root will be of value by interfering maxillary and mandibular fibres section of sensory root proximal to ganglion prevents regeneration of nerve.

DIPLOIC VEINS

Diploic veins drain blood from diploë. These veins drains into dural venous sinuses. These veins look valves. Four cells of diploic veins usually drain to nearest venous sinuses. These are as follow:

a) **A frontal diploic vein** pass through supraorbital foramen to end in supraorbital vein.

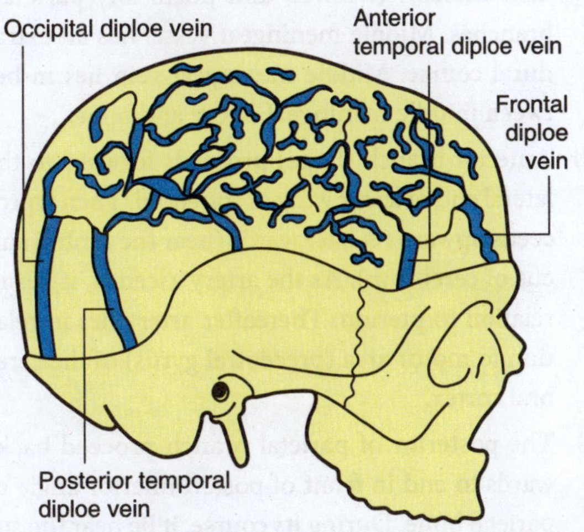

Fig. 6.18: Diploic veins of the skull

b) **An anterior temporal diploic vein** ends in sphenoparietal sinus.

c) **A posterior temporal diploic vein** join the transverse sinus.

d) **An occipital diploic vein** join transverse sinus usually. (Fig. 6.18)

MIDDLE MENINGEAL ARTERY (Fig. 6.19)

It is an important branch of first part of maxillary artery.

Origin: It arises from the first part of maxillary artery in the infratemporal fossa.

Course:

a) It runs in the infratemporal fossa upwards between sphenomandibular ligament and lateral pterygoid muscle. The artery passes through the loop formed by two roots of auriculotemporal nerve. Then artery lie on lateral surface of tensor veli palatini muscle.

b) Then it enters the cranial by passing through foramen spinosum. Here it is accompanied by nervous spinosus (meningeal branch of mandibular).

c) In the cranial cavity (middle cranial fossa) it runs forwards and laterally in a groove on the squamous part of temporal bone and ends by dividing into anterior (frontal) and posterior (parietal) branches. Middle meningeal vessel has an extradural course. Middle meningeal vein lies in between middle meningeal artery and bone.

d) Anterior branch (large) proceeds forward to the lateral end of lesser wing of sphenoid. Then it proceeds upwards & backwards (near the central sulcus of cerebrum). As the artery ascends, it lies in relation to pterion. Thereafter artery lies in relation to motor area (precentral gyrus) of the cerebral cortex.

e) The posterior of parietal branch proceed backwards to end in front of posteroinferior angle of parietal bone. During its course, it lie near the superior temporal sulcus and about 4cm above the zygomatic arch and external acoustic meatus.

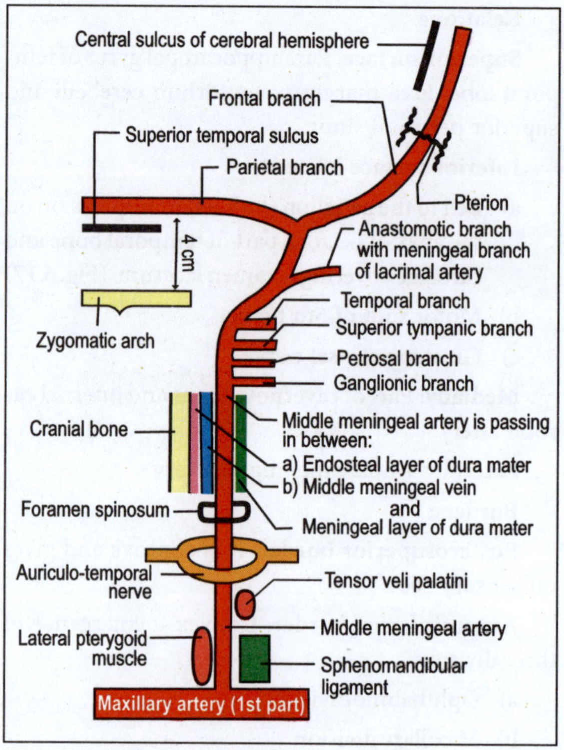

Fig. 6.19: Course, relations and branches of middle meningeal artery

Branches: Besides the two terminal anterior and posterior branches, the middle meningeal artery gives give branches within the cranial cavity:

1. Ganglionic branches (to trigeminal ganglion)
2. Anastomotic branch (with recurrent meningeal branch of lacrimal artery).
3. Temporal branches for the temporal region.
4. Superior tympanic branch supply tympanic (middle ear) cavity.
5. Petrosal branch supply middle ear cavity.

Applied anatomy: In case of fracture skull of the temporal region or separation of dura from the bone without fracture there will be haemorrhage from this artery and a subdural haematoma will be formed and it may compress the motor area causing paralysis of the opposite side. This is to be relieved by trephining the skull at pterion usually and by application of ligature of the bleeding vessels.

chapter 7

DEEP STRUCTURES OF THE NECK

AT A GLANCE

- *Thyroid gland—*
  - *Situation, shape, weight, different parts,*
  - *Lobes*
    - *Number, Shape, Parts, Measurement, Apex, Base, Surfaces, Borders*
  - *Isthmus*
    - *Surfaces, borders*
  - *Pyramidal lobe*
  - *Capsules*
  - *Blood supply, lymphatic drainage*
  - *Support of gland*
  - *Development*
  - *Nerve supply*
  - *Applied anatomy*
- *Parathyroid gland*
- *Subclavian arteries*
- *Common carotid arteries*
- *Internal carotid artery*
- *External carotid artery*
  - *Superior thyroid artery, Facial artery*
  - *Occipital artery, Posterior auricular artery, Superficial temporal artery, Maxillary artery*
- *Internal jugular vein*
- *Sympathetic nerve (Cervical part)*
- *Cervical plexus*
- *Lymphatic drainage of head & neck*
- *Lateral vertebral muscles*
- – *Scalenus anterior, Scalenus median, Scalenus posterior*
- *Trachea*
- *Oesophagus*

Deep structures of the neck are arranged as follows:

a) Cervical viscera: Thyroid, parathyroid, thymus, trachea and oesophagus.

b) Nerves, blood vessels and lymphatics:
   - Last four cranial nerve (IXth, Xth, XIth and XIIth cranial nerves)
   - Carotids (common, external and intern and subclavian arteries)
   - Internal jugular vein and subclavian vein
   - Lymphatics of head and neck

c) Scalene muscles

THYROID GLAND

The word **"Thyroid"** means an oblong shield shaped organ. It is the most vascular of all endocrine glands and depends upon raw materials external environments for production of secretion.

Situation: It is situated in front and sides of the neck and ***opposite fifth to seventh cervical*** and ***first thoracic vertebrae.***

Shape: More of less 'H' shaped horizontal part represents isthmus and two vertical limbs two lateral lobes.

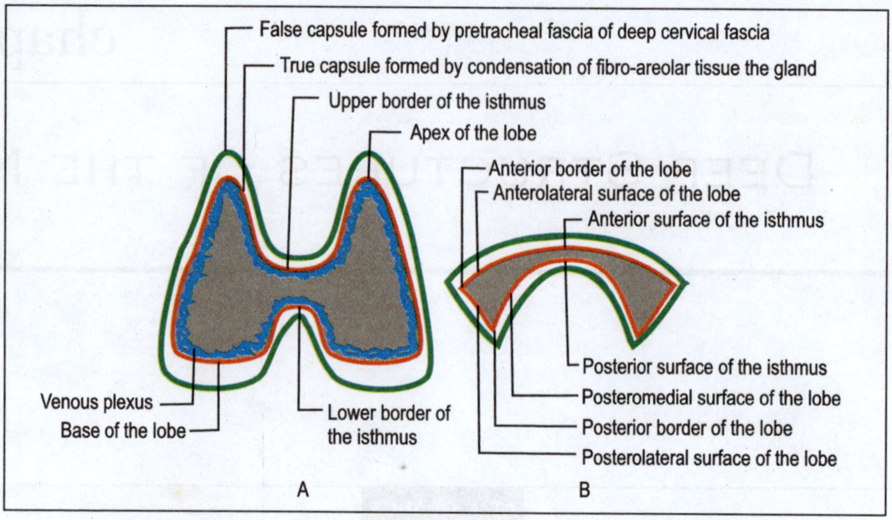

Fig. 7.1: Showing the capsules of the thyroid gland along with base, apex, surfaces and borders of lobes and also showing isthmus (borders & surfaces) of the thyroid gland A: Coronal section thyroid gland; B: Transverse section

Weight: Varies from 20 to 30gms. Average 25gms weight and size more in female specially during menstruation and pregnancy.

Capsules: Two:

1. **Outer false capsule**: It is derived from the pretracheal layer of deep cervical fascia by splitting to enclose the gland. The false capsule is thickened to form **ligament of Berry** which connect the medial surface of thyroid lobe to the cricoid cartilage. Due to this connection (ligament of Berry) the thyroid gland moves during deglutition.
2. **Inner true capsule**: It is formed by condensation of fibro-areolar element of the gland. Venous plexus lies deep to true capsule. (Fig. 7.1)

   [**Note** – In case of prostate venous plexus lies in between two capsules]

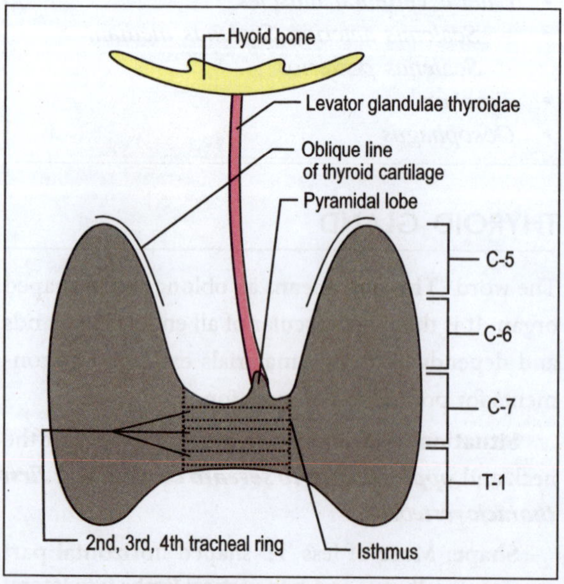

Fig. 7.2: Thyroid gland as seen from front

Features

Consists of (a) Two lateral lobes: (right and left); (b) One isthmus connecting the two lobes (Fig. 7.2)

LATERAL LOBES

Number: Two – (right and left)

Shape: Conical or pyramidal

Extent: It extends from oblique line of thyroid cartilage above to sixth tracheal ring below.

Different parts of lateral lobe

1. Apex; 2. Base; 3. Three surfaces and two borders.

Dimensions or measurements

Length: 5cm; Width: 3cm; Thickness: 2cm.

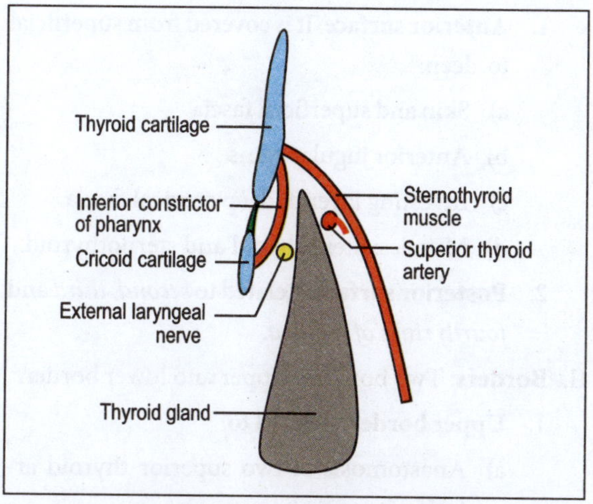

Fig. 7.3: Apex of the lobe of the thyroid gland is in between sternothyroid and inferior constrictor of pharynx

1. **Apex of lateral lobe:**
   a) Situated and directed upwards and laterally at the oblique line of thyroid cartilage.
   b) Lies between inferior constrictor medially and sternothyroid laterally.
   c) Upper limit of the apex (lateral lobe) is determined by the attachment of sternothyroid and it cannot grow further upwards.
   d) Apex of the lateral lobe separate superior thyroid artery and external laryngeal nerve. (Fig. 7.3)
2. **Base of lateral lobe:**
   a) Situated at the level of fifth of sixth tracheal ring.
   b) Related to inferior thyroid artery and recurrent laryngeal nerve which may pass in front or behind or may pass in between the divisions of artery. [*Surgeon should ligate the artery away from the gland*].

Surfaces, borders of lateral lobe and their relations

Three surfaces:

I. **Anterolateral or superficial surface**: Convex covered by muscles from deep to superficial:
   1. Sternothyroid
   2. Sternohyoid

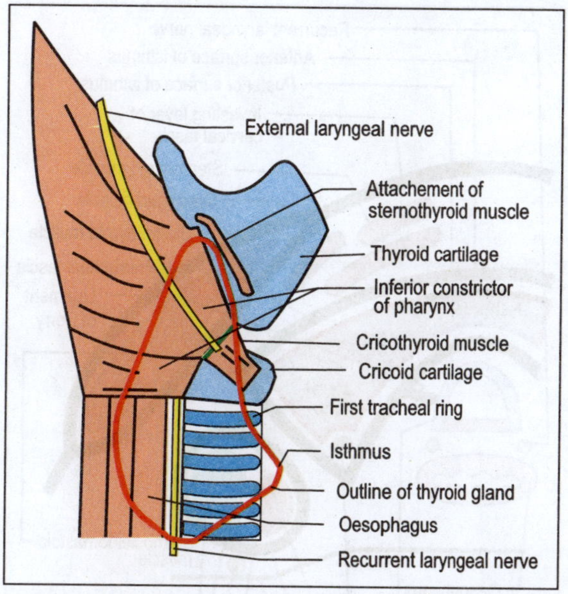

Fig. 7.4: Deep relations of the lobe of the thyroid gland

   3. Superior belly of omohyoid
   4. Lower part by sternocleidomastoid (anterior border)

II. **Posteromedial surface**: Related to
   1. Two tubes:
      a) Larynx continued as trachea (Fig. 7.4)
      b) Pharynx continued as oesophagus
   2. Two muscles: Inferior constrictor and cricothyroid
   3. Two nerves: External laryngeal and recurrent laryngeal. (Fig. 7.5)
   4. Two cartilages: Thyroid and cricoid cartilages.

III. **Posterolateral surface**: Related to carotid sheath and its contents (internal jugular vein laterally, common carotid artery medially and vagus nerve in between them in a posterior plane).

   Ansa cervicalis is embedded in the anterior wall of carotid sheath. Cervical sympathetic chain lies posterior to carotid sheath.

Borders: Two:

I. **Anterior border**: It separates superficial from posterolateral surface.

   Related to: anterior branch of superior thyroid artery.

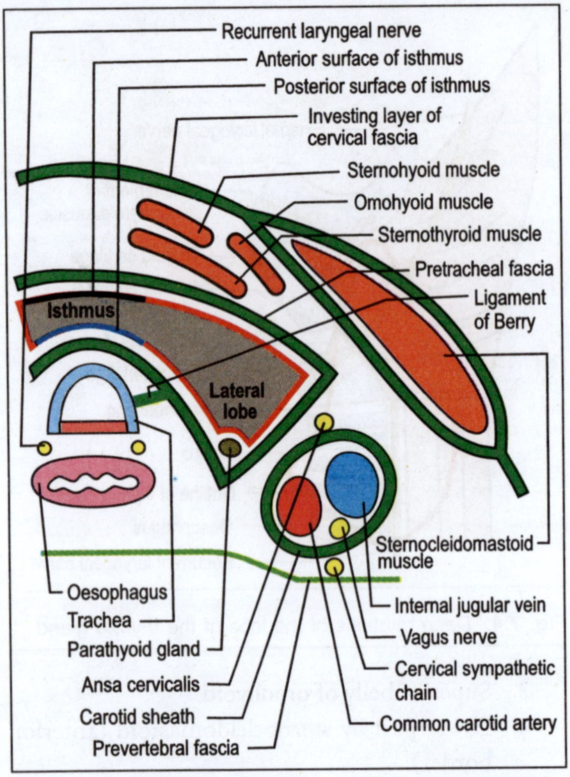

Fig. 7.5: Relations of the isthmus (anterior & posterior surfaces) and lateral lobe (anterolateral, posteromedial & posterolateral surface) of the thyroid gland

II. **Posterior border**: It separates posteromedial from posterolateral surface.

Related to

a) Anastomosis of superior and inferior thyroid arteries

b) Upper and lower parathyroid glands.

c) Thoracic duct on left side.

Isthmus

It is the part of the gland situated in the middle line and connects the lower parts of two lateral lobes. [Isthmus may be absent]

Measurement: Transverse and vertical diameters: 1.25cm

Surface and Borders

I. **Surface**: Two:

1. **Anterior surface**: It is covered from superficial to deep:

   a) Skin and superficial fascia

   b) Anterior jugular veins

   c) Investing layer of deep cervical fascia

   d) Muscles: Sternohyoid and sternothyroid.

2. **Posterior surface**: Related to *second, third* and *fourth rings of trachea.*

II. **Borders**: Two borders: Upper and lower border.

1. **Upper border**: Related to

   a) Anastomosis of two superior thyroid arteries.

2. **Lower border**: Related to:

   a) Inferior thyroid veins emerge out

   b) Entrance of arteria thyroidea ima.

Pyramidal lobe of thyroid gland

Occasionally pyramidal lobe projects from the upper border of isthmus usually to the left of the midline. Occasionally it is connected to the hyoid bone (body) by fibromuscular band called **levator glandulae thyroideae.** (Fig. 7.2)

Blood supply:

Arterial supply: It is supplied by:

1. *Superior thyroid branch of external carotid artery* and enters the gland superficially. *It accompanies by external laryngeal nerve.* At the apex of lobe superior thyroid artery divides into anterior and posterior branches. The anterior branch descends along the anterior border. Anterior branch continue along the upper border of isthmus to anastomose with anterior branch of opposite side.

   The posterior branch descends along the posterior border to anastomose with ascending branch of inferior thyroid artery.

2. *Inferior thyroid artery branch of thyrocervical trunk* and enters the gland from its deep surface. *It is closely related to recurrent laryngeal nerve.*

   After arising from thyrocervical trunk the inferior

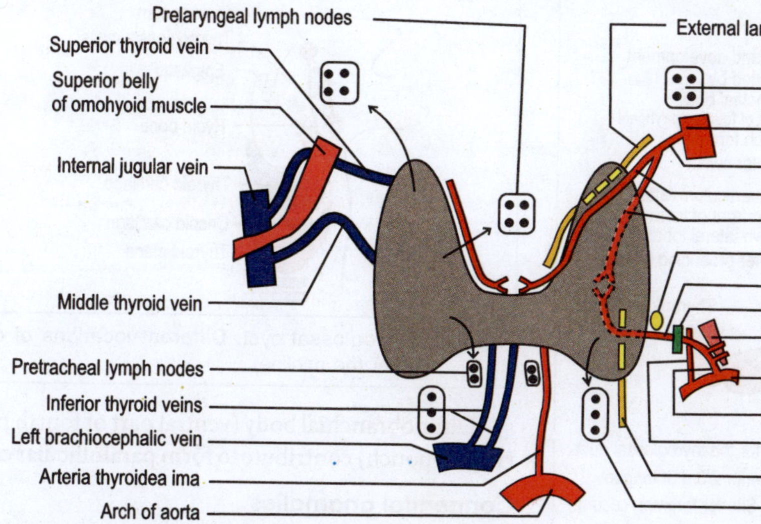

Fig. 7.6: Blood supply and lymphatic drainage of thyroid gland

thyroid artery ascends along the medial border of scalenus anterior, then the artery forms a loop (behind carotid sheath and in front of vertebral artery) which lies below the middle cervical sympathetic ganglion to reach the thyroid gland. In the process the artery presents variable relations with recurrent laryngeal nerve. It gives few branches and one ascending branch run along posterior border to anastomoses with posterior division of superior thyroid artery.

3. *Arteria thyroidea ima*: Occasional branch of arch of aorta or brachiocephalic artery and when present it supplies '**Isthmus**'. (Fig. 7.6)
4. *Accessory thyroid arteries*: These are *branches of oesophageal* and *tracheal arteries* and *enter the posteromedial surface.*

Venous drainage: Veins arise from venous plexus (lies below the true capsule). The veins do not accompany arteries. Venous drainage involves following veins:

1. **Superior thyroid vein**: Emerges from upper pole of the gland and lies at the outer border of the superior belly of the omohyoid and ends in *internal jugular vein* (sometimes in common facial vein).
2. **Middle thyroid vein**: Emerges from middle of lateral lobe and lies on the medial border of the superior belly of omohyoid muscle and ends in *internal jugular vein.*
3. **Inferior thyroid veins**: Emerges from lower border of isthmus and ends in *left brachiocephalic vein.*
4. **Fourth thyroid vein** (Kocher's) may emerge from lower pole and ends into *internal jugular vein.*

Lymphatic drainage:

Lymphatics of thyroid gland consist of two sets (ascending & descending lymphatics) and each set is again divided into medial and lateral.

I. **Ascending lymphatics (Vessels)**
   1. *Medial*: Drain into prelaryngeal lymph nodes situated on the cricothyroid membrane.
   2. *Lateral*: Drain into the *jugulo-digastric group of deep cervical lymph nodes.*

II. **Descending lymphatics:**
   1. *Medial*: Drain into *pretracheal* group on the trachea and lower deep cervical lymphnodes.
   2. *Lateral*: Drain into *glands of recurrent chain on the recurrent laryngeal nerve.*

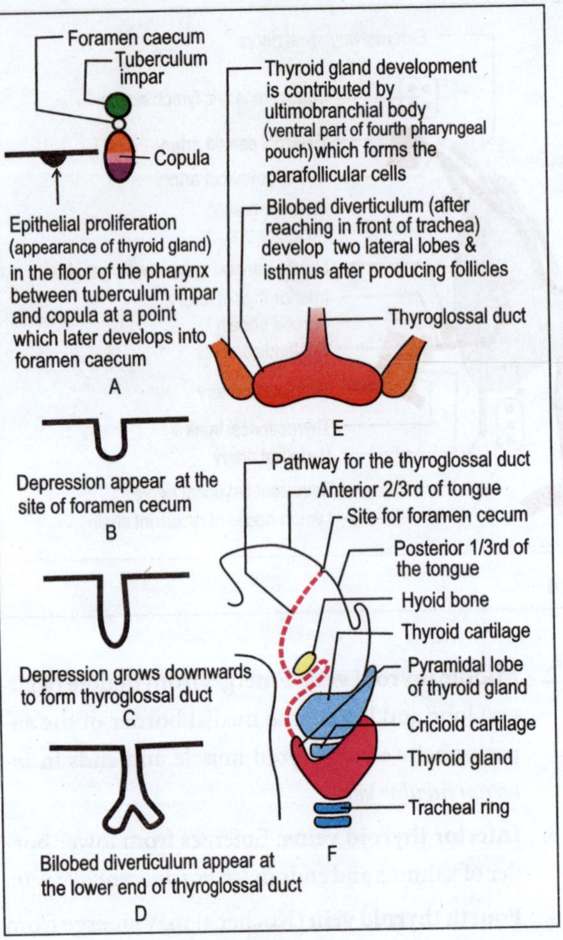

Fig. 7.7: Development of thyroid gland (A, B, C, D, E & F)

DEVELOPMENT OF THYROID GLAND

Thyroid gland appear between the **tuberculum impar** and **copula** as an epithelial proliferation in the floor of pharynx. Later on **foramen caecum** develop in between tuberculum impar and copula at the site of epithelial proliferation.

Thyroglossal duct appear as diverticula in the foramen caecum.

Thyroglossal duct runs downwards in front of the hyoid bone and ascend little behind the hyoid bone.

Subsequently, **thyroglossal duct (bilobed diverticulum)** descend in front of laryngeal cartilages (thyroid and cricoid) to reach its final position in front of trachea and form lateral lobe and isthmus. It forms thyroid follicles (Fig. 7.7).

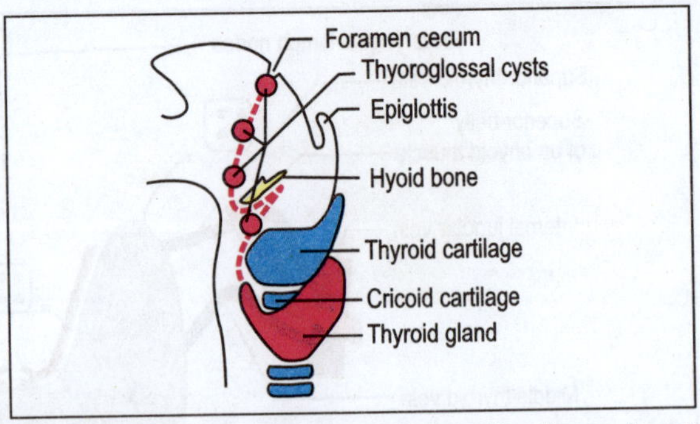

Fig. 7.8: Thyroglossal cyst. Different locations of cyst (near the midline)

Ultimobranchial body (ventral part of fourth pharyngeal pouch) contribute to form parafollicular cells.

Congenital anomalies

1. **Thyroglossal cyst or fistula**: The thyroglossal cyst may be at any point in the migratory pathway of thyroid gland in the midline of the neck. Sometimes thyroglossal cyst rupture, then fistula arises which is connected to the outside by **thyroglossal fistula.** 50% of the thyroglossal cysts are close to hyoid bone (Fig. 7.8).
2. **Anomalies of shape:**
   a) **Agenesis:** Absence of isthmus or one of the lobes.
   b) **Pyramidal lobe**: It usually arises in the upper part of isthmus (left side). It may arise from right or left lobe.
3. **Abnormal positions of thyroid:**
   a) **Lingula thyroid:** It may present just below mucosa.
   b) **Intralingual:** In the tissues of tongue.
   c) **Suprahyoid:** In the midline just above hyoid bone.
   d) **Infrahyoid:** Below hyoid bone.
4. **Ectopic thyroid tissue:** In addition to normal thyroid, ectopic thyroid tissue has been reported in the tongue, larynx, trachea, oesophagus, pleura, ovaries.

MICROSCOPIC FEATURES OF THYROID GLAND

1. Thyroid gland is invested by capsule which sends connective tissue inside the gland and divides the gland into several lobules (Fig. 7.9)

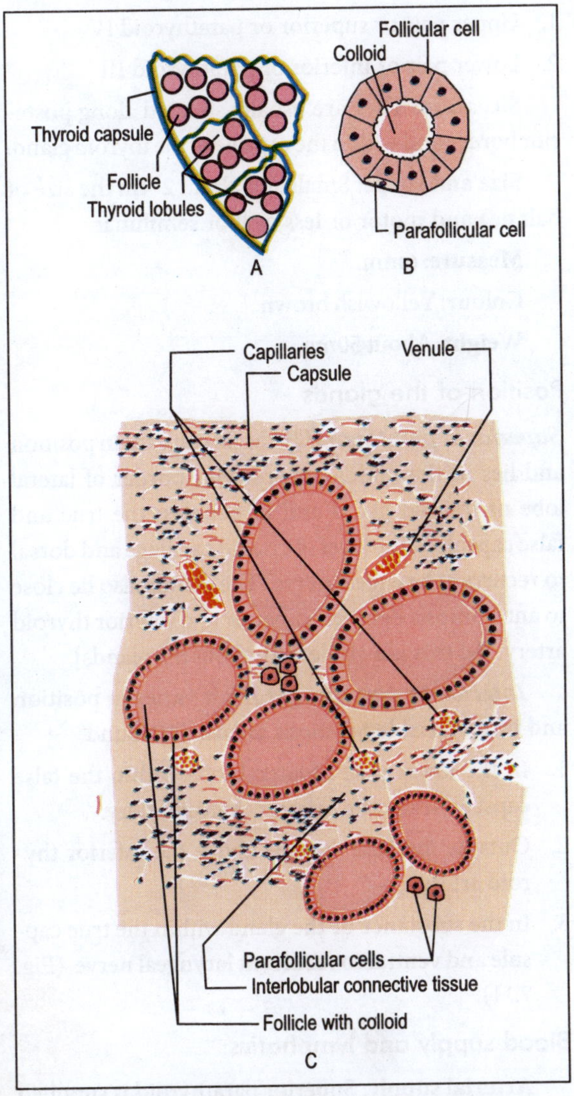

Fig. 7.9: A – Arrangement of thyroid follicles; B – Thyroid follicle with parafollicular cell; C – Microscopic features of the thyroid gland

2. Parenchyma of the gland within lobules contain follicles:
   a) A follicle is made up of follicular cells resting basement membrane.
   b) The follicle has a cavity which is filled with colloid.
   c) The follicular cells are cuboidal cells when they are moderately active. The follicular cells are squamous when they are inactive, the cells are columnar when they are highly active.
   d) Follicular cells secrete two hormones called thyroxine (T_4) and triiodothyronine (T_3), which play an important role in maintaining the basal metabolic rate, growth and development.

Parafollicular cells or C-cells or clear cells

1. These cells are polyhedral or oval.
2. They are present in between the follicular cells and the basement membrane. Some of cells lie in the spaces between follicles.
3. Parafollicular cells secrete calcitonin. It plays an important role in calcium metabolism by the following action:
   a) Decreased absorption of calcium in gut.
   b) Increased urinary secretion of calcium in the kidney.
4. Interlobular connective tissue contain capillaries & venules.

NERVE SUPPLY OF THYROID GLAND

Both sympathetic and parasympathetic.

1. *Sympathetic*: Post ganglionic fibres from superior, middle and inferior cervical ganglia and pass along the perivascular coat to the gland. Function of sympathetic is *mainly vasomotor and recent conception is that it also as: controls regulation of synthesis of hormone due to certain stimuli.*
2. *Parasympathetic*: From vagus and recurrent laryngeal nerves.

APPLIED ANATOMY

1. During operation for removal of thyroid gland:
   a) Superior thyroid artery is ligated close to gland to avoid injury to external laryngeal nerve which accompanies the artery. The nerve leaves the artery at the apex of lateral lobe of the gland.
   b) Inferior thyroid artery is ligated away from the gland to avoid injury to recurrent laryngeal nerve which is intimately related with the artery close to gland. The nerve either passes in front or behind the artery or passes through the divisions of the artery.

c) Ligature is also applied to blood vessels in between the two capsules to avoid excessive bleeding and it is advantageous that trunks of blood vessels are found in the space between the true and false capsule.

d) In surgical removal of the gland the gland is removed along with true capsule and along with venous plexus which lies deep to true capsule and this is done to avoid excessive bleeding.

e) **Suspensory ligament of Berry** must be cut during removal of thyroid gland for mobilisation of the gland because these ligaments anchor the gland.

2. Thyroid gland moves with deglutition because the false capsule is attached to cricoid cartilage through ligament of Berry..
3. Any growth of thyroid gland tends to grow backward due to thin capsule posteriorly and compress trachea and oesophagus leading to
   - Dyspnea (due to pressure on trachea)
   - Dysphagia which is difficulty of swallowing (due to pressure on oesophagus).
4. Any enlargement of thyroid gland is **goitre** and may cause **hypothyroidism** [**cretinism** before puberty and **myxoedema**] and **hyperthyroidism** (thyrotoxicosis or exophthalmic goitre).
5. During operation of partial removal of thyroid gland the posterior parts of both the lateral lobes are usually left (not removed) in order to avoid simultaneous removal of parathyroids.
6. During enlargement of thyroid there may be embarrassment of heart. The anatomical fact is that the pretracheal fascia of deep cervical fascia forming outer false capsule of the thyroid gland and inferiorly pretracheal fascia attached to pericardium. Enlargement of thyroid gland will stretch the pretracheal fascia. The stretching of pretracheal layer may pull the fibrous pericardium causing embarrassment of heart.

PARATHYROIDS (Fig. 7.10)

Two pairs of endocrine glands. Number – four:

1. Upper pair or superior or parathyroid IV
2. Lower pair or inferior or parathyroid III

Situation: They are usually situated along posterior border and within the capsule of the thyroid gland.

Size and shape: Small and about 2-4m the size of half pea and motor or less oval or semilunar

Measure: 6mm.

Colour: Yellowish brown.

Weight: About 50mg.

Position of the glands

Superior or parathyroid IV: Most constant in position and lies in the middle of posterior border of lateral lobe of thyroid gland and in between the true and false capsule at the level of cricoid cartilage and dorsal to recurrent laryngeal nerve. The glands also lie close to anastomosis between superior and inferior thyroid artery. [So this is a guide to find out the glands].

Inferior or parathyroid III: It varies in position and three variable positions are usually found.

1. In the lower pole of lateral lobe within the false capsule below the inferior thyroid artery.
2. Outside the false capsule above the inferior thyroid artery.
3. In the substance or the gland within the true capsule and ventral to recurrent laryngeal nerve. (Fig. 7.11).

Blood supply and lymphatics:

Arterial supply: Superior parathyroid is supplied by branch of superior thyroid artery. Inferior parathyroid is supplied by branch of inferior thyroid artery.

Venous drainage: Parathyroid gland is drained by thyroid veins.

Lymphatic drainage: The lymph vessels from parathyroid gland accompanies the lymph vessels of thyroid gland.

Nerve supply

Sympathetic: From superior and middle cervical sympathetic ganglia and vasomotor in function.

DEVELOPMENT

Endodermal in development.

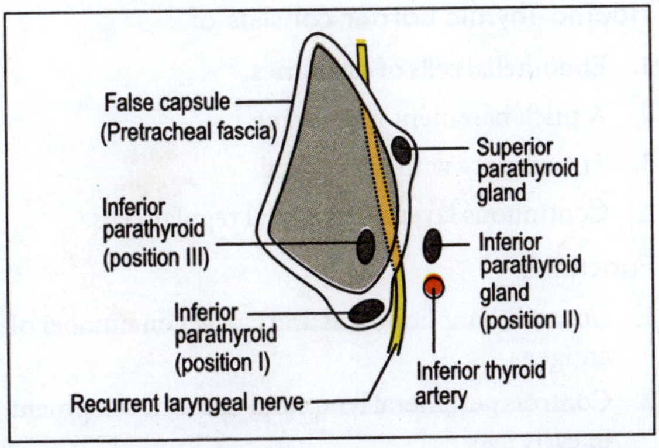

Fig. 7.10: Showing variable positions of inferior parathyroid gland

Superior parathyroids are developed from fourth pharyngeal pouch and so called as **parathyroid IV**.

Inferior parathyroids are developed from third pharyngeal pouch and so called **parathyroid III.**

SECRETORY ACTIVITIES OF GLANDS

Controlled by calcium level in the blood. Low level stimulates and high level depress the secretion of the gland.

MICROSCOPIC FEATURES OF PARATHYROID GLAND

1. Invested by fibrous capsule which gives septa (processes) within the substance of the gland and divided and subdivide into lobules.
2. Cells of the gland form anastomotic cords or groups of cells supported by fibres with sinusoidal capillaries.
3. Cells are of two types: (Fig. 7.11)
   a) **Chief or principal cells**: (Secrete parathormone hormone). Chief cells are polygonal, plenty and small.
   b) **Oxyphil cell**: In small quantity. Cytoplasm is eosinophilic. Oxyphil cells increases as age increases. Cells are large.

Function

Chief cells secrete **parathormone (PTH)** which increases the blood calcium level by

1. Increased absorption of calcium from the gut.
2. Increasing the mobilization of calcium from bone

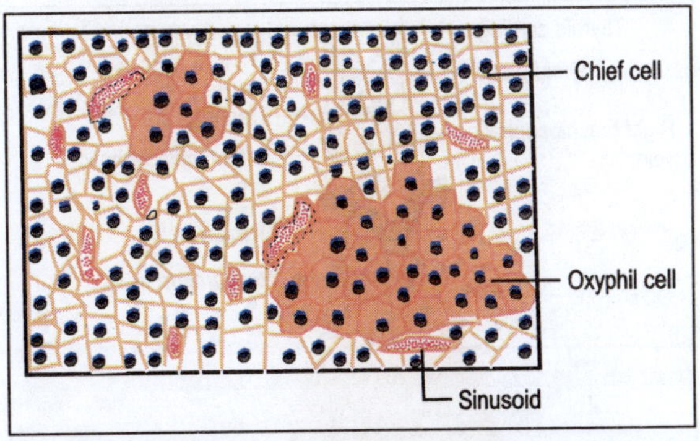

Fig. 7.11: Microscopic features of parathyroid gland

3. Decreased excretion of calcium in the urine by kidney.

APPLIED ANATOMY

1. Hyperparathyroidism (due to tumour causes hypersecretion of gland and results in Osteitis fibrosa cystica (softening with formation of cysts in the bone – finally bowing fracture occurs) and formation of renal stone.
2. Hypoparathyroidism: It usually occurs due to removal of gland accidentally and caused tetany and increased neuromuscular activities.

THYMUS

It is a lymphoid organ.

Situation: In the lower part of the neck, anterior and superior mediastinum of thorax and lies on pericardium, great vessels of superior mediastinum and trachea. (Fig. 7.12)

Age changes: Well developed at birth and grows upto puberty and then undergoes gradual atrophy and replacement by fat.

Weight: 10-15gm at birth may increase upto 20 or 30gm after midadult age.

Different lobes: Two lobes which are of unequal sizes and connected by fibroareolar tissue.

Blood supply:

Arterial supply: Branches of internal thoracic and inferior thyroid artery supply the thymus.

Venous drainage: Veins drainage to the left brachiocephalic, internal thoracic and inferior thyroid veins.

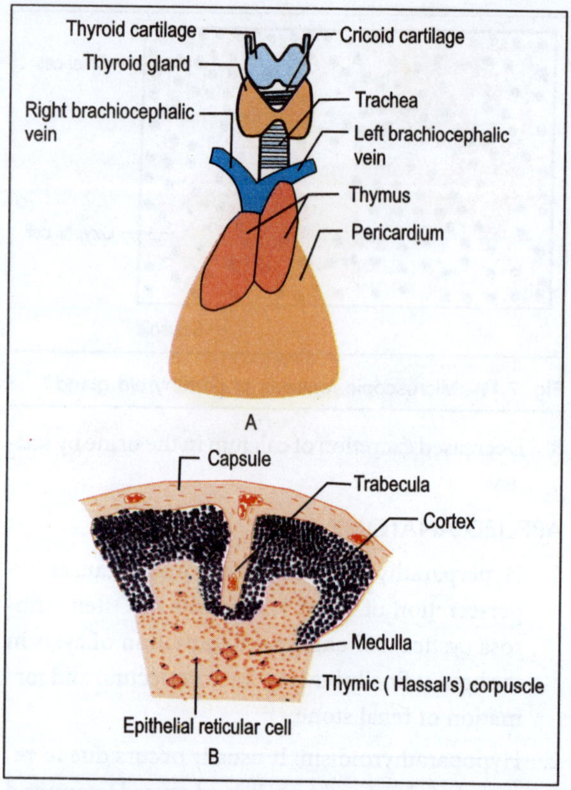

Fig. 7.12: (A) Position of thymus; (B) Microscopic features of thymus

Nerve supply: Sympathetic from stellate ganglion and vasomotor in function.

Capsule of thymus is supplied by phrenic nerve and descendens cervicalis.

Microscopic features: (Fig. 7.12)

1. The thymus is covered by connective tissue capsule from which trabeculae arises. The trabeculae extend inside the thymus to subdivide into numerous incomplete lobules.
2. Each lobule consist of outer dark staining cortex and inner light staining medulla.
3. Cortex contains aggregation of T lymphocytes.
4. Medulla: Medulla of neighbouring lobules shows continuity. Medulla contain epithelial reticular cells and Hassal's corpuscles.

Development:

It is endodermal in development and from ventral part of third pharyngeal pouch and migrate caudalwards towards thorax.

Haemo-thymic barrier consists of

1. Endothelial cells of capillaries.
2. A thick basement membrane.
3. Tissue space with tissue fluid.
4. Continuous layer of epithelial regular cells.

Functions

1. Controls lymphopoiesis and can act on number of antigens.
2. Controls peripheral lymphoid tissue development in early age.
3. Lymphocytes of cortex control autoimmunity.
4. Medulla secretes
   a) Lymphopoietin which stimulates production of lymphocytes in all region.
   b) Competence inducing factor which is responsible for competency of new lymphocytes to act with antigen.

APPLIED ANATOMY

1. Hyperplasia causes myasthenia gravis: a condition of gross fatiguability of voluntary muscles.
2. Involution occurs as a result of hyperactivity of adrenal cortex or injections of cortisone. Involution may be delayed in case of removal of adrenal gland.
3. When thymus enlarge it may press on trachea, oesophagus, great vessels and nerves in the neck and thus results in hoarseness of voice, cough, dysphagia and also cyanosis.

SUBCLAVIAN SYSTEM OF ARTERIES

This system of arteries are mainly for the upper limb but some parts of neck, brain are also supplied by it [a part of abdomen also gets supply].

Origin: Right subclavian artery arises from division of brachiocephalic trunk behind right sternoclavicular joint.

Whereas left subclavian artery arises directly from arch of aorta.

Course:

1. Right consists of cervical part and left consists of thoracic and cervical part. The course of cervical part of each artery is the same.

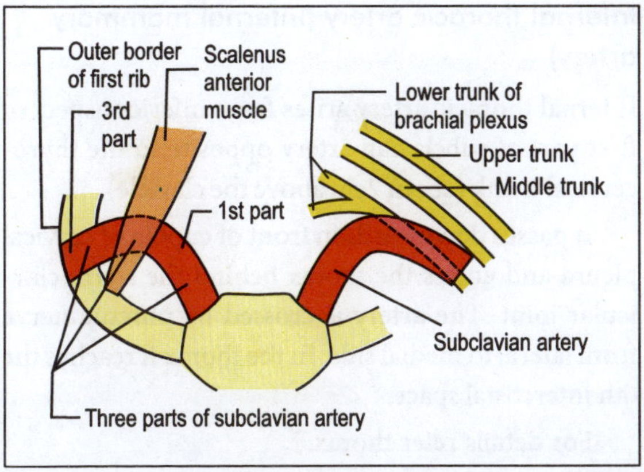

Fig. 7.13: Showing the parts of the subclavian artery and relation of brachial plexus with the subclavian artery

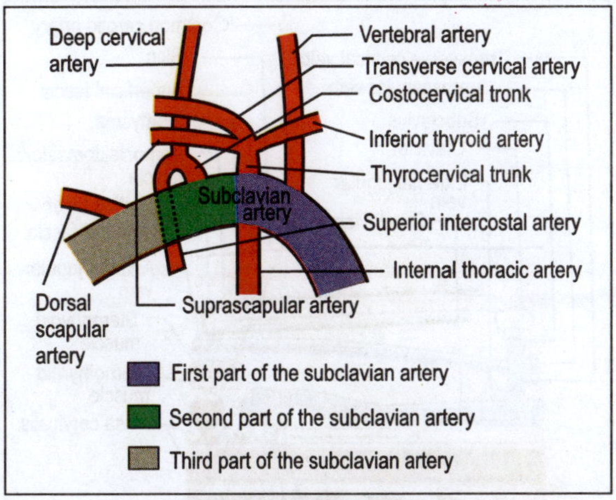

Fig. 7.14: Branches of suclavian artery

2. Thoracic part of left: It runs upwards on the mediastinal pleura and makes groove on the left lung and enters the neck by passing behind the sternoclavicular joint.
3. Cervical parts of both the arteries:
   A. Each artery runs in a curved manner over the cervical pleura and apex of lung with a convexity upwards and extends from sternoclavicular joint to outer border of first rib.
   B. **Division of the artery**: Divided into three parts by scalenus anterior which crosses it.

      First part: Part from origin to medial border of the scalenus anterior. (Fig. 7.13)

      Second part: Behind the scalenus anterior.

      Third part: Part from lateral border of the muscle to termination.

Branches of subclavian artery (Fig. 7.14)

From the first part:

1. Vertebral artery
2. Internal thoracic artery
3. Thyrocervical trunk
   - Inferior thyroid artery
   - Transverse cervical artery
   - Suprascapular artery
4. Costocervical trunk (on left side)

From second part:

1. Costocervical trunk (on right side)

From third part: Dorsal scapular artery.

C. **Relations**:

First part:

a) ***In front*** (immediate): From medial to lateral – common carotid artery, ansa subclavia, cardiac branches of sympathetic and vagus nerves, vertebral and internal jugular veins, left phrenic nerve and thoracic duct (left side).

Further superficially: Sternothyroid, sternohyoid, anterior jugular vein and sternocleidomastoid. (Fig. 7.15)

b) ***Behind***: Suprapleural membrane covering the pleura, apex of lung, ansa subclavia and right recurrent laryngeal nerve.

Second part:

a) ***In front***: Scalenus anterior and structures in front of the muscle are phrenic nerve (right side), subclavian vein, transverse and suprascapular arteries, sternocleidomastoid muscle.

b) ***Behind***: Suprapleural membrane, cervical pleura covering apex of lung, lower trunk of brachial plexus.

c) ***Above***: Upper and middle trunks.

Third part:

a) ***In front***: Suprascapular and transverse cervical vessels, nerve to subclavius, subclavian vein, external jugular and anterior jugular veins. Investing layer of deep cervical fascia, subclavius,

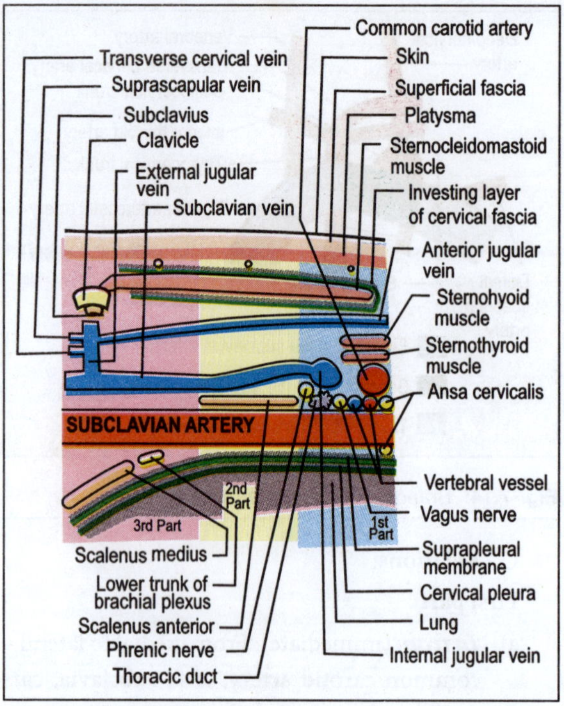

Fig. 7.15: Relations of subclavian artery

clavicle (middle third), posterior border of the sternocleidomastoid.

b) ***Behind***: Scalenus medius, lower trunk of brachial plexus, suprapleural membrane covering cervical pleura with apex of the lung.

c) ***Above***: Inferior belly of the omohyoid, upper and middle trunk.

d) ***Below***: First rib.

Termination: At the outer border of the first rib it continues as axillary artery.

Development

Right subclavian: From three sources:

1. Right fourth arterial arch
2. Part of dorsal aorta
3. Right seventh intersegmental artery.

Left subclavian: From one source: left seventh intersegmental artery.

Branches of subclavian artery

Vertebral artery

Described in chapter 8.

Internal thoracic artery (Internal mammary artery)

Internal thoracic artery arises from inferior aspect of first part of subclavian artery opposite to the thyrocervical trunk (about 2cm above the clavicle).

It passes downwards in front of cupola of cervical pleura and enters the thorax behind the sternoclavicular joint. The artery is crossed by phrenic nerve from lateral to medial side. In the thorax it reaches the 6th intercostal space.

For details refer thorax.

Thyrocervical trunk

It arises from upper aspect of first part of subclavian artery just lateral to the origin of vertebral artery. It immediately divides into three branches:

1. Inferior thyroid artery
2. Superficial cervical and
3. Suprascapular artery

1. **Inferior thyroid artery**: It ascends in relation to medial border of scalenus anterior, and arches medially to C_7 vertebra between vertebral vessels (behind) and carotid sheath with its contents (in front). Loop of the artery is related middle cervical sympathetic ganglion. On reaching the posterior surface of lateral lobe of the thyroid gland, the antery divides into ascending and descending branches. Ascending branch anastomoses with posterior branch of superior thyroid artery in the posterior border of lateral lobe of the thyroid gland. Close to the base of the lateral lobe of the thyroid gland inferior thyroid presents variable relations with recurrent laryngeal nerve.

Other branches:

a) **Ascending cervical artery** ascends medial side of phrenic nerve on the transverse process of cervical vertebrae. The artery act as guide to phrenic nerve. It supplies prevertebral muscles ad gives spinal branches to the vertebral canal.

b) **Inferior laryngeal branch** accompanies recurrent laryngeal nerve and supplies the laryngeal muscles and mucous membrane below vocal cord.

c) **Tracheal, oesophageal and pharyngeal branches** supply trachea, oesophagus and pharynx.

2. **Superficial cervical artery**: It reaches the posterior triangle in front of brachial plexus after crossing scalenus anterior and phrenic nerve. It ascends beneath the trapezius to anastomose with a branch of occipital artery.
3. **Suprascapular artery**: It reaches the suprascapular ligament after crossing scalenus anterior and clavicle to anastomoses with circumflex scapular artery and dorsal scapular artery.

Costocervical trunk:

It arises from the posterior aspect of first part of the subclavian artery on the left side or second part of the right subclavian artery. The artery arches backward above the copula of the pleura and on reaching the neck of first rib and transverse process of C_7 vertebra it divides into deep cervical and superior intercostal arteries.

1. **Deep cervical artery** ascends behind the transverse process of C_7 vertebra. It passes between semispinalis capitis and semispinalis cervicis and anastomoses with branch of the occipital artery.
2. **Superior intercostal artery** descends in front of neck of upper two ribs. It gives two (upper) intercostal (posterior) arteries to the first two intercostal space.

Dorsal scapular artery:

t arises from the third part of the subclavian artery. It reaches the medial border scapula after passing in between brachial plexus and beneath levator scapulae. The artery helps to form scapular anastomoses. **Superficial cervical** and **dorsal scapular arteries** arises from thyrocervical trunk (in 33%, those two arteries arise as a **transverse cervical artery**).

APPLIED ANATOMY OF SUBCLAVIAN ARTERY

Cervical rib is a extra rib which arises from cervical vertebra and anteriorly fused with first rib. This may press the brachial plexus and subclavian artery. The patient is asked to extend, abduct & lateral rotation of the affected arm; also ask the patient to take a deep breaths. The test is positive, if there is marked decrease of the radial pulse (**Adson's test**).

SUBCLAVIAN VEIN

It is the continuation of axillary vein from outer border of first rib to the medial border of scalenus anterior where it joins internal jugular vein to form corresponding brachiocephalic vein.

Relation:

Anteriorly: Clavicle and subclavians muscle.

Posteriorly: Scalenus anterior, phrenic nerve and subclavian artery.

Below: First rib.

Tributaries:

1. External jugular vein
2. Dorsal scapular vein
3. Thoracic duct on the left side and right lymphatic duct, at the junction of internal jugular vein subclavian vein.
4. Anterior jugular vein sometimes.

CAROTID SYSTEM

It consists of **common carotid arteries** and its two divisions: **external and internal carotid arteries.**

[The word **carotid** means heavy sleep as there is an idea that deep sleep is caused by pressure on carotid arteries].

COMMON CAROTID ARTERY

Two: Right and left.

Origin: They differ on two sides: **Right** arises as one of the terminal division of brachiocephalic artery behind sternoclavicular joint whereas the left arises as a direct branch from arch of aorta in the superior mediastinum of the thorax. (So left consists of thoracic and cervical parts).

Course:

1. In the neck the course of the two arteries are same.
2. It ascends on each side of the front of neck within carotid sheath from behind the sternoclavicular joint and passes in front of transverse processes of lower four cervical vertebrae and undercover of anterior border of sternocleidomastoid muscle to the level of upper border of thyroid cartilage.
3. The lower part of artery lies deeper under cover of sternohyoid, sternothyroid and superior belly of omohyoid and the upper part lies superficial only under cover of sternocleidomastoid muscle.

Termination: It terminates at the level of upper border of thyroid cartilage and opposite the disc between 3rd and 4th cervical vertebrae by dividing into external and internal carotid arteries.

Characteristics at the point of division (Termination): Presence of carotid sinus and carotid body.

Carotid sinus: A dilatation at the termination of common carotid or at the beginning of internal carotid artery structurally tunica media is thin but adventitia is thick and innervated by 9th nerve and sympathetic and acts as **pressure receptor** and thus regulates pressure in the cerebral arteries.

Carotid body: A small reddish body lies behind the point of division of common carotid artery and supplied by 9th, 10th and sympathetic nerves. It acts as **chemoreceptor** and influenced by O_2 and CO_2 contents or blood].

Relations:

1. **Anteriorly**
   a) Skin, superficial fascia, platysma, investing of deep cervical fascia. (Fig. 7.16)
   b) Sternocleidomastoid (in upper part) and (in lower part) in addition sternohyoid, sternothyroid, superior belly of omohyoid.
   c) Descendens hypoglossi and ansa cervicalis in front of carotid sheath.
   d) Crossed by sternocleidomastoid branch of occipital artery, superior and middle thyroid veins and anterior jugular veins.

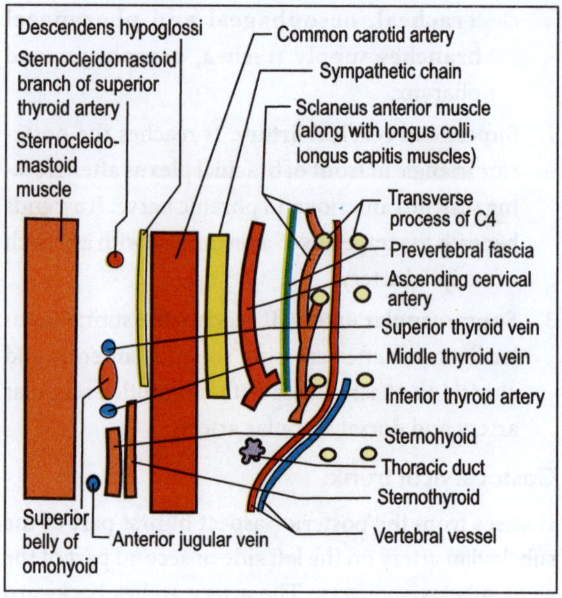

Fig. 7.16: Relations of the common carotid artery

2. **Posteriorly**
   a) Transverse processes of lower four cervical vertebrae and prevertebral muscles covered by prevertebral fascia, sympathetic trunk behind posterior wall of carotid sheath.
   [The artery can be compressed on the carotid tubercle of 6th cervical – about 4cm above sternoclavicular joint].
   b) Vertebral vessels in the lower part and crossed by inferior thyroid artery and thoracic duct on left side.
   c) Carotid body at the point of division.
3. **Laterally**: Internal jugular vein and vagus nerve in a posterior plane.
4. **Medially**: Larynx continued as trachea, pharynx continued as oesophagus, recurrent laryngeal nerve and thyroid gland.

Development: Developed from third arterial arch (ventral part) on each side.

APPLIED ANATOMY

If one common carotid artery is ligated the collateral circulation may be formed by

1. Anastomosis between superior thyroid branch of

external carotid and inferior thyroid branch of subclavian artery.

2. Anastomosis between descending branch of occipital with transverse cervical and deep cervical branches of subclavian.
3. In the middle anastomosis between the branches of external carotid artery of each side.

INTERNAL CAROTID ARTERY

It is one of the terminal branches of common carotid artery and supplies the major part of cerebral hemisphere, eye and its accessory organs, forehead and nose.

Origin: Arises at the bifurcation of common carotid at the level of upper border of thyroid cartilage opposite C_3 and C_4 vertebrae.

Course: Divided into four parts: Cervical, petrous, cavernous and cerebral.

I. **Cervical part**:
1. From origin to base of skull at the carotid canal through which enters the skull and continues as petrous part.
2. It will be within the carotid sheath.
3. **Relations**: (Fig. 7.17)
   a) **Posteriorly**: Upper three cervical vertebrae (transverse processes), prevertebral fascia covering prevertebral muscles, superior cervical sympathetic ganglions crossed by superior laryngeal nerve and close to base internal jugular vein and last four cranial nerves.
   b) **Anteriorly**: (i) In the lower part – it will be crossed by hypoglossal nerve, facial and lingual veins, posterior belly of digastric and stylohyoid muscles, occipital and posterior auricular arteries. (ii) In the upper part – covered by parotid gland with external carotid artery, styloid process and its attached muscles and 9th nerve, pharyngeal branch of 10th cranial nerve.

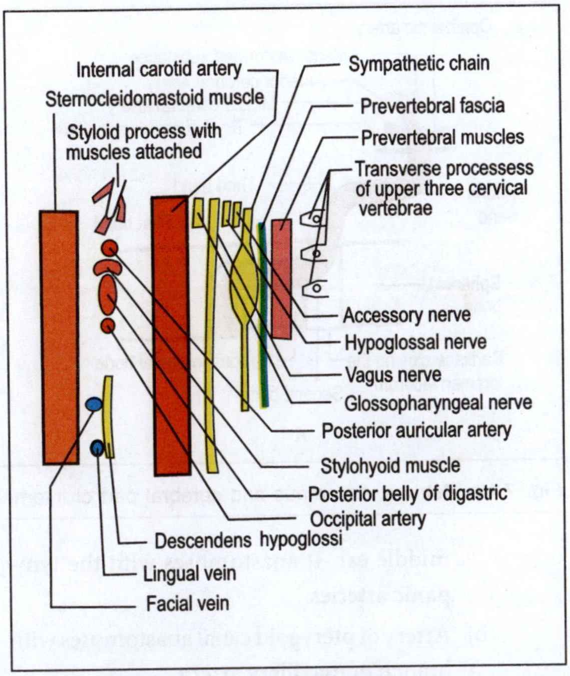

Fig. 7.17: Relations of internal carotid artery

   c) Medially: Pharynx, ascending pharyngeal artery and superior laryngeal nerve.
   d) Laterally: Internal jugular vein and vagus nerve in between artery and vein.
4. This part has no branches.

II. **Petrous part** (Fig. 7.18)
1. It lies within the carotid canal and it first passes upwards and then changes its direction medially at right angle.
2. It emerges at the apex of petrous part and at the posterior part of foramen lacerum.
3. Then it passes upwards and medially above the cartilage covering foramen lacerum.
4. Relations:
   a) Surrounded by sympathetic plexus.
   b) Above and behind: Middle ear and cochlea.
   c) Front and lateral: Auditory tube and tensor tympani muscle.
   d) Trigeminal ganglion: Lies above.
5. **Branches**:
   a) **Carotico-tympanic branch**: It enters the

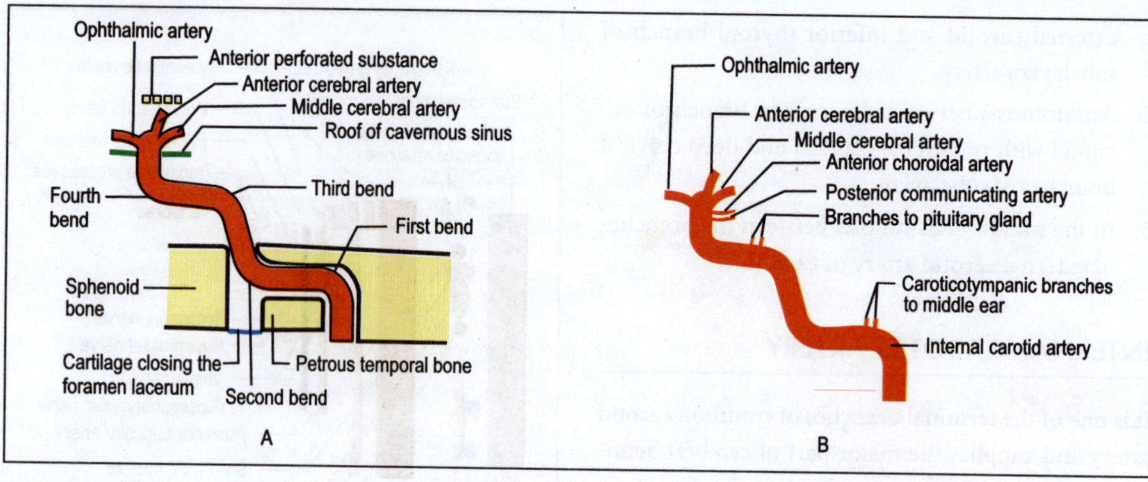

Fig. 7.18: Petrous, cavernous and cerebral part of internal carotid artery. A – Course; B – Branches

middle ear. It anastomoses with the tympanic arteries.

b) Artery of pterygoid canal anastomoses with branch of maxillary artery.

III. **Cavernous part**

1. It begins from foramen lacerum and passes upwards to the medial aspect of lingula of sphenoid bone and enters cavernous sinus.
2. In the cavernous sinus it is situated in a sulcus on each side of sella turcica and runs forward.
3. Within the sinus it lies on the inferomedial wall separated from blood by endothelium.
4. **Relations in the sinus**: Abducent nerve inferolateral to artery.
5. Finally the part ends by piercing the dura mater forming the roof of sinus between middle and anterior clinoid process.
6. **Branches:**
   a) Cavernous branches: Supplies the hypophysis and the trigeminal ganglion.
   b) Hypophyseal branches: Supply the hypophysis.
   c) Meningeal artery: Supply the dura mater of anterior cranial fossa.

IV. **Cerebral part**:

1. This part begins from the roof of cavernous sinus.
2. It at first runs backward along the roof of cavernous sinus in the subarachnoid space and lies below optic nerve.
3. Ultimately it runs upward on the side of optic chiasma and reaches anterior perforated substance.

   Here it ends by dividing into anterior and middle cerebral arteries.
4. **Branches**: (a) Superior hypophyseal; (b) Ophthalmic artery; (c) Posterior communicating; (d) Anterior choroid; (e) Anterior cerebral artery; (f) Middle cerebral artery.

Carotid siphon: A 'U' shaped bend with convexity forward is formed by internal carotid artery during its passage through cavernous sinus. Its function is to maintain a regular flow of blood to the brain by damping down the pulsation of artery.

EXTERNAL CAROTID ARTERY

It is the main artery of the head and neck region and supplies outer aspect of the head, face and greater part of neck (structures in front part of neck).

Origin: It is one of the terminal branches of common carotid artery and arises as a result of bifurcation of common carotid artery at the level of upper border of thyroid cartilage and opposite the disc between third and fourth cervical vertebrae.

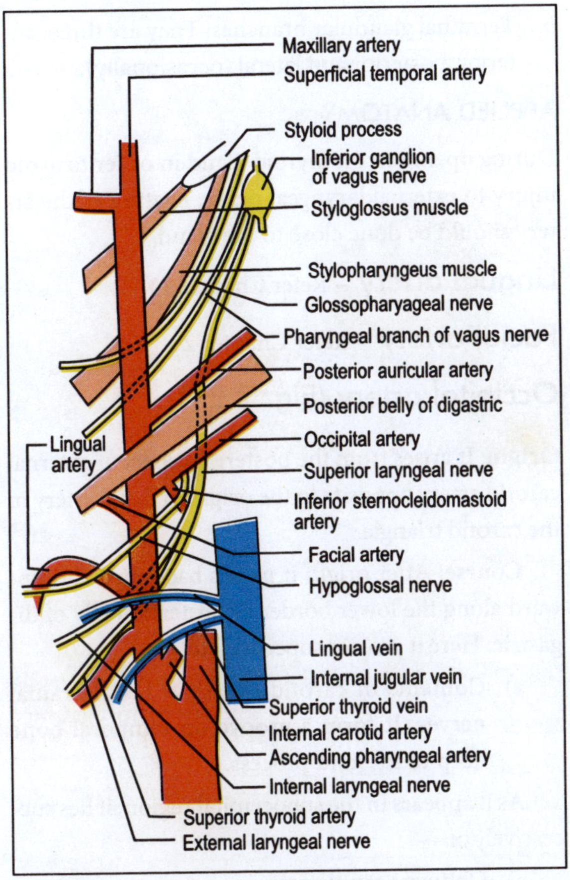

Fig. 7.19: Relations of external carotid artery

Course: After origin it passes upwards, forwards and then backwards and enters the substance of parotid gland.

At the site of origin the external carotid artery lies anteromedial to internal carotid artery. Its course like the italic '*f*' shaped.

Termination: In the substance of parotid gland at the level of the neck of mandible it terminates by dividing into maxillary and superficial termporal branches.

Relations:

I. **In the carotid triangle**

1. **Superficial**
   a) Covered by skin, superficial fascia, platysma and deep fascia and crossed by—
   Nerves: Cervical branch of facial nerve, hypoglossal nerve. (Fig. 7.19)
   b) Veins: Facial, lingual and superior thyroid veins.
   c) Muscles: Overlapped by anterior border of sternocleidomastoid muscles.
2. **Deep**
   a) Wall of pharynx with constrictor muscles of pharynx.
   b) Superior laryngeal nerve with its two division: external and internal laryngeal nerves.
   c) Ascending pharyngeal artery.

II. **Above the carotid triangle**: Posterior belly of digastric and stylohyoid lie superficial to artery.

III. **Within the substance of parotid gland**: Superficially: Retromandibular vein and facial nerve and its branches.

IV. **Deep to parotid**: Internal carotid artery and six structures separating it from external carotid artery:

a) Styloid process of the temporal bone
b) Styloglossus
c) Stylopharyngeus
d) A part of the parotid gland
e) Glossopharyngeal nerve
f) Pharyngeal branch of the vagus.

Other structures deep to internal carotid as superior laryngeal nerve and superior cervical sympathetic ganglia.

Branches: 'External' consists of '8' letters–

E X T E R N A L – so branches are eight:
1 2 3 4 5 6 7 8 (Fig. 7.20)

A. **From the front part**: Three from below upwards
   1. Superior thyroid artery
   2. Lingual artery
   3. Facial artery
B. **From medial side**: One
   4. Ascending pharyngeal artery
C. **From behind**: Two
   5. Occipital artery, and
   6. Posterior auricular artery
D. **Terminal branches**: Two
   7. Superficial temporal, and
   8. Maxillary

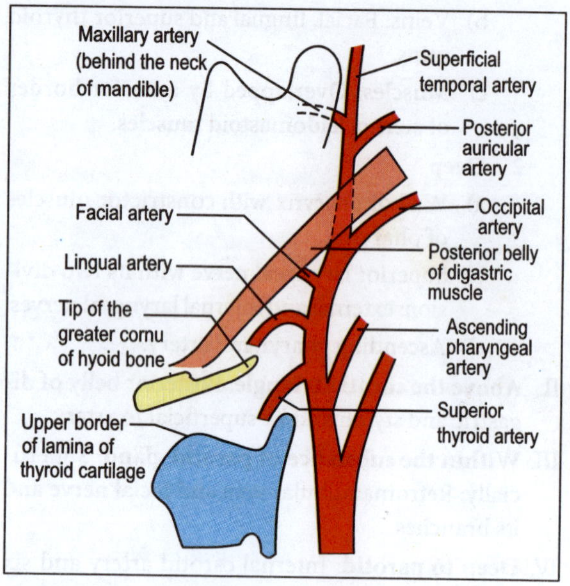

Fig. 7.20: Branches of external carotid artery

Development: It is developed from an outgrowth from third arterial arch.

Superior Thyroid Artery

It arises from front and at the level of greater cornu or hyoid bone.

Course: It runs downwards and forwards – accompanied by external laryngeal nerve (which lies posteromedial to artery). It lies on inferior constrictor and passes deep to omohyoid, sternohyoid and sternothyroid muscles and finally reaches the upper pole lateral lobe thyroid gland. Here it ends by dividing into terminal branches and lie superficial to gland and the nerve passes deep to gland.

Branches:

1. Infrahyoid: anastomoses with artery of opposite side.
2. Superior laryngeal: It pierces the thyrohyoid membrane along with internal laryngeal nerve and anastomosis with inferior laryngeal branch of inferior thyroid artery.
3. Cricothyroid branch: Anastomosis with fellow of opposite side.
4. Sternocleidomastoid branch: Supply to the muscle.
5. Terminal glandular branches: They are three: anterior, posterior and lateral (occasionally).

APPLIED ANATOMY

During operation on thyroid gland in order to avoid injury to external laryngeal nerve, ligature of the artery should be done close to the gland.

Lingual artery – Refer Chapter 13

Facial artery – Refer Chapter 2

Occipital artery (Fig. 7.21)

Origin: It arises from the posterior aspect of external carotid artery opposite to the origin of facial artery in the carotid triangle.

Course: After origin it passes backward and upward along the lower border of posterior belly of digastric. Here it crosses superficial to

a) Contents of carotid sheath & last 4 cranial nerves. It form a groove on temporal bone deep to mastoid process.

As it appears in the suboccipital region, it lies successively on—

a) Obliquus capitis superior
b) Semispinalis capitis

Ultimately it pierces trapezius and accompanies greater occipital nerve and reaches the posterior aspect of scalp.

Terminates: It terminates by giving branches to posterior part of scalp.

Branches:

1. Upper and lower sternocleidomastoid branches: Upper branch accompanies spinal accessory nerve. Lower branch is hooked by hypoglossal nerve.
2. Mastoid branch: It supplies mastoid air cells after entering the cranial cavity through mastoid foramen.
3. Meningeal branch: It enters the posterior cranial fossa through jugular foramen to supply dura mater.
4. Muscular branch supply the adjoining muscles.

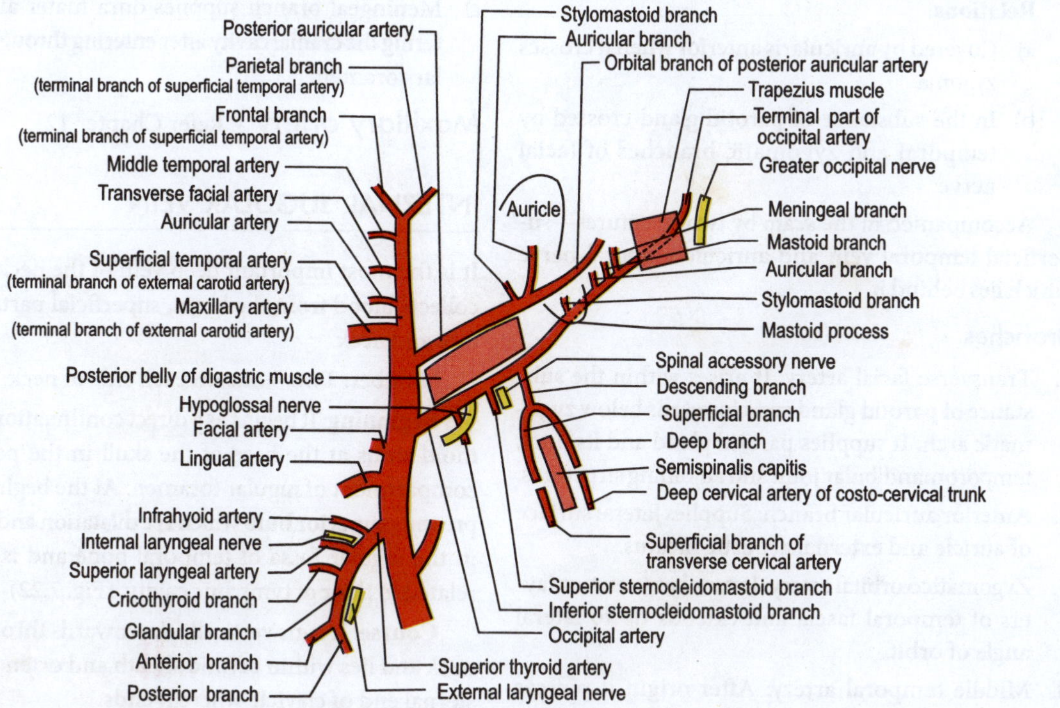

Fig. 7.21: Courses and branches of superior thyroid artery, posterior auricular artery, occipital artery and superficial temporal artery of external carotid artery

5. Auricular branch (occasionally) supply auricle.
6. Descending branches – superficial and deep: Superficial branch anastomoses with superficial branch of transverse cervical artery (superficial to semispinalis capitis). Deep branch anastomoses with deep cervical artery deep to semispinalis capitis.
7. Occipital branches

Posterior auricular artery

1. It arises from posterior aspect of external carotid above the origin of occipital.
2. It passes backward along the upper border of posterior belly of digastric.
3. It lies under cover of parotid and superficial to styloid process of temporal bone.
4. It terminates in between auricle and mastoid process by dividing into occipital and auricular branches.
5. **Branches**—
   a) **Stylomastoid artery** supplies facial nerve, middle ear and mastoid air cells.
   b) Auricular branch supplies both surfaces of auricle.
   c) Occipital branch supplies scalp above and behind auricle.

Superficial temporal artery

It is one of the terminal branches of external carotid artery.

Origin: It arises as a result of division of external carotid artery within the substance of parotid gland behind the neck of mandible.

Course: After origin it crosses posterior root of zygomatic process of temporal bone and in front of auricle.

Termination: It terminates about 5cm above the posterior root of zygomatic process by dividing into anterior and posterior branches.

Relations:

a) Covered by auricularis anterior when it crosses zygoma

b) In the substance of parotid gland crossed by temporal and zygomatic branches of facial nerve.

Accompanied in the scalp by two structures—superficial temporal vein and auriculotemporal nerve which lies behind it.

Branches

1. Transverse facial artery: It arises within the substance of parotid gland runs forwards below zygomatic arch. It supplies parotid gland and its duct, temporomandibular joint and adjoining structures.
2. Anterior auricular branch: Supplies lateral surface of auricle and external acoustic meatus.
3. Zygomatico orbital artery: It runs between two layers of temporal fascia and extends up to lateral angle of orbit.
4. Middle temporal artery: After origin it pierces temporal fascia and supplies temporalis muscle.
5. Anterior or frontal branch: It supplies muscle and skin of frontal region and anastomoses with branches of ophthalmic artery.
6. Posterior or parietal: It supplies skin of auricle.

APPLIED ANATOMY

1. Its pulsation is readily felt at the preauricular point as it lies here deep to skin and superficial fascia. So it serves useful purpose to all physicians, specially surgeons or anaesthetists, when radial pulse is not available.
2. During injury to scalp and bleeding is continuing this preauricular point can be compressed against the bone to stop bleeding from scalp and temporal region.

Ascending pharyngeal artery

It is the first branch of the external carotid artery. It (slender artery) ascend upward vertically (side of pharynx) towards base of skull.

Branches

a) Pharyngeal branches supplies pharyngeal wall.

b) Inferior tympanic branch supplies tympanic cavity.

c) Meningeal branch supplies dura mater after entering the cranial cavity after entering through jugular foramen.

Maxillary artery – Refer Chapter 12

INTERNAL JUGULAR VEIN

It is the most important deep vein of the neck which collects blood from the brain, superficial parts of the face and neck.

Number: Two – one on each side of neck.

Beginning: It begins as a direct continuation of sigmoid sinus at the base of the skull in the posterior compartment of jugular foramen. At the beginning it presents **superior bulb** which is a dilatation and lodged in the jugular fossa of temporal bone and is closely related to floor of tympanic cavity. (Fig. 7.22)

Course: It runs vertically downwards through the neck and lies within carotid sheath and extends up to sternal end of clavicle where it ends.

End: It ends behind the sternal end of the clavicle by uniting with the subclavian vein and forming brachiocephalic vein (innominate) of the corresponding side.

It presents **inferior bulb** (dilatation) at its termination and is provided with pair of valves.

Relations: (Fig. 7.23)

1. **In front**

a) Sternocleidomastoid muscle: more or less overlap and cover.

b) Crossed by superior belly of omohyoid and posterior belly of digastric. (Fig. 7.23)

c) In the lower part: sternohyoid, sternothyroid and anterior jugular veins.

d) In between digastric and omohyoid: crossed by occipital and sternocleidomastoid branches of superior thyroid artery and occipital artery deep cervical group of lymph nodes, inferior root of ansa cervicalis (descendens cervicalis).

e) In the upper part: Posterior auricular artery, accessory nerve (may be behind), parotid gland and styloid process with muscles attached to it.

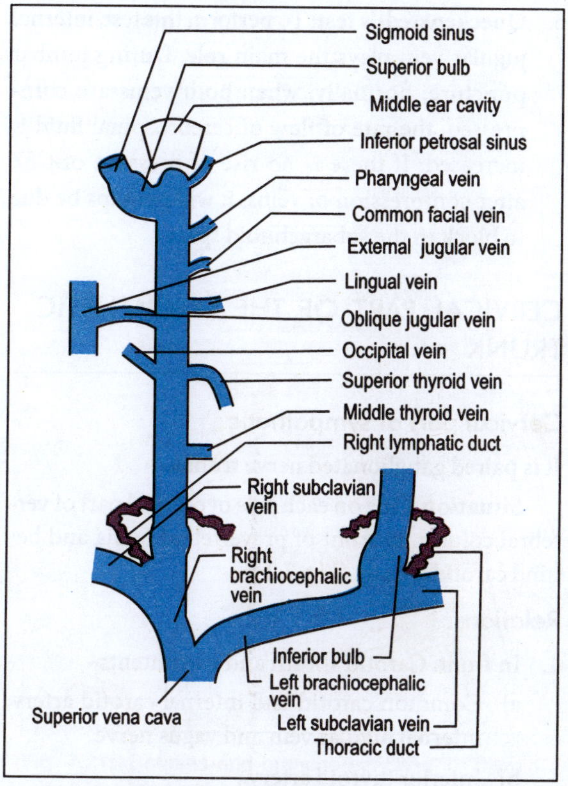

Fig. 7.22: Tributaries and termination of internal jugular vein

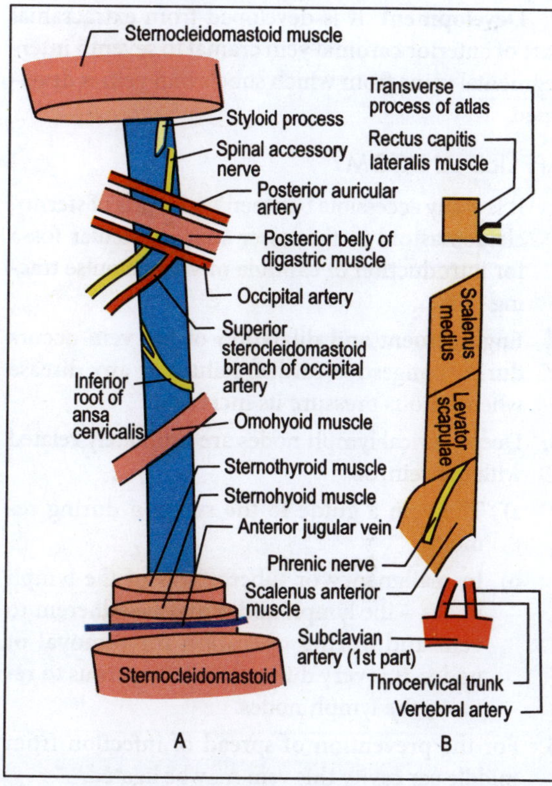

Fig. 7.23: Relations of internal jugular vein. A – Anterior relations; B – Posterior relations

2. **Behind**
   a) Transverse process of the atlas.
   b) Levator scapulae and scalenus medius.
   c) Cervical plexus of nerves.
   d) Scalenus anterior with phrenic nerve.
   e) Thyrocervical trunk, inferior thyroid artery, first part of subclavian artery.
   f) Thoracic duct on left side and right lymphatic duct on right side.
   g) Rectus capitis lateralis.
   h) First part of subclavian artery.
3. **Medially**
   a) Internal carotid artery in the upper part and common carotid artery in the lower part.
   b) Vagus nerve lies in between artery and vein in a posterior plane.
   c) In the uppermost part at the base of skull-internal carotid artery in front, internal jugular vein behind and 9th, 10th, 11th and 12th cranial nerves lie between them tributaries.

Tributaries (Fig. 7.22)

1. Inferior petrosal sinus (first tributary, sometimes cochlear vein may open into it and may be first tributary)
2. Pharyngeal veins
3. Common facial vein
4. Lingual vein
5. Superior thyroid vein
6. Middle thyroid vein (often 4th thyroid or Kocher's vein)
7. Occipital vein (sometimes)
8. **Thoracic duct** (on left side) and right lymphatic duct (on right side) opens at the junction of internal jugular and subclavian vein.

Communications

a) With external jugular by oblique jugular vein
b) With cavernous sinus by inferior petrosal sinus.

Development: It is developed from extracranial part of anterior cardinal vein cranial to seventh intersegmental veins from which subclavian vein is developed.

APPLIED ANATOMY

1. It is easily accessible between two heads of sternocleidomastoid in the lesser supraclavicular fossa for introduction of cannula of venous pulse tracing.
2. Engorgement and dilatation of the vein occurs during congestive cardiac failure or any disease when venous pressure its increased.
3. Deep cervical lymph nodes are intimately related with the vein. So
   a) The vein a guide to the surgeon during removal.
   b) In malignancy or tuberculosis of the lymph nodes – the lymph nodes may be adherent to vein and during operation for removal of nodes, it is very difficult and dangerous to remove the lymph nodes.
5. For the prevention of spread of infection from middle ear cavity this vein may be ligated.
6. **Queckenstedt's test**: To perform this test, internal jugular vein plays the main role. During lumbar puncture, normally, when both veins are compressed, the rate of flow of cerebrospinal fluid is increased. If there is no rise of pressure of CSF after compression of veins, it will perhaps be due to block in the subarachnoid space.

CERVICAL PART OF THE SYMPATHETIC TRUNK

Cervical part of sympathetic

It is paired ganglionated nerve trunks.

Situation: One on each side of cervical part of vertebral column in front of prevertebral fascia and behind carotid sheath. (Fig. 7.24)

Relations:

1. In front: Carotid sheath and its contents–
   a) Common carotid and internal carotid artery, internal jugular vein and vagus nerve.
   b) Inferior thyroid artery.

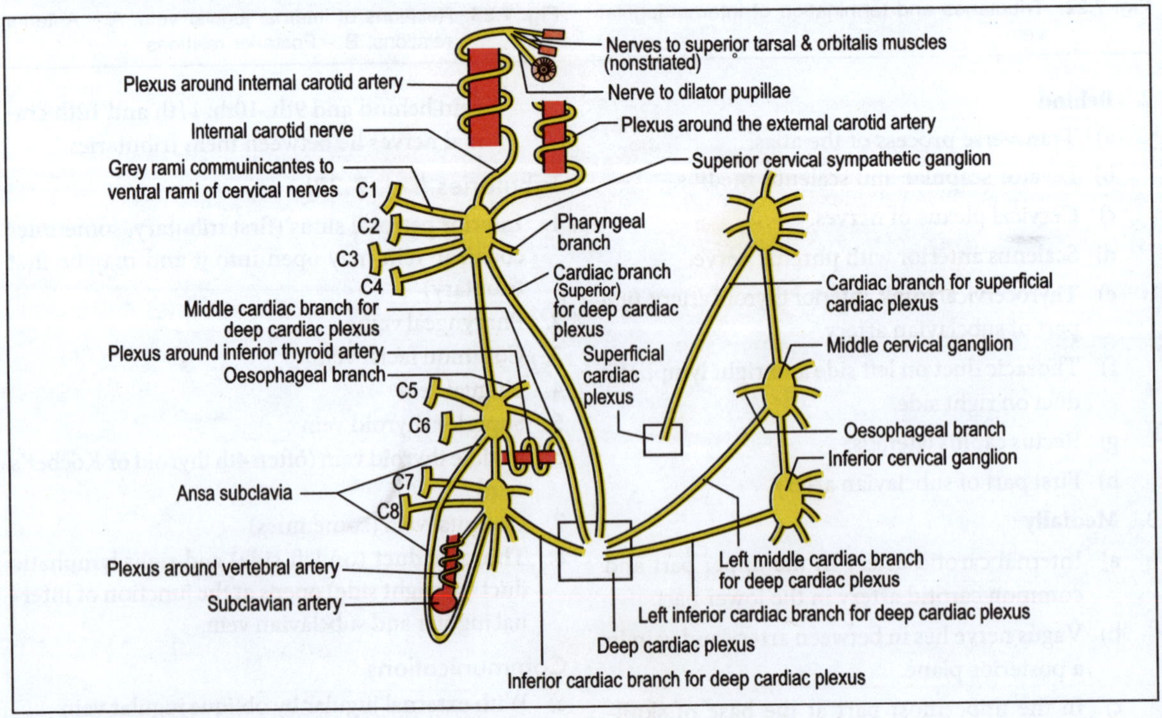

Fig. 7.24: Cervical sympathetic trunk with its branches

2. Behind: Prevertebral fascia covering longus capitis and cervicis muscles. Transverse processes of lower six cervical vertebrae.

Characteristics of formations

1. No white rami communicates but grey rami communicates are present and sent to all cervical spinal nerves.
2. The cervical part of the trunk is formed by first (T_1) to fourth (T_4) segments of spinal cord i.e., thoracic spinal nerves which pass upwards to the neck.

Ganglia: Three ganglia are present. They are superior, middle and inferior. [Though there are eight spinal nerves – the presence of 3 ganglia is due to fusions of the ganglia].

SUPERIOR CERVICAL GANGLIA

It is the largest of the three ganglia of the cervical part of the sympathetic trunks and corresponds to upper four cervical nerves.

Shape: Spindle shaped.

Size: 2.5cm long.

Formation: By fusion of upper four cervical ganglion.

Situation: Just below skull, in front of transverse processes of C_2 and C_3 vertebrae.

Relations:

In front: Carotid sheath and internal carotid artery.

Behind: Prevertebral fascia covering longus capitis.

Connections:

With IX, X, XI and XIIth cranial nerves.

Branches:

A. All the branches carry post ganglionic fibres and some sensory fibres.

B. Preganglionic fibres come from upper 3 or 4 thoracic spinal nerves.

I. a) Upper four cervical nerves by grey rami communicates.

II. a) Laryngopharyngeal: These branches supply carotid body and form pharyngeal plexus with 9th and 10th nerve.

b) Cardiac branches: Right cardiac nerve takes part in deep and left cardiac nerve in superficial cardiac plexus.

III. They form plexuses around common carotid artery, external carotid artery and its branches.

The plexuses of facial artery give sympathetic root to submandibular ganglion and otic ganglion.

IV. It forms internal carotid nerve forming plexus around internal carotid artery and supply dilator pupillae. Some fibers form deep petrosal nerve which passes through pterygopalatine ganglion. Some fibers pass to the ciliary ganglion. It also supply extraocular nonstriated muscles.

MIDDLE CERVICAL GANGLION

It is the smallest of three cervical sympathetic ganglia and formed by the fusion of two ganglia (5th + 6th cervical).

Size and shape: About pin's head.

Situation: Situated in the lower part of the neck and in front of transverse 6th cervical vertebra, behind carotid sheath and above inferior thyroid artery.

Connection with inferior cervical ganglion: Connected by two filaments – anterior and posterior. They pass in front and behind subclavian artery.

The anterior one loops below the subclavian artery and forms ansa subclavia.

Branches: Two groups:

1. Lateral: To 5th and 6th cervical spinal nerves by grey rami communicates.
2. Medial
   a) Branches to thyroid gland through inferior thyroid artery.
   b) Tracheal and oesophageal branches.
   c) Cardiac branch to deep cardiac plexus.

INFERIOR CERVICAL GANGLION

It is intermediate in size and lowermost cervical ganglion and formed by the fusion of C_7 and C_8 ganglia.

It may sometimes be fused with first thoracic ganglion and then known as **stellate** (because of star shaped) or **cervicothoracic ganglion**.

Situation: Situated between the transverse processes of seventh cervical and neck of first rib.

Size and shape: Irregular in shape, about the size of small pea-like and larger than the middle ganglion.

Branches:

1. To C_7 and C_8 cervical spinal nerves by grey rami communicates.
2. Cardiac branch to deep cardiac plexus.
3. Vertebral branch forming plexus around vertebral artery.
4. Subclavian branch forming plexus around subclavian artery.

APPLIED ANATOMY

Injury to cervical sympathetic involving upper 2 and 3 thoracic segments which supply head and neck after relaying in superior cervical ganglion. Thus, will cause **'Horner's syndrome'**:

Manifestations are:

a) Ptosis (drooping of upper eyelid)

b) Constriction of pupil (due to paralysis of dilator pupillae)

c) Enophthalmos (retraction of eyeball)

d) Anhydrosis absence of the sweating on the half of the face and head.

CERVICAL PLEXUS

It is nerve plexus situated on the surface of levator scapulae and scalenus medius beneath the prevertebral layer of deep cervical fascia and undercover of sternocleidomastoid.

Relations: In front:

1. Sternocleidomastoid
2. Carotid sheath
3. Prevertebral fascial

Formation: It is formed by ventral primary rami of upper four cervical nerves.

So the first to fourth cervical nerves form roots.

Each divide into upper and lower branches except the first. They are connected with each others as C_1, with C_2, and so on. Thus, they form three loops.

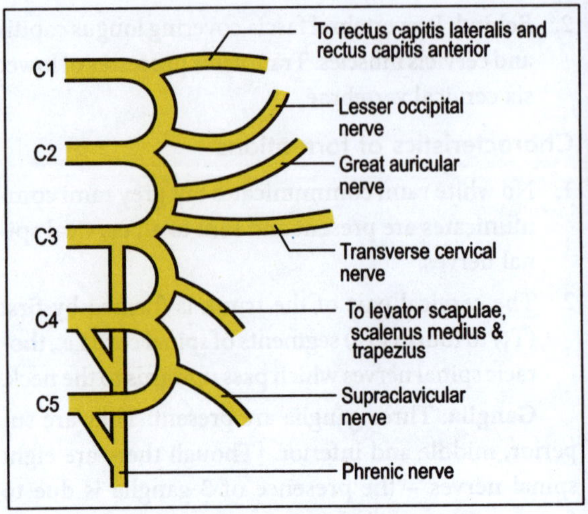

Fig. 7.25: Cervical plexus with its branches

Branches:

I. **Superficial**: Four cutaneous branches:

A. Three ascending branches

1. **Lesser occipital**: Root values/C_2
2. Great auricular $C_{2,3}$
3. Transverse cutaneous nerve of neck $C_{2,3}$

B. **One descending branch**: Supraclavicular nerve $C_{3,4}$

II. **Deep branches**: (Fig. 7.25)

A. Communicating

1. Grey rami from superior cervical sympathetic ganglion to each of four roots (C_1 – C_4 nerves).
2. A branch from C_1 to hypoglossal nerve.
3. A branch from C_2, C_3 to sternocleidomastoid and branches from C_3-C_4 to trapezius (communicate with spinal accessory nerve).

B. **Muscular branches**: Two groups

Medial:

1. Rectus capitis anterior $C_{1,2}$
2. Rectus capitis lateralis C_1, C_2
3. Longus capitis $C_1 - C_3$
4. Longus colli $C_3 - C_8$
5. Descendens cervicalis or strap muscles ($C_1 - C_3$)
6. Phrenic nerve $C_{3,4,5}$

Lateral:

1. To sternocleidomastoid $C_{2,3}$
2. Trapezius $C_{3,4}$
3. Levator scapulae $C_{3,4,5}$
4. Scalenus medius $C_{3,4}$

LYMPHATIC DRAINAGE OF HEAD & NECK

Lymph nodes of head and neck region are classified mainly into two groups:

I. Terminal
II. Outlying.

I. **Terminal groups**: Deep cervical lymph nodes.

II. **Outlying groups or peripheral lymph nodes**: The outlying groups are again arranged into two circles:

a) Outer circle,
b) Inner circle,

Drainage of lymph

1. All the lymph of head and neck ultimately drain into deep cervical nodes either directly or indirectly by being filtered through outlaying nodes.
2. All the lymph is finally collected in the lower part of deep cervical nodes.
3. The collected lymph from the lower part of deep cervical nodes (efferents from these nodes) form jugular trunks.
4. Left jugular trunk ends in thoracic duct or may end in junction of left internal jugular and left subclavian vein. Right jugular trunk ends in the junction of internal jugular and subclavian vein of the right side or may ends in right lymphatic duct.

I. TERMINAL: Deep cervical group of lymph nodes

These are the ultimate draining centre of the all the lymph from head and neck region.

Arrangement and situations: They are arranged and situated as a vertical chain deep to sternocleidomastoid muscle along internal jugular vein.

Different groups: They are subdivided into **two groups** by division of common carotid artery or intermediate tendon of omohyoid muscle.

They are:

1. **Jugulo-digastric or superior group**
   a) They mostly lie near the internal jugular vein.
   b) **Jugulo-digastric group** – main group of nodes of the superior group and situated in the triangular area bounded by posterior belly of digastric, facial vein and internal jugular vein. (Fig. 7.26)
   c) Jugulo-digastric group consists one large and few small lymph nodes.
   d) Afferents: (Jugulo-digastric) from posterior third of tongue, palatine tonsil.

   Efferents: (from superior deep cervical as a whole) – drain into inferior group of deep cervical or directly into jugular trunks.

2. Inferior group or **Jugulo-omohyoid** is the main group.
   a) This group mainly lies deep to sternocleidomastoid and extend to subclavian triangle and also is related to subclavian vessels and brachial plexus. Jugulo-omohyoid consisting of one node lies either on or above intermediate tendon of omohyoid.

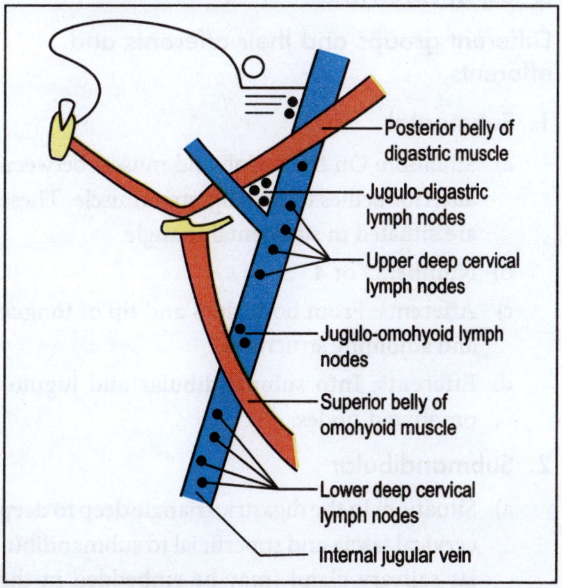

Fig. 7.26: Deep cervical lymph nodes

b) Afferents: Directly from tongue and indirectly through superficial nodes like submental, submandibular and upper deep cervical group.

c) **Virchow's glands**: Some lymph nodes of this group extend in front of scalenus anterior and on the left side is known as Virchow's gland. The importance of this node is that it is enlarged during malignant condition of stomach. The testicular and oesophageal carcinoma usually effect these lymph nodes.

II. Outlying or superficial lymph nodes

(a) OUTER CIRCLE:

The lymph nodes of this circle are arranged in a circular manner and extend from chin in front to occipital region behind.

Constituent group: The circle consist of (Fig. 7.28)

1. Submental
2. Submandibular
3. Buccal
4. Preauricular or parotid
5. Postauricular or mastoid
6. Occipital lymph
7. Anterior cervical lymph nodes
8. Superficial cervical

Different groups and their afferents and efferents

1. Submental

a) Situation: On the mylohyoid muscle between anterior bellies of two digastric muscle. These are situated in submental triangle.

b) Number: 3 or 4

c) Afferents: From both sides and tip of tongue and adjoining structures.

d) Efferents: Into submandibular and jugulo-omohyoid nodes.

2. Submandibular

a) Situation: In the digastric triangle deep to deep cervical fascia and superficial to submandibular salivary gland (may be embedded in the substance) of the gland.

b) Number: 3 in number

[When this lymph node is infected and form an abscess – the marginal mandibular branch of facial nerve may be cut when incision is given to drain the abscess or for removal of the node].

c) Afferents

1. Centre of forehead
2. Cheek and angle of mouth
3. Upper lip
4. Lateral part of lower lip
5. Frontal, maxillary and ethmoidal sinuses
6. Submental lymph nodes.

d) Efferents: Partly into Jugulo-digastric and mainly into Jugulo-omohyoid nodes.

3. Buccal: Actually belonging to submandibular group.

a) Situation: On the buccinator in relation to facial view.

b) Afferents: From lower eyelid and part of cheek.

c) Efferents: Into upper deep cervical group.

4. Preauricular or parotid lymph nodes (Fig. 7.27)

a) Situation: Situated partly in superficial fascia or partly in deep fascia and one or two in the substance of parotid gland. The nodes lying front of tragus are the preauricular.

b) Number: About 5 or 6.

c) Afferents:

1. Upper part of forehead and temporal region.
2. Lateral aspect of scalp
3. Anterior wall of external acoustic meatus
4. Parotid gland
5. Nasopharynx, posterior part of nose and tympanic cavity (deep node).

d) Efferents: Into upper deep cervical group.

5. Post auricular or mastoid node

a) Situation: Situated superficial to sternocleidomastoid and mastoid process and deep to au-

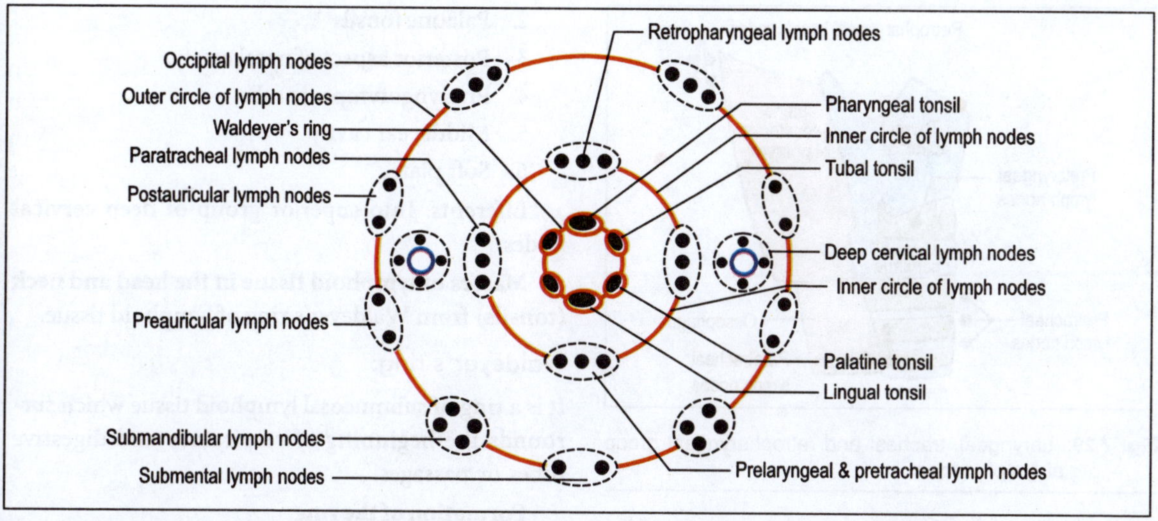

Fig. 7.27: Diagram showing superficial and deep groups of lymph nodes and Waldeyer's ring

ricularis posterior.

b) Afferents: From
   1. Upper part of inner surface of auricle
   2. Posterior wall of external acoustic meatus.

c) Efferents: Into upper deep cervical lymph nodes.

6. Occipital nodes (Fig. 7.28)

a) Situation: At the apex of posterior triangle superficial to trapezius and in close relation with occipital artery.

b) Efferents: To supraclavicular nodes.

7. Anterior cervical nodes

They are detached lymph nodes of outer circle.

a) Situation: Lie along anterior jugular vein and superficially. Suprasternal node belongs to this group, and lies in the suprasternal space. They are the extension of submental lymph group.

b) Afferents: From skin or anterior part of neck and anterior triangular region.

c) Efferents: Into lower deep cervical group of lymph nodes.

8. Superficial cervical nodes:

They are detached part of outer circle and part of parotid lymph nodes.

a) Situation: Lie superficial to sternocleidomastoid and on the side of external jugular vein.

b) Afferent: From
   1. Lobule of auricle
   2. Floor of external acoustic meatus
   3. Angle of jaw
   4. Lower part of parotid gland.

c) Efferents: To upper and mainly into lower deep cervical group of lymph nodes.

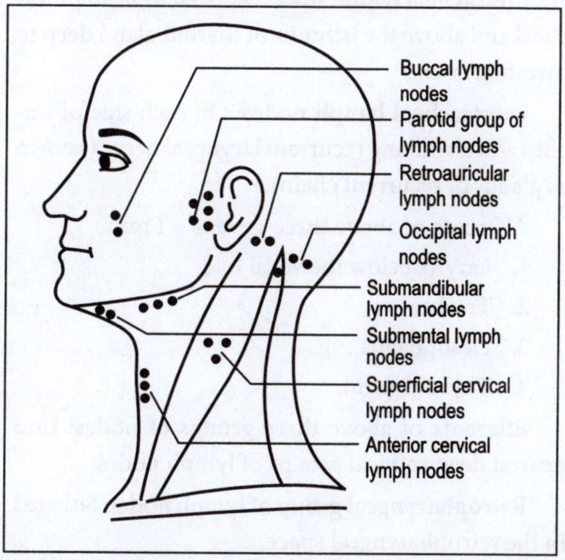

Fig. 7.28: Superficial group of lymph nodes of head and neck

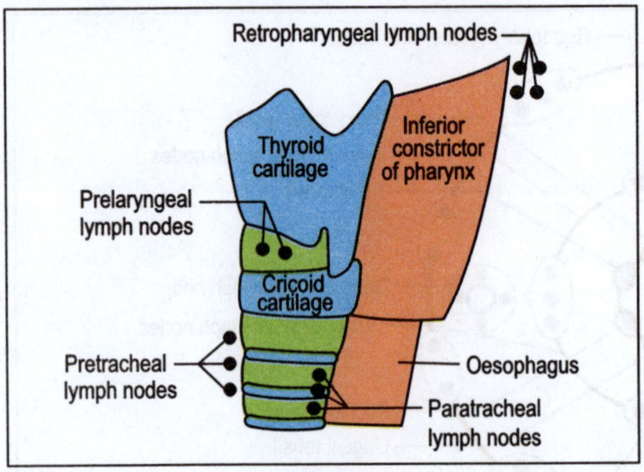

Fig. 7.29: Laryngeal, tracheal and retropharyngeal group of lymph nodes

(b) INNER CIRCLE OF OUTLYING LYMPH NODES

The inner circle consists of lymph nodes which are arranged in circular manner around the supper part of respiratory and alimentary tracts.

It consists of

1. Pretracheal and prelaryngeal group.
2. Paratracheal group.
3. Retropharyngeal group.

Prelaryngeal lymph node: Situated in front of conus elasticus deep to investing fascia. (Fig. 7.29)

Pretracheal lymph node: Situated in front of tracheal and above the isthmus of thyroid gland deep to investing fascia.

Paratracheal lymph nodes: On each side of trachea and also along recurrent laryngeal nerve (known as glands of recurrent chain).

Afferents of above three groups – From

1. Larynx below the vocal fold.
2. Trachea
3. Oesophagus
4. Thyroid gland.

Efferents of above three groups of nodes: Into nearest deep cervical groups of lymph nodes.

Retropharyngeal group of lymph nodes: Situated in the retropharyngeal space.

Afferents – From

1. Pharynx
2. Palatine tonsils
3. Posterior aspect of nasal cavity.
4. Pharyngotympanic tube
5. Middle ear cavity
6. Soft plate.

Efferents: Into superior group of deep cervical nodes.

Masses of lymphoid tissue in the head and neck (tonsils) from Waldeyer's ring of lymphoid tissue.

Waldeyer's ring:

It is a ring of submucosal lymphoid tissue which surrounds the beginning of respiratory and digestive tubes or passages.

Formation of the ring:

In front and below: Lingual tonsils (encapsulated masses of lymphoid tissues in the submucosa of posterior one third of tongue).

On each side: Palatine tonsils

Behind and on each side: Tubal tonsils.

Above and behind: Nasopharyngeal tonsil.

Function:

a) Filters tissue fluid coming from inner circle of lymph nodes.

b) It prevents entry of infecting organisms from outside and acts as police guards at the entrance of important tracts of the body.

LATERAL VERTEBRAL MUSCLES

Three muscles scalenus anterior, medius and posterior are situated on the lateral side of neck and extend in a ladder like manner from upper two ribs to transverse processes of cervical vertebrae.

Scalenus anterior (Fig. 7.30)

Situated deeply at the side of neck behind sternocleidomastoid. The scalenus anterior is an important muscle at the root of the neck which divides the subclavian artery into three parts.

Origin: From anterior tubercles of transverse processes of third, fourth, fifth and sixth cervical vertebrae. (Fig. 7.30)

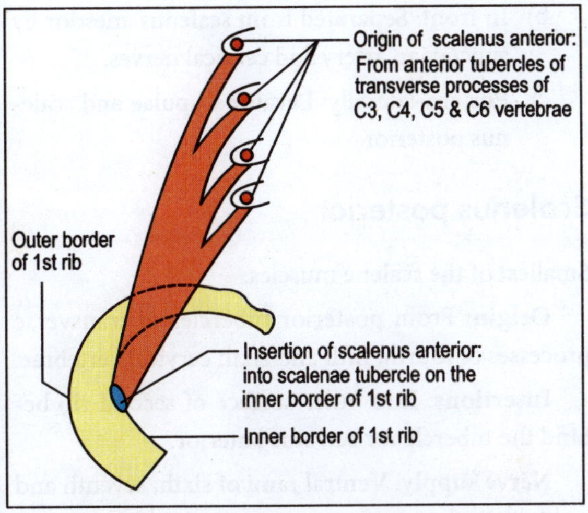

Fig. 7.30: Origin and insertion of scalenus anterior

Insertion: The muscle fibers descends vertically and form a flat narrow tendon. The tendon is inserted into scalene tubercle on the inner border of first rib and also into ridge on the upper surface.

Nerve supply: Ventral rami of fourth, fifth and sixth cervical nerve.

Actions:

A. Acting from below: Bending of vertebral column forwards or lateral if acting unilaterally and may rotate to the apposite side.

B. It acting from above: Elevation of first rib and acts as accessory muscle of respiration.

Relations:

Anterior:

1. Clavicle, subclavius, carotid sheath
2. **Two muscles**
   a) Sternocleidomastoid
   b) Inferior belly of omohyoid
3. **Three arteries** (Fig. 7.31)
   a) Transverse cervical
   b) Suprascapular
   c) Common carotid
4. **Three veins**
   a) Anterior jugular
   b) Subclavian
   c) Internal jugular
5. **Two nerves**
   a) Phrenic
   b) Vagus

Posterior: Suprapleural membrane; cervical pleura; roots of brachial plexus; subclavian artery, scalenus medius.

Medial border forms lateral boundary of scaleno-vertebral triangle which contain vertebral artery, inferior thyroid artery, sympathetic trunk.

Lateral border is related to trunks of brachial plexus.

The upper part of scalenus anterior is related to ascending cervical artery and longus capitis.

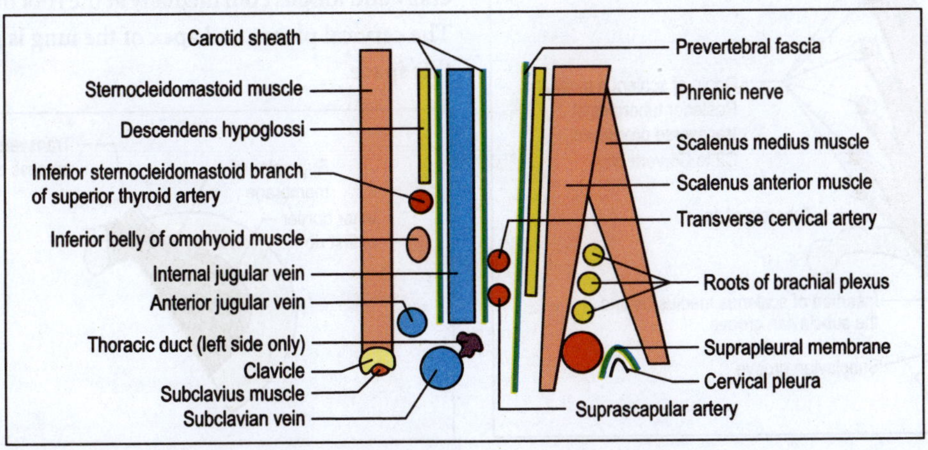

Fig. 7.31: Relations of scalenus anterior muscle

APPLIED ANATOMY

Hypertrophy of scalene anterior muscles compress lower trunk of brachial plexus affecting hypothenar muscles and progressive wasting of intrinsic muscles of hand and absence of radial pulse (due to compression of subclavian artery).

Scalenus medius

Largest and strongest of scalene muscles.

Origin: From posterior tubercles of transverse processes of third to seventh cervical vertebrae and transverse process of axis. (Fig. 7.32)

Insertion: Into upper surface of the first rib behind the groove for subclavian artery.

Nerve supply: Ventral rami of third to eight cervical nerves.

Action:

1. Lateral flexion of cervical part of vertebral column.
2. Elevation of first rib acting as accessory muscle of respiration.
3. Stabilisation of neck.

Relation:

a) Antero-laterally: Sternomastoid, clavicle, omohyoid.

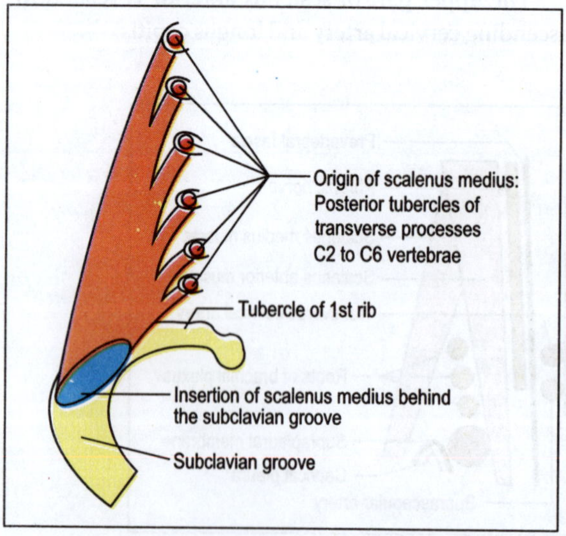

Fig. 7.32: Origin and insertion of scalenus medius

b) In front: Separated from scalenus anterior by subclavian artery and cervical nerves.

c) Postero-laterally: Levator scapulae and scalenus posterior.

Scalenus posterior

Smallest of the scalene muscles.

Origin: From posterior tubercles of transverse processes of fourth, fifth and sixth cervical vertebrae.

Insertions: Into outer surface of second rib behind the tubercle for serratus anterior.

Nerve supply: Ventral rami of sixth, seventh and eight cervical nerves.

Action:

a) Lateral flexion of cervical part of vertebral column

b) Elevation of second rib

c) Stables the neck

Scalenus minimus or Sibson's fascia

Scalenus minimus is related to cervical pleura. Suprapleural membrane is degenerated part of scalenus minimus muscle. (Fig. 7.33)

Scaleno-vertebral triangle

It is a triangular space between scalenus anterior laterally and longus colli medially at the root of the neck. The cervical pleura and apex of the lung is present in this space.

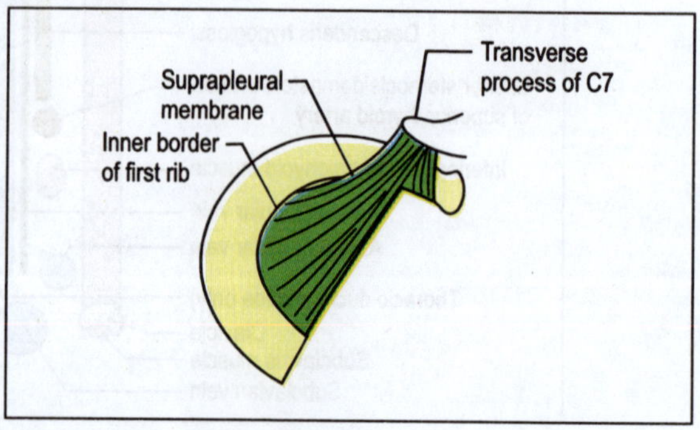

Fig. 7.33: Suprapleural membrane

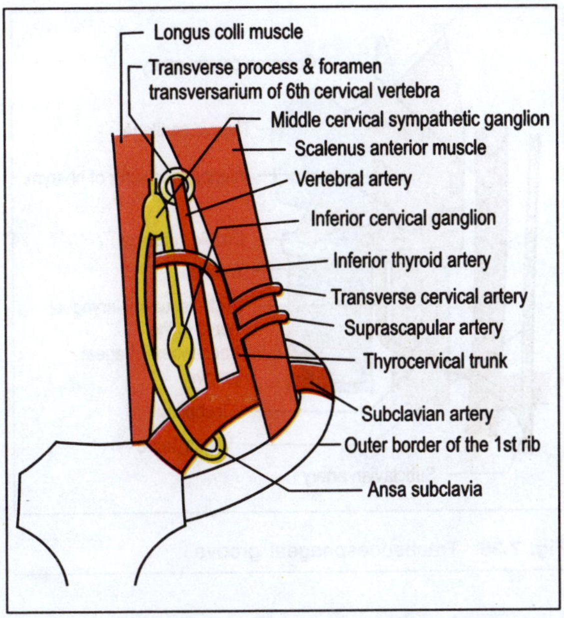

Fig. 7.34: Scaleno-vertebral triangle and its contents

Boundaries:

Medially: Longus colli muscle

Laterally: Medial border of scalenus anterior (Fig. 7.34).

Apex: Transverse process of the C_6 vertebra.

Base: First part of subclavian artery.

Posterior wall or floor (above downward)

a) Transverse process of C_7 vertebra
b) Ventral ramus of C_8 nerve
c) Neck of first rib
d) Cervical pleura.

Contents

1. **First part of the vertebral artery**: Vertebral artery with vein extend vertically upwards to enter the foramen transversarium of C_6 from the base of triangle to the apex.
2. **Cervical part of sympathetic trunk: Middle cervical ganglion** lies above the loop of inferior thyroid artery. **Inferior cervical ganglion** lies behind the vertebral artery.

   Ansa subclavia is a connection between middle and inferior cervical ganglion which loops in front, below and behind the first part of subclavian artery.
3. **Thyrocervical trunk** lies in the medial part of triangle.

TRACHEA

Trachea is the continuation of larynx at the lower border C_6 vertebra (lower border of cricoid cartilage). The trachea descends vertically downwards and divide into right and left principal bronchii.

Dimension: Length – 10-11cm

External diameter – 2cm male; 1.5cm female.

Parts: Two parts – (a) Cervical – 7cm long; (b) Thoracic – 3-4cm.

Structure:

- Consist of 16-20 'C' shaped ring of cartilage.
- Posteriorly gap is filled by involuntary muscles trachealis.
- Absence of cartilage in the posterior aspect allows the expansion of oesophagus dump deglutition.

Relations:

Cervical part

Anteriorly

- Skin, superficial fascia containing anterior jugular veins, jugular, venous arch (suprasternal space).
- Investing layer of deep cervical fascia. (Fig. 7.35)
- Sternothyroid & sternohyoid muscles.
- Isthmus of thyroid gland in front of 2nd, 3rd & 4th trachea ring.
- Inferior thyroid veins, arteria thyroidea ima, and remains of thymus
- Left brachiocephalic veins.

From superficial to deep.

Posteriorly: Oesophagus, recurrent laryngeal nerve.

On each side – lobe of thyroid gland

- Carotid sheath with its contents.

Thoracic part: Refer thorax.

Blood supply:

Arterial supply: Inferior thyroid arteries.

Venous drainage: Drain to left brachiocephalic vein.

Lymphatic drainage: Drain into pre & paratracheal lymph nodes.

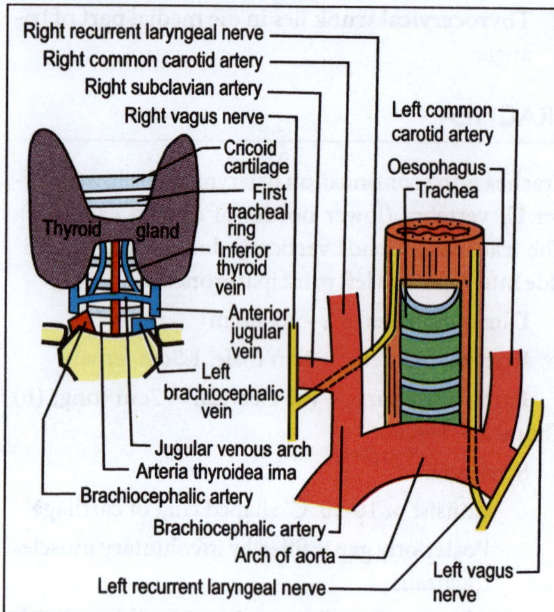

Fig. 7.35: Relations of trachea and oesophagus

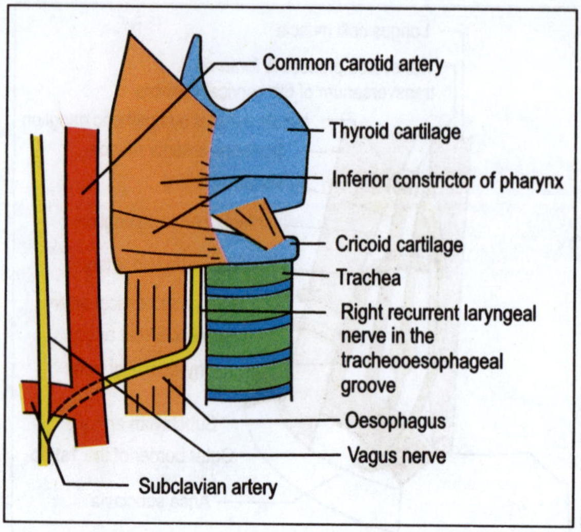

Fig. 7.36: Tracheooesphageal groove

Nerve supply:

Parasympathetic: Through recurrent laryngeal nerve branch of vagus nerve.

Sympathetic: Derived from middle cervical ganglion.

OESOPHAGUS

Oesophagus is the continuation of laryngopharynx at the lower border of C_6 vertebra (lower border of cricoid cartilage). Pharyngo-oesophageal junction is the narrowest part of the digestive tube.

Parts: Three part – Cervical, thoracic & abdominal.

Relations of cervical part (from lower end of C_6 vertebra to superior border of manubrium sterni)

Anteriorly: Trachea, recurrent laryngeal nerve.

Posteriorly: Prevertebral muscles, vertebrae.

On each side: Lobe of thyroid gland, Carotid sheath.

Blood supply: *Arterial supply* – Inferior thyroid artery.

Venous drainage – Drain into inferior thyroid vein & left brachiocephalic vein.

Lymphatic drainage: Drain in pretracheal & deep cervical lymph nodes (Fig. 7.36).

PHRENIC NERVE

This is a mixed nerve.

Origin: It arises from third, fourth & fifth cervical nerves (arises chiefly from fourth cervical nerve).

Course & relations:

1. It is formed at the level of the upper border of the thyroid cartilage (at the lateral border of scalenus anterior).
2. The nerve crosses the scalenus anterior from its lateral border to its medial border.
3. The nerve lies anterior to the prevertebral fascia, inferior belly of omohyoid, transverse cervical artery, suprascapular artery.
4. After leaving the anterior surface of scalenus anterior, the nerve descends behind the first costal cartilage & brachiocephalic vein.
5. On the left side the nerve leaves the anterior surface of the scalenus anterior at a higher level.
6. The nerve descends in front of the first part of subclavian artery.
7. It supplies the muscles of the diaphragm; it also carry sensory fibers from the diaphragm. (Fig. 7.37)

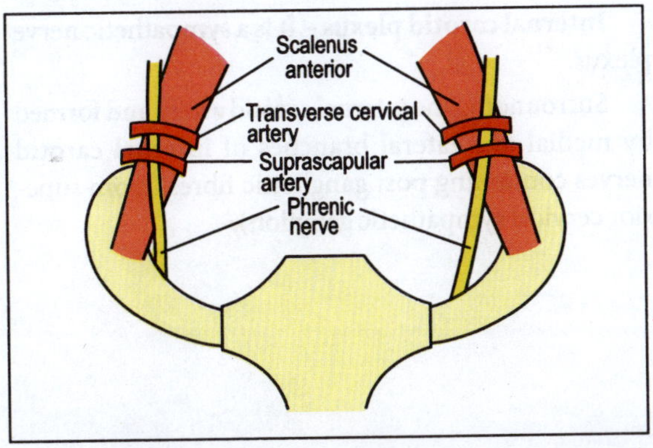

Fig. 7.37: Phrenic nerves of both sides (Note: The left phrenic nerve leaves the anterior surface of scalenus anterior at higher level)

SPECIAL CHARACTERISTICS OF FLOW OF BLOOD IN INTERNAL JUGULAR VEIN

1. It should be noted that blood from superficial cerebral veins pass through superior sagittal sinus, right transverse sinus, right sigmoid sinus and finally right internal jugular vein, successively.
2. Blood from deep cerebral veins pass successively through great cerebral vein, straight sinus, left transverse sinus, left sigmoid sinus and ultimately into left internal jugular vein.

STYLOID APPARATUS (Fig. 7.38)

The following structures (styloid apparatus) are:

1. **Muscles**:
   a) **Styloglossus**
   Origin: From the tip of styloid process.
   Insertion: Side of tongue (posteriorly).
   Action: Draws the tongue posterosuperiorly.
   Nerve supply: Hypoglossal nerve.
   b) **Stylohyoid**
   Origin: From the mid part of styloid process (posteriorly).
   Insertion: Hyoid bone (body).
   Action: Draws hyoid bone upwards.
   Nerve supply: Facial nerve.
   c) **Stylopharyngeus**
   Origin: From the base of the styloid process.
   Insertion: Posterior border of the lamina of thyroid cartilage.
   Action: Draws the larynx upwards during deglutition.
   Nerve supply: Glossopharyngeal nerve.
2. **Ligaments**:
   a) **Stylohyoid ligament**: It lies between lesser cornu of hyoid to the tip of the styloid process.
   b) **Stylomandibular ligament**: It lies between angle of the mandible and posterior part of the styloid process. This ligament is part of investing layer of deep cervical fascia.

FEATURES OF CERVICAL SYMPATHETIC

1. It consists of internal carotid nerves on each side.
2. It arises from upper part of superior cervical ganglion of sympathetic trunk.

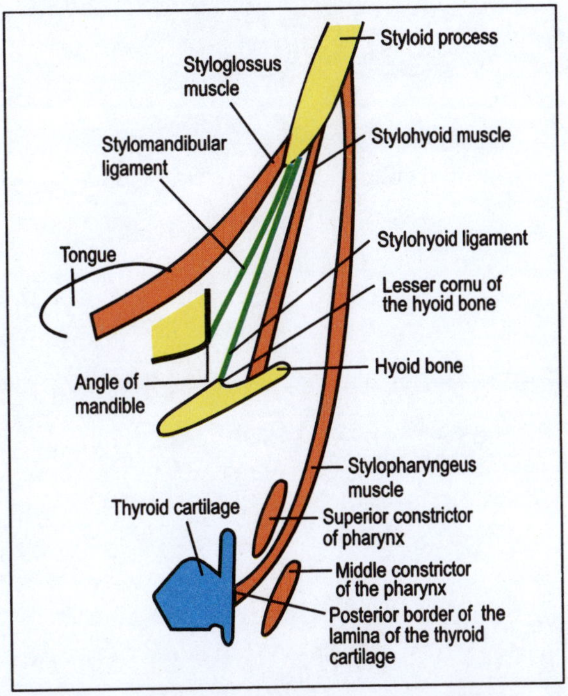

Fig. 7.38: Structures attached to styloid process

3. It contains postganglionic fibres.
4. It enters the cranial cavity through carotid canal and terminates.
5. It terminates by dividing into medial and lateral branches which form internal carotid plexus.

Internal carotid plexus – It is a sympathetic nerve plexus.

Surrounding the internal carotid artery and formed by medial and lateral branches of internal carotid nerves containing post ganglionic fibres (from superior cervical sympathetic ganglion).

chapter 8

THE PREVERTEBRAL REGION

AT A GLANCE

- *Longus colli*
- *Longus capitis*
- *Rectus capitis lateralis*
- *Rectus capitis anterior*
- *Vertebral artery*
- *Craniovertebral joint*
- *Atlanto-axial joint*
- *Lateral atlanto-axial joint*
- *Ligament connecting the axis with occipital bone*

THE PREVERTEBRAL MUSCLES

The prevertebral muscles are longus colli, longus capitis & rectus capitis anterior. The muscles are covered by prevertebral fascia. The muscles are supplied by ventral rami of cervical plexus. The muscles flex the neck, and the head on neck.

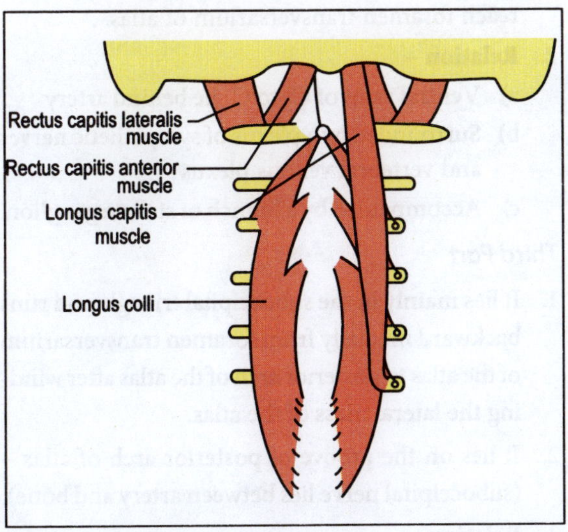

Fig. 8.1: Prevertebral muscles

LONGUS COLLI

It extend from body of T_3 vertebra to the anterior tubercle of atlas. It is attached to the transverse processes of third to sixth cervical vertebra.

Nerve supply: C_2-C_6 (Ventral rami).

Action: Flexes the cervical vertebrae.

LONGUS CAPITIS

It is attached to anterior tubercles of the third to sixth cervical transverse processes and to the base of the skull on either side of pharyngeal tubercle.

Nerve supply: Ventral rami of C_2-C_6

Action: Flexes the head.

RECTUS CAPITIS ANTERIOR

It is attached to anterior surface of the lateral mass of the atlas to the base of skull (anterior of occipital condyle).

Nerve supply: Ventral rami of $C_{1,2}$

Action: Flexes the head.

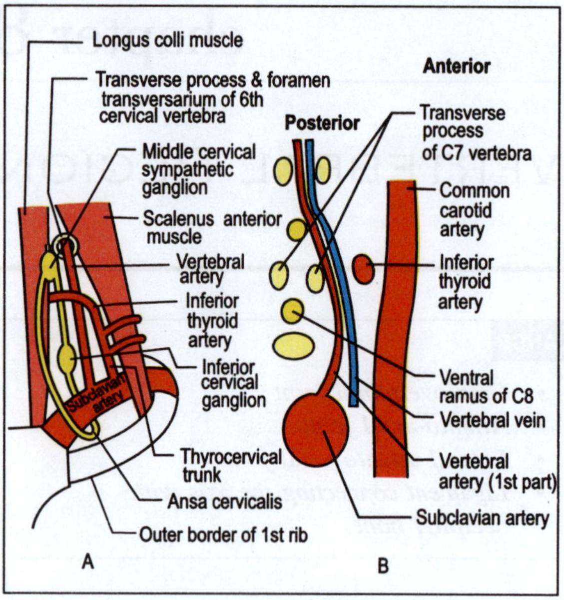

Fig. 8.2: First part of the vertebral artery. A – in scaleno-vertebral triangle; B – Relations (anterior & posterior)

RECTUS CAPITIS LATERALIS

It is a short, flat muscle.

Origin: From upper surface of transverse process of atlas.

Insertion: Into inferior surface of jugular process of the occipital bone.

Nerve supply: C_1 and C_2 (ventral rami)

Action: Flexes head laterally.

VERTEBRAL ARTERY

They are two main arteries on each side which supply the brain, spinal cord, meninges, muscles of the region and bones.

Origin: From posterosuperior part of first part of subclavian artery.

Termination: It ends within cranial cavity at the lower border of pons by uniting with opposite artery and form *basilar artery*.

Course and relations

The course is divided into four parts:

1. ***First or cervical part***: Part from origin to foramen transversarium of 6th cervical vertebra.

First Part

1. Extends from origin to foramen transversarium of sixth cervical vertebra.
2. It passes upwards ad backwards through scalenovertebral triangle between longus colli and scalenus anterior.
3. **Relation**–
   A. *In front* –
      a) Carotid sheath containing common carotid artery
      b) Vertebral vein
      c) Inferior thyroid artery
      d) Thoracic duct on left side.

   B. *Behind* –
      a) Transverse process of seventh cervical vertebra
      b) Ventral rami C_7 and C_8
      c) Inferior cervical or stellate ganglion.

Second Part

1. It starts from foramen transversarium of C_6 and passes through the foramina of transverse process of upper six cervical vertebrae. It runs vertically upwards to axis then upwards and laterally to reach foramen transversarium of atlas.
2. **Relation** –
   a) Ventral rami of C_2 to C_6 lie behind artery
   b) Surrounded by a plexus of sympathetic nerves and vertebral venous plexus
   c) Accompanied by a branch of stellate ganglion.

Third Part

1. It lies mainly in the suboccipital triangle and runs backward medially from foramen transversarium of the atlas to posterior arch of the atlas after winding the lateral mass of the atlas.
2. It lies on the groove of posterior arch of atlas – (suboccipital nerve lies between artery and bone).
3. **Relation**–
   a) *In front* – Lateral mass of atlas

b) *Behind* – Semispinalis capitis
c) *Medially* – Ventral rami C_1
d) *Laterally* – Rectus capitis lateralis
e) *Below* –Suboccipital nerve (Dorsal rami of C_1) and posterior arch of atlas.

Third part ends below lower arched border of the posterior atlanto-occipital membrane to enter the vertebral canal to continue as 4th part.

Fourth Part

1. Extends from posterior atlanto-occipital membrane at the posterior arch of the atlas to lower border of the pons.
2. It pierces the dura, arachnoid in the vertebral canal in front of 12th cranial nerve and runs medially towards the medulla (after passing through foramen magnum) and finally reaches at the lower border of the pons and unites with the opposite vertebral artery to form trunk of the **basilar artery**.

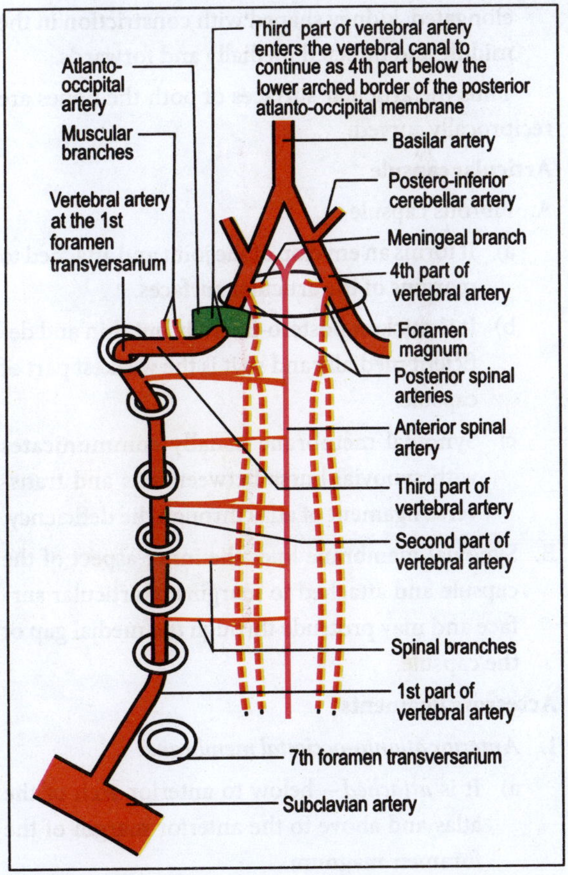

Fig. 8.3: Course and branches of vertebral artery

BRANCHES OF VERTEBRAL ARTERY

A. ***Branches in neck (Cervical)***

1. *Spinal branches* (supply upper five or six segments of spinal cord), enter the vertebral canal through the intervertebral foramina.
2. *Muscular branches* (supply muscles of suboccipital triangle).

B. ***Cranial branches***

1. *Meningeal* branches supply meninges of posterior cranial fossa.
2. *Posterior spinal* artery runs downward to divide into two branches. One lie in front of dorsal root of spinal nerve & other run behind the dorsal roots of spinal nerves.
3. *Anterior spinal* artery descends & unite with opposite artery to form anterior median spinal artery which supplies the area medial to hypoglossal nerve including pyramid of medulla oblongata.
4. *Postero inferior cerebellar artery* winds around olive to supply:
   a) lateral area of medulla oblongata which includes nucleus ambiguus, lateral spinothalamic tract, & nucleus of trigeminal nerve.
   b) inferior vermis and inferolateral part of cerebellar hemisphere.
5. *Medullary.*

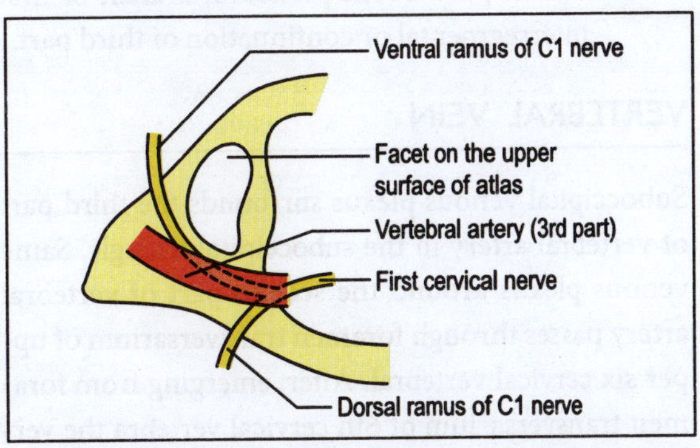

Fig. 8.4: Relations of 3rd part of the vertebral artery with superior surface of atlas

APPLIED ANATOMY

1. *Stealing of blood from brain through vertebral artery of opposite side* by subclavian artery occurs when subclavian artery is obstructed proximal to origin of vertebral artery.
2. *In the event of obstruction* posterior communicating artery connecting vertebrobasilar system of arteries with internal carotid artery and also forms a part of circle of Willis and so it is an important channel of collateral circulation.
3. Involvement anterior spinal nerve leads to impairment of movement (volitional) of contralateral side for the problem in the cortico-spinal tract. Due to involvement of hypoglossal nerve leads to ipsilateral loss of tongue movement. This is known as **'medial medullary syndrome'**.
4. Involvement of posterior inferior cerebellar artery produces loss of pain and temperature of same side of face, paralysis of vocal cord, soft palate & pharyngeal muscles of ipsilateral side. This is known as **'lateral medullary syndrome'**.

Development: Four parts are form four sources – so composite in origin.

1. *First part*: From dorsal branch of seventh intersegmental artery.
2. *Second part*: From the postcostal anastomosis between upper six intersegmental arteries.
3. *Third part*: From spinal branch of first intersegmental artery.
4. *Fourth part*: From preneural branch of first intersegmental or continuation of third part.

VERTEBRAL VEIN

Suboccipital venous plexus surrounds the third part of vertebral artery in the suboccipital triangle. Same venous plexus around the second part of vertebral artery passes through foramen transversarium of upper six cervical vertebral. After, emerging from foramen transversarium of 6th cervical vertebra the vertebral venous plexus become single vertebral vein. Each vertebral vein ends in brachiocephalic veins.

CRANIOVERTEBRAL JOINT

They include

1. Atlanto-occipital
2. Atlantoaxial
3. Ligaments connecting axis with the occipital bone.

ATLANTO-OCCIPITAL JOINT

These are paired joints.

Type – Synovial

Subtype – Ellipsoidal (polyaxial)

Bones taking part in the joint: Occipital condyles above and superior articular facets of atlas below:

Articular surfaces

a) of occipital condyles are convex.

b) of superior articular facets of atlas are concave, elongated, kidney shaped with constriction in the middle and directed medially and forwards.

Thus the articular surfaces of both the bones are reciprocally curved.

Articular capsule

A. Fibrous capsule

   a) It forms an envelop of the joint and attached to margins of the articular surfaces.

   b) It is thickest postero-laterally but thin and deficient medially and so it is the weakest part of capsule.

   c) Synovial membrane usually communicates with synovial bursa between axis and transverse ligament of atlas through the deficiency.

B. Synovial membrane lines the inner aspect of the capsule and attached to margins of articular surface and may protrude through the medial gap of the capsule.

Accessory ligaments

1. *Anterior atlanto-occipital membrane*

   a) It is *attached* – below to anterior arch of the atlas and above to the anterior margin of the foramen magnum.

   b) It fuses with capsule laterally

c) It is strengthened by anterior longitudinal ligament anteriorly

2. *Posterior atlanto-occipital membrane*
   a) It is attached – below to upper border of posterior arch of the atlas and above to posterior margin of foramen magnum.
   b) Laterally fuses with capsule
   c) On each side it arches over groove for vertebral artery and forms an opening for vertebral artery and first cervical nerve.

Arterial supply – Vertebral artery

Nerve supply – First cervical nerve

Movement – The movements are

a) Flexion

b) Extension

c) Slight lateral flexion

Axis of movements

a) Flexion and extension (nodding) movements occur around a transverse axis.

b) *Lateral flexion* – around an antero-posterior axis.

Muscles responsible for these movements

Flexion

a) Rectus capitis anterior

b) Longus capitis and

c) Sternocleidomastoid

Extension

a) Rectus capitis posterior major and minor

b) Obliquus capitis superior

c) Splenius capitis

d) Sternocleidomastoid

e) Upper part of trapezius

Lateral flexion

a) Rectus capitis lateralis

b) Semispinalis capitis

c) Splenius capitis

d) Sternocleidomastoid

e) Upper part of trapezius.

Maintenance of head in position during erect posture

The line of gravity of the weight of a head (average 7 lbs) usually passes in front of atlanto-occipital joints. It is the traction caused by extensor muscles (particularly semispinalis capitis) which is responsible to keep the head in proper position.

ATLANTOAXIAL JOINTS

Composite joints of three well separated joints between atlas and axis. They are

1. Median atlantoaxial and

2 & 3. Two lateral atlantoaxial

All these joints move as one unit and produce rotation of atlas with skull on axis.

Median atlantoaxial

Type – Synovial

Subtype – Pivot (uniaxial)

[**Characteristic of pivot** – one ring and an axis within it. Either ring will rotate around the pivot which is fixed or axis will rotate within fixed ring. (Fig. 8.5)

In atlantoaxial joint axis is fixed ring rotates but in superior radio ulnar joint – also a pivot joint – the axis head of radius rotates within fixed annular ligament].

Bones taking part

1 . *Odontoid process of axis*

2. *Anterior arch of atlas*

Articular surface – An oval facet on anterior surface of dens (odontoid process) articulate with oval facet on the posterior surface of anterior arch of atlas.

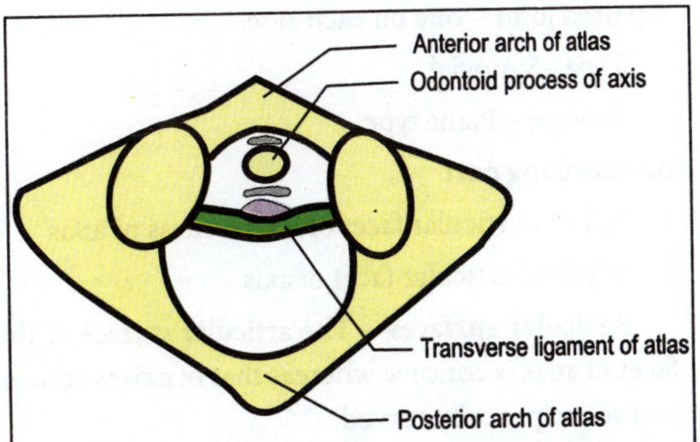

Fig. 8.5: Atlanto-axial joint (superior view)

Formation of pivot joint

1. Axis or pivot is the odontoid process of axis.
2. Ring – Formed by anterior arch of atlas in front and transverse ligament of atlas behind. In case of movement of rotation pivot is fixed and the ring moves (rotation).

Characteristic – It has two separate synovial cavities an anterior and posterior – anterior smaller and posterior larger.

Capsule and synovial membrane

a) A loose capsule is present in the anterior part of the joint and is lined by synovial membrane.
b) Posterior larger part is a synovial cavity termed bursa.

Ligaments – mainly transverse ligament of atlas and other ligaments are associated with the axis and not directly concerned with the joint.

Transverse ligament of atlas

a) It is attached on each side to the medial surface of lateral mass of atlas.
b) In median plane it is prolonged upwards to basilar part of occipital and downwards to body of axis and so forms cruciate ligament.
c) It lies on a groove in the posterior surface of odontoid process of axis and prevents backward dislocation of the process.

Other ligaments are ligaments connecting axis to occipital bone – as alar ligaments and apical ligament.

Lateral atlanto-axial joint

A paired joint – one on each side.

Type – Synovial

Subtype – Plane type

Bones taking part

1. Inferior articular facet of lateral mass of atlas
2. Superior articular facet of axis.

Articular surfaces – The articular surface of the facet of atlas is concave whereas that of axis is convex and so reciprocally curved.

Capsule

a) Attached to margins of articular surface
b) It is *lean, loose* and *lax* and so allow forward and backward movement during rotation of atlas.
c) It is supported by capsular, lateral part of anterior longitudinal ligament and ligamentum flavum.

Nerve supply – By second cervical nerve.

Movements – Rotatory movements of the atlas with skull on the axis around a *vertical axis.*

In the initial stage alar ligaments are relaxed whereas when full range is reached it is checked by anterior part of the ligament on the side of rotation and posterior part of ligament on the opposite side.

Muscles responsible for the movement

1. Obliquus capitis inferior
2. Rectus capitis posterior major
3. Splenius capitis
4. Sternocleidomastoid of opposite side.

Ligaments connecting the axis with the occipital bone

Four ligaments. They are:

1. **Apical ligament** (Figs. 8.6 and 8.7)
   a) It is the ligament connecting the tip of odontoid process below to upper surface of basilar part of occipital bone near the anterior margin of foramen magnum.
   b) It lies in front of upper band of cruciate ligament.
   c) Morphologically it represents remnant of notochord, (other remnant is nucleus pulposus) so it is ectodermal derivative.
2. **Cruciate or cruciform ligament**
   a) It consists of two bands, *strong horizontal* and *vertical band.*
   b) *Horizontal band* is known as *transverse ligament of atlas* which extends between the tubercles on the medial side of lateral mass of atlas and passes behind the odontoid process in a groove separated by bursa. It is converted by a loose fibrous capsule.

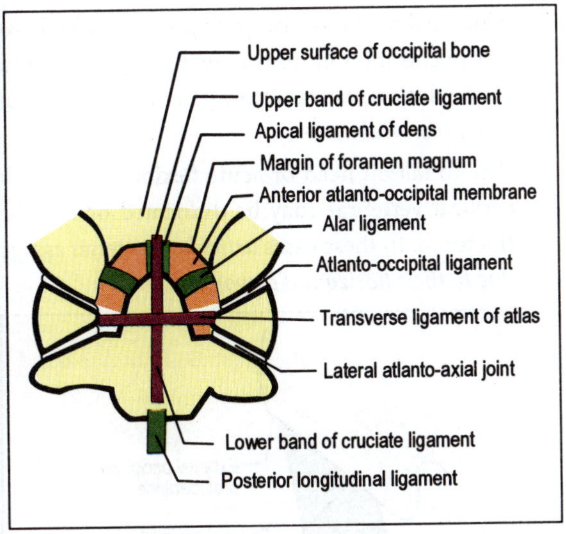

Fig. 8.6: Atlanto-occipital joint and atlanto-axial joint (from behind)

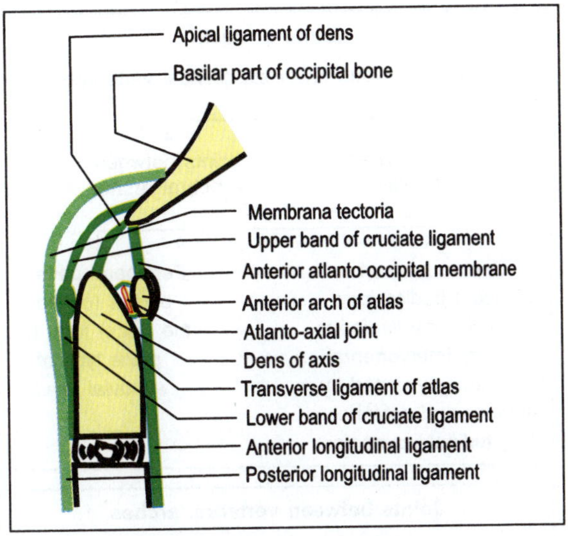

Fig. 8.7: Ligaments connecting axis with occipital bone and atlanto-axial joints

c) *Vertical band* consists of *upper* and *lower* bands which are prolonged upwards and downwards from the upper and lower margins of transverse ligament at the level of odontoid process respectively.

Upper band – attached above to the upper surface of basilar part of occipital bone in between apical ligament and membrana tectoria.

Lower band – attached below to the posterior surface of body of axis.

d) Functionally

i) It supports both atlanto-axial and atlanto-occipital joints and

ii) prevents dislocation of the odontoid process.

3. **Membrane tectoria**

a) It is a ligament situated within vertebral canal.

b) It is attached below to posterior surface of body of axis and above to upper surface of basilar part of occipital bone.

c) It covers the axis, transverse ligament, apical and upper band of cruciate ligaments.

d) *It represents upward continuation of posterior longitudinal ligament.*

Alar ligament

a) They are paired ligaments – one on each side.

b) It is attached below on each side of tip of odontoid process and above to the tubercles on the medial aspect of condyles of occipital bone.

c) These ligaments are very strong and check the rotation and flexion of head by acting on atlanto-axial joints. They are *known as check ligaments.*

They are relaxed during extension of head.

Applied anatomy

1. *After hanging,* death occurs due to

a) *rupture of transverse ligament of atlas*

b) *fracture of odontoid process or separation of axis from* 3rd *cervical vertebra.*

c) after the *dislocation of atlas occurs and cause compression of spinal cord and medulla with fatal results* – death.

2. *Pathological dislocation of atlas from axis* may occur due to softening or relaxation of transverse ligament of atlas *following infection of pharynx.*

Joints of neck

Joints between lower six cervical vertebrae
↓
- Joints between bodies
  ↓
  - Central parts of adjacent bodies form *secondary cartilaginous joints* by intervertebral discs strongly united by anterior and posterior longitudinal ligaments
  - Peripheral parts of bodies (outside the discs) form two plane type of *synovial joints*
- Joints between vertebral arches

Joints between vertebral arches
↓
- Articular processes of adjacent vertebrae form plane synovial *joints*
- Laminae of adjacent vertebrae are connected by ligamentum *flavum and form fibrous type of* joints
- Spines of adjacent vertebrae are connected by ligamentum *nuchae* (Fig. 8.8) *and interspinous* ligaments and form fibrous *type of joints*

Applied anatomy of joints of cervical vertebrae

1. **Cervical spondylosis**: In old age degenerative changes or any injury may cause rupturing of annulus fibrosus with prolapse of nucleus pulposus which is known as disc prolapse or **spondylosis** (more common in lumbar region). This cervical spondylosis cause *radiating pain due to compression of cervical nerves.*
2. Due to fall on head or acute flexion of the neck cervical vertebrae may be dislocated or may be fractured. In these cases *articular processes escape due to their horizontal disposition.*

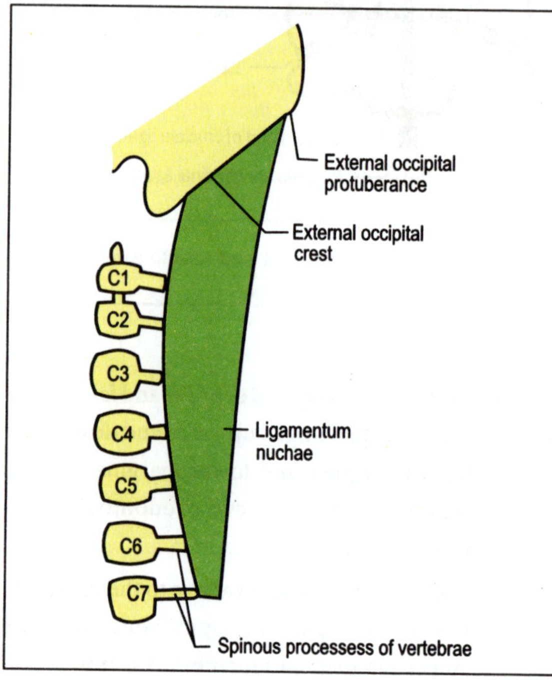

Fig. 8.8: Ligamentum nuchae

chapter 9

THE ORBIT

AT A GLANCE

- *Boundaries of orbit*
- *Superior orbital fissure*
- *Inferior orbital fissure*
- *Attachments of tendinous ring*
- *Periorbita*
- *Fascia bulbi*
- *Check ligaments*
- *Suspensory ligament of eyeball*
- *Extrinsic muscles of eyeball*
- *Opthalmic artery*
- *Opthalmic nerve*
- *Ciliary ganglion*

Orbits are a pair of bony pyramid (four sided) with a base (orbital margin) and apex with optic canal. Orbits are situated on either side of nasal cavity. Nasal cavities separates the medial walls of the orbits. Medial walls of both orbits are parallel and 2.5cm apart, lateral walls of the both orbits meet with each other at a right angle. (Fig. 9.1)

Orbit (height: 35mm; breadth: 40mm) contains eyeballs, extraocular muscles, nerves, blood vessels, lymphatics and fat, lacrimal gland, & fascia bulbi.

BOUNDARIES OF THE ORBIT

It is four-sided (roof, floor, medial wall, lateral wall) pyramid, base (orbital margin) and apex with optic canal.

Floor:

- Three bones form floor. Bones are:
  a) Orbital surface of body of the maxilla
  b) Orbital surface of zygomatic bone (anterolaterally)
  c) Orbital process of palatine bone (postero-medially).

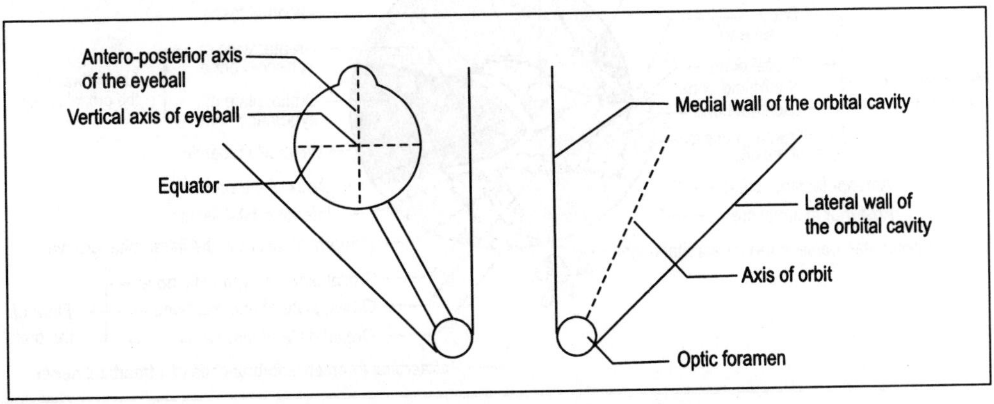

Fig. 9.1: Various axes of orbit and eyeball with medial and lateral walls of orbit

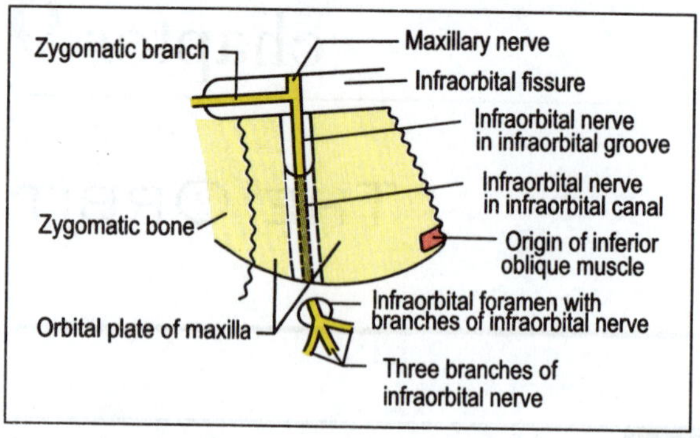

Fig. 9.2: Floor of the orbit

- It contains infraorbital groove and canal (containing infraorbital nerve and vessels).
- Origin of inferior oblique muscle (near the lacrimal groove (Fig. 9.2)

Roof:

- Two bones forms roof. Bones are
  a) Orbital plate of frontal bone (in front)
  b) Orbital surface of the lesser wing of sphenoid (behind)
- Anterolateral part of roof is having fossa for lacrimal gland.
- Anteromedial part is having spine for pulley for superior oblique muscle.
- Optic canal is present in the posterior most of the roof.

Medial wall (thinnest):

- Four bones form the medial wall.
- Bones are (before backwards):
  a) Frontal process of the maxilla
  b) Lacrimal bone
  c) Orbital plate of ethmoid bone
  d) Body of sphenoid.
- Anterior lacrimal crest is present in the frontal process of maxilla.
- Posterior lacrimal crest is present in the lacrimal bone.
- Lacrimal fossa is between anterior and posterior lacrimal crest.
- Anterior and posterior ethmoidal foramina (for transmitting anterior & posterior ethmoidal vessels & nerves) lies at the junction medial wall and roof (Fig. 9.3).

Lateral wall:

- Two bones from lateral wall (strongest). Bones are:
  a) Orbital surface of zygomatic bone (in front)
  b) Greater wing of sphenoid (behind)
- There are two small foramina (for transmitting zygomatico facial and zygomatico temporal nerves).

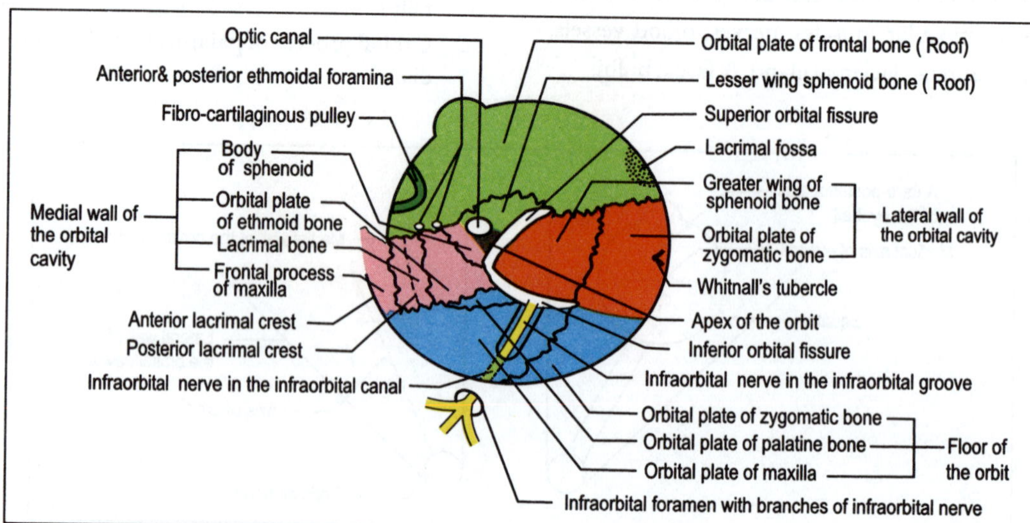

Fig. 9.3: Boundaries of the orbit

- An elevation just behind lateral margin and below frontozygomatic suture is known as Whitnall's tubercle. It gives attachment of lateral check ligament, lateral palpebral ligament.

Base of orbit (orbital margin)

Supraorbital margin: Formed by frontal bone and presents a notch or foramen at the junction of lateral two thirds & medial one-third.

Infraorbital margin: Formed by zygomatic bone (laterally) and maxilla (medially); it is continuous with anterior lacrimal crest.

Medial orbital margin: It is ill defined margin. It is formed by frontal bone and maxilla.

Lateral orbital margin: Formed by frontal process of zygomatic bone and zygomatic process of frontal bone.

Apex of the orbit:

Bony part in between optic canal and superior orbital fissure.

SUPERIOR ORBITAL FISSURE (Fig. 9.4)

Boundaries

Superiorly – Lesser wing of sphenoid.

Inferiorly – Greater wing of sphenoid.

Medially – Body of sphenoid.

Superior orbital fissure is divided into 3 compartments by common tendinous ring:

1. *Lateral compartment (above & lateral to common tendinous ring)*

   Structures passing through—

   a) Recurrent meningeal branch of lacrimal artery
   b) Lacrimal nerve
   c) Frontal nerve
   d) Trochlear nerve
   e) Superior ophthalmic vein

2. *Intermediate compartment* (within common tendinous ring)

   Structures passing through—

   a) Superior and inferior divisions of oculomotor nerve
   b) Nasociliary nerve lies between two divisions of oculomotor nerve.
   c) Abducent nerve lies lateral to inferior division of oculomotor nerve.

3. *Medial compartment* (below and medial to common tendinous ring)

   Structure passing through—

   a) Inferior ophthalmic vein.

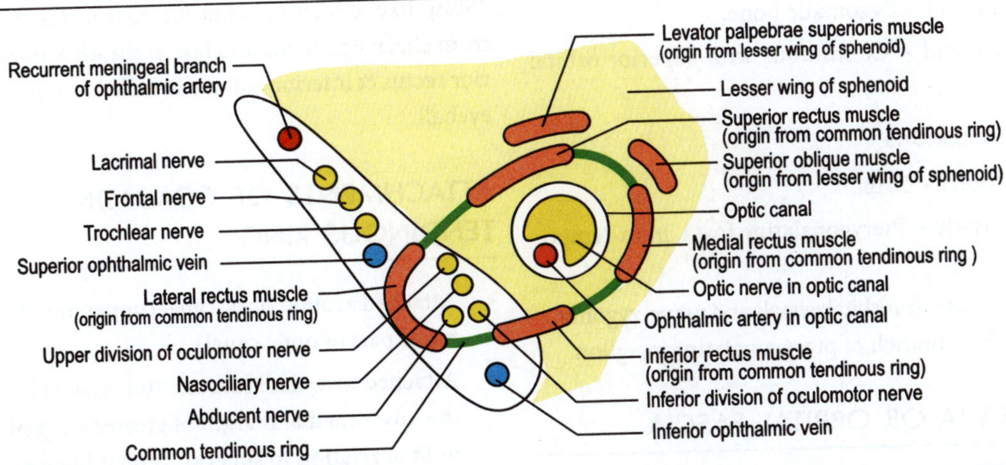

Fig. 9.4: Superior orbital fissure and common tendinous ring

RELATIONS OF THE ORBIT

The relations of orbit are as follows:

Above – Anterior cranial fossa.

Below – Maxillary air sinus.

Medially – Ehtmodial air sinus.

Laterally – Temporal fossa.

CONTENTS OF THE ORBIT

The structures in the orbits are as follows:

1. Eyeball
2. Muscles
3. Fascia bulbi
4. Nerves: optic, oculomotor with ciliary ganglion, trochlear nerve, ophthalmic, abducent.
5. Ophthalmic artery.
6. Ophthalmic vein
7. Lacrimal gland
8. Orbital fat

INFERIOR ORBITAL FISSURE

Boundaries

Anteromedially – Maxilla.

Postero laterally – Greater wing of sphenoid.

Lateral end – Zygomatic bone.

Medial end – Continuous with superior orbital fissure.

Communications

Anteriorly – Orbit.

Posteriorly – Pterygopalatine fossa, infra-temporal fossa.

Transmits infraorbital vessels and nerve, zygomatic nerve, orbital branch of pterygopalatine ganglion.

PERIORBITA OR ORBITAL FASCIA

Periosteum or periorbita loosely envelops the orbit. It is continuous at the margins of the orbit as orbital septa into upper & lower eyelids. It forms lacrimal fascia at the lacrimal fossa and it also sends an extension to hold the fibrous pulley for superior oblique muscles. It also bridges over inferior orbital fissure where nonstriated orbitalis muscle is present. (Fig. 9.5)

FASCIAL SHEATH OF THE EYEBALL

The **fascia bulbi** or **Tenon's** capsule enclosed major part eyeball. **Anteriorly** it is attached mean the limbus to the sclera. **Posteriorly** it is continuous with dura mater covering optic nerve.

Structures piercing the fascia bulbi

1. Four recti & two oblique muscles of eyeball
2. Ciliary vessels and nerve.

CHECK LIGAMENTS

Medial check ligament: is an extension from fascia covering medial rectus muscle and attaches to the posterior lacrimal crest of the lacrimal bone.

Lateral check ligament is an extension from fascia covering lateral rectus muscle and is attached to Whitnall's tubercle of zygomatic bone.

SUSPENSORY LIGAMENT OF EYEBALL

"Sling-like" structure is contributed from fascial sheath from check ligaments and fascial sheath around inferior rectus & inferior oblique muscles. It supports the eyeball.

ATTACHMENTS OF COMMON TENDINOUS RING

- Attached around optic canal (upper, medial & inferior part of optic canal)
- Attached to a small tubercle (tubercle of Zinn) on the lower medial margin of greater wing of sphenoid in relation to superior orbital fissure.
- It encloses the optic canal and intermediate part of the superior orbital fissure.

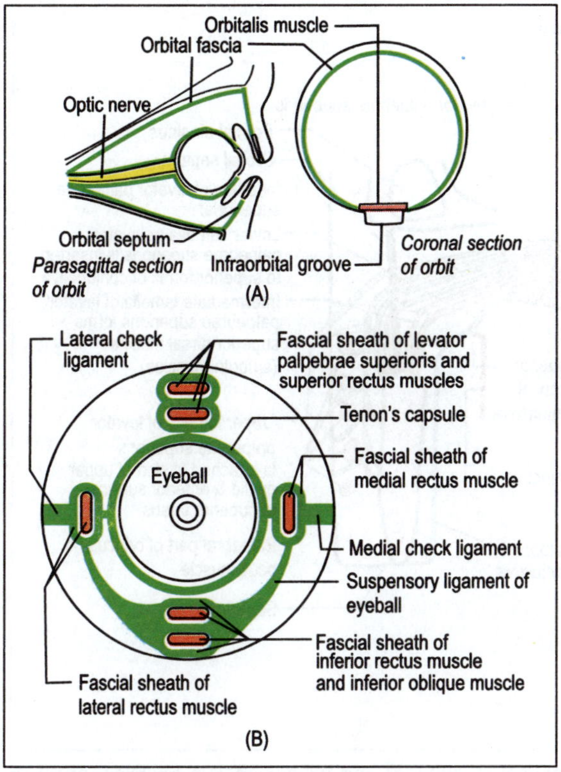

Fig. 9.5: (A) Orbital fascia, orbitalis muscle; (B) Facial sheath of eyeball with ligaments

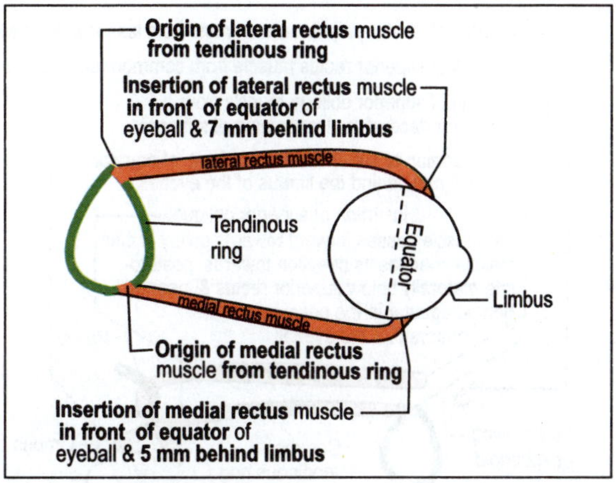

Fig. 9.6: Origins & insertions of medial & lateral rectus muscles

EXTRAOCULAR MUSCLES

The extraocular muscles are divided into two types: (A) Voluntary muscles; (B) Involuntary muscles

A. VOLUNTARY MUSCLES:

Recti muscles

Origin: From corresponding margins of common tendinous ring.

The lateral rectus takes origin by two heads. Small tendinous head arises from the orbital surface of the greater wing of the sphenoid. Abducent nerve passes in between the two heads.

Insertion: Into the sclera behind sclerocorneal junction (limbus) in front of equator and at an average distance:

a) Medial rectus – 5mm (Fig. 9.6)
b) Inferior rectus – 6mm
c) Lateral rectus – 7mm
d) Superior rectus – 8mm

Oblique muscle

1. **Superior oblique** (Fig. 9.7)

Origin: Arises from the under surface of the lesser wing of sphenoid superomedial to common tendinous ring.

Insertion: The muscle proceeds forward at the junction of medial wall & root of the orbit and forms tendon which passes through fibrocartilaginous pulley. From the pulley muscle changes its direction towards backward & laterally below the superior rectus muscle and inserted into sclera behind the equator in the posterosuperior quadrant.

2. **Inferior oblique** (Fig. 9.7)

Origin: Arise from orbital surface of maxilla, near the lacrimal groove.

Insertion: The muscle is inserted into sclera in the posterosuperior quadrant below the superior oblique. The muscle passes, initially, posterolaterally (below the inferior rectus) & then turns postero-superior-laterally under cover of lateral rectus.

Levator palpebrae superioris

It lies between roof of the orbit & superior rectus.

Origin: The muscle arises from under surface of the lesser wing of sphenoid above the common tendinous ring, as narrow tendon. (Figs. 9.7 and 9.8)

Course: As it passes forward it becomes broad & fleshy.

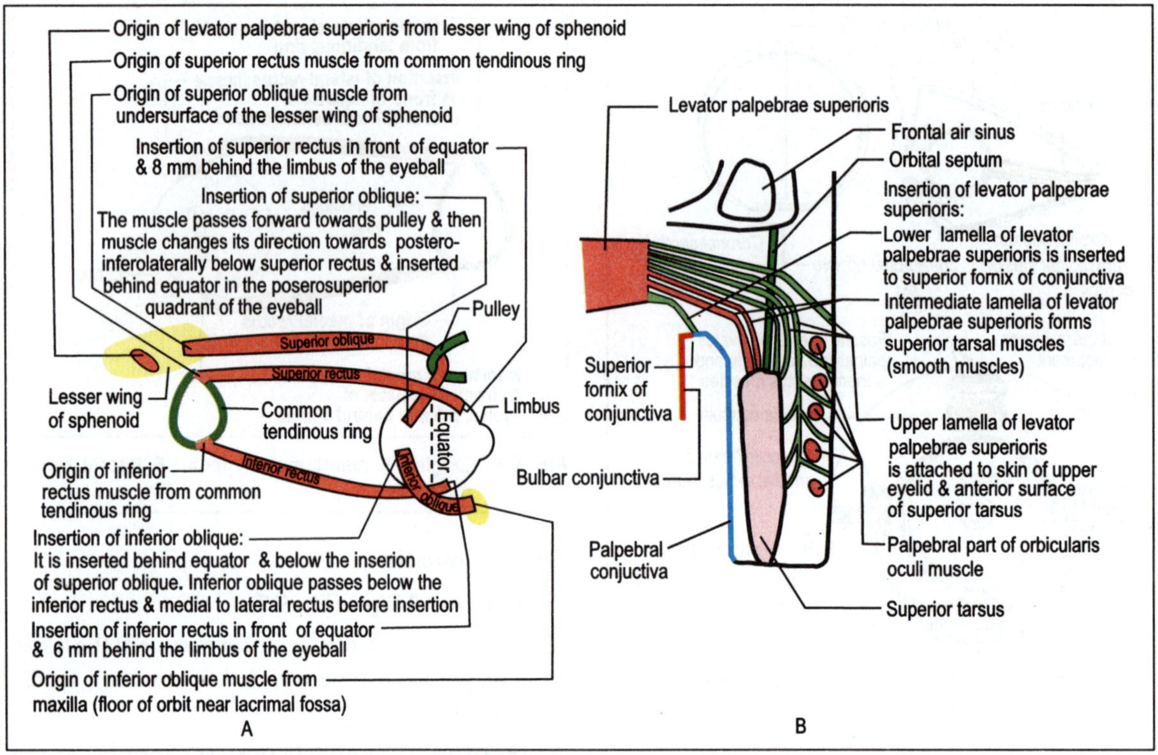

Fig. 9.7: A – Origin and insertions of superior rectus, inferior rectus, superior and inferior oblique muscles, origin of levator palpebrae superioris; B – Insertion of levator palpebrae superioris muscle

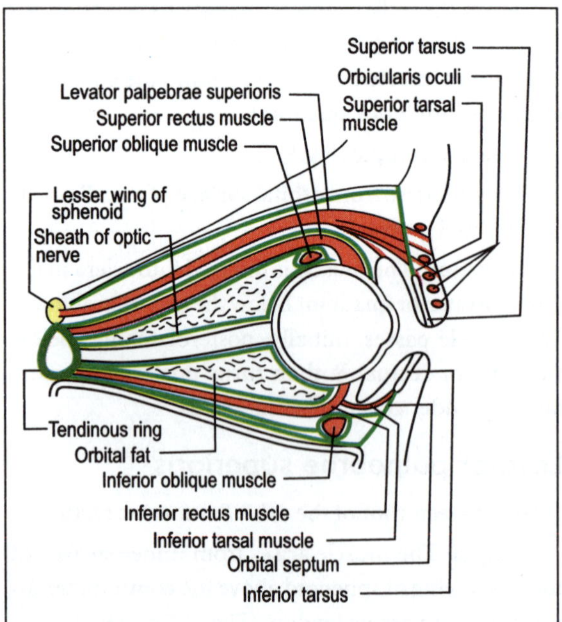

Fig. 9.8: Sagittal section of the orbital cavity

Insertion: Terminal part of flat tendon divides into three lamellae.

a) Upper lamella is inserted on the skin of upper eyelid and anterior surface of superior tarsus.
b) Intermediate lamella becomes nonstriated **superior tarsal muscle** to be inserted in the upper margin of the superior tarsus.
c) The lower lamella is inserted into the superior fornix of conjunctiva.

Nerve supply: It is supplied by oculomotor nerve. Superior tarsus is supplied by postganglionic sympathetic fibers.

Action: It elevates the upper eyelid.

(B) INVOLUNTARY MUSCLES

The muscles are superior tarsal, inferior tarsal and orbitalis.

NERVE SUPPLY OF EXTRAOCULAR MUSCLES

All the extraocular muscles are supplied by the oculomotor nerve except lateral rectus and superior oblique muscles. Lateral rectus is supplied by abducent nerve (sixth cranial nerve) and superior oblique is supplied by trochlear nerve (fourth cranial nerve), [S.O. (Superior oblique) – 4 (IVth cranial nerve); L. R. (Lateral rectus) – 6 (VIth cranial nerve). So the formula to remember the nerve supply will be S.O. 4; L.R. 6]. (Fig. 9.9).

Involuntary muscles are supplied by postganglionic sympathetic fibers from superior cervical sympathetic ganglion.

TABLE 9.1: Actions of individual muscles

Muscle	In primary position	Abducted eye	Adducted eye
Superior rectus	Elevation, adduction, intortion	Elevation only	Intortion only
Inferior rectus	Depression, adduction, extorsion	Depression only	Extorsion only eye
Superior oblique	Depression, abduction, intorsion	Intortion only	Depression only
Inferior oblique	Elevation, abduction, extorsion	Extorsion only	Elevation only
Medial rectus	Adduction only		
Lateral retus	Abduction only		

Actions of individual muscles

Superior rectus: Elevation, adduction, intorsion

Inferior rectus: Depression, adduction, extorsion

Superior oblique: Depression, abduction, intortion

Inferior oblique: Elevation, abduction, extortion

Medial rectus: Adduction

Lateral rectus: Abduction. (Fig. 9.10)

APPLIED ANATOMY

Nerve involvement will lead to unilateral paralysis of individual muscle producing **strabismus or squint** (deviation of eye in different direction) which produces **diplopia** (double vision).

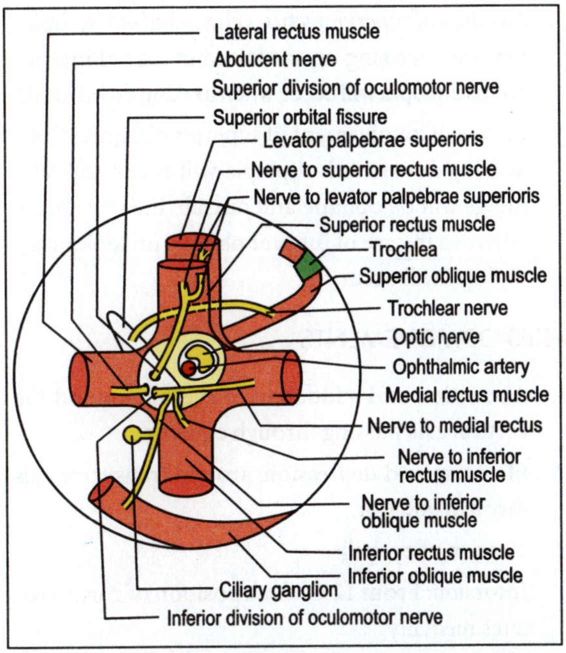

Fig. 9.9: Extraocular muscles with their nerve supply

1. *Internal strabismus*: Due to paralysis of lateral rectus – diplopia will be present if one looks to paralysed side.
2. *External squint*: Due to paralysis of medial rectus and is characterised by presence of diplopia.

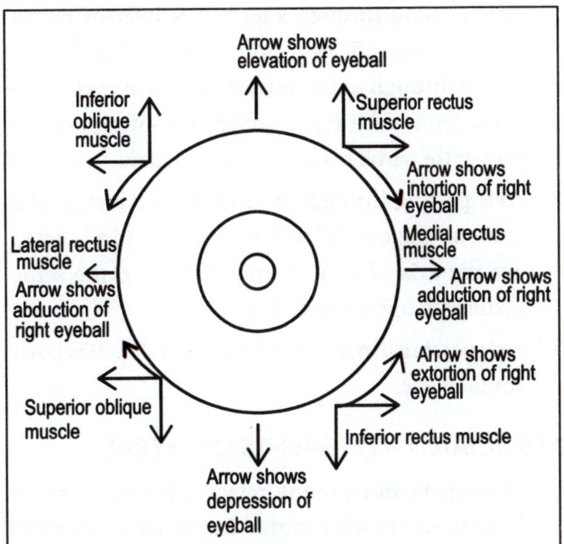

Fig. 9.10: Scheme to show the actions of the extraocular muscles

3. *Paralysis of superior rectus* is characterised by diplopia when looking upwards and in case of inferior rectus diplopia will occur when looking downwards.
4. In case of involvement of superior oblique: When looking downwards diplopia will occur and false image will be oblique and outside the true image where as in case of inferior oblique on looking up diplopia will occur.

AXES OF MOVEMENTS

1. Abduction and adduction of eyeball: around the vertical axis passing through equator.
2. Elevation and depression: around transverse axis through equator.
3. Torsion of eyeball:

   Intorsion: From 12 O'clock position of cornea rotates medially.

   Extorsion: From 12 O'clock position of cornea rotates laterally.

   Movements occur around antero-posterior axis passes from anterior pole to posterior pole of the eye.

AXES OF MUSCLES

1. Axis passing through superior & inferior rectus make an angle 25° away from the optical axis which passes through anteroposterior pole of eyeball. In abducted eye the axis of superior & inferior rectus stay in the same plane with optical axis.
2. Axis passing through superior & inferior oblique make an angle of 51° with optical axis. In adducted eye the axis of oblique muscle stay in the same plane with optical axis. (Fig. 9.11)
3. Axis passing through medial & lateral recti is horizontal plane.

ASSOCIATED MOVEMENTS OF EYEBALL

1. **Conjugate movement** refers bilateral fixation (which occurs after motor coordination of eyes) on a single object.

   Horizontal conjugate gaze is controlled by oculomotor nerve and abducent nerve.

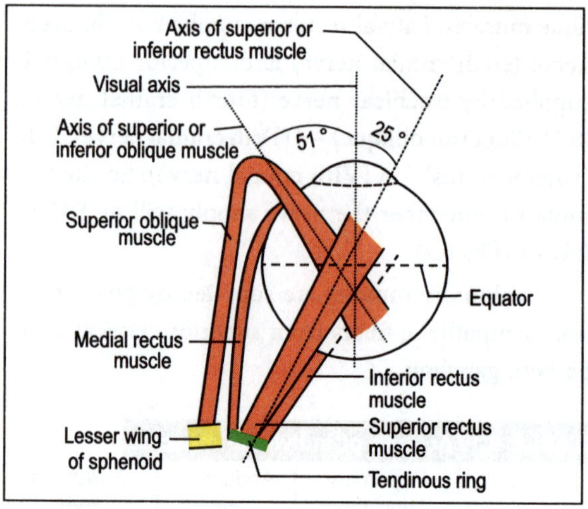

Fig. 9.11: Axes passing through superior oblique and superior rectus muscle

   Vertical conjugate gaze is controlled by oculomotor nerve and trochlear nerve.

2. Vergence movements: It is the simultaneous movement in opposite directions of eyes in order to obtain single binocular vision. Vergence movements are connected to accommodation of the eye.

   Convergence is the simultaneous inward movements of eyes (towards each other) in order to maintain single binocular vision.

   Divergence is the simultaneous outward movements of eyes away from each other in order to maintain single binocular vision.

MOVEMENTS AND RESPONSIBLE MUSCLES

1. Elevation or upward rotation: Superior rectus and inferior oblique.
2. Depression or downwards rotation: Superior oblique and inferior rectus.
3. Medial rotation or adduction: Medial rectus, superior and inferior recti.
4. Lateral rotation or abduction: Lateral rectus and superior oblique and inferior oblique.
5. Intortion: Superior oblique and superior rectus.
6. Extortion: Inferior oblique and inferior rectus.

OPTIC NERVE

Origin: Axons of ganglion cells form the optic nerve which emerges from eyeball 3 or 4mm nasal to its posterior pole. The nerve is about 4cm, out of which 25mm are intraorbital, 5mm intracanalicular (within optic canal) and 10mm intracranial. The entire nerve enclosed in three meningeal sheaths.

The optic nerve reaches the middle cranial fossa after passing through optic canal and forms optic chiasma with opposite optic nerve.

Relation in the orbit

1. Near the optic canal, the nerve is closely surrounded by recti muscles. The ciliary ganglion lies between optic nerve and the lateral rectus.
2. Central artery and vein of retina pierces the optic nerve (inferomedially) about 1.25cm behind the eyeball.
3. The optic nerve is crossed superiorly by the superior ophthalmic vein, ophthalmic artery and nasociliary nerve (before backward).

   Refer chapter 20 for further details.

OCULOMOTOR NERVE

Oculomotor nerve (two divisions) enter the orbit through middle compartment of superior orbital fissure.

The upper division supply superior rectus and levator palpebrae superioris.

The lower divisions supply, inferior rectus, medial rectus and inferior oblique.

Nerve to inferior oblique gives a branch to ciliary ganglion. Refer chapter 20 for further details.

CILIARY GANGLION

It is one of the parasympathetic ganglion. It is functionally connected with oculomotor nerve and topographically with nasociliary nerve.

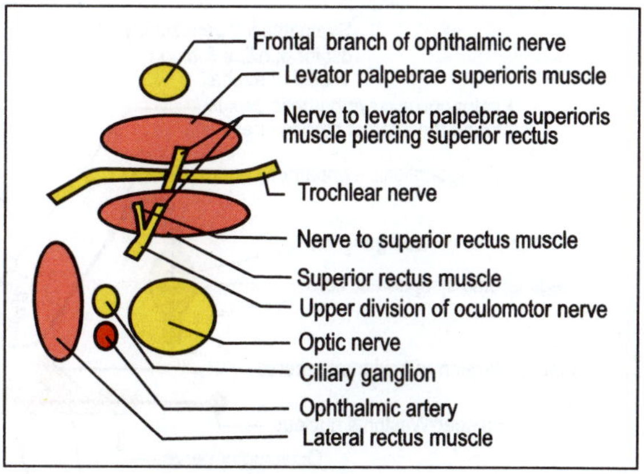

Fig. 9.12: Showing the locations of the frontal nerve, frontal nerve, superior division of oculomotor nerve & ciliary ganglion

Location: The ganglion is situated near the apex of the orbit, between optic nerve and lateral rectus. Sometimes, medial to ganglion, ophthalmic artery is present. (Fig. 9.12)

Connection: Three roots.

Motor root: From **Edinger Westphal nucleus** preganglionic fibre (parasympathetic part) originate & then travels along the oculomotor nerve to reach the ganglion through nerve to inferior oblique muscle. Preganglionic fibres synapse in the ganglion & postganglionic fibres reach the eyeball through short ciliary nerve to supply ciliaris muscles & sphincter pupillae. (Fig. 9.13)

Sensory root: These nerve arises from eyeball pass through the ganglion without interruption. It conveys pain, touch & thermal sensations from eyeball (through nasociliary nerve).

Sympathetic root is the postganglion fibres from superior cervical sympathetic part through plexus around internal carotid artery which reaches the ganglion & passes through the ganglion without interruption to reach the blood vessels of eyeball & dilator pupillae muscle.

Branches: Short ciliary branches (8-10) from the anterior border of the ganglion around the optic nerve. On reaching the eyeball, they further divide into 15-20 branches piercing sclera until they reach the concerned areas.

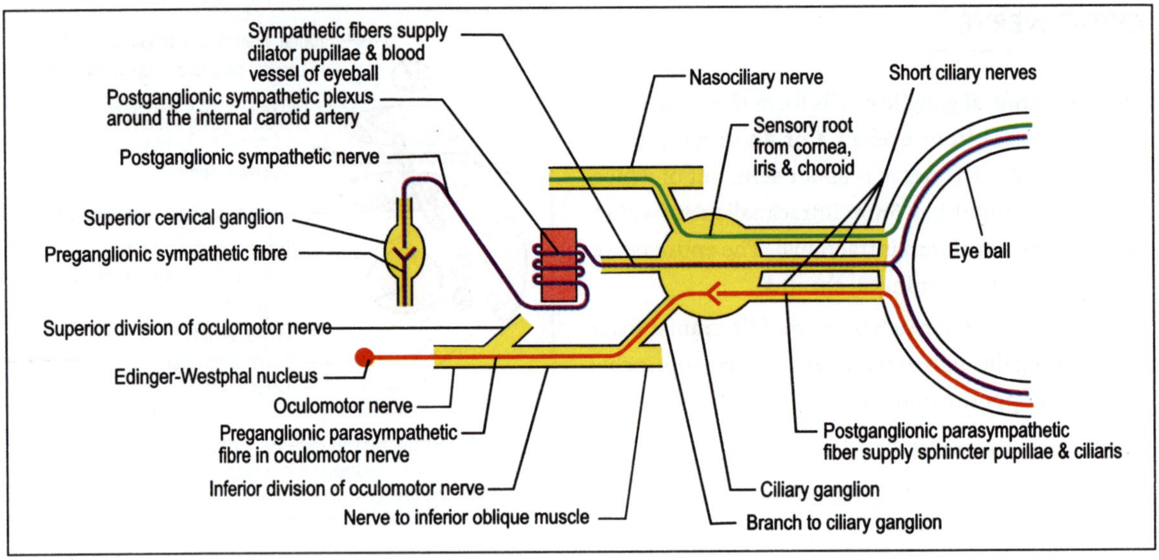

Fig. 9.13: Showing connections with ciliary ganglion

Short ciliary nerves contain postganglionic parasympathetic fibres, sensory fibres & sympathetic fibres.

TROCHLEAR NERVE

Trochlear nerve supplies superior oblique muscle after entering the orbit through superior orbital fissure. Refer chapter 20 for further details.

OPHTHALMIC NERVE (Fig. 9.14)

1. It is one of the divisions of trigeminal nerve
2. It is purely a sensory nerve.
3. Arises from the convex anterior margin of trigeminal ganglion.
4. After origin it lies on the lateral wall of cavernous sinus below 4th cranial nerve and above maxillary divisions.
5. In the anterior part of cavernous sinus it terminates by dividing into (i) frontal, (ii) lacrimal; (iii) nasociliary.

Frontal nerve

1. Largest branch of ophthalmic nerve. It originates at the
2. It is a sensory nerve.
3. It enters the orbit through lateral part of superior orbital fissure outside the common tendinous ring lateral to trochlear nerve. It lies on the levator palpebrae superioris.
4. It terminates in the midway between base and apex of the orbit by dividing into: (a) supraorbital nerve and (b) supratrochlear nerve.
   a) **Supraorbital nerve**: It passes through supraorbital notch or foramen and terminates by distributing following structures: (i) upper eyelid and conjunctiva; (ii) deep to frontalis divides into medial and lateral branches which pierce the muscles and supply skin of scalp and forehead up to lambdoid suture, mucous membrane of frontal sinus and pericranium.
   b) **Supratrochlear**:
      1. It passes forward above the trochlea of superior oblique muscle of eyeball and then emerges from orbit medial to supra orbital foramen and accompanied by supratrochlear vessels.
      2. It supplies the conjunctiva, skin of upper eyelid and lower part of forehead.

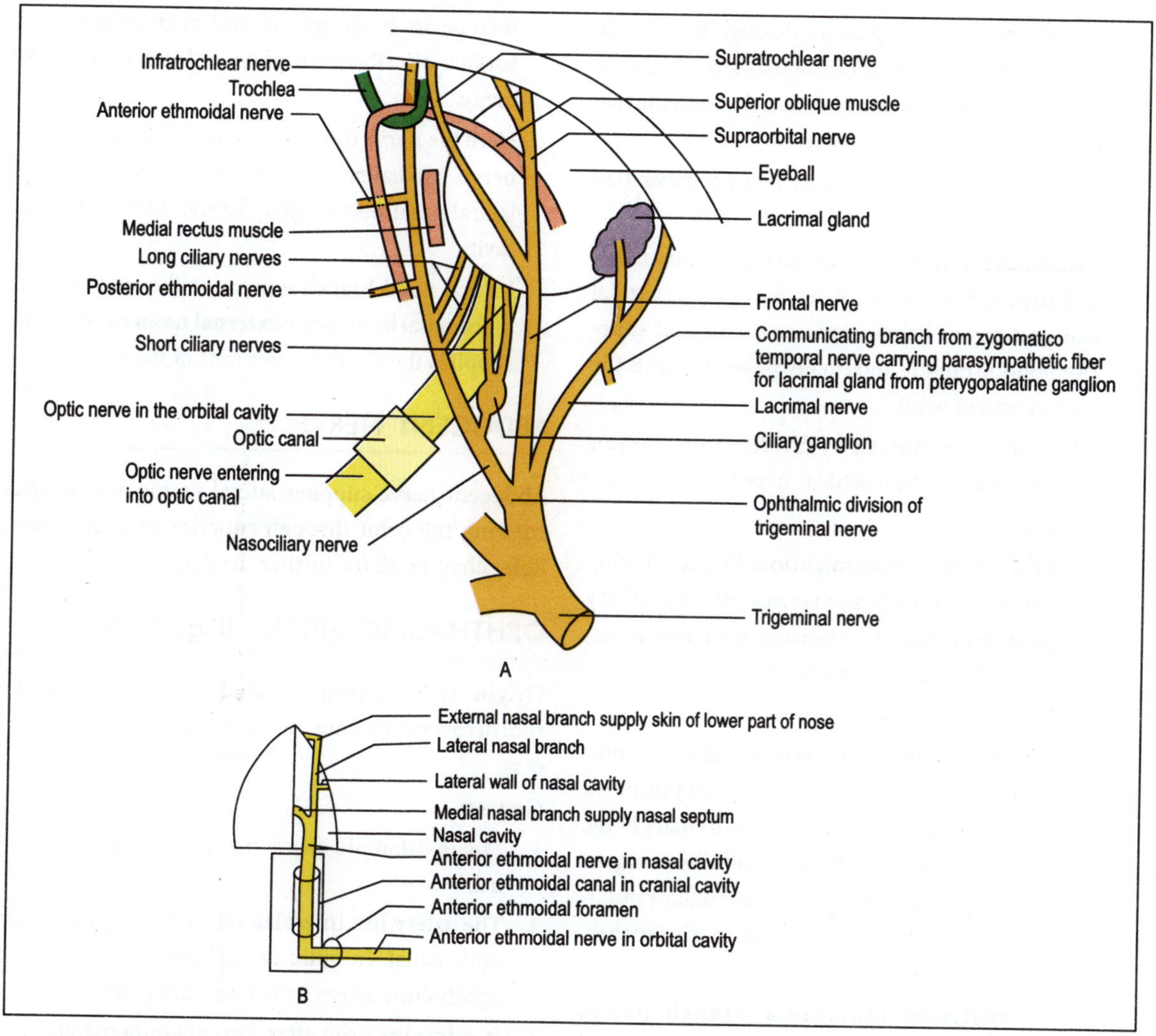

Fig. 9.14: (A) Course and branches of ophthalmic nerve; (B) Course and branches of anterior ethmoidal nerve

Lacrimal Nerve

1. Smallest of the branches of ophthalmic nerve and sensory nerve.
2. It passes to orbit through lateral compartment of superior orbital fissure out side common tendinous ring and lateral to frontal nerve.
3. In the orbit it passes above lateral rectus accompanied by lacrimal artery and receives a twig from zygomaticotemporal branch which carries post ganglionic secretomotor fibres for lacrimal gland.
4. It gives branches to lacrimal gland and conjunctiva.
5. Finally it pierces orbital septum and ends in the skin of lateral part upper eyelid.

Nasociliary nerve

1. It is sensory nerve and one of the three branches of ophthalmic nerve.
2. Origin: It arises from the ophthalmic nerve in the anterior part of cavernous sinus.

3. It enters the orbit by passing through the middle compartment of superior orbital fissure within the common tendinous ring and then through the two heads of lateral rectus muscle.
4. Within superior orbital fissure it lies between two rami (divisions) of oculomotor nerve.
5. **Within orbit**: It at first lies lateral to optic nerve and then crosses above it from lateral to medial side and passes below superior rectus and superior oblique muscle and finally passes towards the medial wall of orbit.
6. Ultimately it terminates by dividing into anterior ethmoidal and infratrochlear nerve.
7. **Branches:**
   A. **Branches of communication**: Before crossing the optic nerve a branch arises and joins ciliary ganglion forming its sensory root and sometimes also sympathetic root.
   B. **Branches of distribution**
      a) **Long ciliary branches** two or three in number and arise during crossing of optic nerve and distribute sensory fibers to ciliary body, iris, cornea and usually contains postganglionic sympathetic fibres for dilator pupillae. These fibres carries pain, touch and thermal sensations from eyeball.
      b) **Posterior ethmoidal branch** passes through posterior ethmoidal foramen and distributes to ethmoidal and sphenoidal air sinuses.
8. **Terminal branches**: The nasociliary nerve ends by dividing into **infratrochlear** and **anterior ethmoidal nerve** near anterior ethmoidal foramen.

   Intratrochlear: It passes below the pulley for superior oblique muscle and escapes out of orbit near medial canthus of the eye. It supplies skin of eyelids, upper part of nose, conjunctiva, lacrimal sac and caruncle.

   Anterior ethmoidal: It is the terminal branch of nasociliary nerve and passes through anterior ethmoidal foramen and enters the cranial cavity and then passes in the groove and canal on the upper surface of cribriform plate and enters the nasal cavity.

   Here the nerve divides into medial & lateral nasal nerve. Medial nasal nerve supply nasal septum & lateral nasal nerve supply lateral wall of the nasal cavity.

   Lateral nasal branch emerge at the lower border of the nasal bone as the **external nasal nerve** which supplies the skin of lower part of the nose.

ABDUCENT NERVE

Abducent nerve supplies lateral rectus muscle after entering the orbit through superior oribital fissure. Refer chapter 20 for further details.

OPHTHALMIC ARTERY (Fig. 9.15)

Origin: It arises from internal carotid artery at the roof of cavernous sinus, medial to anterior clinoid process.

Course:

1. The ophthalmic artery passes to rough optic canal.
2. The artery lies inferolateral to optic nerve in the optic canal. In optic canal, both optic nerve and ophthalmic artery lie within dura mater.
3. It enters the orbit after piercing dura mater.
4. It passes forward lateral and above to optic nerve. At this place nasociliary nerve lies behind the artery.
5. The artery passes towards medial wall of orbit between medial rectus & superior oblique muscle.

Termination:

1. At the medial angle of eye, the artery divides into two terminal branches:
   a) Supratrochlear artery
   b) Dorsal nasal artery.

Branches of ophthalmic artery:

1. **Central artery of retina:** It arises from ophthalmic

artery below the optic nerve. It pierces the dural sheath 1.25cm behind the eyeball. It reaches optic disc through the central part of the nerve. The nerve supply 6-7 layers of retina. The central artery is an end artery and blindness occur in obstruction of the artery.

2. **Posterior ciliary arteries**: These arteries (long and short) pierce sclera around optic nerve.

   Long posterior ciliary arteries (usually 2) reach he margin of iris, to anastomose with anterior ciliary arteries to supply iris & ciliary body. Anterior ciliary arteries are the branches of muscular branches of four recti.

   Short posterior ciliary arteries (usually 7) forms capillary plexus in the choroid to supply choroid and 3-4 layers of retina by diffusion.

3. **Lacrimal artery**: It runs forward in the upper border of lateral rectus and supplies lacrimal gland, eyelids & conjunctiva. It gives following branches:
   a) Lateral palpebral arteries – one for each lid.
   b) **Zygomatic branch** – divides into **zygomatico facial & zygomaticotemporal branch.**
   c) **Recurrent meningeal artery** – It passes through superior orbital fissure to anastomoses with branches of middle meningeal artery. It also supply muscles of the orbit.

4. **Posterior ethmoidal artery**: It passes through posterior ethmoidal foramen to supply posterior ethmoidal sinuses.

5. **Anterior ethmoidal artery**: It enters the cranial cavity through anterior ethmoidal foramen, then enters the nasal cavity. It supplies anterior & middle ethmoidal air sinuses, anterosuperior part of septum & lateral wall of nasal cavity.

6. **Supraorbital artery**: It enters the scalp through supraorbital notch or foramen to supply skin of scalp.

7. **Medial palpebral artery** supply both the eyelids.

8. **Supratrochlear artery** supply skin of the scalp.

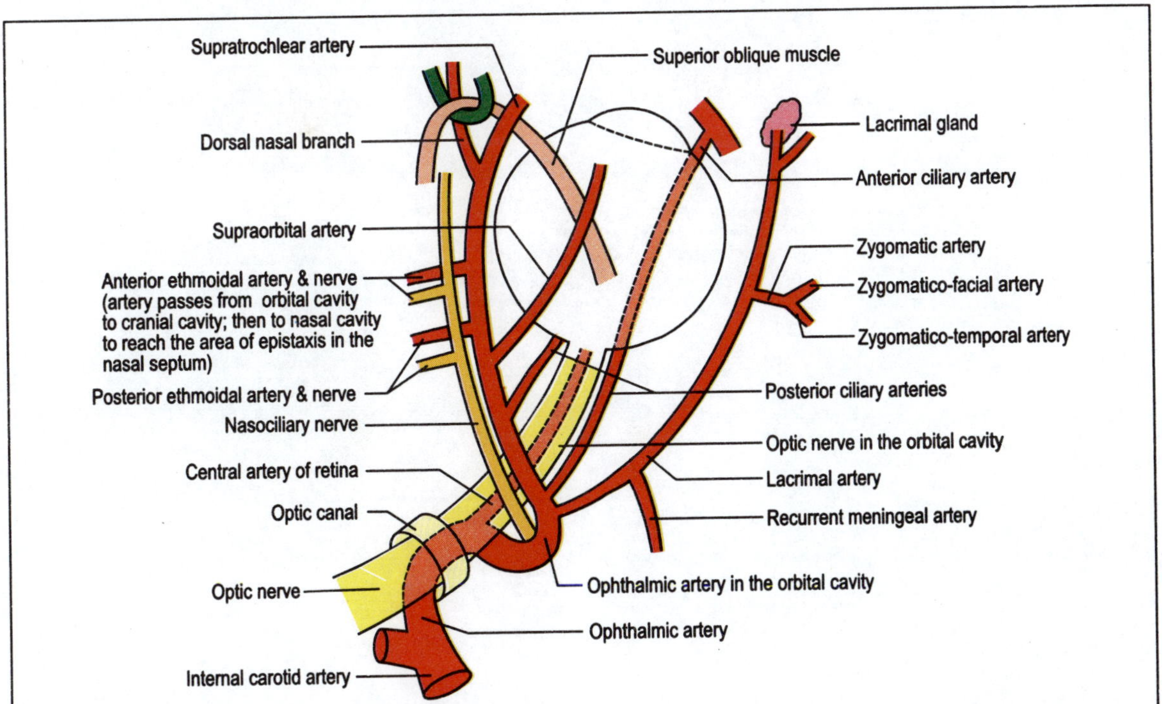

Fig. 9.15: Course and branches of the ophthalmic artery

9. **Dorsal nasal artery** supply upper part of nose & anastomoses with terminal part of facial artery at the medial angle of the eye.

OPHTHALMIC VEINS

Venous drainage of the orbit id done by two veins.

Superior ophthalmic vein, joins the supraorbital vein with cavernous sinus & passes through superior orbital fissure.

Inferior ophthalmic vein begins at the floor of the orbit. It drains from lower orbital muscles lacrimal sac & lower eyelid. It drains to cavernous sinus directly or after joining superior ophthalmic veins.

chapter 10

Parotid Region

AT A GLANCE

- *Parotid region*
- *Parotid gland: Capsules; Shape; Features – Base, Apex, Surfaces (superficial, antero medial & postero-medial), Borders (anterior & posterior), Different processes of parotid gland, Structures within gland; Relations; Parotid duct; Blood supply of gland, Lymphatic drainage; Nerve supply of gland; Applied anatomy; Microscopic features*

PAROTID REGION

Largest serous salivary gland lies in the parotid region. The parotid gland lies in the region.

Boundaries of the parotid region (Fig. 10.1).

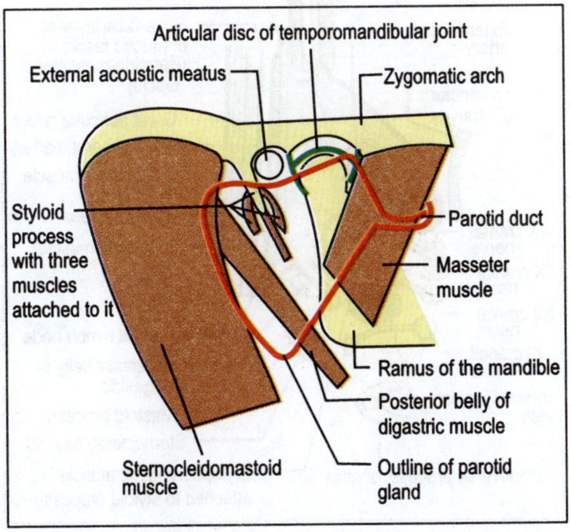

Fig. 10.1: Showing the parotid region

A. *In front*: Ramus of the mandible, anterior border of masseter (laterally), and medial pterygoid muscle (medially).
B. *Behind*: Mastoid process and sternocleidomastoid muscle.
C. *Above*: External acoustic meatus, zygomatic arch and posterior part of temporomandibular joint.
D. *Below*: Posterior belly of digastric and stylohyoid muscle.
E. *On the inner aspect or medially*: Styloid process and muscles attached to it (stylohyoid, styloglossus and stylopharyngeus muscles).

PAROTID GLAND

Type: Serous type.

Capsules: The gland is covered by outer false capsule and inner true capsule.

1. ***Outer false capsule***: It is formed by investing layer of deep cervical fascia. Investing layer of deep fascia splits into superficial lamina or layer & deep lamina or layer.

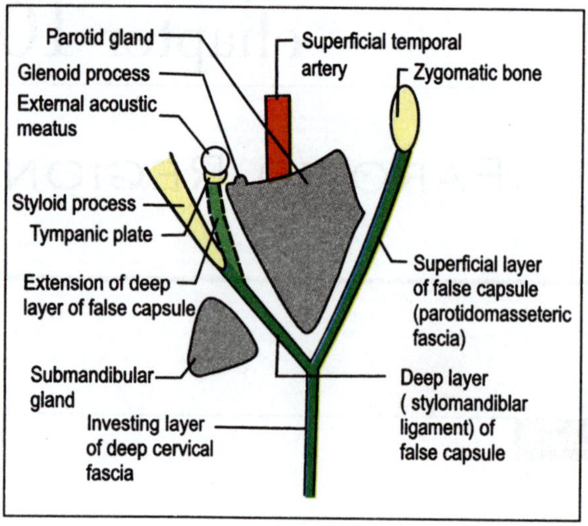

Fig. 10.2: Capsules of parotid gland

a) **The superficial lamina** or **layer** is known as **parotidomasseteric fascia** which is strong thick, and a very tense and tough and attached to lower border of zygomatic arch and covers superficial surface, and adherent to the gland. Superficial layer blends with epimysium of the masseter to form parotidomasseteric fascia.

b) The deep layer (thin) is attached to angle of mandible, styloid process and tympanic plate. The part of the deep layer or lamina between styloid process & angle of mandible is known as stylomandibular ligament which separates parotid from submandibular salivary gland.

2. ***Inner true capsule***: Formed by condensation of the fibrous stroma of the gland (Fig. 10.2).

Presenting parts (External features)

The gland presents like a inverted pyramid. The *apex* of the pyramid is directed downwards. The gland has four surfaces & three borders: (Fig. 10.3)

Surfaces: (1) Superior surface or base; (2) Superficial surface; (3) Anteromedial surface; (4) Posteromedial surface.

Borders: (1) Anterior, (2) Posterior; (3) Medial.

Apex

1. Directed downwards and extends beyond the posterior belly of digastric up to upper part of carotid triangle.

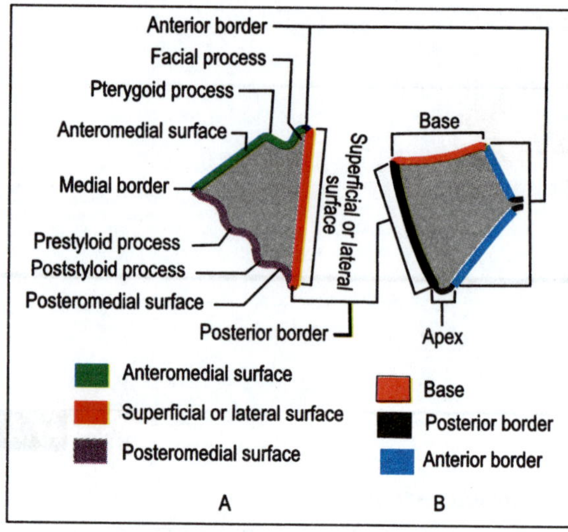

Fig. 10.3: Showing borders, surfaces & processes of parotid gland. A – Transverse section; B – Section of the parotid gland shoing base, apex, anterior & posterior border

2. Structures emerging through the apex include:
   a) Anterior and posterior division of retromandibular vein. (Posterior division of retromandi-

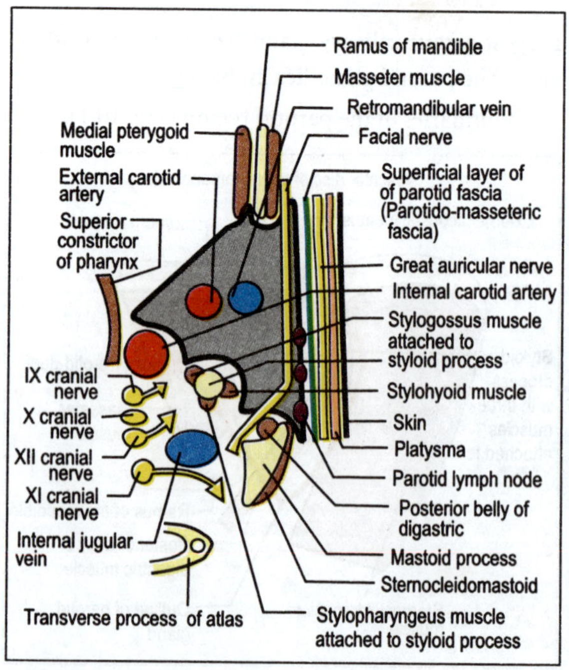

Fig. 10.4: Relations of the parotid gland

bular vein joins with posterior auricular vein forming external jugular vein).

b) Cervical branch of facial nerve

Surfaces (Fig. 10.4)

Base or superior surface

1. It is the upper end or upper surface of the gland and is concave.
2. Related to external acoustic meatus and posterior aspect of temporomandibular joint.
3. Structures passing through this part are
   a) Superficial temporal vessels
   b) Auriculotemporal nerve
   c) Temporal branch of facial nerve.

A. **Superficial (lateral) surface**: Largest surface from outside inwards covered by –

1. Skin.
2. Superficial fascia with great auricular nerve (supplying skin of angle of mandible) and superficial or preauricular parotid lymph nodes.
3. Platysma.
4. Superficial layer of parotid fascia (parotidomasseteric) fascia.
5. Deep parotid lymph nodes embedded in the gland. (Fig. 10.4)

B. **Anteromedial surface**: It is grooved by the ramus of mandible and related to:

1. Masseter (postero inferior part)
2. Posterior border of ramus of mandible
3. Capsule of temporomandibular joint
4. Branches of facial nerve emerge at the outer lip of the groove
5. Maxillary artery comes out at the inner lip of the groove and medial to neck of mandible.
6. Medial pterygoid muscle.

C. **Posteromedial surface**: An extensive surface moulding over the mastoid and the styloid process with structures attached to them.

Related to–

1. Mastoid process with sternocleidomastoid and posterior belly of digastric.
2. Transverse process of atlas with rectus capitis lateralis.
3. Styloid process with muscles and ligaments and all attached to it.
4. Deep to styloid process: Internal carotid artery in front and internal jugular vein behind and 9th, 10th, 11th and 12th cranial nerves between vein and artery.
5. Structures piercing this surface
   a) Facial nerve (after emerging from stylomastoid foramen) in the upper part
   b) External carotid artery in the groove of the lower part (before the artery pierces the gland)

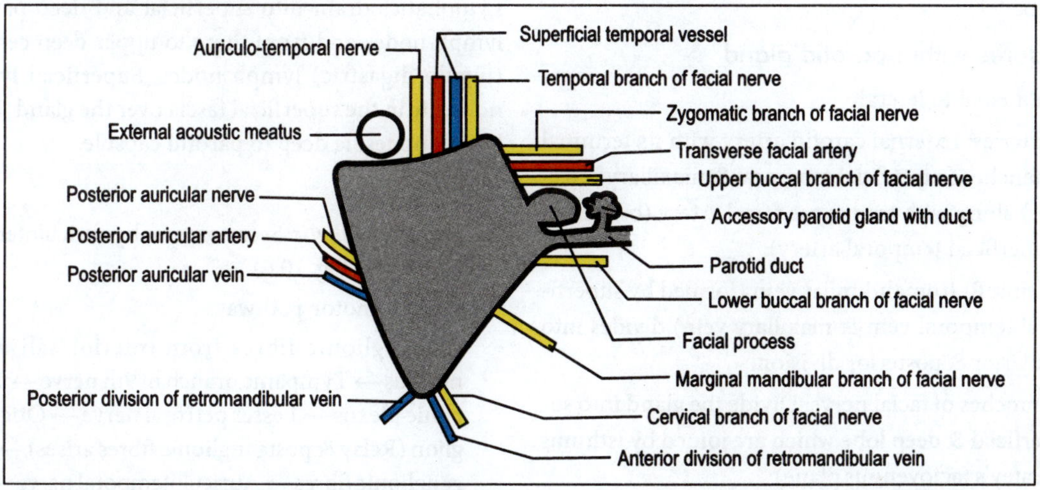

Fig. 10.5: Structures emerging from base, anterior border, apex & posterior border of the parotid gland

Borders

A. **Anterior border**: (Fig. 10.3 & Fig. 10.5)
   1. It separates superficial surface from antero-medial surface
   2. It rests on masseter and extends from front part of the base to the apex.
   3. Structures emerging from this border are from above downwards:
      a) Zygomatic branch of facial nerve
      b) Transverse facial vessels
      c) Upper buccal branch of facial nerve
      d) Accessory parotid gland with duct when present
      e) Parotid duct
      f) Lower buccal branch of facial nerve
      g) Marginal mandibular branch of facial nerve.

B. **Posterior border**:
   1. It separates the superficial surface from posteromedial surface
   2. It lies on sternocleidomastoid
   3. Posterior auricular vessels and nerve emerge deep to this border.

C. **Medial border**: It separates anteromedial from postero-medial surfaces. It is also known as *pharyngeal border* as it is related to lateral wall of pharynx.

Structures within parotid gland

From medial to lateral

a) Arteries: External carotid artery with its terminal branches (superficial temporal & maxillary arteries) along with transverse facial artery (branch of superficial temporal artery).

b) Veins: Retromandibular vein (formed by superficial temporal vein & maxillary vein) divides into anterior & posterior division.

c) Branches of facial nerve: Divide the gland into superficial & deep lobe which are joined by isthmus (Patey's faciovenous plane)

   Process (accessory) of the gland: Facial process, pterygoid process, glenoid process, pre- & post-styloid process.

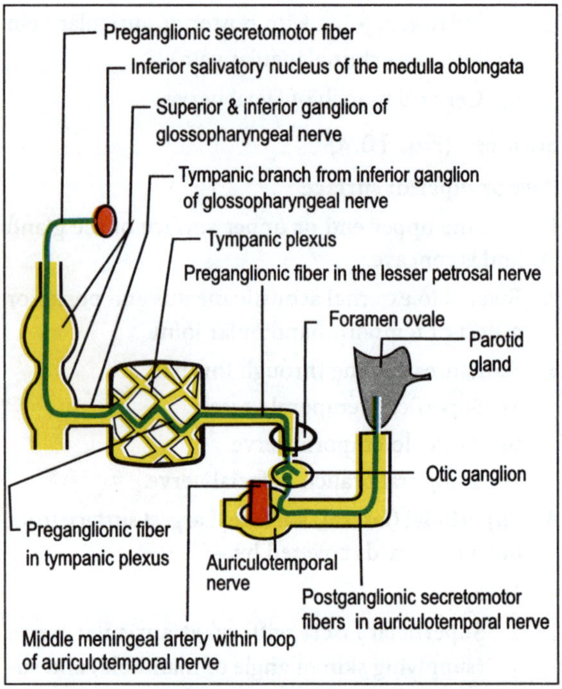

Fig. 10.6: Secretomotor pathway for parotid gland

Blood supply of parotid gland

Arteries are from branches of external carotid and veins drain into external jugular vein.

Lymphatics:

Lymphatics drain into superficial and deep parotid lymph nodes and from there to upper deep cervical (jugulo-digastric) lymph nodes. Superficial lymph nodes lie in the superficial fascia over the gland. Deep lymph nodes lie deep to parotid capsule.

Nerve supply

1. *Parasympathetic*: Secretomotor by auriculotemporal werve. (Fig. 10.6)

   [Secretomotor pathway:

   Preganglionic fibres from inferior salivatory nucleus → Tympanic branch of 9th nerve → Tympanic plexus → Lesser petrosal nerve → Otic ganglion (Relay & postganglionic fibres arises) → Post ganglionic fibres → Auriculotemporal nerve → Parotid gland]

2. *Sympathetic*:
   a) *Vasomotor by post ganglionic fibres from superior cervical ganglion through plexus around external carotid artery.*
3. *Sensory*: By auriculotemporal branch of posterior division of mandibular nerve.

APPLIED ANATOMY

1. Inflammatory swellings are very painful due to
   a) Very tense character of parotidomasseteric fascia and
   b) Also *pressure on branches of facial nerve lying on superficial plane.*
2. **Parotid abscess** may be due to spread of infection from mouth cavity or due to infection of parotid lymph nodes. **Parotitis** (due to **mumps**) is usually due to viral infection.

   Horizontal incision by Hilton's method usually is method of choice for draining the pus in parotid abscess in order to avoid facial nerve injury.
3. Parotid growth always tend to grow on the deeper aspect where the capsule is weak upper part stylomandibular ligament (which extend from styloid process to tympanic plate).
4. In complete removal of the gland the process adopted is following the nerve from behind forwards and the gland is removed in two parts—superficial & deep and nerve to be preserved between the two parts.
5. Auriculotemporal nerve and great auricular nerve are sometimes injured due to penetrating wound. During regenerations of those nerves, secretomotor fibers of auriculotemporal nerve grow & join the great auricular nerve, through which the fibres reach the sweat glands in the face. When the patients eat then secretions comes out from the sweat glands in the face. This syndrome is known as **Frey's syndrome**.

PAROTID DUCT

Parotid duct (Also known as Stenson's duct): (Fig. 10.7): It is a thick walled duct which carries secretion of the parotid gland to vestibule of mouth.

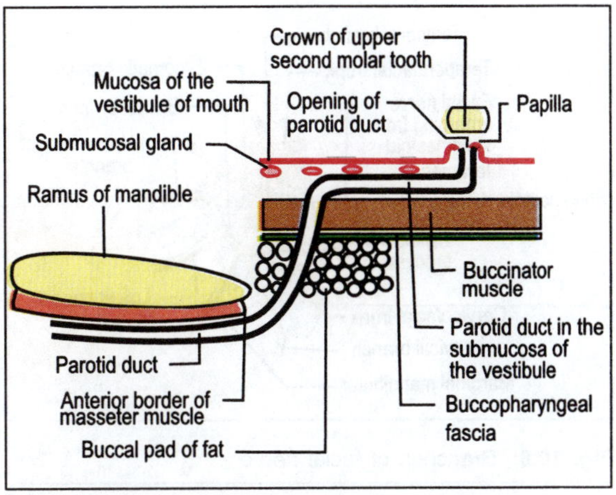

Fig. 10.7: Course & relations of parotid duct

Formation: Formed within the substance of the gland by the union of the two vertical duct (formed by ductules).

Length: 5cm; **Width**: 3mm

Size: About the size of a *crow quill.*

Course

A. Parotid duct is formed by the union of two vertical ducts within the gland.
B. *Point of emergence*: From the middle of anterior border of the parotid gland.
C. It at first runs forwards on the masseter muscle between upper & lower buccal nerves and at the anterior border of the muscle it sharply *bends* medially and pierces successively buccal pad of fat, buccopharyngeal fascia and buccinator muscle. Then it again forms *another bend* and runs forwards between fibres of buccinator and mucous membrane of cheek.

   Finally it forms a *third bend* medially and pierces the mucous membrane and enters the vestibule of mouth and ends.
D. *End*: It ends by opening on the summit of a raised papilla opposite the *crown (projected part of tooth) of upper second molar tooth within the vestibule of mouth.*

Structure of the ducts: Broadly two layers

1. Outer fibroelastic coat with smooth muscles.
2. Inner mucous membrane lined by simple cubical epithelium.

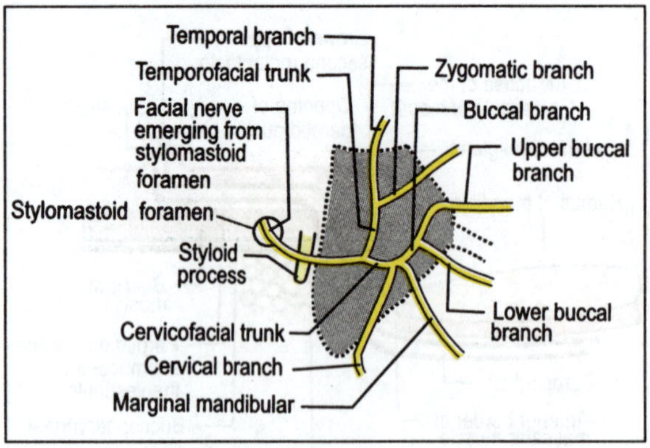

Fig. 10.8: Branches of facial nerve

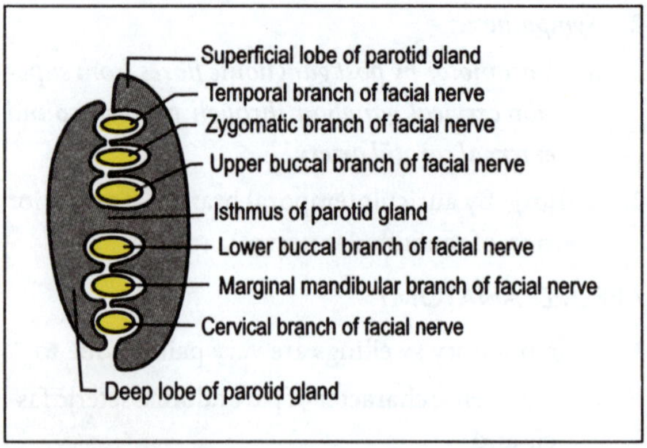

Fig. 10.9: Lobes of the parotid gland

Development: Ectodermal from proximal part of the outgrowth from the angle of stomodeum (Primitive mouth).

DIFFERENT PROCESSES OF THE PAROTID GLAND

1. *Accessory parotid gland and duct*: A small part of gland may be detached from the main gland and is usually situated between zygomatic arch above and parotid duct below.
2. *Facial process*: A triangular projecting part lying superficial to masseter along the parotid duct.
3. *Pterygoid process*: A triangular part between ramus of mandible and medial pterygoid muscle and projecting from deep part of gland.
4. *Glenoid process*: Process of the gland lying between external acoustic meatus and capsule of temporomandibular joint.
5. *Pre and post styloid process*: A groove is formed in the gland by styloid process, prestyloid process is the part in front of the groove and related to internal carotid artery.

   Post-styloid process is the part behind the groove and may be related to internal jugular vein.

STRUCTURES WITH IN GLAND (PASS THROUGH THE GLAND)

From superficial to deep: Structure are arranged in three plane. From superficial to deep, structures are: (1) Facial nerve, (2) Retromandibular rein; (3) External carotid artery.

1. ***Superficial or nervous plane***: Facial nerve emerges from stylomastoid foramen (about 2.5cm deep to midpoint of anterior border of mastoid process) and runs downwards and forward for about 1cm & then the nerve pierces the posteromedial surface of the parotid gland. Within the gland, the nerve passes about 1cm (superficial to retromandibular gland) before dividing into temporofacial and cervico-facial-trunks. The temporofacial subdivides into temporal & zygomatic branches. The cervico facial trunk subdivides into buccal, marginal mandibular and cervical branches.

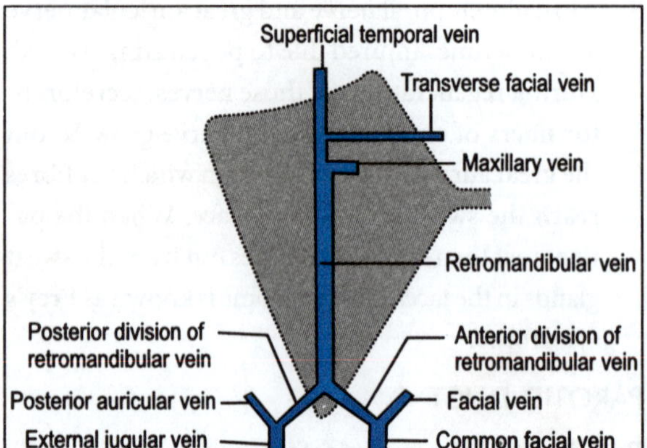

Fig. 10.10: Veins in parotid gland

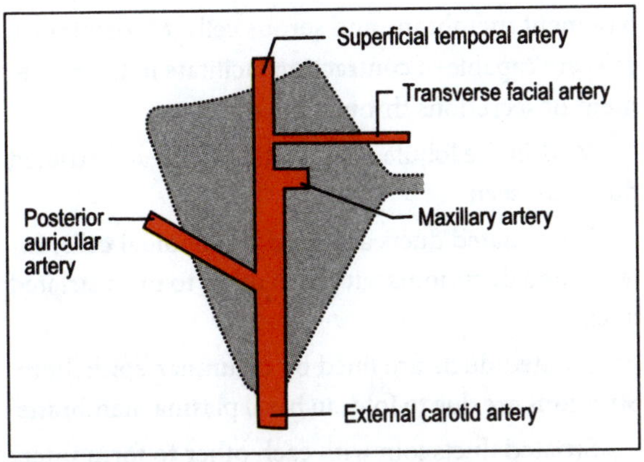

Fig. 10.11: Arteries within parotid gland

Five terminal branches (temporal, zygomatic, buccal, marginal mandibular & cervical) of facial nerve is like goose feet and so this pattern is known as pes anserinus. **Branches of facial nerve divide the gland into superficial and deep part or lobes.** Superficial and deep parts or lobes are connected through isthmus of glandular tissue and the gland appears H-shape in coronal section. Removal of parotid gland with tumour is possible leaving nerve intact as the branches of the nerve lie in between superficial & deep part or lobes. (Fig. 10.8 & Fig. 10.9)

2. ***Intermediate or venous plane*.** Retromandibular vein occupies intermediate zone of gland and its formation by superficial temporal and maxillary veins and ends by dividing into anterior and posterior divisions. Anterior division unites with facial vein to form common facial and posterior division unites with posterior auricular vein to form external jugular vein (Fig. 10.10).
3. ***Arterial plane*.** External carotid artery lie in the deep zone of the gland after piercing posteromedial surface and divide in the substance of gland into superficial temporal and maxillary artery. Superficial temporal here gives transverse facial branch (Fig. 10.11).

Development: The gland is *ectodermal* in development and from *distal expanded end of the out growth from the angle of primitive mouth* (stomodeum) and it undergoes division and subdivision and form *acini* and *duct system*.

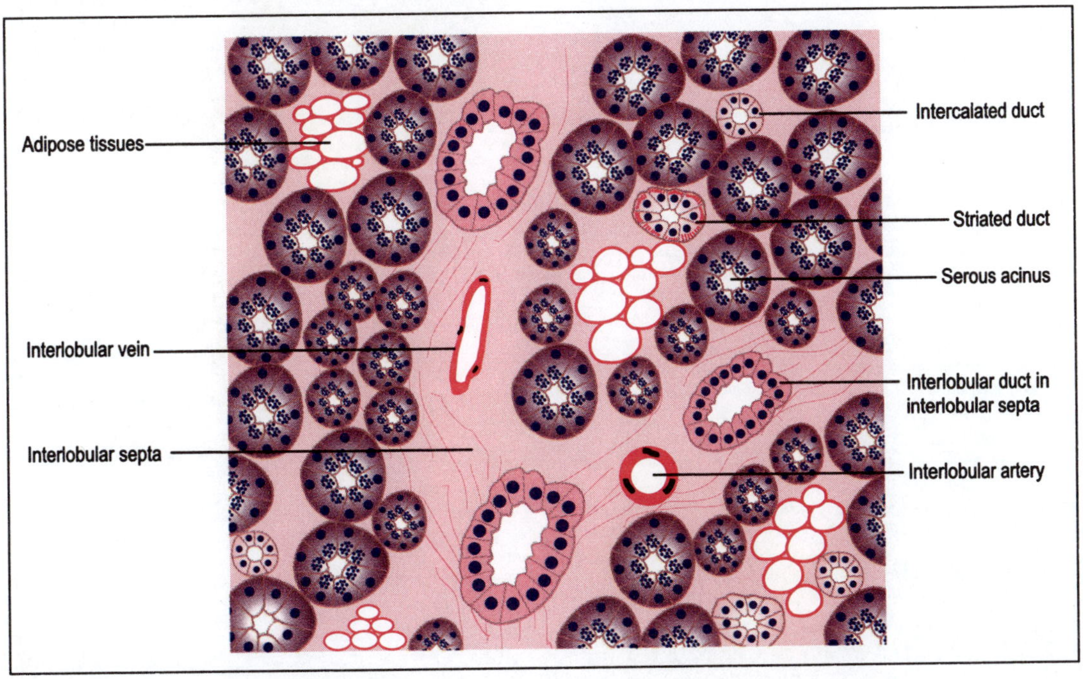

Fig. 10.12: Histology of parotid gland

HISTOLOGY OF PAROTID GLAND

Parotid gland is invested by the capsule (connective tissue) which enter into the gland to divide into numerous lobules. (Fig. 10.12)

This is a compound, acinar, serous exocrine gland.

Secretory tissue or the parenchyma of the gland is divided by irregular connective tissue. Interlobular connective tissue contains blood vessels, nerves and interlobular excretory duct. Interlobular duct is lined by tall columnar epithelium.

Secretory tissue consists of mainly serous acini. The serious acini are lined by pyramidal cells. Rounded nucleus is placed in the basal half of cell. Basophilic zymogen granules are present in the supranuclear portion. Myoepithelial cells are present in between basement membrane and serous cells. Myoepithelial cells are capable of contraction facilitate in the movement of secretions through the ducts.

Within the lobule, many intercalated and striated ducts are seen.

Intercalated ducts are lined by cuboidal cells. Intercalated ducts joins with each other to form striated duct.

Striated ducts are lined by columnar epithelium. Striations are due to folds in basal plasma membrane.

Striated ducts join with each other to form interlobular duct.

Interlobular duct joins with each other to form parotid duct.

Adipose tissues are present in between secretory tissues.

chapter 11

Pharyngeal Apparatus

AT A GLANCE

- *Introduction pharyngeal apparatus*
- *Derivatives of pharyngeal arched*
- *Derivatives of pharyngeal pouches*
- *Pharyngeal clefts*
- *Branchial cyst & fistula*
- *First arch syndrome: Treacher Collins syndrome; Pierre Robin syndrome*

PHARYNGEAL APPARATUS

- **Pharyngeal apparatus** form the neck and some structures of head region. It starts developing between the stomatodaeum and pericardial cavity. Pharyngeal apparatus consist of pharyngeal arches, pharyngeal pouch and pharyngeal clefts.
- **Pharyngeal arches or branchial arches**: A series of mesodermal thickening lined on outside by ectoderm and on inside by endoderm. There are six arches initially, but soon fifth arch disappear.
- **Structures of a pharyngeal arch**: Each pharyngeal arch is having three layers:

  Outside: Lined by ectoderm.

  Inside: Lined by endoderm.

  Intermediate: Mesoderm (derived from paraxial, lateral plate mesoderm and neural crest cells).

Components of pharyngeal arches

The mesenchymes of each pharyngeal arch forms following components:

a) Skeletal component
b) Muscular component
c) Arterial component
d) Nerve supply

Pharyngeal pouch

There are outward bulging of endoderm (internally) in between pharyngeal arches which are known as pharyngeal pouch or endodermal pouch (internally).

Pharyngeal cleft or ectodermal cleft

Depressions (ectodermal) externally in between arches are known as pharyngeal cleft.

Pharyngeal cleft is present at the same site of pharyngeal pouch.

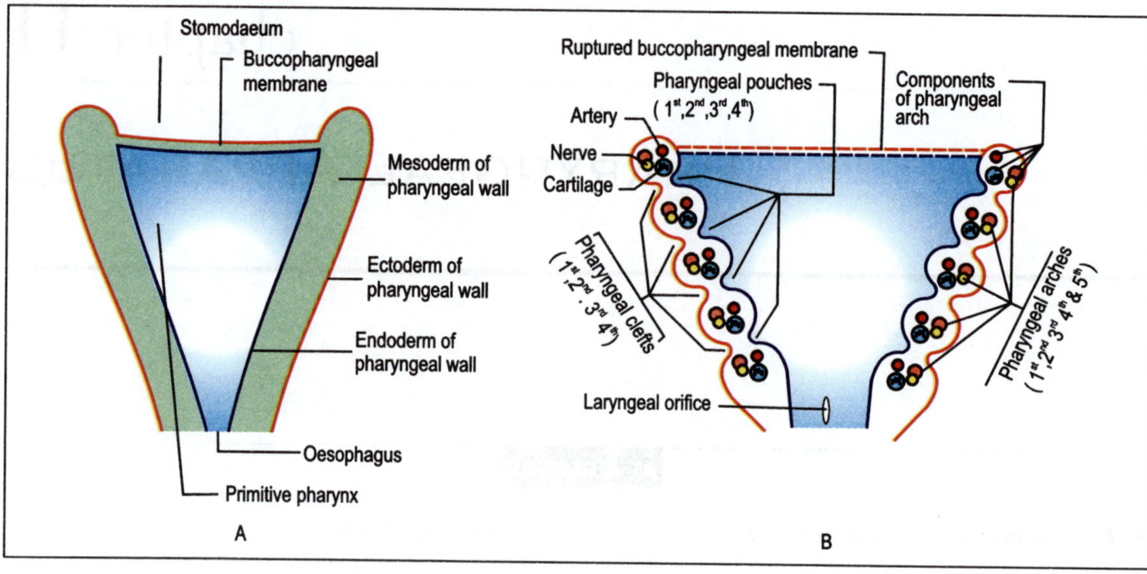

Fig. 11.1: Coronal section of primitive pharynx. A – Before formation of pharyngeal arches; B – After formation of pharyngeal arch

Structures of pharyngeal pouch and pharyngeal cleft

Bilaminar membrane

- Ectoderm (externally) close to each other.
- Endoderm (internally) close to each other.
- No mesoderm.
- Mesoderm appear, in the latter part of development in the 1st pharyngeal cleft which sill produce tympanic membrane.

PHARYNGEAL ARCHES

Pharyngeal arches grow ventrally and fuse with each other to form floor of the developing pharynx.

DERIVATIVES OF PHARYNGEAL ARCHES OR BRANCHIAL ARCHES

FIRST PHARYNGEAL ARCH OR MANDIBULAR ARCH (Fig. 11.1)

Skeletal derivatives

Cartilage of first pharyngeal arch is called **Meckel's cartilage. Dorsal end** of the Meckel's cartilage is related with developing ear and forms **malleus** and **incurs.**

- **Middle part** of the Meckel's cartilage forms **anterior ligament of malleus** and **sphenomandibular ligament.** (Fig. 11.2)
- **Ventral part** of the cartilage disappear.

First pharyngeal arch also develop maxillary prominence (its mesenchyme gives rise mandible, maxilla, zygomatic bone and squamous part of temporal bone.

Muscular derivatives

Muscles are:

- Muscles of mastication (temporalis, masseter, and pterygoids, and
- Anterior belly of digastric, mylohyoid, tensor tympani and tensor palatini.

Nerves of first arch

Mandibular nerve is nerve of first branchial arch.

Lingual branch of mandibular nerve is the posttramatic branch of first arch.

Chorda tympanic nerve (branch facial nerve) is the pretrematic branch of first arch.

Artery of first arch: Maxillary artery.

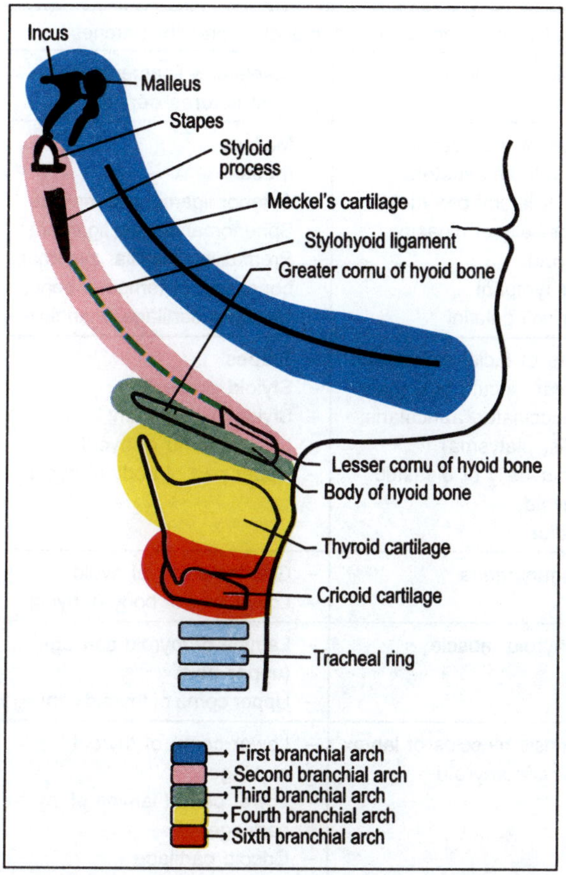

Fig. 11.2: Structures formed by the cartilaginous components of the pharyngeal arches

SECOND PHARYNGEAL OR BRANCHIAL ARCH

Skeletal derivatives

Cartilage of second pharyngeal arch is **hyoid arch** (also known as Reichert's cartilage).

Cartilage of second arch forms the following:

1. Stapes
2. Styloid process of the temporal bone
3. Stylohyoid ligament
4. Lesser cornu & superior part of the body of hyoid bone.

Muscular derivatives:

The muscles are:

- Stapedius
- Stylohyoid
- Posterior belly of digastric
- Auricular muscles
- Muscles of facial expression

Nerve of second arch

Facial nerve is the nerve of second pharyngeal or branchial arch.

Chorda tympani (branch of facial nerve) is the pretrematic nerve of first arch.

Artery of second arch: Hyoid and stapedial arteries.

THIRD PHARYNGEAL OR BRANCHIAL ARCH

Skeletal derivatives

Cartilage of third pharyngeal arch forms:

- Greater cornu of hyoid
- Lower part of the body of hyoid

Muscular derivatives

The only muscle is stylopharyngeus

Nerve of third pharyngeal or branchial arch

Nerve of the third pharyngeal muscle is glossopharyngeal nerve.

Arteries of third arch:

a) Common carotid artery
b) Internal carotid artery

FOURTH PHARYNGEAL ARCH

Skeletal derivatives

- Upper cornu of thyroid cartilage
- Upper part of lamina of thyroid cartilage.

Muscular derivatives

- Cricothyroid muscle

Artery of fourth pharyngeal arch

- Left side: Arch of aorta from the left common carotid artery to the left subclavian artery.
- Right side: Right subclavian artery (proximal part).

Table 11.1: Structures derived from skeletal and muscular components of pharyngeal or branchial arches

Pharyngeal or branchial arch	Nerve of the arch	Muscles derived	Skeletal & ligamentous structures derived
1. First (Mandibular arch)	Mandibular nerve	– Muscles of mastication (temporalis, masseter, medial & lateral pterygoids) – Anterior belly of digastric – Mylohyoid – Tensor tympani – Tensor veli palatini	– Malleus – Incus – Anterior ligament of malleus – Sphenomandibular ligament – Premaxilla, maxilla, zygomatic bone, part of temporal bone, Meckle's cartilage, mandible
2. Second (Hyoid arch)	Facial nerve	– Muscles of facial expression (orbicularis oculi, orbicularis oris, buccinator, auricularis, frontalis, platysma) – Posterior belly of digastric – Stylohyoid, – Stapedius	– Stapes – Styloid process – Stylohyoid ligament – Lesser cornu of hyoid – Upper part of body of hyoid
3. 3rd	Glossopharyngeal nerve	– Stylopharyngeus	– Greater cornu of hyoid – Lower part of body of hyoid
4. 4th	Superior laryngeal nerve	– Cricothyroid muscle	– Lamina of thyroid cartilage (upper part) – Upper cornu of thyroid cartilage
5. 6th	Recurrent laryngeal nerve	– All intrinsic muscles of larynx except cricothyroid	– Lower cornu of thyroid cartilage – Lower part of lamina of thyroid cartilage – Cricoid cartilage • Arytenoid cartilage • Corniculate cartilage • Cuneiform cartilage

Nerve of the fourth pharyngeal arch

- External laryngeal nerve branch of superior laryngeal nerve

FIFTH PHARYNGEAL ARCH

It disappear in early stage

SIXTH PHARYNGEAL ARCH

Skeletal derivatives

- Lower cornu of thryroid cartilage
- Lower part of lamina of thyroid cartilage
- Cricoid cartilage
- Arytenoid cartilage
- Corniculate cartilage
- Cuneiform cartilage

Muscular derivative

- All the intrinsic muscles of larynx except cricothyroid.

Artery of sixth pharyngeal arch

- Left side: Left pulmonary artery and ductus arteriosus.
- Right side: Right pulmonary artery.

Nerve of the sixth pharyngeal arch

- Recurrent laryngeal nerve

PHARYNGEAL POUCHES

There are four pair of pouches. These pouches are lined by endoderm. Endodermal lining of the pouches give rise to important organs. Fifth pouch is rudimentary. (Fig. 11.3)

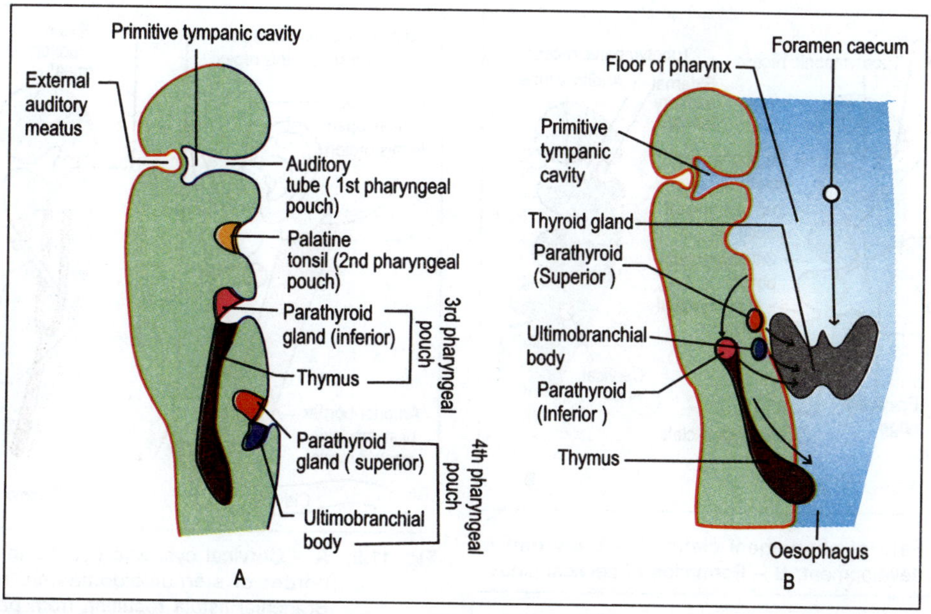

Fig. 11.3: Pharyngeal pouches: A – Structures formed by pouches; B – Migration of structures of the pouches

First pharyngeal pouch:

First pharyngeal pouch forms **tubotympanic recess**, which comes in contact with ectodermal lining of first pharyngeal cleft. The distal part of tubotympanic recess widens to form **middle ear cavity** and **mastoid antrum**.

Tubotympanic recess also form proximal part of auditory tube; and also form tympanic membrane which comes in contact with first pharyngeal cleft.

This pouch lies in between first and second arch.

Second pharyngeal pouch:

The endoderm of second pharyngeal pouch proliferates and form bud that invade to surrounding mesoderm. The buds are secondarily invaded by mesoderm to form **palatine tonsil**. Part of the pouch remains as **tonsillar fossa.**

Second pharyngeal pouch lies in between second and third arches.

Third pharyngeal pouch:

The distal extremity of the third pharyngeal pouch differentiate into dorsal part and ventral part.

Endoderm of the dorsal part give rise to **inferior parathyroid gland.** Endoderm ventral part proliferate to form **thymus.**

Third pharyngeal pouch lies in between second and fourth pharyngeal pouch.

Fourth pharyngeal pouch

Endoderm of the fourth pharyngeal pouch differentiate into ventral and dorsal part.

Endoderm of the ventral part of fourth pharyngeal pouch give rise to **ultimo branchial body.** Cells of the ultimo branchial body incorporate into the thyroid gland and give rise to **parafollicular** cells.

Endoderm of the dorsal part of the fourth pharyngeal pouch gives rise **superior parathyroid gland.**

PHARYNGEAL CLEFT OR GROOVE

There are four pairs of pharyngeal cleft.

First pharyngeal cleft give rise to external auditory meatus and outer layer (ectodermal) of tympanic membrane.

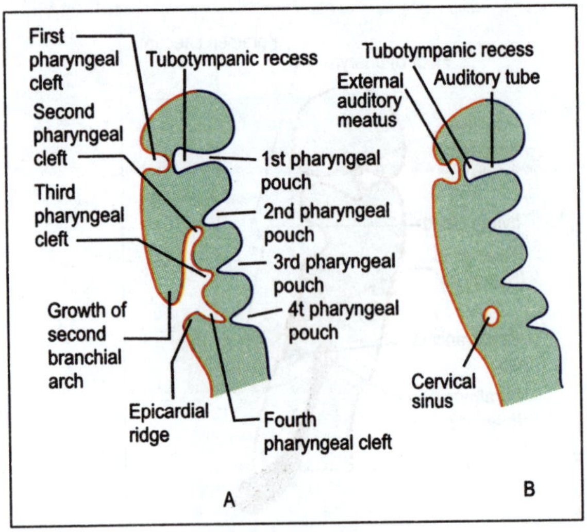

Fig. 11.4: Fate of pharyngeal clefts: A – Early part of development; B – Formation of cervical sinus

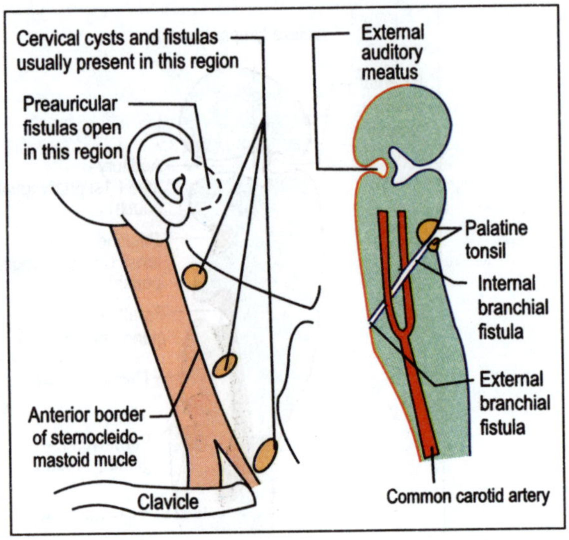

Fig. 11.5: A – Cervical cyst and fistulas in the anterior border of sternocleidomastoid muscle; B – Branchial fistula resulting from persistence of part of second pharyngeal pouch and second pharyngeal cleft

Second, third and fourth pharyngeal cleft: The mesenchyme of second pharyngeal arch grows rapidly downward, overlaps second, third and fourth pharyngeal cleft and fuses with epicardia ridge. Second, third and fourth cleft join with other to form slit like cavity—cervical sinus (lined by ectoderm) get buried under surface and eventually disappears in normal condition as neck develops. (Fig. 11.4)

BRANCHIAL CYST

The mesenchyme of the second pharyngeal arch grows rapidly downwards over second, third and fourth pharyngeal clefts to fuse with epicardial ridge. Second, third and fourth pharyngeal cleft join with each other to form cervical sinus. It (cervical sinus) lie deep to second arch. Cervical sinus is lined by ectoderm. As the neck develops cervical sinus disappear normally, but sometimes cervical sinus fails to obliterate, eventually it forms branchial cyst.

Branchial cyst appears along the anterior border sternocleidomastoid at the following points:

1. Below and behind of angle of mandible.
2. At the junction of the upper one-third and lower two-third. (Fig. 11.5)

BRANCHIAL FISTULA

Branchial fistula is formed after the rupture of branchial cyst. Branchial fistula (external) is usually found along the anterior border of sternocleidomastoid.

Internal branchial fistula opens into the tonsillar sinus of pharyngeal membrane in the second pharyngeal cleft second pharyngeal pouch and passes between internal and external carotid arteries.

FIRST ARCH SYNDROMES

Due to lock of migration of neural crest cells into first pharyngeal arch, there develops first arch syndrome.

First arch syndromes (few) are Treacher Collins syndrome, Pierre Robin syndrome and DiGeorge syndrome.

TREACHER COLLINS SYNDROME

It is an autosomal dominant trait (due to autosomal dominant gene). It occurs in 1/85,000 births.

Clinical presentation:

- Molar hypoplasia (due to small zygomatic bone)
- Mandibular hypoplasia.
- Deformed external ear.

PIERRE ROBIN SYNDROME

It is an autosomal recessive disorder and occurs in 1/85,000 birth.

Clinical presentations:

- Small mandible (micrognathia)
- Cleft palate

DIGEORGE SYNDROME

This is due to deletion of long arm of chromosome 22. It occurs in 1/25,000 births.

Clinical presentations:

- Thymus and parathyroid glands are absent.
- Fish mouth deformity (shortened philtrum).

WHY RIGHT RECURRENT LARYNGEAL NERVE HOOKS BELOW RIGHT SUBCLAVIAN ARTERY AND LEFT RECURRENT LARYNGEAL NERVE HOOKS BELOW LIGAMENTUM ARTERIOSUM?

During the early part of development, the right recurrent laryngeal nerve (nerve of 6th pharyngeal arch)

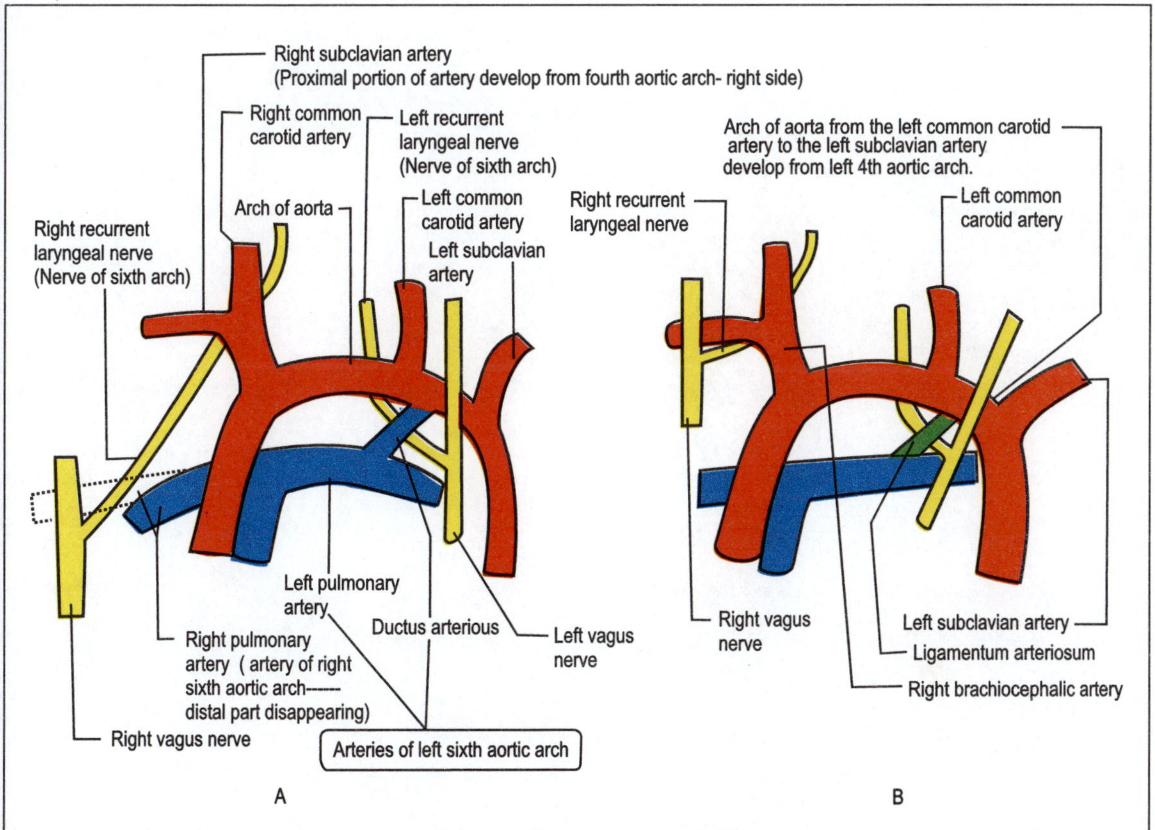

Fig. 11.6: A – Right recurrent laryngeal nerve (nerve of 6th pharyngeal arch) hooks below distal part of right pulmonary artery (artery of right 6th aortic arch) and left recurrent laryngeal nerve hooks below ductus arteriosus (artery of left 6th aortic arch); B – After disappearance of distal part of right pulmonary artery the right recurrent nerve ascends up and hooks below right subclavian artery (artery of right 4th aortic arch). Left recurrent laryngeal nerve remains in place and hooks around the ligamentum arteriosum (remnant of ductus arteriosus)

hooks below right pulmonary artery (artery of right 6th aortic arch). Left recurrent laryngeal nerve (nerve of 6th pharyngeal arch) hooks below ductus arteriosus (artery of 6th aortic arch).

During early development 5th arch disappear completely.

After the disappearance of distal part of right pulmonary artery, the right recurrent laryngeal nerve ascends up and hooks around the right subclavian artery (artery of right 4th aortic arch). On the left, the nerve remains in place and hooks around ligamentum arteriosum (remnant of ductus arteriosus—artery of 6th aortic arch)(Fig. 11.6).

chapter 12

TEMPORAL AND INFRATEMPORAL REGIONS

AT A GLANCE

- *Temporal region*
- *Infratemporal region*
- *Pterygopalatine fossa*
- *Muscles of mastications*
- *Maxillary artery with its branches*
- *Mandibular nerve with its branches*
  - *Applied anatomy*
- *Maxillary nerve*
- *Pterygopalatine ganglion*
- *Otic ganglion*
- *Temporomandibular joint*

TEMPORAL REGION

Boundaries: (Fig. 12.1)

In front: Frontal process of zygomatic bone.

Behind: Supramastoid crest.

Superiorly: Superior temporal line.

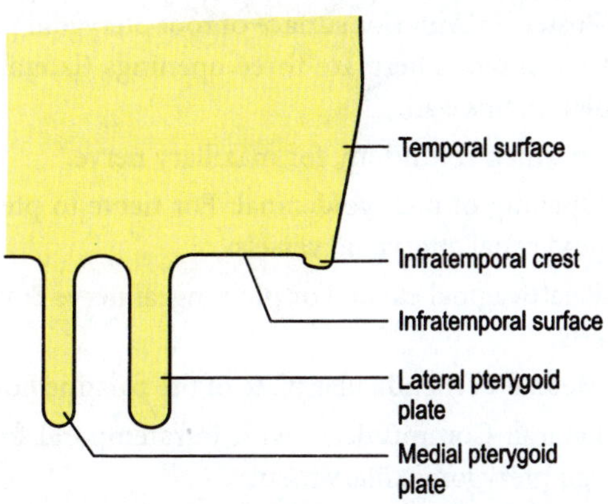

Fig. 12.1: Infratemporal & temporal surface of the sphenoid bone (Coronal section)

Inferiorly: Communicate with infratemporal fossa through deep to zygomatic arch.

Floor: Parts of parietal, frontal, temporal and greater wing of sphenoid bone. Pterion is present here. Temporalis muscle is attached here.

Contents:

1. Temporalis muscle and its covering fascia.
2. Deep temporal nerve and vessels.
3. Superficial temporal vessel.
4. Auriculo temporal nerve.

Temporal fascia: It is strong fascia which covers the temporalis muscle and attached to the superior temporal line. It splits into two layer just above the zygomatic arch and attached to outer and inner margin of zygomatic arch. Deep surface gives origin to temporalis muscle. Superficial surface is closely related galea aponeurotica. Superficial surface is related to superficial temporal vessels, auriculotemporal nerve and temporal branch of facial nerve. Auricularis anterior and auricularis superior takes origin from superficial surface.

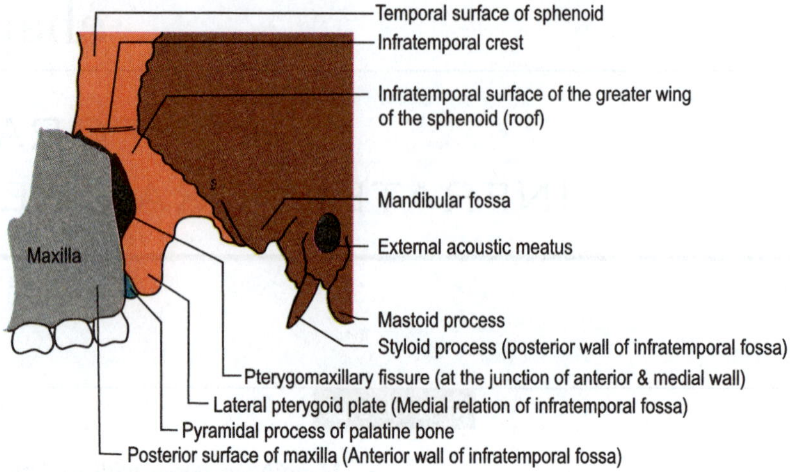

Fig. 12.2: Temporal & infratemporal fossa

INFRATEMPORAL REGION (Fig. 12.2)

This region lies below zygomatic arch.

Boundaries:

Anteriorly: Posterior surface of body of the maxilla.

Posteriorly: Styloid process.

Medially: Lateral pterygoid plate with pyramidal process of the palatine bone. It is separated from anterior wall by pterygomaxillary fissure.

Laterally: Ramus of the mandible with its coronoid process.

Superiorly: Infratemporal surface of greater wing of sphenoid. Foramen spinosum and foramen ovale can be seen in this surface.

Inferiorly: Open and continuous with spaces around pharynx and oesophagus.

Communications of the region

Anteriorly: With the orbit through inferior orbital fissure.

Medially: With pterygopalatine fossa through pterygomaxillary fissure.

Superolaterally: With temporal fossa through the space medial to zygomatic arch.

Superiorly: With middle cranial fossa through foramina ovale & spinosum.

Contents:

1. Medial & lateral pterygoid muscle.
2. Mandibular nerve and its branches, otic ganglion with its connections, chorda tympani nerve.
3. Maxillary artery (1st & 2nd part) & its branches & accompanying veins pterygoid venous plexus.
4. Maxillary nerve with posterior superior alveolar nerve. (Fig. 12.2)

PTERYGOPALATINE FOSSA (Fig. 12.3)

Deep to pterygomaxillary fissure, there lies pterygopalatine fossa.

Boundaries:

Anterior: Posterior surface of maxilla.

Posterior: Anterior surface of root pterygoid process sphenoid. There are three openings (lateral to medial) in this wall:

1. Foramen rotundum, for maxillary nerve.
2. Opening of pterygoid canal: For nerve to pterygoid canal, pterygoid vessels.
3. Palatovaginal canal: For pharyngeal nerve & vessels.

Medial: Perpendicular plate of the palatine bone.

Lateral: Communicate with infratemporal fossa though pterygomaxillary fissure.

Superiorly: Body of sphenoid (medial part) and lateral part inferior orbital fissure (through which the fossa communicate with orbit).

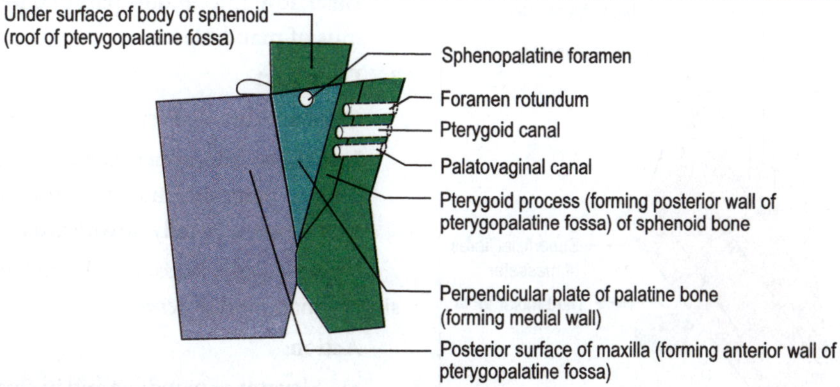

Fig. 12.3: Pterygopalatine fossa

Inferiorly: Where anterior and posterior wall meets.

Contents:

1. Maxillary nerve & its branches with pterygopalatine ganglion.
2. Maxillary artery (third part) and its branches.

MUSCLES OF MASTICATION (Fig. 12.4)

There are four muscles of mastication: Masseter, temporalis, medial and lateral pterygoid muscles.

Masseter: A quadrilateral muscle covering the ramus of mandible.

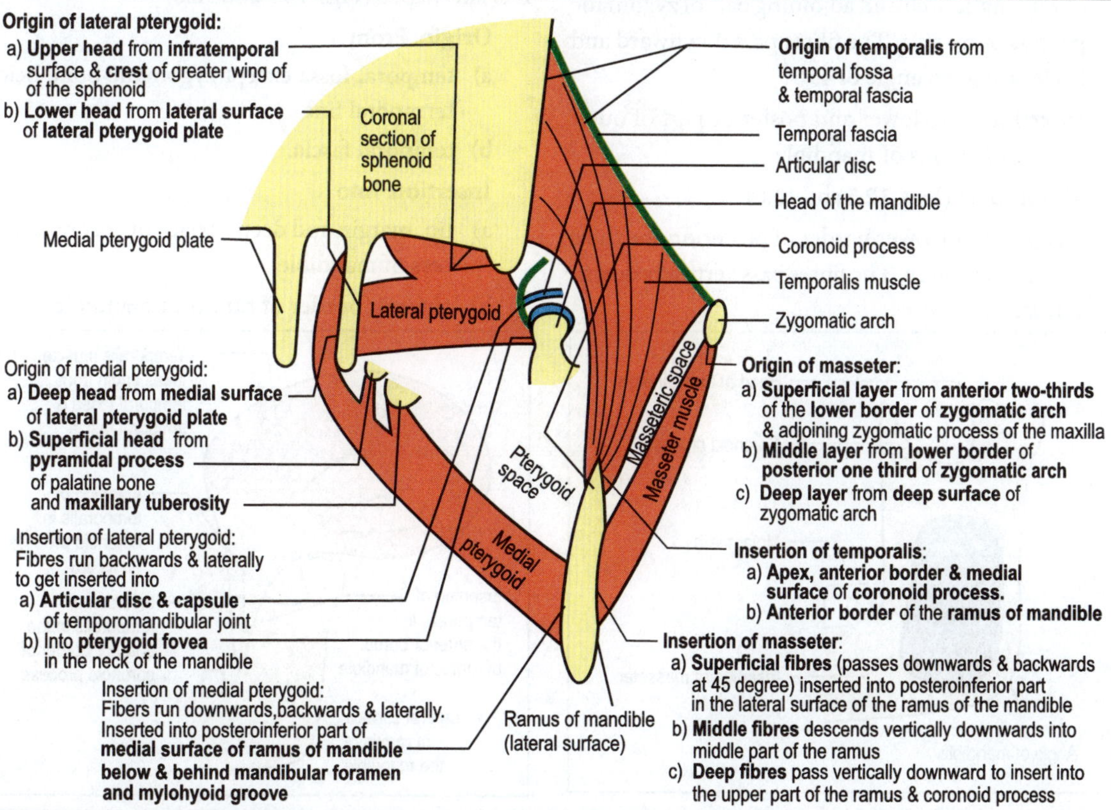

Fig. 12.4: Muscles of mastications (origins & insertions) in coronal section

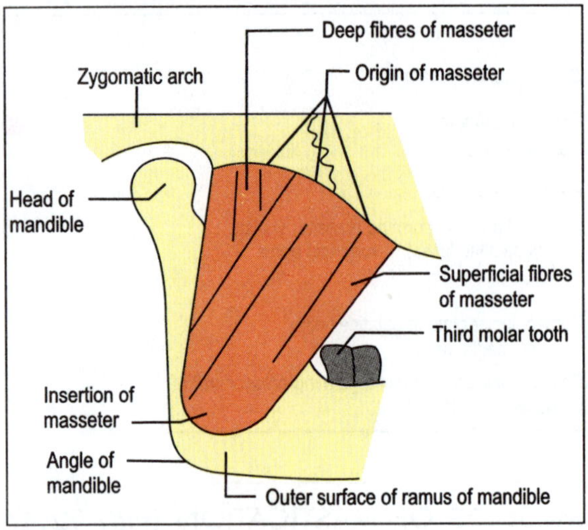

Fig. 12.5: Masseter muscle

Different parts: Three:

1. **Superficial part**

   Origin: From anterior two thirds of lower border of zygomatic arch and adjoining part of zygomatic process of maxilla. The fibres pass downward and backward at an angle of 45°.

   Insertion: Into lower and posterior part of outer surface of ramus of mandible.

2. **Middle part** (Figs. 12.5 and 12.6)

   Origin: From lower border of posterior one third of zygomatic arch. The fibres pass vertically downwards.

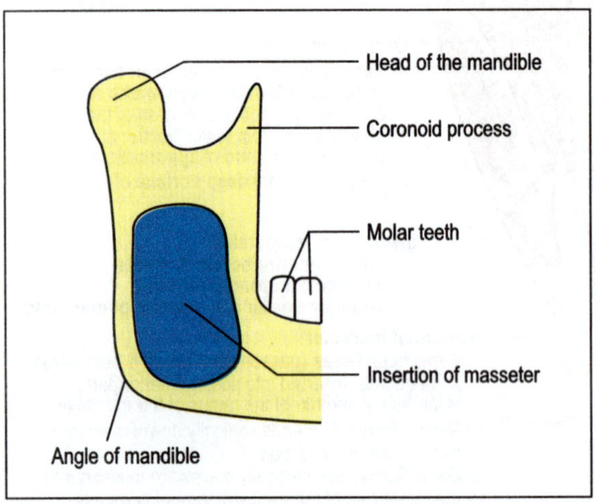

Fig. 12.6: Insertion of the masseter

   Insertion: Into middle part of outer surface of ramus of mandible.

3. **Deep part**

   Origin: From deep surface of zygomatic arch.

   Insertion: Into upper part of outer surface of ramus of mandible and its coronoid process. The fibres pass vertically downwards.

   Nerve supply: Masseteric branch of anterior division of mandibular nerve.

   Action:

   a) Elevator of mandible and in closing the mouth.

   b) Superficial fibres – protractor.
      Deep fibres – retractor of mandible.

Applied anatomy:

Trismus or locked jaw is a condition due to tonic spasm of both masseters specially occurs in tetanus.

Temporalis:

It is fan shaped (Figs. 12.7 and 12.8)

Origin: From

a) temporal fossa except zygomatic bone below termporal line

b) temporal fascia.

Insertion: Into

a) tip, margin and deep surface of coronoid process of mandible

b) anterior border of ramus of mandible.

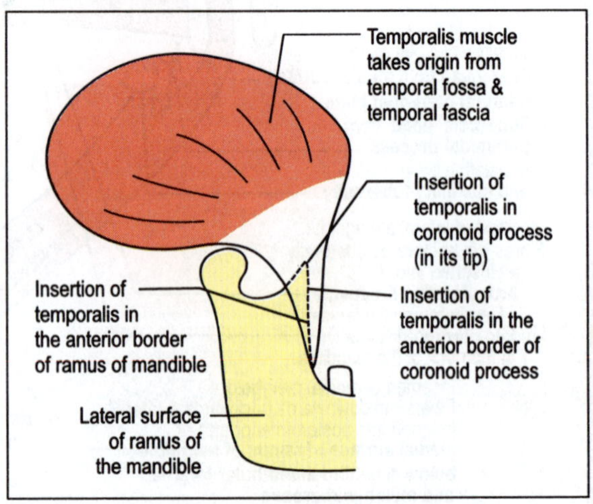

Fig. 12.7: Temporalis muscle

Table 12.1: Muscles of mastication

Muscle	Origin	Insertion	Nerve supply	Action
1. Masseter: Quadrilateral, covers the outer surface of ramus of mandible, has three layers.	1. Superficial layer: From lower border of zygomatic arch (anterior 2/3rd) & adjoining part of zygomatic process of maxilla. Fibres passes downwards & backward at an angle of 45° 2. Middle layer: From lower border (posterior 1/3rd) of the zygomatic arch. Fibres pass vertically downward 3. Deep layer: From deep surface of zygomatic arch	1. Superficial layer into lower and posterior part of the outer surface of ramus of mandible. 2. Middle layer into middle of the mandibular ramus 3. Deep layer – into upper, and anterior part of the lateral surface of the ramus of mandible (fibers pass vertically downwards)	Masseteric nerve, a branch of anterior division of mandibular nerve	a) Elevate the mandible. b) Superficial fibres help in protraction
2. Temporalis: Fan shaped muscle, lie in the temporal fossa	a) From the floor of the temporal fossa below the inferior temporal line except zygomatic bone b) From temporal fascia: Anterior fibres pass vertically, middle obliquely, posterior fibres horizontally. All fibres converge and pass through gap deep to zygomatic arch	Inserted into tip, medial surface and anterior border of coronoid process. Also into anterior border of ramus of the mandible	Two deep temporal branches from anterior division of mandibular nerve	1. Elevates the mandible 2. Both side temporalis helps in side to side grinding movement 3. Posterior fibres retract the protruded mandible
3. Medial pterygoid – Quadrilateral & consist of superficial & deep head	a) Superficial head: From tuberosity of maxilla and pyramidal process of palatine bone b) Deep head: From medial surface of lateral pterygoid plate. Fibers passes downwards, backwards & laterally	Fibres are inserted by tendinous lamina into roughened area on the medial surface of the ramus and angle of the mandible, below and behind mandibular foramen and mylohyoid groove	Nerve to medial the pterygoid, branch of the main trunk of mandibular nerve	– Elevate the mandible – Protrude the mandible & alternate contraction (in combination with lateral pterygoid) produce side to side chewing movements
4. Lateral pterygoid: Key muscle of infratemporal region. Conical, has upper & lower heads	a) Upper head: From infratemporal surface & crest of greater wing of the sphenoid b) Lower head: From the lateral surface of lateral pterygoid plate. Fibers proceed backward and laterally and converge to form a tendon	To a pterygoid fovea (depression) in front of neck of the mandible and partly to the capsule and articular disc of temporomandibular joint	A branch of the anterior division of mandibular nerve	– Depress the mandible to open the mouth – In combination with medial pterygoid of both side protrude the mandible – Upper head act for chewing & lower head protrude the mandible – Lateral & medial pterygoid of both side when contract alternately produce side to side chewing movement

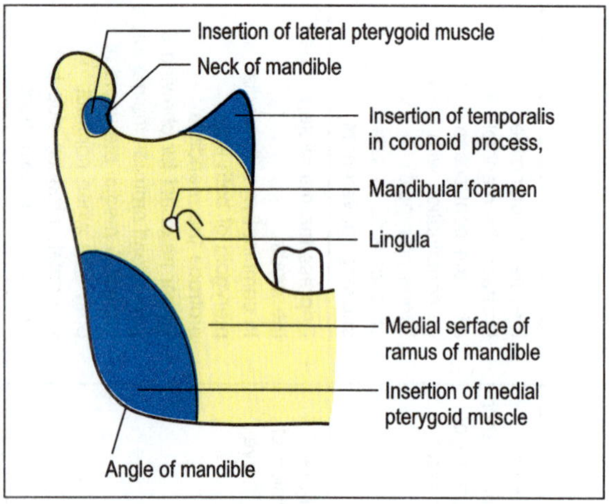

Fig. 12.8: Insertions of the lateral pterygoid, temporalis and medial pterygoid muscles

Nerve supply: Deep temporal branches of anterior division of mandibular nerve.

Action:

a) Elevates the mandible quickly and closes the mouth

Table 12.2: Relations of pterygoids (medial & lateral)

Medial pterygoid	Lateral pterygoid
Lateral surface: – Lateral pterygoid muscle – Sphenomandibular ligament – Maxillary artery – Inferior alveolar vessels & nerve – Lingual nerve – A portion of parotid gland – Masseter – Ramus of the mandible – Tendon of the temporalis **Medial surface**: – Tensor veli palatini – Superior constrictor of pharynx – Styloglossus & stylopharyngeus – Submandibular gland	**Superficial**: (outside inwards) Masseter, ramus of mandible, tendon of temporalis, maxillary artery **Deep**: Mandibular nerve, chorda tympani nerve, middle meningeal artery, sphenomandibular ligament, deep head of medial pterygoid **Upper border**: Deep temporal & masseteric nerve **Lower border**: Lingual nerve, inferior alveolar nerve, middle meningeal artery, sphenomandibular ligament **In between two heads of muscle**: a) Maxillary artery (junction of 2nd & 3rd part) b) Buccal nerve

b) Posterior fibres act as retractor of protruded mandible.

c) Muscles of both sides help in side to side grinding movement.

Pterygoid muscles – Lateral and Medial

Lateral pterygoid:

It is key muscle of infratemporal fossa. Short thick muscles with two heads.

Origin:

a) Upper head: From infratemporal surface and crest of greater wing of sphenoid bone.

b) Lower head: From lateral surface of lateral pterygoid plate of sphenoid bone.

Insertion: The fibres of two heads run backward and laterally to form tendon which is inserted into:

a) **Pterygoid fovea** in front of neck of the mandible.

b) Articular capsule and disc of temporomandibular joint.

Relations: Superficial from outside inwards:

a) Masseter (Fig. 12.9)

b) Ramus of mandible

c) Maxillary artery

d) Temporalis (may pass tendon deep to it)

Deep:

a) Mandibular nerve and branches

b) Chorda tympani nerve

c) Medial pterygoid muscle

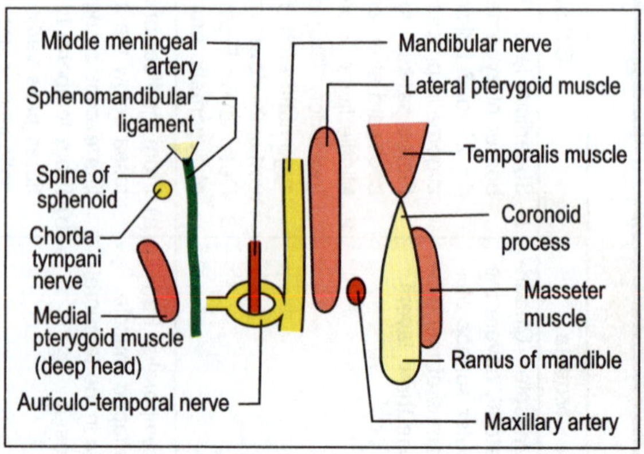

Fig. 12.9: Relations of the lateral pterygoid muscle

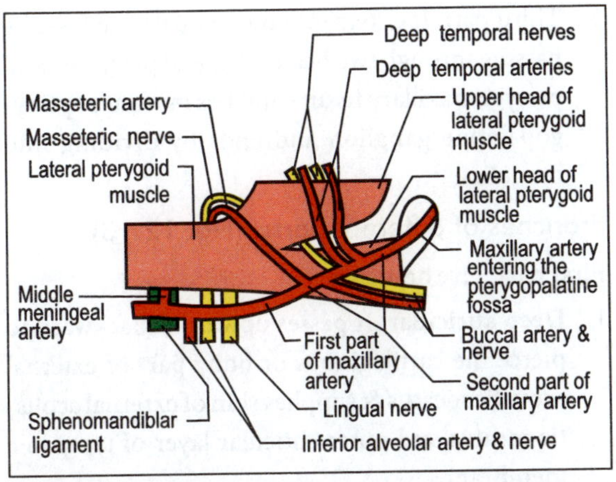

Fig. 12.10: Relations of upper & lower borders of the lateral pterygoid muscle

d) Sphenomandibular ligament
e) Middle meningeal artery. (Fig. 12.10)

Upper border: Deep temporal and masseteric branches of mandibular nerve.

Deep temporal and masseteric vessels

Lower border:

a) Middle meningeal artery
b) Lingual and inferior alveolar nerves
c) Sphenomandibular ligament.

In between two heads of muscle pass

a) Maxillary artery
b) Buccal nerve

Action:

1. Depressions of mandible by pulling forward the head along with articular disc and thus opens the mouth.
2. Protrusion of mandible by the action of lateral and medial pterygoid of both sides. Lower head helps in protrusion. Upper head act for chewing.
3. Side to side chewing movements by alternate action of both the pterygoids of one side with that of other side.

Nerve supply: By a branch of anterior division of mandibular nerve.

Medial pterygoid:

It is a thick quadrilateral muscle.

Origin: By two heads

a) Deep head: From the medial surface of lateral pterygoid plate.
b) Superficial head: From tuberosity of maxilla and lateral surface of pyramidal process of palatine bone.

Insertion: The fibers run downwards, backwards & laterally to be inserted by a tendinous lamina into posteroinferior part of the medial surface of the ramus of the mandible in between mandibular foramen, mylohyoid line & angle of the mandible.

Nerve supply: A branch from the trunk of mandibular nerve before division [This branch also supplies tensor veli palatini and tensor tympani muscle].

Relation: (Fig. 12.11)

A. Lateral surface: Ramus of mandible separated by
   a) Lateral pterygoid
   b) Sphenomandibular ligament
   c) Maxillary artery
   d) Inferior alveolar vessels and nerve
   e) Lingual nerve
   f) A process of parotid gland.

B. Medial surface: (a) Tensor veli palatini and superior constrictor separated by stylopharyngeus and styloglossus. (b) Submandibular gland.

Action:

1. Elevation of mandible
2. Protrusion when act with lateral pterygoid.
3. Side to side chewing movement by alternate action of both pterygoids.

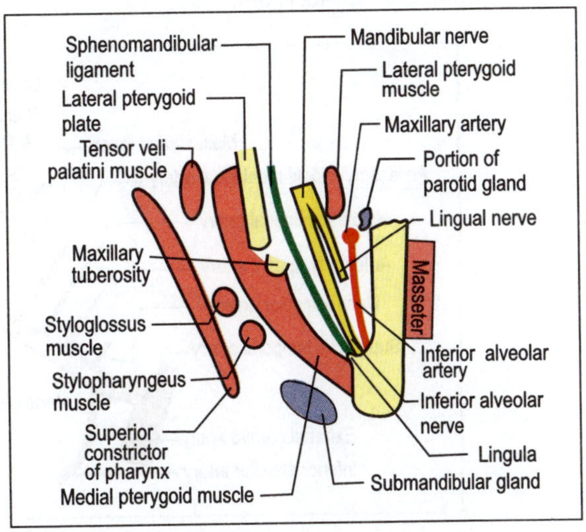

Fig. 12.11: Relations of medial pterygoid muscle

MAXILLARY ARTERY (Fig. 12.12)

It is one of the larger terminal branch of external carotid artery and is also called internal maxillary artery.

Origin: It arises as a result of division of external carotid artery behind the neck of mandible within the substance of parotid gland.

Parts: the course is divided into **three parts**. The three parts are demarcated by lateral pterygoid muscle.

1. First part of mandibular part: From origin to lower border of lateral pterygoid. It lies between the sphenomandibular ligament and the neck of the mandible laterally. The auriculo-temporal nerve lies above the artery.
2. Second part of pterygoid part: From the lower border of lateral pterygoid to the upper border of the lower haed of lateral pterygoid.
3. Third part or pterygopalatine part: Part in the pterygopalatine fossa.

Course of different parts:

1. First part: It passes horizontally forwards between neck of mandible and sphenomandibular ligament and lies parallel and little below the auriculotemporal nerve and reaches the lower border of lateral pterygoid.
2. Second part: It runs upwards – either superficial or deep to lateral pterygoid.
3. Third part: It enters into pterygopalatine fossa by passing through two heads of lateral pterygoid and pterygomaxillary fissure and lies in front of pterygopalatine ganglion and ends by dividing into branches.

Branches of different parts: (Fig. 12.13)

First part: Five branches

1. **Deep auricular**: It passes upward & backward to pierce the cartilaginous or bony part of external acoustic meatus & supplies skin of external acoustic meatus and outer cuticular layer of tympanic membrane.
2. **Anterior tympanic**: It enter into tympanic cavity through petrotympanic fissure and supplies inner mucous layer of tympanic membrane and anastomoses with following arteries and forms a **'Vascular circle'** around this aspect of tympanic membrane.
   a) Posterior tympanic branch of stylomastoid artery
   b) Small branches from artery of pterygoid canal
   c) Caroticotympanic branch of internal carotid artery.
3. Middle meningeal artery: It is the largest meningeal branch supplying dura mater, trigeminal ganglion skull bones etc. It enters the cranial cavity through foramen spinosum.

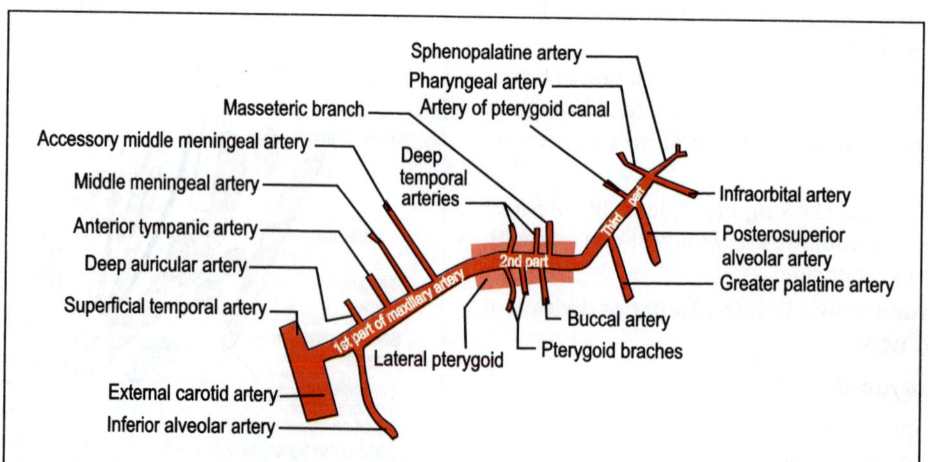

Fig. 12.12: Maxillary artery with its branches

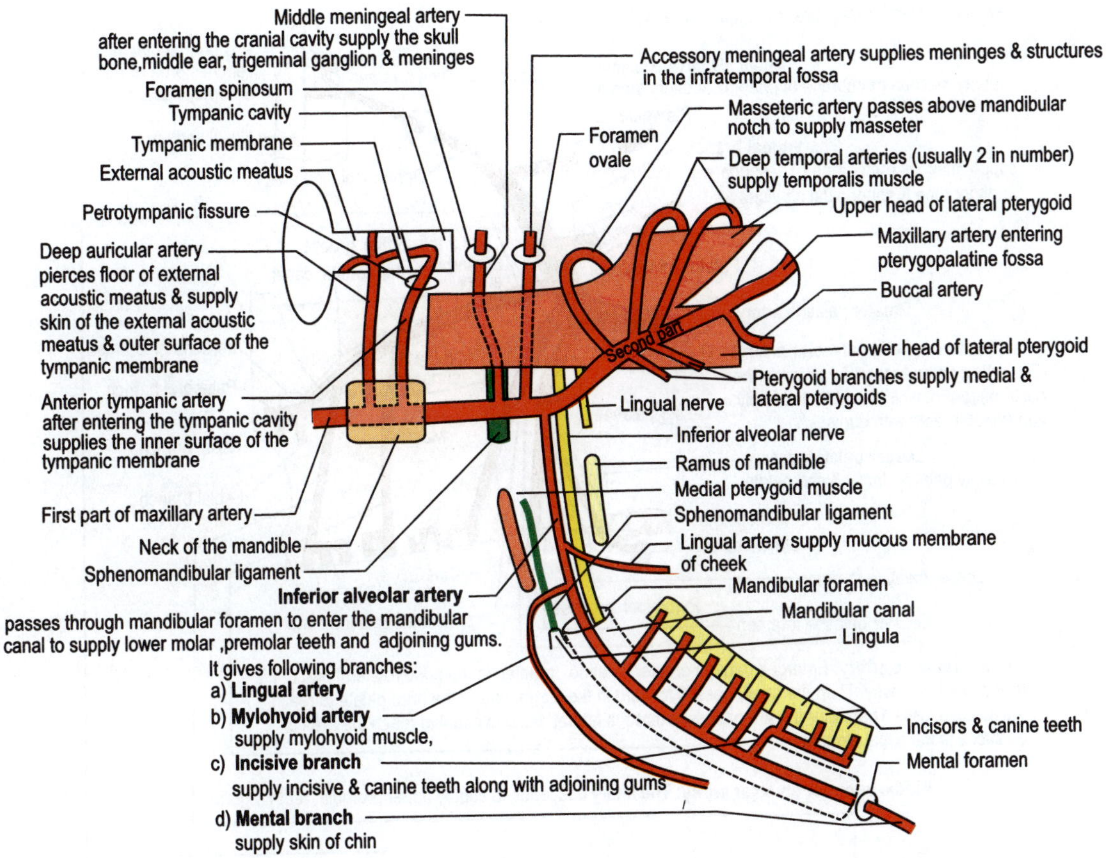

Fig. 12.13: Courses & branches of first & second part of the maxillary artery

Refer chapter 6 for details.

4. **Accessory meningeal artery**: It also supply dura mater after entering the cranial cavity through foramen ovale. It supplies meninges and structures in the infratemporal fossa.
5. **Inferior alveolar artery**: It passes downwards in between sphenomandibular ligament & ramus of mandible. Both vessels & nerve enter the mandibular canal through mandibular foramen, supply lower molar & premolar teeth and gums. It divides into mental & incisive branches. The mental artery supply the skin of the chin after emerging through mental foramen. The incisive artery supply the canine and incisor teeth and adjoining gums.

Before entering mandibular foramen, it divides into lingual & mylohyoid branches. Lingual branch supplies mucous membrane of cheek (accompanies the lingual nerve). The mylohyoid branch supplies mylohyoid muscle after piercing the sphenomandibular ligament (accompanies the mylohyoid nerve).

Second part: Four muscular branches:

1. **Deep temporal**: Usually two in number, passes upwards in between temporalis & bone to supply temporalis.
2. **Masseteric**: It passes above the mandibular notch to supply masseter.
3. **Pterygoid**: Supply medial & lateral pterygoids.

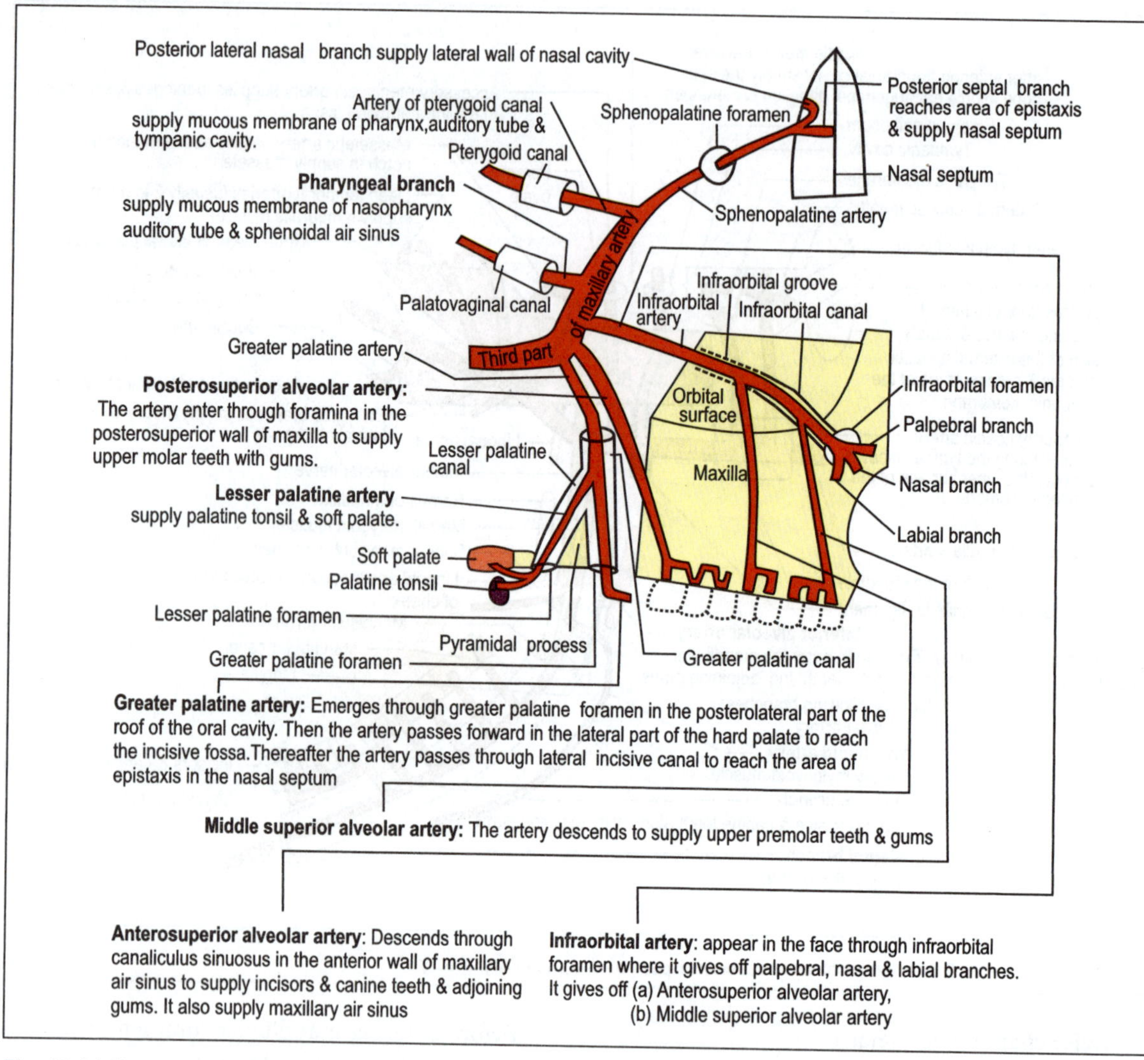

Fig. 12.14: Courses & branches of third part of the maxillary artery

4. **Buccal**: Supplies buccinator accompanies the nerve. (Passes in both between both heads of lateral pterygoids).

Third part: **Six branches**: (Fig. 12.14)

1. **Posterior superior alveolar**: It passes through pterygomaxillary fissure. It (after dividing into branches) enters through the foramina on the posterior surface of the body of maxilla. It supplies upper molar and adjoining gums; it also supply mucous membrane of maxillary air sinus.
2. **Infraorbital**: The artery passes through inferior orbital fissure, infraorbital groove and canal to appear in the face through infraorbital foramen (accompanied corresponding nerves). Infraorbital artery gives **middle superior alveolar artery** in the infraorbital groove & supply premolar teeth and adjoining gums. In the orbital canal, infraorbital artery gives **anterosuperior alveolar artery** which supply incisors & canine teeth, and adjoining gums. In the face, it gives off (after emerging from infraorbital foramen) branches to supply lacrimal sac, side of nose and upper lip.

Table 12.3: Branches of maxillary artery

Branches	Foramen, fissure etc.	Distribution
A. **First part (Mandibular part):**		
1. Deep auricular: Passes upward and backwards.	– Pierces cartilaginous or bony part of external acoustic meatus	– Supplies skin of external acoustic meatus and outer surface of tympanic membrane
2. Anterior tympanic	– Enters tympanic cavity through petro-tympanic fissure.	– Supplies inner surface (mucous membrane) of tympanic membrane
3. Middle meningeal	– Passes through foramen spinosum to enter cranial cavity	– Supplies dura mater, skull bones, trigeminal ganglion, middle ear, tensor tympanic
4. Accessory meningeal	– Passes through foramen ovale	– Supplies pterygoids & meninges
5. Inferior alveolar	– Enters the mandibular canal through mandibular foramen	– Supplies the lower teeth, adjoining gums & mylohyoid muscles
B. **Second part**		
1. Masseteric	– Passes laterally through masseteric notch	– Supply masseter
2. Deep temporal – two in number	– Ascends between the temporalis & bone	– Supply temporalis
3. Pterygoids		– Supply medial & lateral pterygoids
4. Buccal	– Passes between two heads of lateral pterygoid	– Supply buccinator
C. **Third part**		
1. Postero-superior alveolar artery	– Enters through the foramina on the posterior surface of the body of the maxilla	– Supply upper molar teeth & adjoining gums; maxillary air sinus
2. Infraorbital artery: It divides into	– Inferior orbital fissure	– Some orbital muscles, lacrimal sac, side of nose & upper lip
a) Middle superior alveolar artery	– It (while on the infraorbital groove) descends downwards in the anterior wall of maxillary air sinus	– It supplies premolar teeth & adjoining gums
b) Anterior superior alveolar artery	– It (while in infraorbital canal) descends in the anteromedial part of the maxillary air sinus	– It supplies incisors and canine & adjoining gum, and maxillary air sinus
3. Greater palatine artery:	– It descends through greater palatine canal and emerge in the hard palate through greater palatine foramen.	– Upper jaw gums
	– Lesser palatine artery is a branch from greater palatine artery in the greater palatine canal and emerge through lesser palatine foramina on the pyramidal process of palatine bone	– Supplies soft palate and palatine tonsil
4. Pharyngeal artery: It passes backwards	– Through palatovaginal canal (inferior aspect of body of sphenoid bone)	– It supplies mucous membrane of nasopharynx, auditory tube & sphenoidal air sinus
5. Artery of pterygoid canal: It runs backwards	– Through pterygoid canal	– It supplies pharynx, auditory tube, tympanic cavity
6. Sphenopalatine artery:	– Sphenoplatine artery enter nasal cavity through sphenopalatine foramen. – It divides into:	
	a) Posteromedial branch	– Posteromedial branch supply nasal septum and help to forms anastomoses in Little's area
	b) Posterolateral branches: Ramify over conchae & meatus.	– Posterolateral branches supply sphenoidal & ethmoidal sinuses and lateral wall of nasal cavity

3. Greater palatine artery: It descends vertically to enter the greater palatine canal.
   a) **Greater palatine artery** passes through greater palatine canal to appear in the posterolateral part of the roof of the oral cavity through greater palatine foramen. Then it passes forward in lateral groove in the hard palate to reach the incisive fossa. Terminal part of the greater palatine artery passes upwards through lateral incisive canal to reach Little's area of the nasal septum.
   b) **Lesser palatine artery** arises from greater palatine artery (within greater palatine canal). Then the lesser palatine artery passes through lesser palatine canal in pyramidal process of palatine bone and appear in the oral cavity through lesser palatine foramina to supply soft palate and palatine tonsil.
4. **Pharyngeal artery**: It passes posteriorly through palatovaginal canal to supply nasopharynx, auditory tube and sphenoidal air sinus.
5. **Artery of pterygoid canal**: It passes posteriorly through the pterygoid canal & supplies pharynx, auditory tube, and tympanic cavity.
6. **Sphenopalatine artery**: It is the continuation of maxillary artery. It enters the nasal cavity through sphenopalatine foramen, and divides into postero-medial & postero lateral nasal branches.

   Postero medial branch passes forwards & downwards in the nasal septum, and reach the Little's area to anastomoses with terminal part of greater palatine artery.

   Postero lateral nasal branch supplies the lateral wall of nasal cavity, sphenoidal & ethmoidal air sinus.

   Pterygoid venous plexus: This plexus lie on lateral pterygoid muscle. The plexus drains into maxillary vein.

MANDIBULAR NERVE (Fig. 12.15)

It is the largest division of trigeminal nerve.

Type: Mixed (motor & sensory root).

Developmental: It is the nerve of first branchial arch.

Origin: Larger sensory root arises from convex aspect of trigeminal ganglion and immediately leaves the cranial cavity to enter infratermporal fossa through foramen ovale.

Smaller motor root arises from pons and passes through foramen ovale.

Formation of trunk: The two roots unite to form the trunk of the mandibular nerve just below the foramen ovale.

Course: The united trunk in the infratemporal fossa lies in between tensor veli palatine medially and lateral pterygoid laterally.

Termination: In the infratemporal fossa it terminates by dividing into small anterior and a large posterior divisions which give branches for distribution.

Branches:

I. From the trunk, i.e., before division:
   1. **Nervous spinous** or meningeal branch: It enters into the cranial cavity along with middle meningeal artery through foramen spinosum and divides into two branches and supplying duramater of middle and cranial fossa and mucous membrane of mastoid air cells.
   2. **Nerve to medial pterygoid**: Nerve to medial pterygoid pass through otic ganglion and supplies medial pterygoid. The nerve to medial pterygoid also supplies tensor tympani and tensor veli palatini.

II. **From the anterior divisions**
   A. Motor branches:
      1. **Deep temporal branch**: Usually two in number and pass between the skull and upper border of lateral pterygoid and enters the deep surface of temporalis.
      2. **Nerve to lateral pterygoid**: Supplies lateral pterygoid.

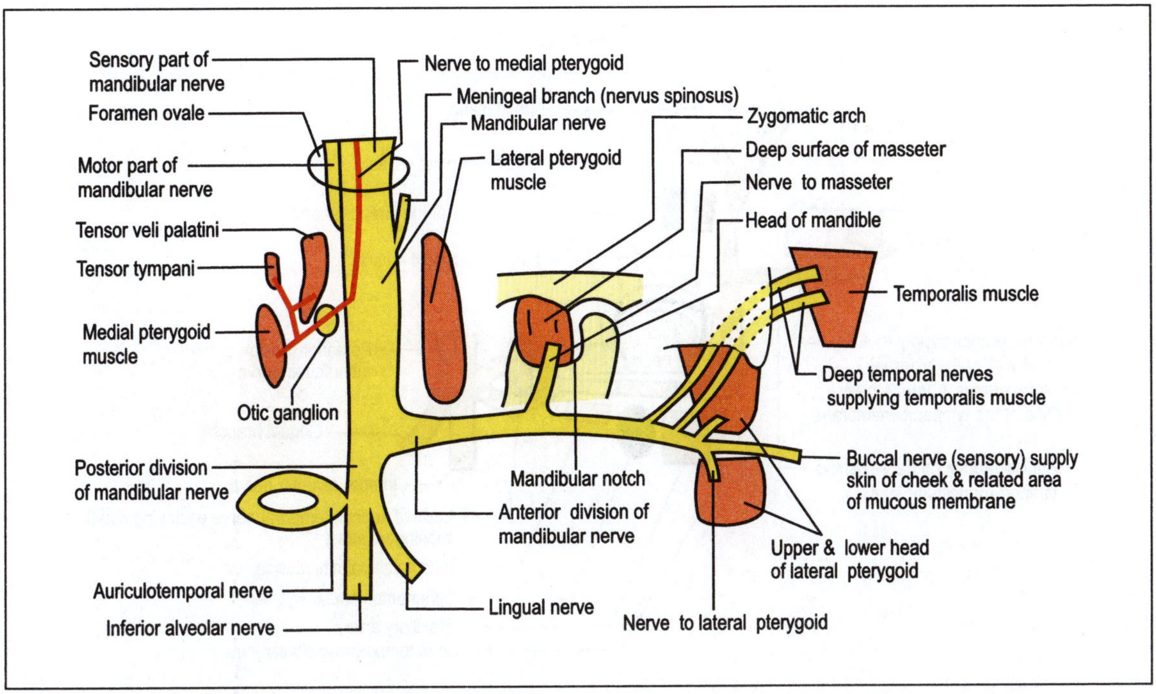

Fig. 12.15: Scheme to show course, relations & branches of the mandibular nerve; also showing course relations & branches of anterior division of mandibular

3. **Masseteric branch**: It emerges laterally, just in front of temporomandibular joint and passes through mandibular notch accompanied by masseteric vessels and enter deep suface of masseter muscle. It also supplies temporomandibular joint.

B. **Buccal branch**: It is the only sensory branch of anterior division. It passes between the two heads of the lateral pterygoid muscle, passes downwards & forwards, appear at the anterior border of masseter. It supplies the skin & mucous membrane related to the buccinator; but not the muscle.

III. **Posterior division**: It is having three sensory branches: (1) Auriculotemporal nerve; (2) Lingual nerve; (3) Inferior alveolar.

1. **Auriculotemporal**: Its origin is characteristic. It arises by two roots and through which middle meningeal artery passes. It then passes backwards under cover of lateral pterygoid on the surface of tensor veli palatini and then passes between the sphenomandibular ligament and neck of mandible. It lies above the maxillary artery. Behind the neck of the mandible it passes upwards. Behind the temporomandibular joint it ascends posterior to superficial temporal vessel. Over the root of zygoma it terminates by dividing into superficial temporal and auricular branches (Fig. 12.16).

Branches:

a) Auricular branches: Supply skin of tragus, roof & anterior wall of external acoustic meatus and part of external surface of tympanic membrane.

b) Temporal branch: Supplies the skin of the temple.

c) Articular branch: Supply the temporomandibular joint.

d) Secretomotor fibres to parotid gland.

2. **Lingual nerve**: It is a sensory nerve for mucous

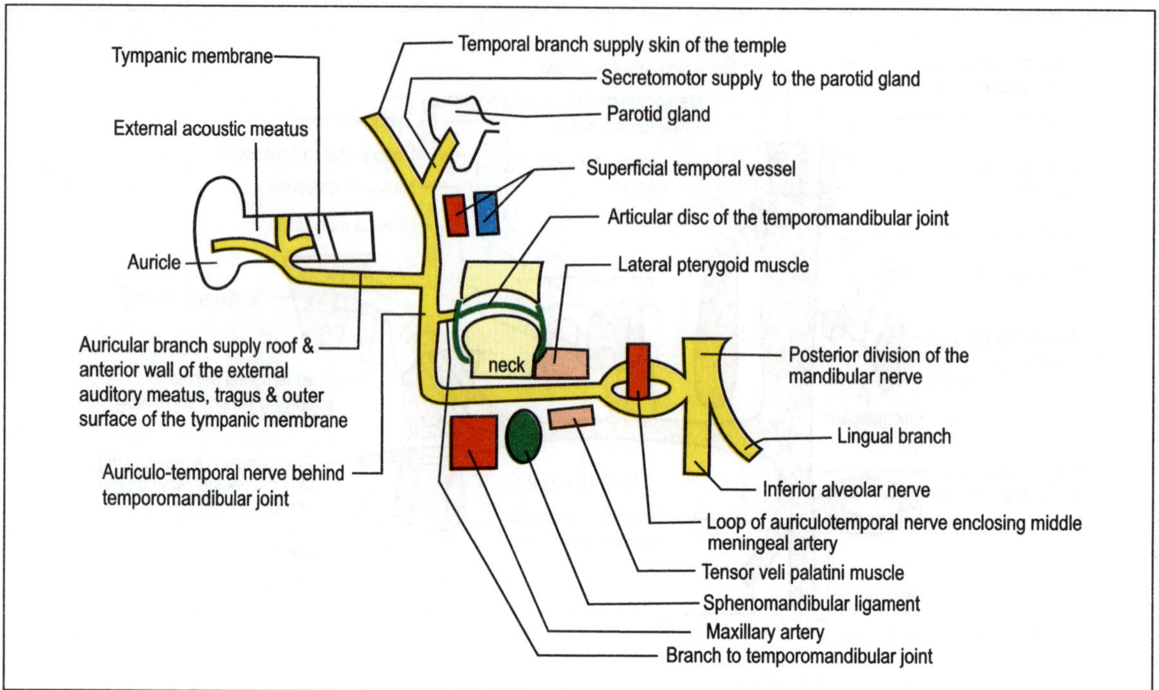

Fig. 12.16: Scheme to show course, relations & branches of the auriculotemporal nerve

membrane of anterior-2-3rd of tongue, floor of mouth and gum. (Fig. 12.17)

Origin: From the posterior division of mandibular nerve in the infratemporal fossa.

Course: After origin it passes between tensor veli palatini and lateral pterygoid and then between lateral and medial pterygoids; and about 2cm below the skull in this part chorda tympani nerve joins it. It passes between ramus of mandible and medial pterygoid and comes in direct contact with mandible medial to the third molar tooth, between the origins of superior constrictor of pharynx and mylohyoid. After that it crosses styloglossus and runs on the lateral surface of hyoglossus but deep to mylohyoid and also lies above deep part of submandibular gland and its duct. Finally it lies on the genioglossus. Here the nerve presents, intimate relation with submandibular duct (first above, then lateral, then below & finally medial to duct), and the lingual nerve divides into terminal branches.

Termination: It terminates by dividing branches undercover of mucous membrane of tongue.

Distribution: Branches supply

a) Mucous membrane of floor of the mouth
b) Lingual surface of gum
c) Mucous membrane of anterior 2-3rd of tongue except vallate papilla.
d) It also carries secretomotor fibres for submandibular & sublingual salivary glands.

3. **Inferior alveolar nerve**: It is the large terminal branch of posterior division of mandibular nerve (Fig. 12.18).

Course: It runs downwards between medial pterygoid and ramus of mandible. Then enters mandibular foramen and the mandibular canal along with inferior alveolar artery. Thereafter the inferior alveolar nerve runs through the mandibular canal as far as mental foramen and terminates by dividing into mental and incisive branch.

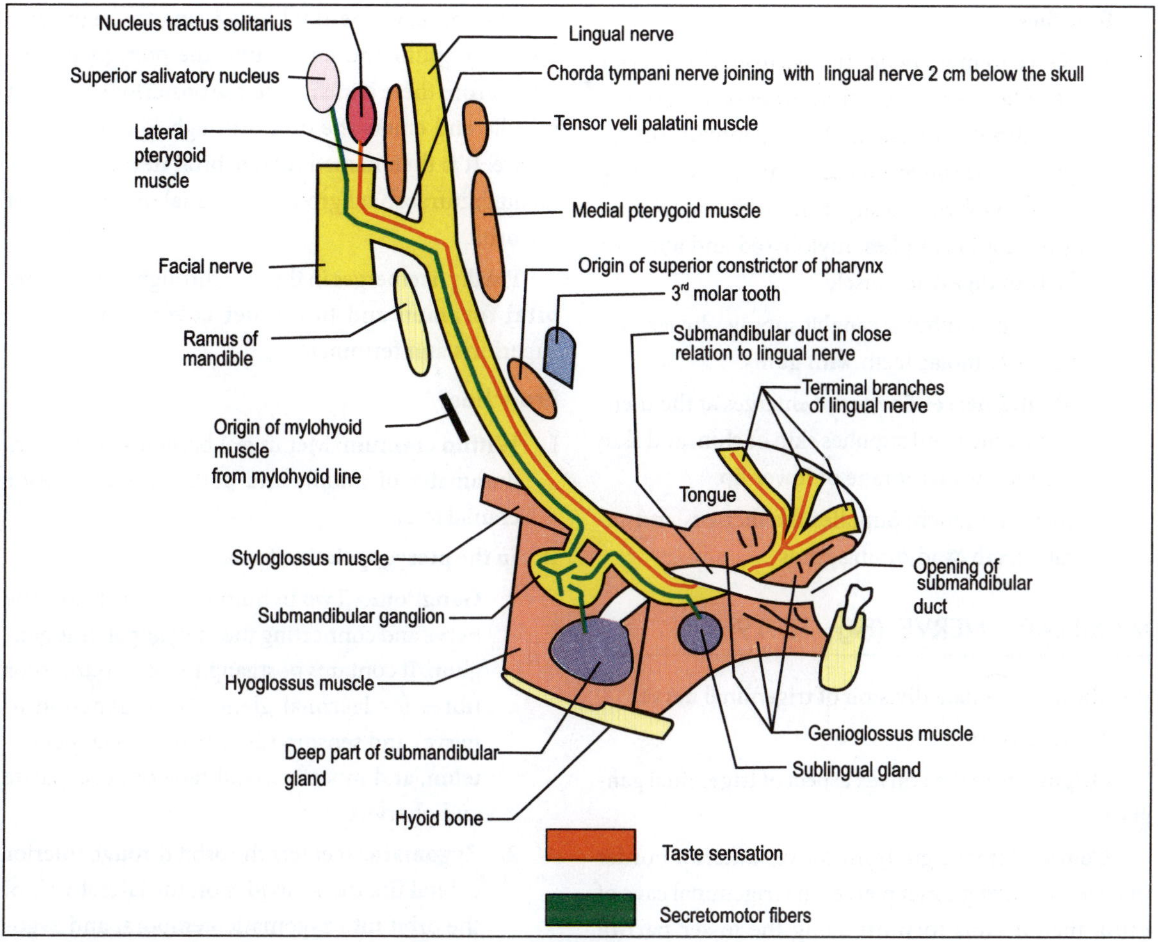

Fig. 12.17: Course, relations & branches of the lingual nerve

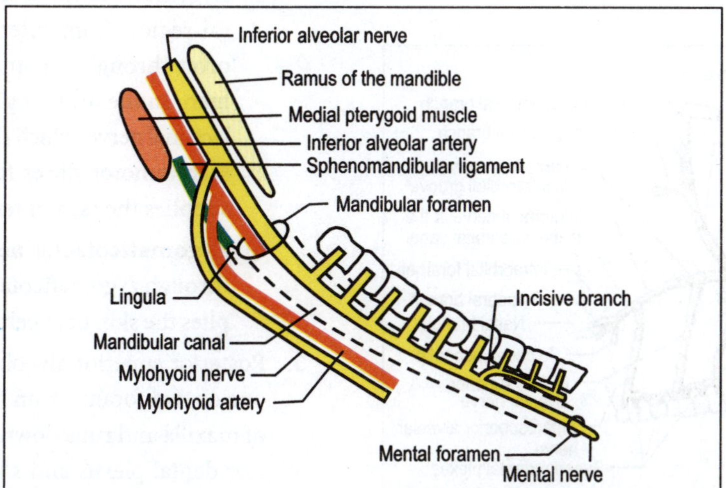

Fig. 12.18: Course, relations and branches of the inferior alveolar nerve

Branches:

1. Nerve to mylohyoid: It arise from the inferior alveolar nerve before the nerve enters the mandibular foramen. The mylohyoid nerve pierces the sphenomandibular ligament along with mylohyoid artery, runs in the mylohyoid groove and supplies, mylohyoid and anterior belly of digastric muscle.
2. In the mandibular canal it supplies lower premolar & molar teeth with gums.
3. **Mental nerve**: The nerve emerges at the mental foramen and supplies skin of chin, and skin & mucous membrane of lower lip.

   Incisive branch: Supplies the incisors and canine teeth & adjoining gums.

MAXILLARY NERVE (Fig. 12.19)

It is the intermediate division of trigeminal nerve.

Type: Sensory.

Origin: From the convex aspect of trigeminal ganglion.

Course: After origin from convex anterior border of trigeminal ganglion it pierces the trigeminal cave of dura; then it runs forward along the lower part of lateral wall of cavernous sinus below the ophthalmic nerve, trochlear and oculomotor nerve.

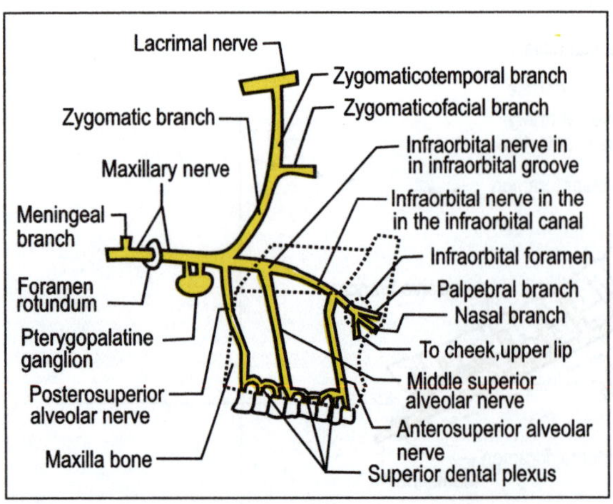

Fig. 12.19: Course and branches of the maxillary nerve

Then it leave the skull by passing through foramen rotundum and enters into the *pterygopalatine fossa*. From there it inclines to the posterior surface of maxilla and enters the orbit through *inferior orbital fissure*. It is then named **infraorbital nerve**. It passes through infraorbital groove and canal on the floor of the orbit.

Finally, it emerges in the face through the **infraorbital foramen** and lies under cover levator labii superioris and terminates.

Branches:

I. **Within cranium**: Meningeal branch – It supplies duramater of middle and partly in the anterior cranial fossa.

II. **In the pterygopalatine fossa**:

1. **Ganglionic**: Two in number and lie below the nerve and connecting the pterygopalatine ganglion. It contains postganglionic secretomotor fibres for lacrimal gland (from ganglion to nerve) and sensory fibres from orbital periosteum, and mucous membrane of nose, palate and pharynx.
2. **Zygomatic**: It enters the orbit through inferior orbital fissure. It divides on the lateral wall of the orbit into zygomaticotemporal and zygomaticofacial nerve.
   a) **Zygomaticotemporal nerve** enters temporal region from inferolateral wall of the orbit through zygomaticotemporal foramen. In the orbit, it gives a branch to join lacrimal nerve, which carries postganglionic secretomotor fibres for lacrimal gland. It supplies the skin of temporal region.
   b) **Zygomaticofacial nerve** enters the face through zygomaticofacial foramen. It supplies the skin of cheek (prominence).
3. Posterior superior alveolar: It passes through one or two foramina on the posterior surface of maxilla and runs downwards to from superior dental plexus and supply mucous membrane of maxillary sinus, vestibule, molar teeth and adjoining gums.

III. **In the infraorbital groove**:

1. **Middle superior alveolar**: It runs downwards & forward in the lateral wall of maxillary air sinus to join superior dental plexus and supplies premolar teeth.
2. **Anterior superior alveolar**: It arises in the middle of infraorbital canal and passes through **canalis sinuosus** in the anterior wall of maxillary sinus and divides into dental & nasal branch. Dental branch joins with superior dental plexus & supply canine and incisor teeth and adjoining gums. Nasal branch appear lateral wall to supply mucous membrane of the same area up to the opening of maxillary air sinus.

IV. **Termination**: It terminates as **infraorbital nerve** in the face by dividing into three branches.

1. **Palpebral**: Supplies skin of lower eyelid.
2. **Nasal**: Supplies skin of ala of nose and movable part of nasal septum.
3. **Superior labial**: Supplies skin and mucous membrane of upper lip.

PTERYGOPALATINE GANGLION (Fig. 12.20)

It is the largest peripheral parasympathetic ganglion.

Topographically it is related to maxillary nerve but functionally related to seventh cranial nerve through greater petrosal nerve.

Situation: It is placed in pterygopalatine fossa and is hanging below maxillary nerve.

Relations:

a) Posteriorly: Pterygoid canal.
b) Medially: Sphenopalatine foramen of perpendicular plate of palatine bone.
c) Above: Maxillary nerve.

Ganglion lies between pharyngeal artery (medially) and artery of the pterygoid canal (laterally).

Size: Larger than pin's head – colour reddish grey in colour.

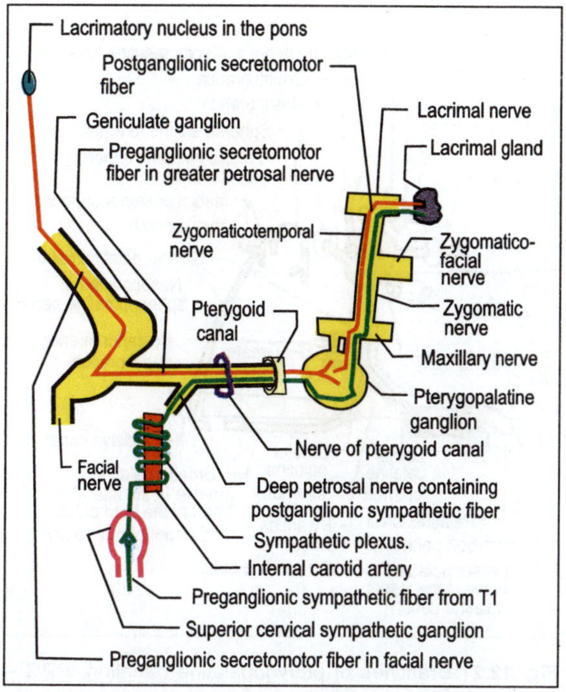

Fig. 12.20: Connections of pterygopalatine ganglion

Root:

I. **Parasympathetic or motor root**: Nerve of pterygoid canal conveys the preganglionic fibers from the lacrimatory nucleus of pons.

Secretomotor pathways for lacrimal gland:

Lacrimatory nucleus of pons → Nervus intermedius of facial nerve → Geniculate ganglion of facial nerve → Greater petrosal nerve → Nerve of pterygoid canal → Relay in pterygopalatine ganglion → Postganglionic fibres join maxillary nerve → Zygomatic branch of maxillary nerve → Zygomaticotemporal nerve → Lacrimal branch of ophthalmic nerve → Lacrimal gland

Some of the postganglionic secretomotor fibres nasal, palatine and pharyngeal glands.

II. **Sympathetic root**: Deep petrosal nerve joins with the greater petrosal nerve to form the nerve of pterygoid canal. Deep petrosal nerve contains postganglionic sympathetic fibres from plexus around internal carotid artery. The fibres pass through the ganglion without relay and distribute vasomotor fibres to lacrimal gland.

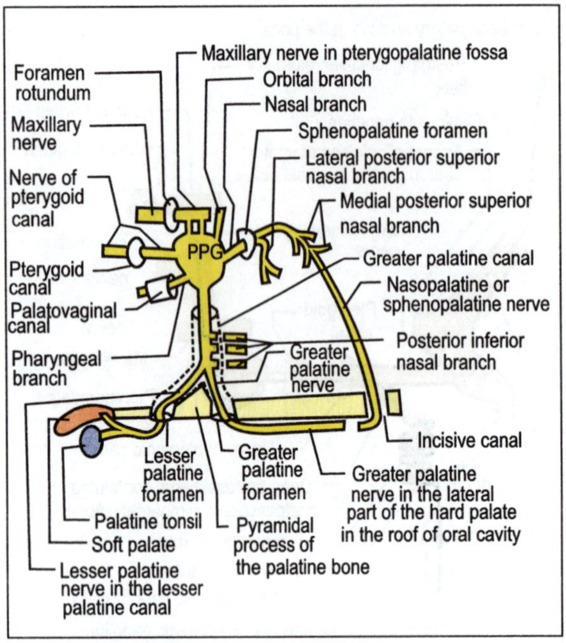

Fig. 12.21: Branches of pterygopalatine ganglion, PPG – Pterygopalatine ganglion

III. **Sensory root**: From maxillary nerve and pass through ganglion without relay.

Branches (Fig. 12.21)

1. **Orbital branches**: Pass through inferior orbital fissure & supply orbitalis, periosteum of orbit.
2. **Palatine branches**: (a) Greater (anterior) and (b) Lesser (middle and posterior). **Greater palatine nerve** descends through greater palatine canal & emerges at the under surface of hard palate through greater palatine foramen. Then it passes forward in the lateral part of the hard palate towards the incisive fossa. Posterior inferior nasal nerve (branches from the canal) supply posteroinferior quadrant of the lateral wall of nasal cavity. Greater palatine nerve supply mucous membrane of hard palate and adjoining gum.

   Lesser palatine nerve descends through greater & lesser palatine canal & appear under surface of hard palate through lesser palatine foramen on the pyramidal process of palatine bone, supply mucous membrane of soft palate & palatine tonsil.
3. **Nasal branches**: Enter the nasal cavity through sphenopalatine foramen & divide into postero-supero-lateral nasal & postero-supero-medial branches.

   Posteromedial superior nasal branches are two or three, one of the branch is long, known sphenopalatine (nasopalatine) nerve lie on vomer. Left nasopalatine nerve passes through anterior incisive foramen to reach roof of mouth, right nasopalatine nerve passes through posterior incisive foramen to roof of the mouth.
4. **Pharyngeal branches**: These branches passes backwards to the nasopharynx through palatovaginal canal. It supplies mucous membrane of nasopharynx posterior to auditory tube.

OTIC GANGLION (Fig. 12.22)

It is peripheral ganglion of the parasympathetic system.

Topographically: It is related to mandibular nerve, but functionally related with glossopharyngeal nerve.

Situation: In the infratemporal fossa just below the foramen ovale.

Size and shape: Small over, flattened (about the size of pin's head).

Colour: Reddish grey.

Relations:

a) **Laterally**: Mandibular nerve.
b) **Medially**: Tensor veli palatini separating cartilaginous part of pharyngotympanic tube.
c) **Posteriorly**: Middle meningeal artery.
d) **Anteriorly**: Medial pterygoid muscle.

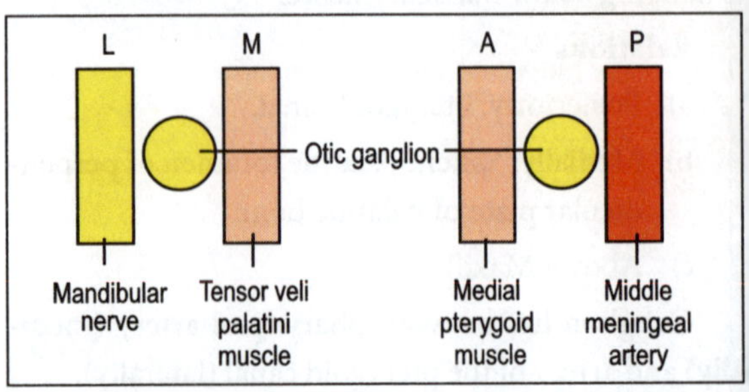

Fig. 12.22: Scheme to show the relations of otic ganglion, L – Lateral, M – Medial, A – Anterior, P – Posterior

Different Roots (Fig. 12.23)

1. Parasympathetic root: From lesser petrosal nerve carrying preganglionic parasympathetic secretomotor fibres for parotid gland. The preganglionic fibres arise from the inferior salivatory nucleus of the medulla oblongata and pass successively through the glossopharyngeal nerve, tympanic branch of glossopharyngeal nerve, tympanic plexus and the lesser petrosal nerve, relay in the otic ganglion, postganglionic fibres joins with the auriculotemporal nerve to supply parotid gland.

   Secretomotor pathways:
   Preganglionic fibres arises from inferior salivary nucleus → Glossopharyngeal nerve → Tympanic branch → Tympanic plexus → Lesser petrosal nerve → Relay in otic ganglion → Postganglionic fibres join auriculotemporal nerve → Parotid gland.
2. **Sympathetic root**: From sympathetic plexus around the middle meningeal artery; it contains postganglionic fibres from superior cervical sympathetic ganglia. Sympathetic fibers passes through otic ganglion to join auriculotemporal nerve & then supply (vasomotor) the parotid gland.
3. **Motor root**: From nerve to medial pterygoid (branch from trunk of mandibular nerve before division) it passes through otic ganglion without relay.

   Development: From neural crest epithelium.

Branches:

1. **Motor**: To medial pterygoid, tensor tympani and tensor veli palatini.
2. **Secretomotor**: A communicating branch to auriculotemporal carrying postganglionic parasympathetic fibres for parotid gland.
3. Two other communicating branches: To chorda tympanic nerve and to nerve of pterygoid canal. These connections provide alternative pathway of taste sensations of the anterior 2/3rd of the tongue & passes to the cell bodies of geniculate ganglion without passing through middle ear.

APPLIED ANATOMY:

1. **Lesion of whole trigeminal nerve**:
   a) Anaesthesia of the corresponding anterior half of scalp, face except the area at the angle of mandible, because of supply by great auricu-

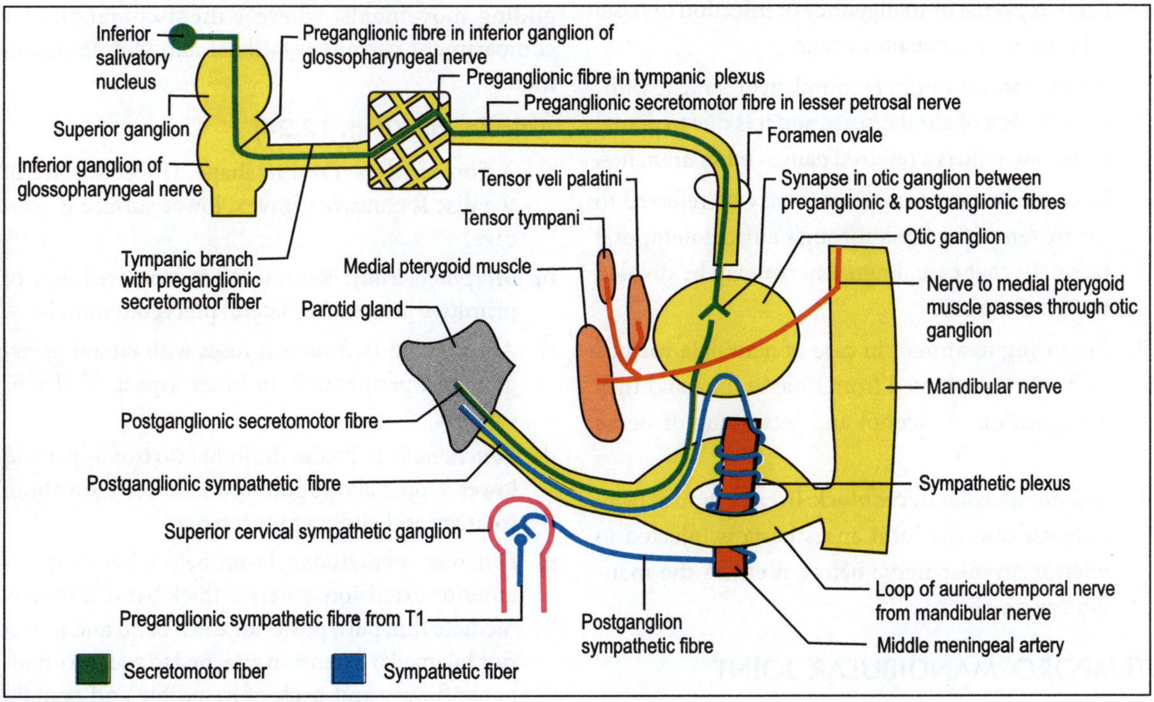

Fig. 12.23: Connections of otic ganglion

lar), cornea, conjunctiva, mucous membrane of nose, mouth, anterior 2-3rd tongue.

b) Paralysis and atrophy of muscles supplied by the nerve and so when patient tries to open the mouth the mandible will be thrust to the paralysed side.

2. **Lesions of any divisions of nerve**: Will cause a limited sensory loss.
3. **Lesion of lingual nerve below the point of joining of chorda tympani** will be loss of general sensation as well as taste sensation of the same half anterior part of tongue.
4. Pain or neuralgia is of very common, pain at first localises to the affected nerve then referred pain occurs in other branches. The best example is in case of dental carries causes referred pain or neuralgia in other branches and relieved by treatment of affected teeth.
5. In case of frontal or ethmoidal sinusitis or glaucoma severe supraorbital pain occurs. It is also a case of referred pain.
6. Maxillary neuralgia may occur in case of maxillary sinus expyema or malignancy or infection of nasal septum or conchae may occur.
7. Patient most commonly complain of earache without any sign of aural disease and it is due to dental caries and pain is a referred pain in other branches.
8. In case of cancer tongue pain may be referred to ear or temporal fossa through auriculotemporal nerve. In that case, lingual nerve may be divided for relief of pain.
9. Regarding treatment in case of neuralgia various methods are adopted from time to time and they are injection of alcohol and sectioning of nerve etc.
10. **Inferior alveolar nerve block**: In extraction of teeth of lower jaw, the local anaesthesia is injected to inferior alveolar nerve before it enters the mandibular canal.

TEMPORO MANDIBULAR JOINT

Also known as **mandibular joint** and they are paired joints one on each side between mandible and base of skull.

Type: Synovial.

Subtype: Bicondylar, as both the joint act as one unit.

Articular surfaces

1. Above: The **upper articular surface** is formed by
   a) Articular tubercle.
   b) Anterior articular part of mandibular fossa of temporal bone.
2. The lower articular surface is formed by the **head** (condyle) of the mandible.

   (Side to side 20mm. Before backwards 10mm.)

   Each condyle is elliptical:

Articular surfaces of both the bone are covered with **fibrocartilage**.

Characteristics of the joint:

It is divided into two joint cavities by an articular disc.

a) Upper: Menisco-temporal

b) Lower: Menisco-mandibular.

Menisco temporal (upper) compartment permits gliding movements, whereas meniscomandibular compartment permits rotational and gliding movements.

Articular disc (Fig. 12.24)

a) A *fibrocartilage*: Oval in shape. Upper surface of the disc is concavo-convex, lower surface is concave.

b) *Morphologically*: Represents degenerated part of primitive insertion of lateral pterygoid muscle.

c) *Attachment*: *In front* – It fuses with lateral pterygoid and peripherally to inner aspect of fibrous capsule.

d) *Functionally* it divides the joint into two upper and lower. Upper allows gliding and lower allows both rotatory and gliding movements.

e) *Different subdivisions*: From before backwards – anterior extension, anterior thick band, an intermediate thin part, posterior thick band and posterior bilamellar extension attached to squamo-tympanic fissure and neck of mandible and contain venous plexus between them.

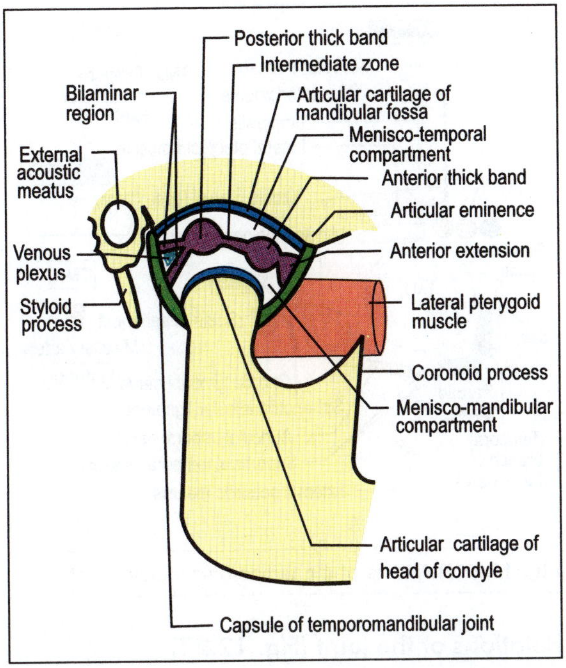

Fig. 12.24: Articular disc of temporomandibular joint

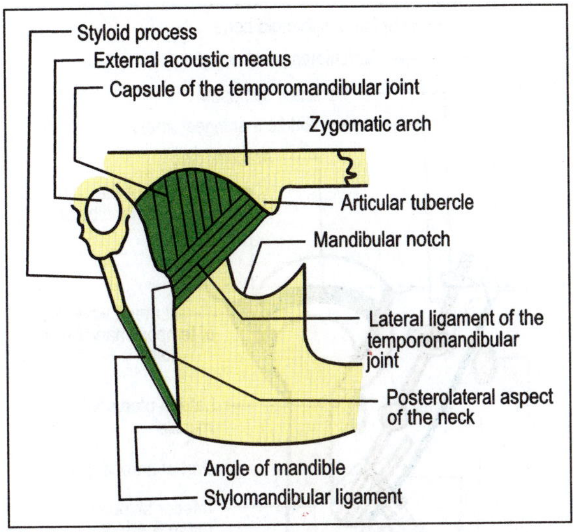

Fig. 12.25: Capsule, stylomandibular ligament & lateral ligament of temporomandibular joint

Ligaments:

The ligaments are: Articular capsule, lateral or temporomandibular ligament, accessory ligament, sphenomandibular & stylomandibular ligament.

Capsular ligament: Consists of outer fibrous capsule and inner synovial membrane lining the capsule.

a) It is the fibrous envelope of the joint
b) Attachment

   Above: Anteriorly to articular tubercle and behind to squamotympanic fissure and margins of articular fossa (Fig. 12.24).

   Below: Around the neck of mandible.

   In front: Fuses with insertion of lateral pterygoid.
c) Texture: Loose above the disc and thick and tense below the disc.
d) Weakest part: Above the disc due to loose character of the capsule.

Head of mandible and disc glide together in the menisco-temporal compartment.

Synovial membrane:

a) It lines the inner aspect of the capsule up to margin of articular cartilages and
b) Also to the neck of capsule
c) It does not cover the articular cartilages.

Accessory ligaments:

1. Lateral or temporomandibular
2. Sphenomandibular
3. Stylomandibular ligaments.

Temporomandibular (lateral) ligament: (Fig. 12.25)

a) It is also known as lateral ligament and covers the lateral aspect of capsule.
b) *Attachment*: From articular tubercle of root of zygoma of temporal bone to posterolateral aspect of the neck of the mandible.
c) Its fibres are directed downwards and backwards.
d) It strengthens the lateral aspect of fibrous capsule.

Sphenomandibular ligament:

It is an accessory ligament of temporomandibular joint but lies away from the capsule medially. (Fig. 12.26)

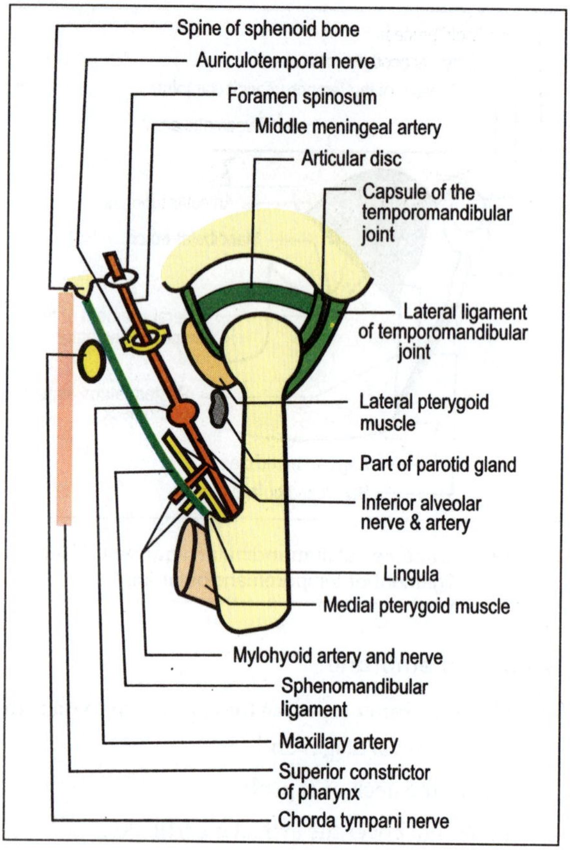

Fig. 12.26: Sphenomandibular ligament with its relations

It is a derivative of Meckel's cartilages [Skeletal element of first branchial arch].

Attachment: *Above* – to spine of sphenoid bones. *Below* to the lingula of mandibular foramen.

It is *pierced by mylohyoid vessels and nerve*.

Relations:

a) *Laterally*: Lateral pterygoid, auriculotemporal nerve, maxillary artery with middle meningeal branch, inferior alveolar vessels and nerve.

b) *Medially*: Medial pterygoid, chorda tympani nerve and wall of pharynx.

Stylomandibular ligament

1. It is an accessory ligament and formed by condensation of investing layer of deep cervical fascia.
2. It extends from styloid process of temporal bone (above) to angle of the mandible (below).
3. It *separates parotid from submandibular salivary glands.*

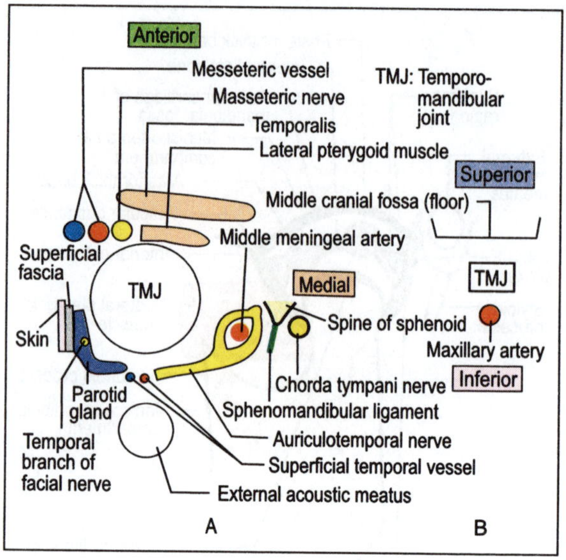

Fig. 12.27: Relations of the temporomandibular joint

Relations of the joint (Fig. 12.27)

1. *In front*: Lateral pterygoid, temporalis and masseteric nerves and vessels.
2. *Behind*: Parotid gland, separating from external acoustic meatus, superficial temporal vessels, auriculotemporal nerve.
3. *Laterally*: Skin, fascia, temporal branch branch of parotid gland.
4. *Medially*: From superficial to deep – Lateral pterygoid, roots of auriculo-temporal nerve with middle meningeal artery, spine of sphenoid with attached sphenomandibular ligament and chorda tympani nerve.

Above: Middle cranial fossa

Below: Maxillary artery and vein

MOVEMENTS OF TEMPORO-MANDIBULAR JOINTS (Fig. 12.28)

Movements are protrusion and retraction, depression, elevation, and side-to-side (chewing) movements.

There are two basic movements:

a) **Gliding movements**: **Menisco-temporal compartment** permits gliding movement in protrusion, retraction and in chewing.

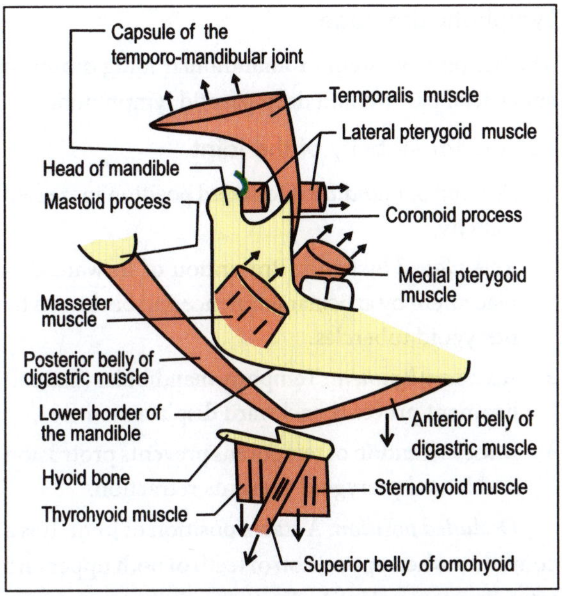

Fig. 12.28: Muscles responsible for movement of temporomandibular joint. The arrows indicate the direction of movements

b) **Rotational movement**: Menisco-mandibular permits rotational movement in
   i) transverse axis: (during elevation and depression)
   ii) vertical axis: (during side-to-side chewing movements).

The **movements at the temporomandibular joint** are (I) Depression and Elevation; (II) Protraction and Retraction; (III) Side to side /chewing

I. (a) **Depression** (opening of mouth)

Mechanism:

1. Movement takes place in the upper (Menisco-temporal) compartment.
2. Head of the mandible along with articular disc glide forward.
3. During the movement, head of mandible rotates forward below the articular disc.

I. (b) **Elevation** (closing of mouth)

Mechanism:

1. Movement takes place in the upper (Menisco-temporal) compartment.
2. Head of the mandible along with articular disc glide backwards.
3. Head of the mandible rotates backward below the articular disc.

Muscles responsible for the movements:

A. *Depression*
   a) Mainly lateral pterygoid of both sides.
   b) Helped of geniohyoid, mylohyoid and digastric muscles.
   c) Gravity helps also.
   d) Infrahyoid muscles help by fixing the hyoid bone.

B. *Elevation* (closing the mouth)
   a) Masseter
   b) Temporalis
   c) Medial pterygoid of both sides. They act as powerful antigravity muscles.

II. **Protraction and retraction:**

a) **Protraction or protrusion:** It is the protrusion of lower teeth beyond upper teeth.

Mechanism:

1. Movement takes place in the *upper (Menisco temporal) compartment.*
2. *In protrusion*: Articular disc and head of mandible together glide forward on the temporal articular surface.
3. During this movement the mandibular teeth proceed beyond maxillary teeth.

b) **In retraction:**

Mechanism:

1. Movement take place in the upper (Menisco-temporal) compartment. Reversal movement of protraction is retraction.
2. Both articular disc and head of the mandible glide backward to keep the mandible in resting position.

Muscles responsible for the movement

A. **Protraction**
   a) Lateral and
   b) Medial pterygoids – both sides.

B. **Retraction:**
   a) Mainly posterior fibres of temporalis helped by

b) Middle and deep fibres of masseter

c) Digastric

d) Geniohyoid muscles.

III. **Chewing or rotatory movements, grinding or side to side movements**

During chewing movements, if head of the right side of the mandible and articular disc glides forwards (as in protraction), then head of left side of the mandible rotates (without gliding) in vertical axis.

Therefore, the chin moves on left side (on which head of the mandible only rotates).

Alternative movements of this kind on both temporomandibular joint will lead to side to side/chewing movements.

Muscles responsible: Lateral and medial pterygoids of one side acting alternately with other side.

Range of movements:

1. *Maximum range of protrusion of mandible*: about 10mm each.
2. *Maximum opening of mouth (Jaw) is* 50mm: Functional range of opening is 40mm.

   Or this 40mm *opening* 25mm *by rotation.* 15mm *by forward gliding.*

Arterial supply:

By branches of superficial temporal and maxillary artery.

Nerve supply:

Auriculo-temporal branch of posterior division and masseteric branch of anterior division of mandibular nerve.

Lymphatic drainage:

The lymph from temporomandibular joing drains to superficial parotid and deep parotid lymph nodes.

Factors for stability of the joint

1. *Position of mandible*: Occluded position increased stability.
2. *Role played by bones*: Prevention of forward displacement by articular eminence and backward by pterygoid tubercles.
3. *Accessory ligament*: Temporo-mandibular (Lateral) ligament prevents backward displacement.
4. *Muscle*: Tendon of temporalis prevents protrusion and lateral pterygoid prevents retraction.

Occluded position: A stable position of joint. It is a condition when opposition of teeth of both upper and lower jaw takes place.]

APPLIED ANATOMY:

1. *Dislocation*: Dislocation of mandible takes place in forward direction and is placed from articular eminence to infratemporal fossa during excessive opening of mouth or during convulsion. It occurs due to sudden spasm of lateral pterygoid. It will result in inability to close the mouth.

   This condition is reduced by pressing the ramus of the mandible downward by a thumb on the last molar teeth and simultaneously chin is elevated to place the head of mandible in its usual position.
2. *Clicking and pain during the movements of the joint* may occur due to *derangement of articular disc.* It ultaimately occurs as a result of over closure or faulty occlusion.

chapter 13

SUBMANDIBULAR REGION

AT A GLANCE

- *Suprahyoid muscles (Digastric, Stylohyoid, Mylohyoid, Geniohyoid)*
- *Submandibular gland—Situation, Different parts–Superficial parts:* (1) *Surfaces (relations); Ends,* (2) *Deep part: Situation; Continuity; Extent; Relations*
- *Microscopic features of submandibular gland*
- *Submandibular duct*
- *Blood & nerve supply of submandibular gland*
- *Lymphatic drainage of submandibular gland*
- *Applied anatomy of submandibular gland*
- *Submandibular ganglion*
- *Sublingual gland with histological features*

The submandibular region contain suprahyoid muscles, submandibular, sublingual salivary glands, vessels, nerves and lymph nodes.

SUPRAHYOID MUSCLES

1. Digastric; 2. Mylohyoid
3. Stylohyoid; 4. Geniohyoid

Digastric muscle (Fig. 13.1)

Consists of two belies united by an intermediate rounder tendon.

Situation: Situated below the body of mandible and extending in angular fashion from mastoid process to chin.

Two bellies: Posterior and anterior (Fig. 13.2)

Posterior belly:

Origin: From mastoid notch of temporal bone.

Course: The muscle passes downward & forward.

Insertion: Inserted into intermediate tendon.

[Intermediate tendon of both the bellies of digastric:

a) It is a tendon in which two bellies end

b) Tendon lies in the triangular gap at the insertion of stylohyoid muscle

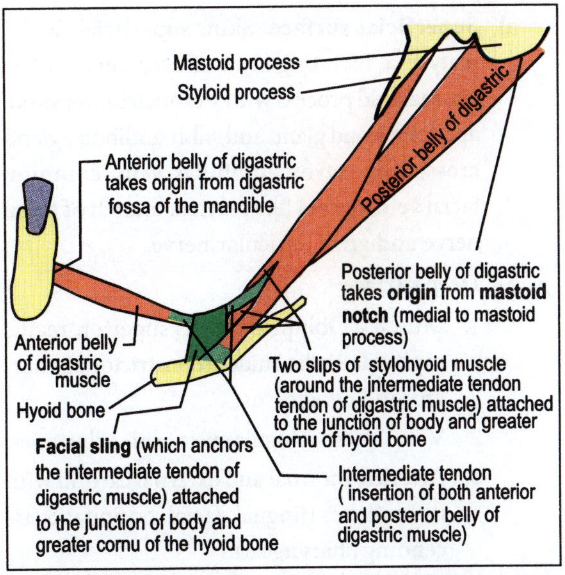

Fig. 13.1: Origin & insertion of the posterior & anterior bellies of digastric muscle along with stylohyoid muscle

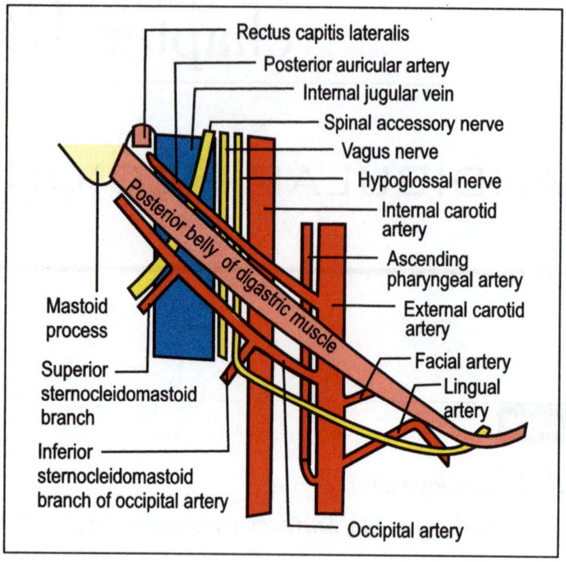

Fig. 13.2: Relations of the posterior belly of digastric muscle

c) It is held to the side of body and greater cornu of hyoid bone by means of an inverted 'U' shaped facial sling (part of deep cervical fascia). Bursa is present in between sling & tendon. Facial sling is attached to hyoid bone at the junction of body and greater cornu.

d) Sometimes it may be absent.

Relations: (Figs. 13.2 & 13.3)

a) **Superficial surface**: Skin, superficial fascia, platysma, investing layer of deep cervical fascia, mastoid process with sternocleidomastoid, apex of parotid gland and submandibular gland crossed by retromandibular vein, common facial vein, nerves like cervical branch of facial nerve and great auricular nerve.

b) **Deep surface**:

1. Muscles: Obliquus capitis superior, rectus capitits lateralis, middle constrictor of pharynx and hyoglossus.
2. Vein: Internal jugular vein with tributaries.
3. Arteries: Internal and external carotid with its branches (lingual, facial, occipital & ascending pharyngeal).
4. Nerves: Vagus, accessory (spinal) and hypoglossal with descendens hypoglossi.

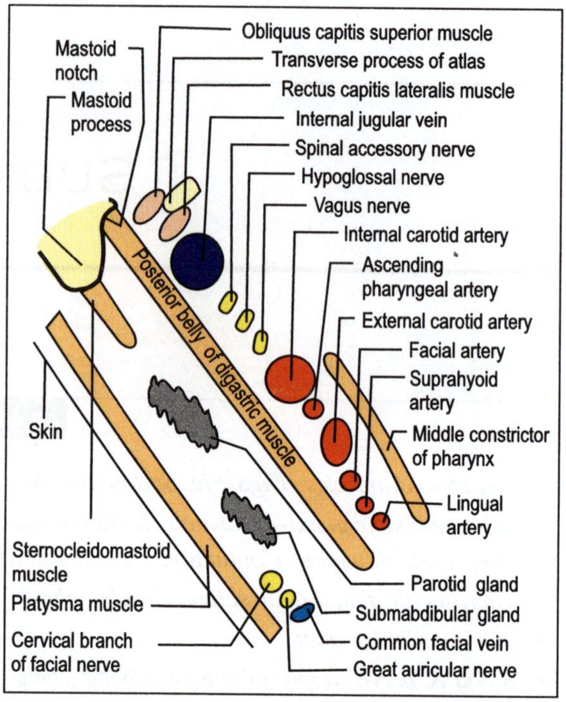

Fig. 13.3: Relations of the posterior belly of digastric muscle after section along the posterior belly of digastric muscle

c) **Upper border**: Stylohyoid muscle and posterior auricular artery. (Fig. 13.4)

d) **Lower border**: Occipital artery along the lower border & it is having upper and lower sternomastoid branches.

Nerve supply: Facial nerve just after coming out of stylomastoid foramen.

Actions:

a) Depressing and retraction of the mandible and opens the mouth.

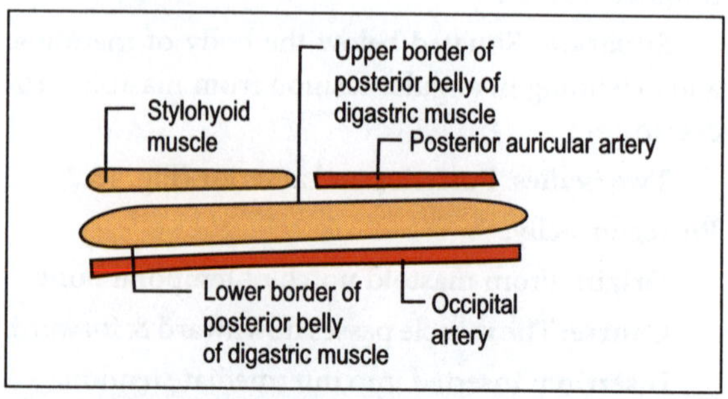

Fig. 13.4: Relations of upper & lower border of the posterior belly of digastric muscle

Important characteristics of posterior belly of digastric:

1. It forms boundaries of two triangles of neck (subdivisions of anterior triangle). Digastric triangle lies below and behind. Carotid triangle above and in front.
2. Three nerves (vagus, spinal accessory and hypoglossal nerve) and three arteries (common carotid, internal and external carotid arteries) pass deep to it.
3. It is a derivative of second arch myotome and supplied by facial nerve.
4. Hypoglossal nerve passes twice deep to it.

Anterior belly

It form boundary of submental triangle.

Origin: From lower border of mandible in the digastric fossa close to median plane at symphysis menti.

Insertion: Into intermediate tendon.

Nerve supply: Nerve to mylohyoid branch of inferior alveolar of mandibular [as it is developed from first arch myotome] nerve.

Action:

1. Depression of mandible during opening of mouth.
2. Elevates hyoid bone. (Fig. 13.1)

Stylohyoid (Fig. 13.5)

A small muscle situated on the upper border of posterior belly of digastric.

Origin: From posterior aspect of styloid process of temporal bone, midway between its tip and base.

Insertion: Into junction of body and greater cornu of hyoid bone. The muscle is having triangular gap (at the insertion) where the intermediate tendon of digastric lie.

Nerve supply: Fascial nerve just after coming out of stylomastoid foramen.

Action:

1. Draws hyoid bone upwards and backwards and thereby elongates the floor of mouth.
2. It can fix the hyoid bone for action of tongue muscles. (Fig. 13.3)

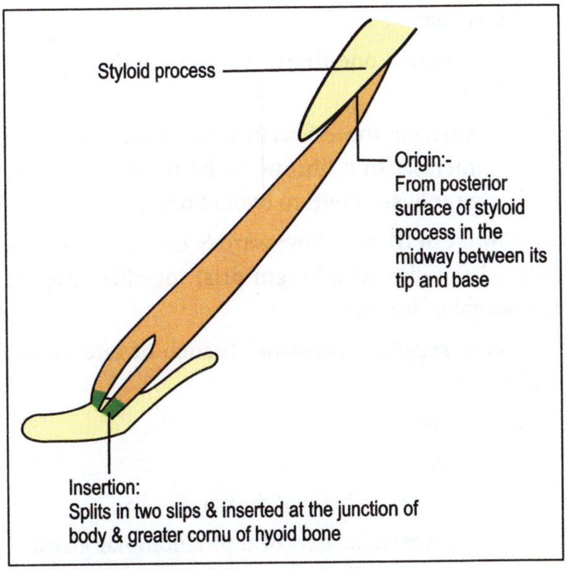

Fig. 13.5: Origin & insertion of stylohyoid muscle

Mylohyoid (Fig. 13.6)

It is a muscle lying deep to anterior belly of digastric and forms floor of oral cavity with fellow of opposite side.

Origin: From mylohyoid line on the inner surface of mandible, extending from last molar tooth to symphysis menti).

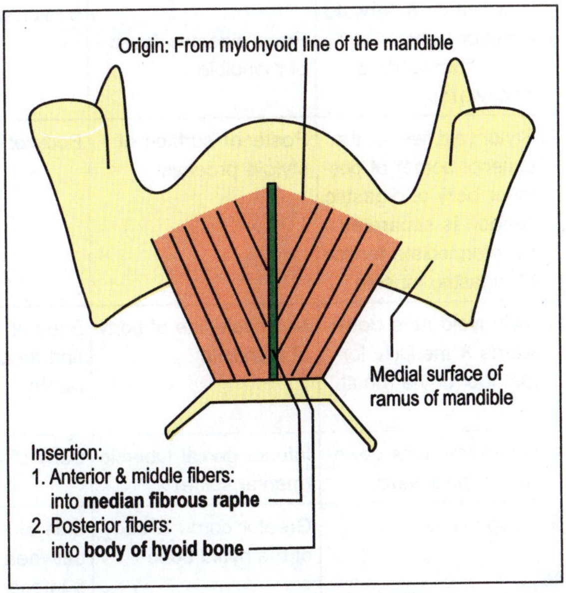

Fig. 13.6: Origin & insertion of mylohyoid muscle

Insertion:

1. Posterior one-fourth fibres to body of hyoid bone.
2. Anterior three-fourth fibres from each side intersect in a fibrous raphe (extending from symphysis menti to hyoid bone).

Course of fibres: Downward & medially two mylohyoid muscles (diaphragm oris) together support the weight of tongue.

Nerve supply: Mylohyoid branch of inferior alveolar nerve.

Relations:

1. Superficial:
   a) Anterior belly of digastric
   b) Superficial part of submandibular gland
   c) Submental vessels
   d) Mylohyoid vessels and nerves.
2. Deep:
   a) Muscles: Hyoglossus, genioglossus, geniohyoid
   b) Between mylohyoid and hyoglossus from above downwards:
      1. Styloglossus
      2. Lingual nerve
      3. Submandibular ganglion
      4. Deep part of submandibular gland with duct and hypoglossal nerve with venae comitantes
   c) On the surface of genioglossus: Lingual nerve, sublingual salivary gland, submandibular duct, third part of lingual artery and hypoglossal nerve.

Actions:

a) Elevation of floor of mouth during first stage of deglutition
b) Depression of mandible
c) Elevation of hyoid bone.

Characteristic: Muscles of both side together form diapharagma oris as it supports the weight of tongue and acts as floor of mouth.

Table 13.1: Suprahyoid muscles

Muscle	Origin	Insertion	Nerve	Action
1. Digastric: Posterior belly runs downwards & forward	Mastoid notch of temporal bone	Intermediate tendon is held to hyoid bone by fibrous pulley	Facial nerve	Elevate hyoid bone
Anterior belly runs downwards & backwards	From digastric fossa of mandible	–do–	Nerve to mylohyoid	Depress the mandible during opening of the mouth
2. Stylohyoid lies on the superior border of posterior belly of digastric. Tendon is separated by intermediate tendon of digastric muscle	Posterior surface of styloid process	Body of hyoid	Facial nerve	Elevates the hyoid bone It helps to fixes the hyoid bone for the action of tongue muscles. It elongate the floor of the mouth
3. Mylohyoid runs downwards & medially forms floor of the mouth	Mylohyoid line of body of mandible	Body of hyoid bone and median fibrous raphe	Inferior alveolar nerve	Elevates the floor of mouth during 1st stage of deglutition and hyoid bone or depress the mandible
4. Geniohyoid runs downwards backwards	Inferior genial tubercle (mental spine)	Body of hyoid	First cervical nerve	Elevates the hyoid bone or depress the mandible
5. Hyoglossus	Greater cornu & body of the hyoid bone	Side of the tongue in between styloglossus & inferior longitudinal muscles of the tongue	Hypoglossal nerve	Depress the sides of the tongue

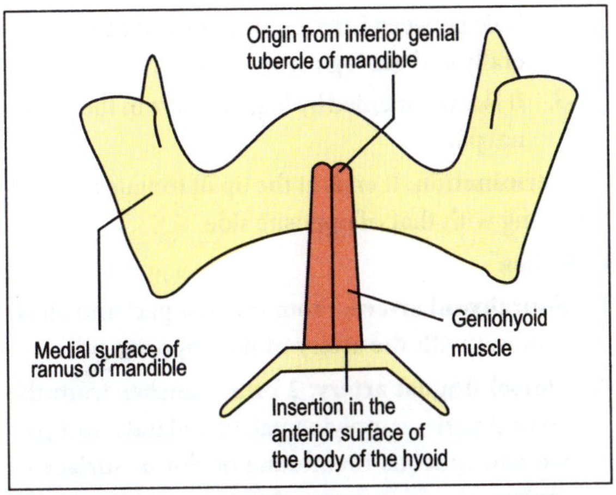

Fig. 13.7: Origin & insertion of the geniohyoid muscle

Geniohyoid (Fig. 13.7)

A narrow muscle situated deep to mylohyoid muscle. (Fig. 13.3)

Origin: From inferior genial tubercles of mandible.

Insertion: To anterior surface of body of hyoid bone.

Nerve supply: First cervical nerve through hypoglossal nerve.

Actions: Elevates the hyoid bone upward and forward and thereby shortens the floor of mouth.

Characteristic: Anatomically related with tongue but morphologically it is the component of suprahyoid group of muscles.

Hyoglossus muscle (Fig. 13.8)

It is a quadrilateral muscle (flat) of the tongue. It lies deep to mylohyoid muscle.

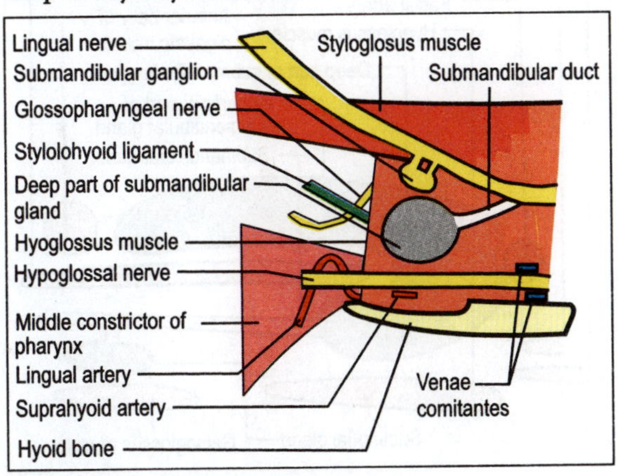

Fig. 13.8: Relations of hyoglossus muscle

Origin: From upper surface of greater cornu and body of hyoid bone

Insertion: Into side of tongue between styloglossus and inferior longitudinal muscle.

Relations:

1. **Superficial relations** (above downward)
   a) Lingual nerve
   b) Submandibular ganglion
   c) Deep part of submandibular gland and submandibular duct
   d) Venae comitantes
   e) Hypoglossal nerve
2. **Deep relations**:
   a) Glossopharyngeal nerve
   b) Stylohyoid ligament
   c) Lingual artery

Nerve supply: Supplied by hypoglossal nerve.

LINGUAL ARTERY (Figs. 13.9 & 13.10)

It is main artery for supply of blood to the tongue.

Origin: It is the second artery arising from front of external carotid artery and opposite the tip of greater cornu of hyoid.

It may arise as a common trunk with facial artery.

Course: Divided into three parts by hypoglossus.

First part: From origin to posterior border of hyoglossus.

Second part: Part deep to hyoglossus.

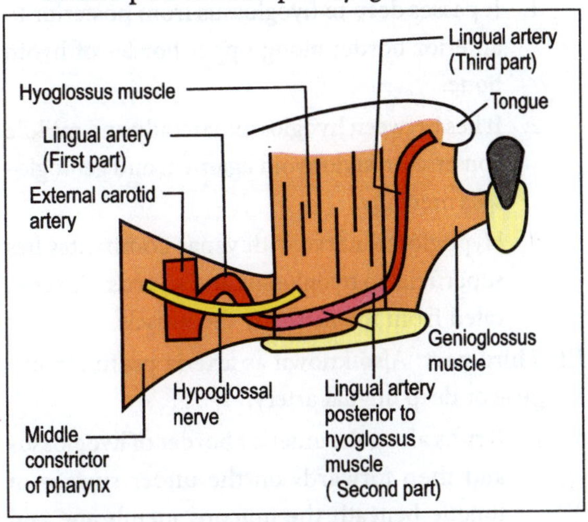

Fig. 13.9: Parts of the lingual artery

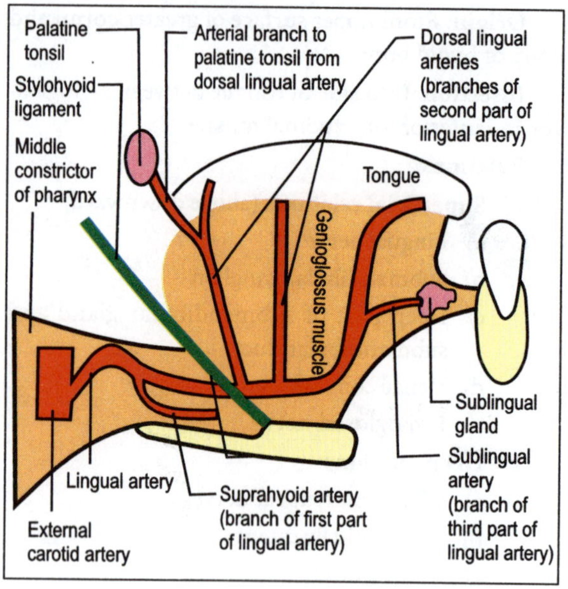

Fig. 13.10: Course & branches of the lingual artery

Third part: Part from anterior border of hyoglossus to termination at tongue & lies on genioglossus.

I. **First part**
   1. Lies in carotid triangle and on the middle constrictor muscle.
   2. Forms a characteristic loop which is crossed by hypoglossal nerve and common facial vein. This loop permits movement of hyoid bone freely.

II. **Second part**
   1. It passes deep to hyoglossus from posterior to anterior border along upper border of hyoid bone.
   2. It lies between hyoglossus laterally and middle constrictor, stylohyoid ligament and genioglossus medially.
   3. Hypoglossal nerve with venae comitantes lies superficial to hyoglossus and so artery is separated from the nerve by the muscle.

III. **Third part**: Also known as arteria profunda linguae or deep lingual artery.
   1. It runs along the anterior border of hyoglossus and then forwards on the under surface of tongue beneath the mucous membrane and on each side of frenulum linguae.
   2. It lie between inferior longitudinal muscle laterally and genioglossus medially.
   3. It is accompanied by lingual nerve in the terminal part.

Termination: It ends at the tip of tongue by anastomosing with that of opposite side.

Branches:
1. **Suprahyoid artery**: From the first part and anastomoses with the artery of the opposite side.
2. **Dorsal lingual artery**: 2 or 3 branches from the second part – supplying palatine glands, soft palate and mucous membrane of dorsal surface of tongue.
3. **Sublingual artery**: From the 3rd part and supplies sublingual gland, mucous membrane of floor of mouth and gums.

APPLIED ANATOMY:

During surgical operation for removal of the tongue the site of ligature will be the first part of the artery before it gives any branch i.e., just after the origin of artery.

SUBMANDIBULAR SALIVARY GLAND

It is the largest and paired mixed type of salivary gland and so is serious (mostly) and mucous (partly).

Situation: In the anterior part of digastric triangle and submandibular fossa of the mandible.

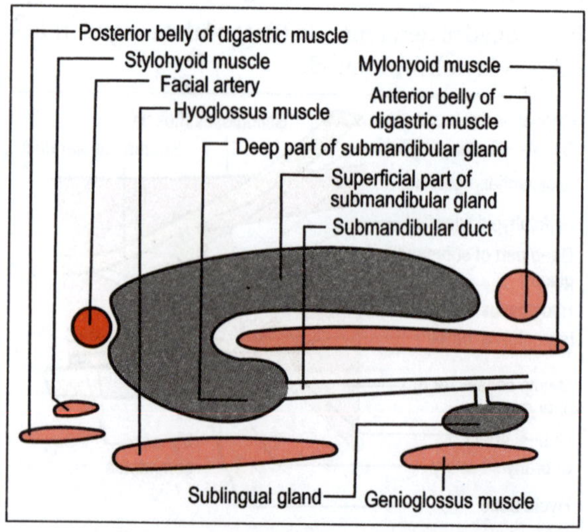

Fig. 13.11: Parts and relations of submandibular gland

Size: About the size of a walnut.

Shape: More or less J shaped.

Weight: About 10 to 20gms.

Different parts: The gland is having two parts: (1) Superficial part; (2) Deep part. (Fig. 13.11)

The gland is divided into two parts by mylohyoid muscle.

Superficial part is continuous with deep part at the posterior border of mylohyoid.

1. **Superficial**: Superficial to mylohyoid and larger part.
2. **Deep**: Deep to mylohyoid and smaller part.

1. **Superficial part of submandibular (salivary) gland**: It is the larger part lying superficial to mylohyoid muscle and more or less occupies the most of digastric triangle and its upper limit extends up to mylohyoid line.

Fascial covering

The investing layer of deep cervical fascia splits into two layers to enclose superficial part of submandibular gland. The superficial layer is attached to inferior border of the mandible after covering inferior surface of the gland. The deep layer (covering the medial surface of the gland) is attached to mylohyoid line. (Fig. 13.12)

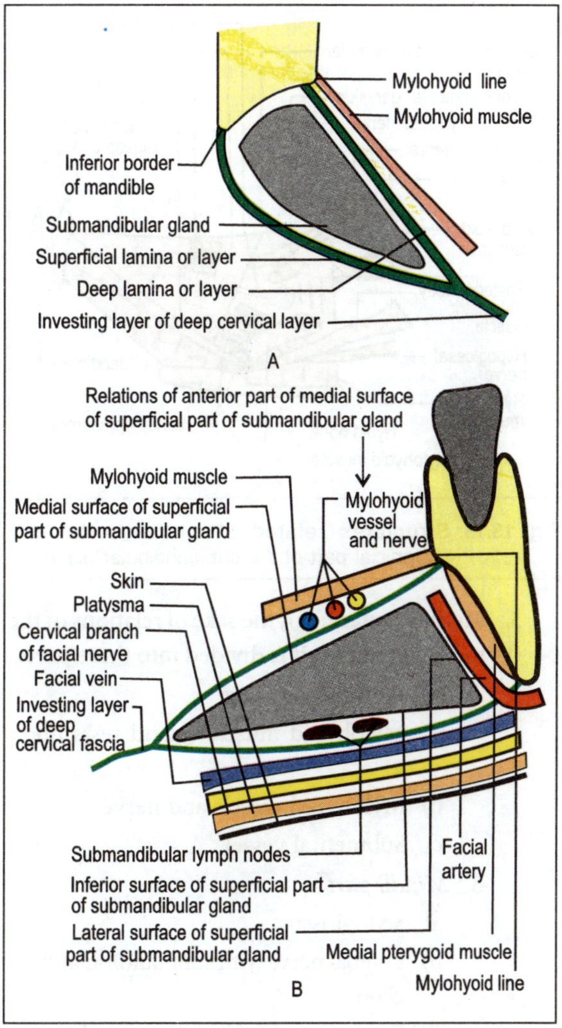

Fig. 13.12: (A) Fascial covering of superficial part of submandibular gland; (B) Relations of inferior surface, lateral surface and part of medial surface of the superficial part of the submandibular gland

Different surfaces and ends of superficial part of submandibular

A. Surfaces: Three – (1) Inferior surface; (2) Lateral surface; (3) Medial surface. (Fig. 13.12)

B. Two ends:
   1. Anterior end: The end extending up to anterior belly of digastric muscle
   2. Posterior end: That end which extends up to stylomandibular ligament.

[This ligament separates the submandibular from parotid gland]. This end presents a groove for facial artery.]

Relations:

1. **Inferior surface**: From superficial to deep
   a) Skin, superficial fascia
   b) Platysma
   c) Cervical branch of facial nerve
   d) Deep cervical fascia
   e) Common facial vein
   f) Submandibular lymph nodes
2. **Lateral surface**: Deep to superficial
   a) Submandibular fossa of the mandible
   b) Insertion of medial pterygoid muscle
   c) Loop of facial artery.

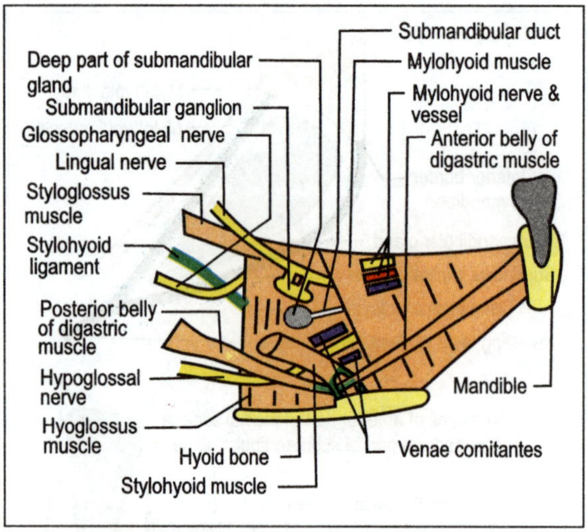

Fig. 13.13: Structures related of medial surface of superficial part of the submandibular gland

3. **Medial surface**: For the sake of relations of the medial surface – it is divided into three parts.
   A. *Front* or *anterior part*
      a) Mylohyoid muscle (gland rests upon it)
      b) Mylohyoid vessels and nerve
      c) Submental vessel
   B. *Middle part*
      a) Styloglossus
      b) Lingual nerve with submandibular ganglion
      c) Deep part of submandibular gland
      d) Submandibular duct
      e) Hypoglossal nerve with vena comitantes and
      f) Digastric tendon (Fig. 13.13)
      g) Stylohyoid
   C. *Posterior part*
      a) Styloglossus, stylopharyngeus
      b) Glossopharyngeal nerve
      c) Posterior belly of digastric
      d) Stylohyoid ligament
      e) Middle constrictor muscle of pharynx
      f) Hypoglossal nerve, and first part of lingual artery.

Deep part of submandibular gland

Situation: Situated in between mylohyoid superficially and hyoglossus deeply.

Size: Small.

Continuity: Continuous with superficial part posteriorly around the posterior border of mylohyoid

Extend: Anteriorly it extends up to posterior part of sublingual gland.

Relations:

A. *Above*: Lingual nerve with submandibular ganglion
B. *Below*: Hypoglossal nerve with vena comitantes.
C. *Laterally*: Mylohyoid.
D. *Medially*: Hyoglossus.

Nerve supply of the gland

1. Parasympathetic. It is secretomotor pathway:

A. **Parasympathetic part**:

Preganglionic secretomotor fiber arises from superior salivary nucleus in the pons
↓
Facial nerve
↓
Chorda tympani nerve
↓
Lingual nerve
↓
Relay in submandibular ganglion
↓
Postganglionic fibers supply sybmandibular gland and sublingual gland

B. **Sympathetic part**:

Preganglionic fiers arises from T_1 segment and relay in superior cervical sympathetic ganglion of cervical sympathetic chain
↓
Postganglionic fibers arises from superior cervical sympathetic ganglion, form plexus around facial artery
↓
Postganglionic fibers passes through the submandibular ganglion to supply the arteries of the submandibular gland and sublingual gland

2. Sympathetic: It is mainly *vasomotor*. [It comes from plexus around fascial artery and carries postganglionic fibres from superior cervical sympathetic ganglion].
3. *Sensory*: From lingual nerve.

APPLIED ANATOMY:

1. When there is an obstruction in the submandibular duct due to stone or growth the gland becomes swollen.
2. Ranula or a cystic swelling in the floor of mouth may be due to obstruction of submandibular duct.
3. Submandibular lymph node may be enlarged and tender when the gland becomes infected. Enlarged submandibular salivary gland may be distinguished by examining by two fingers (bimanually). One finger is to be placed in the floor of mouth and other below the angle of mandible. Whereas a enlarged lymph node can be palpated from superficial aspect just below the angle of mandible.
4. The incision for removal of stone or any growth in submandibular salivary gland is usually given about one inch below the angle of mandible in order to avoid injury to mandibular branch of facial nerve which passes postero-inferior to angle of mandible just before crossing it.
5. *Sialography*: Injecting radio-opaque dye through the opening of submandibular ducts and the duct system of salivary glands will be visualised.

SUBMANDIBULAR DUCT

Also known as Wharton's duct (Figs. 13.11 & 13.14)

Length: 5cm.

Size: About the size of crow quill.

Site of emergence: Emerges from the anterior end of the deep part of the gland.

Course: It runs at first upward and forward between mylohyoid and hyoglossus (lies on hyoglossus) and between lingual nerve above and hypoglossal nerve below.

Here it is *intimately related with lingual nerve which lies at first above, then laterally and loops below the duct and passes medially.*

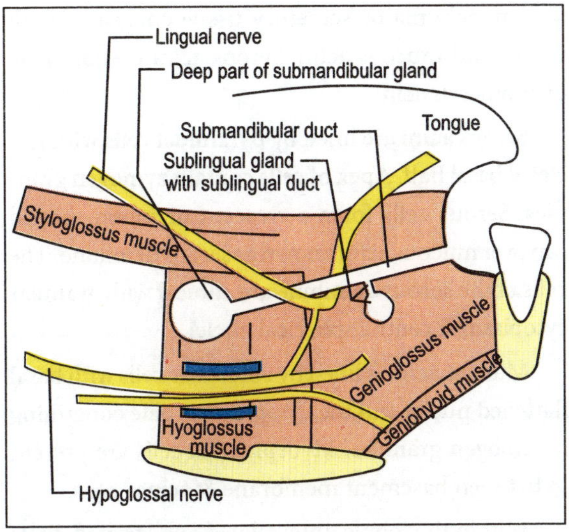

Fig. 13.14: Deep part of submandibular gland with submandibular duct

Then the duct passes between sublingual gland and genioglossus and finally enters the floor of mouth and ends.

Ends: It ends by opening in the floor of mouth on the summit of a sublingual papilla on each side of frenulum of the tongue.

Blood supply of the gland: Arteries by branches of facial and lingual arteries and veins correspond to arteries and drain into common facial or lingual veins and ultimately into internal jugular veins.

Lymphatics of the gland: Into submandibular and then into jugulo-digastric lymph nodes.

HISTOLOGY OF THE SUBMANDIBULAR GLAND (Fig. 13.15)

This is a mixed exocrine gland.

It is invested by the capsule (connective tissue), which enters the gland to divide into several lobules.

The interlobular connective tissue contain blood vessels, nerves and excretory ducts. Interlobular duct is lined by tall columnar epithelium.

Parenchyma or secretory tissue consist of both serous and mucous acini. Serous acini predominate over mucous acini.

Serous acini are lined by pyramidal cells with nuclei at basal half. Apex of cells contain zymogen granules. Serous cells form a crescent or moon-shaped cap over mucous acini known as serous demilune. The cells of the serous demilune are cubical with granular cytoplasm & central spherical nuclei.

Mucous acini is lined by columnar cells with basal flattened nuclei and the cytoplasm is pale containing mucinogen granules. Myoepithelial cells are present in between basement membrane & acinar cells.

Within the lobule, intercalated and striated ducts are present which are lined by cuboidal cells striated ducts are lined by columnar epithelium and striations are due folds in basal plasma membrane. Striated ducts open into interlobular ducts. Interlobular ducts join with each other to form submandibular duct.

SUBLINGUAL SALIVARY GLAND (Fig. 13.16)

It is the smallest of three salivary glands.

Situation: In the sublingual fossa of the mandible in the floor of mouth between mucous membrane and mylohyoid muscle.

Shape: Almond.

Type: Mixed gland – secretion mainly mucous and partly serous.

Weight: 3 to 4gm.

Relations:

In front: Meeting of two glands behind symphysis menti.

Above: Covered with sublingual fold of mucous membrane.

Laterally: Sublingual fossa of mandible.

Medially: Genioglossus and lingual nerve and submandibular duct.

Ducts of the gland: Number – 8 to 20

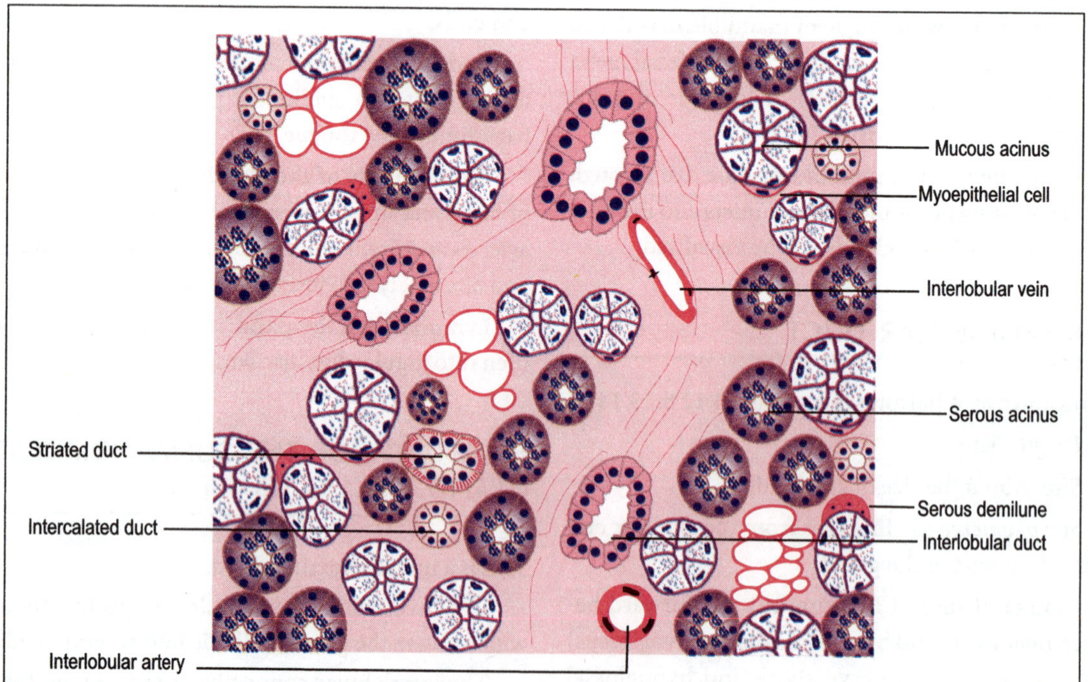

Fig. 13.15: Microscopic features of the submandibular gland

Two groups:

1. **Ducts of Rivinus**: Most of ducts open separately on the floor of mouth.
2. **Duct of Bartholin (Sublingual duct)**: A single duct formed by the union of some duct and open into submandibular duct.

HISTOLOGY OF SUBLINGUAL GLAND

The gland is a mixed exocrine gland having more of mucous acini. (Fig. 13.16)

The gland is invested by capsule (connective tissue) which enters inside the gland to divide the gland into several lobules.

The interlobular connective tissue contain blood vessels, nerves and interlobular duct. Interlobular duct is lined by tall columnar epithelium.

Parenchyma or secretory cells consist of both mucous and serous acini. Mucous acini predominate over serous acini.

Mucous acini is lined by columnar cells with basal flattened nuclei, and the cytoplasm is pale containing mucinogen granules. Serous cells form crescent or moon-shaped cap over mucous acini known as serous demilune. The cells of serous demilune or crescent are cubical, with granular cytoplasm and central spherical nuclei.

Serous acini is lined by pyramidal cells with nuclei at basal half. Supranuclear portion contain numerous basophilic zymogen granules.

Within the lobule intercalated ducts are present, which are lined by cuboidal epithelium.

Interlobular duct joins with each other to form sublingual duct.

SUBMANDIBULAR GANGLION

It is a peripheral ganglion of the parasympathetic system. (Fig. 13.17)

Topographically it is related to lingual nerve.

Functionally: Related to chorda tympani branch of facial nerve.

Situation: Situated on the upper part of superficial surface of hyoglossus muscle and suspended by two roots from lingual nerve.

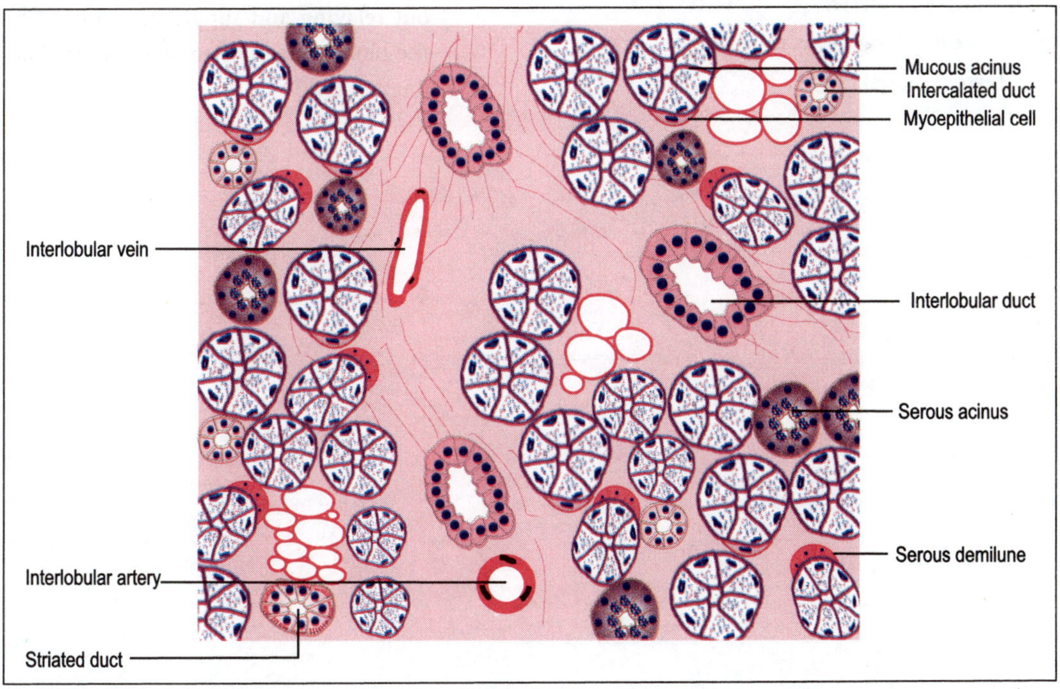

Fig. 13.16: Microscopic features of the sublingual gland

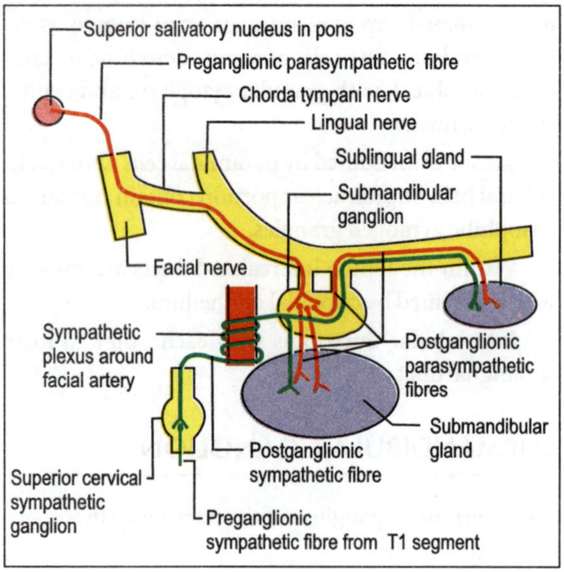

Fig. 13.17: Connections of Submandibular ganglion

Size: Small, fusiform about the size of pin's head.

Relations:

a) **Laterally**: Submandibular salivary gland and mylohyoid muscle.
b) **Medially**: Hyoglossus muscle.
c) **Above**: Lingual nerve.
d) **Below**: Deep part of submandibular salivary gland and its duct.

Roots: It has two roots: (a) **Parasympathetic** and (b) **Sympathetic**

a) **Parasympathetic** or **motor roots**: Preganglionic secretomotor fibres arise from **superior salivary** nucleus in the pons. Then preganglionic secretomotor fibres (parasympathetic part) pass successively through the facial, chorda tympani and lingual nerves. The preganglionic fibres reach the submandibular ganglion where the fibres are relayed. Postganglionic fibres arising from the ganglion supply directly submandibular gland by five or more branches; some postganglionic secretomotor fibres join lingual nerve and supply the sublingual and anterior lingual glands.
b) **Sympathetic root**: Postganglionic sympathetic fibres arises from superior cervical sympathetic ganglion of sympathetic trunk and produces plexus around the facial artery. The fibres passes through submandibular ganglion without relaying and supply vasomotor fibres to the blood vessels of submandibular and sublingual gland.

chapter 14

MOUTH, PALATE AND PHARYNX

AT A GLANCE

- *Mouth—Mouth cavity: Vestibule, Cheeks, Gums; Oral cavity proper; Oropharyngeal isthmus; Sublingual region; Teeth: Parts, Structures & supporting tissue – Enamel, Dentine, Pulp, Cementum; Eruption of tooth; Different surfaces teeth; Characteristic parts of individual parts; Development of teeth*
- *Palate—Different parts; Hard palate; Soft palate: Function, Surfaces & Borders, Composition, Palatine aponeurosis, Muscles, Blood & nerve supply; Development*
- *Pharynx—Situation; Extent, Length, Width; Boundary; Different parts with their features; Important regions of pharynx: Pharyngeal isthmus, Oropharyngeal isthmus, Pyriform fossa; Structures of pharyngeal wall; Blood supply, lymphatics; Nerve supply; Muscles of pharynx (constrictors); Palatine tonsil: Situation, Number, Extension, shape, size, capsule, Features & relations, Structures, Blood supply, Lymphatics, Nerve supply, Development; Applied anatomy*
- *Auditory tube*

MOUTH

Mouth cavity

Mouth cavity extend from lips to the oropharyngeal isthmus (palatoglossal fold and sulcus terminalis) which forms the first part of the digestive tube.

It consist of two parts by alveolar processes, teeth and gums. Two parts are:

1. **Vestibule**: Outer smaller part
2. **Mouth cavity proper**: Inner larger part (Fig. 14.1)

Vestibule of mouth

It is the cleft like space.

Boundary:

Externally: By lips and cheeks

Internally: Teeth and gums

Roof and floor: Reflection of mucous membrane from lips and cheeks to gums.

Communication:

1. With outside by oral aperture.

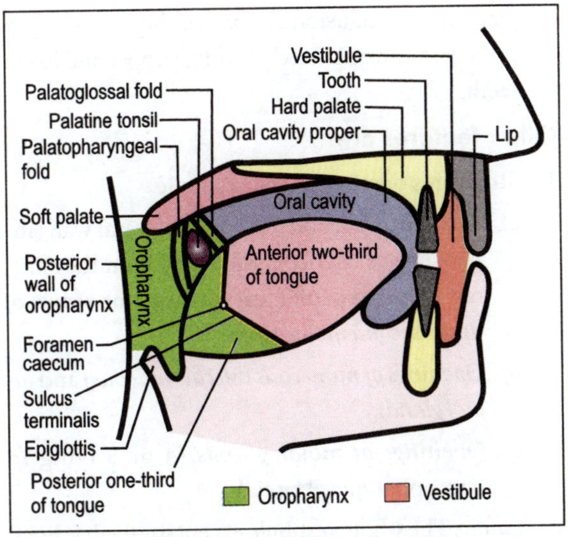

Fig. 14.1: Sagittal section through oral cavity & oropharynx

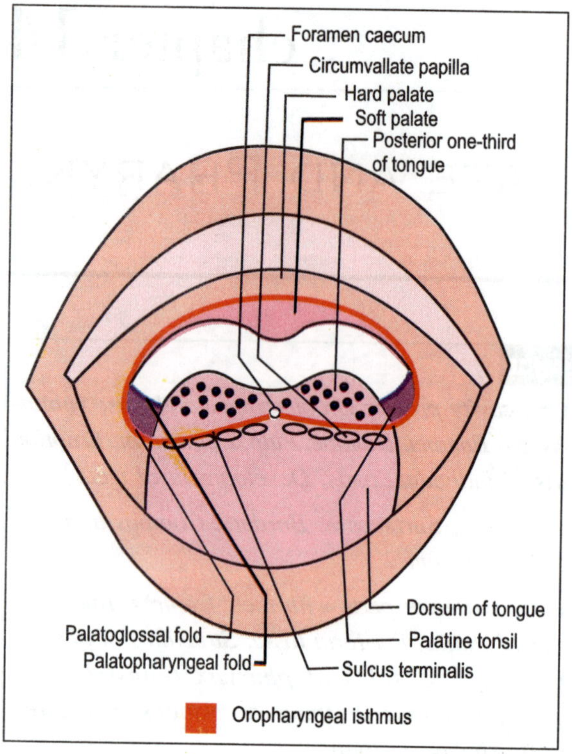

Fig. 14.2: Oral cavity and oropharynx. (Red line indicate oropharyngeal isthmus)

2. With **oral cavity** proper small opening behind third tooth through a gap between the last molar tooth ramus of mandible (retromolar region) and when teeth are in occlusion and when they are in open position it can open freely through upper and lower teeth.

Other features are:

1. Structures opening in the vestibule
   a) *Opening of parotid duct* on the lateral wall (inner surface of cheek) of *vestibule* on the summit of raised papilli just opposite the *crown of upper second molar tooth.*
   b) *Openings of numerous buccal (mucous)* and *labial glands*
   c) *Openings of molar glands* (4 or 5 lying in buccopharyngeal fascia).
2. *Lining*: The whole vestibule except the teeth is lined by mucous membrane.

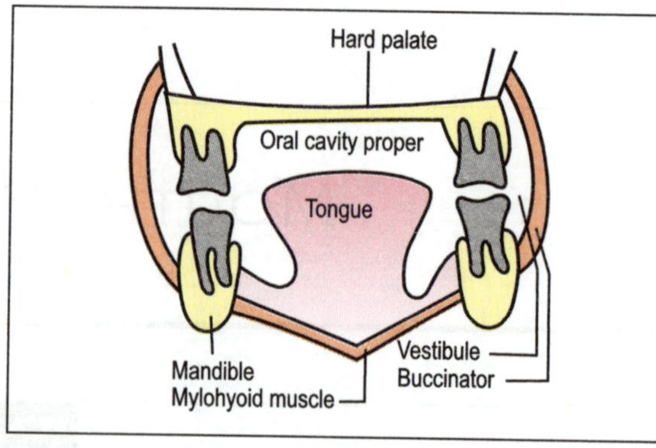

Fig. 14.3: Coronal section of oral cavity

3. *Frenulum of lip*: Fold of mucous membrane between lips and gums.

Lips: They are fleshy movable folds which bound the opening of mouth (oral fissure).

Features:

1. *Vermilion zone*: Reddish part of lip. It is *visible and vascular* through thin most epithelium.
2. *Vermilion border: Mucocutaneous junctional region* (where skin and vermilion zone join).
3. *Philtrum*: A shallow groove in the median part of upper lip (externally).
4. *Frenulum of lip*: Median fold connecting each lip to corresponding gum (internally).
5. *Elements or layers forming lip (composition)*: Each lip is composed of (from outside inwards)
   a) Skin with hair, sebaceous and sweat glands
   b) Subcutaneous tissue
   c) Orbicularis oris
   d) Submucous layer (lamina propria) containing labial glands and arterial circle formed by superior and inferior labial branches of facial artery.
   e) *Mucous membrane*: Lining epithelium is *stratified squamous* (nonkeratinised)
6. *Lymphatics*
   a) *From central part*: To submental lymph node
   b) *Rest of part*: To submandibular lymph nodes.
7. *Blood vessels*: Each lip is supplied by labial branches of facial artery. The labial branches of both side

anastomoses with each other. The corresponding veins drain to facial vein.

8. *Nerve supply*: Upper lip is supplied by labial branch of infraorbital nerve (a branch of maxillary nerve). Lower lip is supplied by mental branch of inferior alveolar nerve (a branch of mandibular nerve).

CHEEKS

Sides of face between angle of mouth to the anterior border of masseter.

Composition:

a) Skin
b) Superficial fascia which contains zygomaticus major and risorius muscles, parotid duct, mucous glands (molar), facial artery and vein, buccal branches of mandibular and facial nerve and buccal pad of fat on buccinator. Buccal pad of fat extends in between buccinator & masseter (pierced by parotid duct).
c) Buccinator covered with buccopharyngeal fascia
d) Submucous with buccal mucous glands
e) Mucous membrane lined by stratified squamous epithelium (non-keratinising)

Lymphatics: Drain into submandibular and preauricular lymph nodes but also partly buccal area into submandibular lymph nodes.

GUM

Also known as gingivae (Fig. 14.4)

Features:

1. Soft tissues covering upper and lower alveolar processes including neck of teeth.
2. Composed of dense and vascular fibrous tissue lined by *stratified squamous epithelium* (thinly keratinised)
3. Parts: Three parts

The gingiva is divided into marginal, attached & interdental areas.

a) **Marginal gingiva**: The marginal gingiva is the terminal edge of gingiva. The marginal gingiva is more translucent than attached gingiva. The marginal gingiva is not having bony support. It surrounds the teeth like collar like fashion. It is pink in colour.

b) **Attached gingiva**: It is continuous with marginal gingiva. It is firm, resilient and tightly bound to underlying periosteum of alveolar bone. The width of gingiva differs in the different areas of facial aspect. It is thickest in the incisor region (3.5-4.5mm in the maxilla, and 33-3.9mm in the mandible); least width in premolar region (1.8-1.9mm). Certain amount of gingiva is necessary for the stability of the underlying root of tooth.

c) **Interdental gingiva**: Inter dental gingiva occupies the gingival embrasure 'V' shaped valleys between adjacent teeth). Inter dental gingiva can be pyramidal or have a depression ('col' shape). Attached gingiva is keratinized. Epithelium in the col consist of marginal gingiva of adjacent teeth, except that it is nonkeratinised. Space between teeth in the anterior region is narrow, so interdental gingiva is minimum.

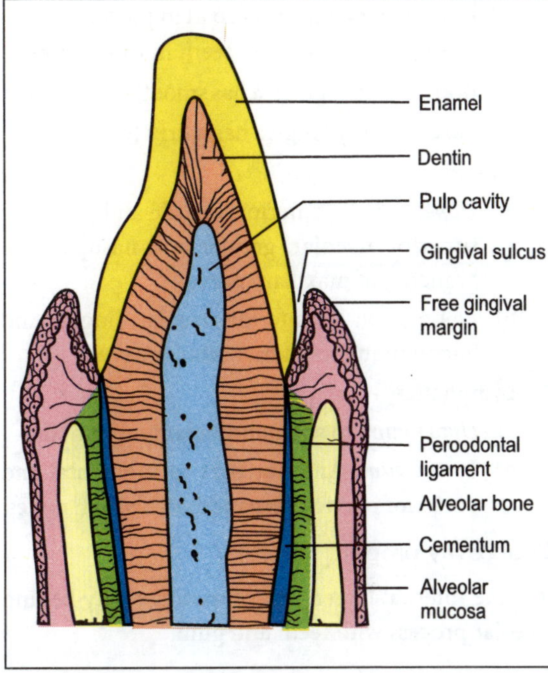

Fig. 14.4: Parts of tooth with gum

Interdental gingiva is broad in posterior teeth due more gap between teeth in this region.

Contour: Healthy gingiva has smooth appearance.

Texture: Healthy gingiva has a firm texture.

4. **Nerves**:
   a) *Upper gum* by anterior, middle and posterior superior alveolar, greater and nasopalatine branches of maxillary nerve.
   b) *Lower gum*: By inferior alveolar, lingual and buccal branches of mandibular nerve.
5. **Lymphatics**:
   a) *Upper gum*: to submandibular lymph nodes
   b) *Lower gum*: Anterior part to submental and posterior part to submandibular lymph nodes.

Oral cavity proper:

It is the internal larger part of mouth cavity behind alveolar process with teeth and gum.

Boundary:

1. *In front and sides*: Alveolar process with teeth gums.
2. *Behind*: Communicates with pharynx through *oropharyngeal isthmus*.
3. *Roof*: By palate (both hard and soft).
4. *Floor*: By tongue behind and sublingual region in front [*sublingual region lies between tongue and floor of mouth*].

Floor of mouth: Formed by both *muscles* and *two muscles form diaphragma oris*.

Oropharyngeal isthmus

Boundary:

1. *Above*: Soft palate
2. *Below*: Dorsal surface of tongue along the sulcus terminalis.
3. *On each side*: Palatoglossal arch (fold of mucous membrane containing palatoglossus muscle).

Sublingual region

Features:

1. *Frenulum of the tongue*: A median mucous fold connecting tongue to floor of mouth.
2. Sublingual papilla: Elevation on each side of lower end of frenulum opening of *submandibular duct* are present here.
3. *Sublingual fold*: A fold extends from sublingual papilla forwards and laterally and overlies sublingual gland. On the edges of the fold *sublingual duct* open. (Fig. 17.3)

Dental anatomy is the field of anatomy which is dedicated to study of structure of human tooth. Dental anatomy is a taxonomical science which is concerned with naming and structures of teeth, which will serve for practical purpose in dental treatment.

There are 20 primary teeth and 28-32 permanent teeth. Third molars or 'wisdom teeth' may or may not grow. Among primary teeth, 10 are found usually in the upper jaw (maxilla) and other 10 in lower jaw. Among permanent teeth 16 are found in upper jaw (maxilla), other 16 are found in lower jaw (mandible). Most of the teeth have special features.

TEETH

Teeth are most important structures concerned for mastication.

Different parts: Three parts–

1. *Root*: Part within the socket of the jaw (hidden)
2. *Crown*: Anatomical crown covered by enamel extends up to clinical crown is the part that projects beyond gum.

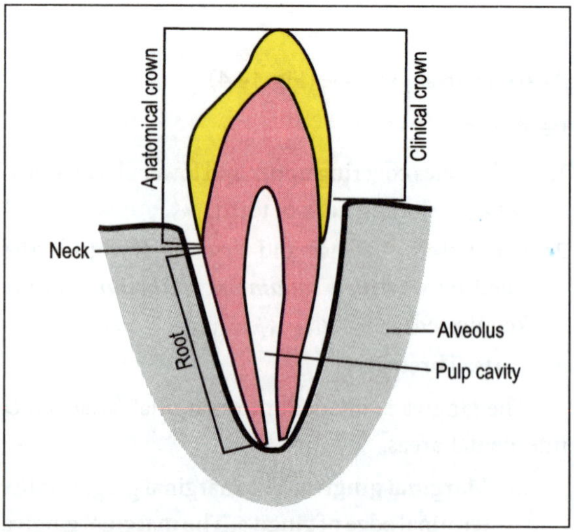

Fig. 14.5: Different types of crown

3. *Neck*: Contricted part between root and crown and encircled by gum (Fig. 14.5).

Other features:

Apical (Alveolar foramen): Pinpoint foramen at the apex of each root leading to wide root canal and finally to tooth or pulp cavity. Pulp cavity is covered by dentine, enamel and cementum (three calcified tissues). Disintegration of one or more dental tissue is known as **caries.**

Structure of teeth and supporting tissues

Structurally teeth are composed of:

1. Enamel
2. Dentin
3. Pulp
4. Cementum
5. Periodental ligament.

1. Enamel:

Enamel covers the anatomic crown of the tooth and is the hardest substance in the human body. It is responsible for translucency and esthetic colour of the tooth. Enamel is susceptible to caries, wear & fracture due to its brittle nature, and stress from occlusion. There is no regeneration after its damage. Loss of enamel require restorative treatment for proper function & form of the tooth. Enamel is developed from ectoderm (ameloblast).

Structure:

- Rods or prisms
- Rod sheath
- Inter prismatic substance
- Enamel lamellae
- Dentino-enamel junction
- Enamel spindle

Rods or prisms:

Number: 5-12 millions

Direction: Wavy course & oriented perpendicular to dentine enamel junction (DEJ)

Rod sheath:

- A thin peripheral layer of rods
- Darken than the rod

Inter prismatic substance

- Occupying the space between prisms or rods
- Less calcified then the rod itself.

Enamel lamellae: Space between enamel rods. They are the weak areas (containing organic material) through which bacteria enter causing caries.

Dentino enamel junction (DEJ): This is the area (30mm) between enamel & dentin. In this area, there is interlocking between enamel projections & depression of dentin.

Enamel spindle: Sometimes odontoblastic process (thickened ends) may cross DEJ to enter enamel. These parts are called enamel spindle.

Function of enamel:

1. Enamel provides a hard, durable shape (esthetic appearance) of the tooth
2. Protects the dentine & pulp.

2. Dentin:

It is usually covered by enamel on the crown and cementum on the root and surrounds entire pulp.

Dentine is derived from dental papilla.

Dentine continues to form throughout life (unlike enamel).

Dentine consist of dentinal tubules which radiate from pulp to the enamel or cementum. Dentinal tubules contain odontoblastic processes from odontoblast.

Canaliculi are connections (lateral) between dental tubules.

Peritubular dentin is mineralized in the walls of dentinal tubules.

Inter tubular dentine: It is present between tubules.

Functions:

1. Flexibility of dentine prevents crack propagation in the brittle enamel.
2. Protect dental pulp.
3. Provides strength & rigidity to the tooth.
4. Initiates the pulpal defense response inspite of the fact that it (dentine) lacks blood supply or nerves.

3. Pulp:

It (connective tissue) is present in the centre of the tooth, occupying the pulp cavity. Morphologically, the pulp is divided into 2 regions: (1) Pulp chamber and (2) Radicular pulp.

1. Pulp chamber: This occupies the pulp chamber in the crown portion of the root.
2. Radicular pulp: This is located in the root portion.

Structure of pulp:

Pulp has 4 distinct layers:

1. Periperal layer: Cell bodies of odontobalst
2. Cell free layer: Has nerve & vessels.
3. Cell rich layer: Has fibroblast, etc.
4. Pulp core: Centre area; Has blood vessels & nerves which enters through apical foramen.

Function:

1. Produces primary & secondary dentine
2. Supply nutrition to dentine through odontoblastic process
3. Protect itself
4. Transmit pain impulse.

4. Cementum:

It is hard tissue formed by cementoblast. It overlaps the root of the tooth. It is avascular & surrounds the apical foramen, and may extend slightly to the inner wall of the pulp canal.

It covers the dentine part of root & cemento-dental junction is smooth. Mostly enamel joins with cementum to form cemento enamel junction (CEJ) which is also known as cervical line.

5. Periodontal ligament

It attaches tooth root to the alveolus. It is having numerous cells, blood vessels, nerves, collagen fibers and ground susbtance.

Functions:

1. Fibers attaches the cementum to the alveolar bone
2. Sensory function: Sensations of touch, pressure, and pain
3. Nutritive: The blood vessels supply nutrients
4. Homeostasis: Cells of periodontal ligament resorb and replace the cementum, alveolar bone and the periodontal ligament.

Eruption or dentition of tooth: Eruption (dentition of tooth) is twice.

Two dentitions

1. **First set: Milk teeth or deciduous teeth.**
2. **Second set: Permanent teeth.**

1. **Deciduous teeth**: 20 *in number*

In each half of jaw they are *five* (5)

Incisors: Two

Canine: One

(Milk) Molars: Two

Dental formula will be

$$\frac{2\quad 1\quad 2 \mid 2\quad 1\quad 2}{2\quad 1\quad 2 \mid 2\quad 1\quad 2}$$

Time of appearance:

Teeth	Central incisor ↓	Lateral incisor ↓	1st Molar ↓	Canine ↓	2nd Molar ↓
Months	6th to 8th month	8th to 10th month	12th to 16th month	16th to 20th month	20th to 24th month

So all teeth appear at the end of second year.

Permanent teeth: After an interval of four years following eruption of deciduous teeth, permanent teeth will appear. Permanent teeth are 32 in number. In each half of the jaw it is 8 (eight) and so 16 in each jaw. (Fig. 14.6).

They are:

A. *Incisors*: Two, central and lateral
B. *Canine*: One
C. *Premolars*: Two-first and second
D. *Molars*: Three-first, second and third.

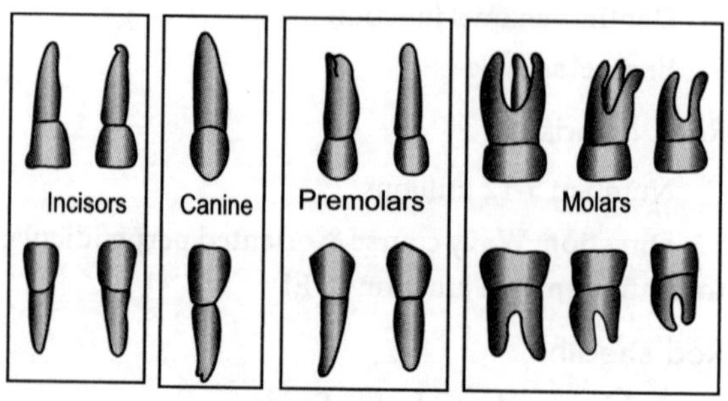

Fig. 14.6: Types of permanent teeth

So **dental formula** will be

$$\frac{3\ 2\ 1\ 2 \mid 2\ 1\ 2\ 3}{3\ 2\ 1\ 2 \mid 2\ 1\ 2\ 3}$$

Time of appearance

Molars → 6 yearly interval

1st: 6th year

2nd: 12th year

3rd: 8th-25th year (wisdom)

Other teeth *from medial to lateral within* 12 *years* (eruption of 2nd molar) except *canine* 11th year.

Teeth	1st Molar ↓	Central incisor ↓	Lateral incisor ↓	1st premolar ↓	2nd premolar ↓	Canine ↓	2nd Molar ↓	3rd Molar ↓
Years	6th	7th	8th	9th	10th	11th	12th	18th

So,

First molar: 6th year

Central incisor: 7th year

Lateral incisor: 8th year

First premolar: 9th year

Second premolar: 10th year

Canine: 11th year

Second molar: 12th year

Third molar (wisdom tooth): 18-24th year

Different groups of teeth:

Two

1. Anterior teeth: Incisors and canines
2. Posterior teeth: Premolars and molars

Different surfaces of teeth (Fig. 14.7): The surfaces named according to the dirction they face. The surface are

1. **Lingual surface**: The surface of the tooth toward tongue.
2. **Facial surface**: Sufaces of the tooth facing check or lips.

   This surface is also known as:

   a) **Labial surface**: The surface of an anterior tooth facing lips.

   b) **Buccal surface**: Surfaces of posterior tooth facing check.

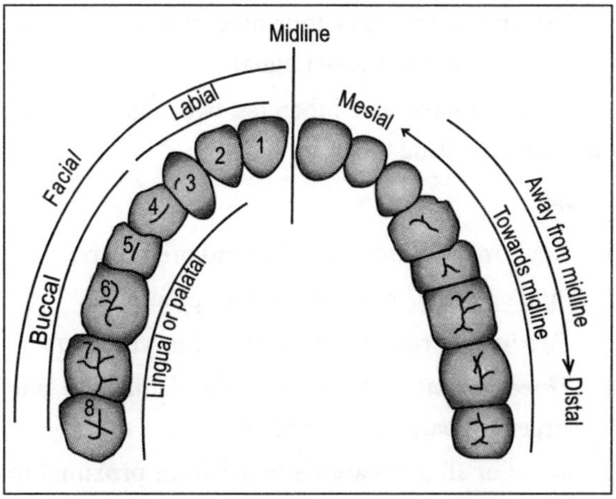

Fig. 14.7: Dental terminology used for surfaces of teeth. 1. Central incisor; 2. Lateral incisor; 3. Canine; 4. First premolar; 5. Second premolar; 6. First molar; 7. Second premolar; 8. Third molar

3. **Proximal surface**: The surface of a tooth that faces adjoining tooth; each tooth has two proximal surfaces:

   a) **Mesial surface**: The surface of a tooth towards midline.

   b) **Distal surface**: The surface of a tooth away from midline.
4. **Occlusal surface**: The masticating or chewing surface of a posterior tooth.
5. **Incisal surface**: Functional edge of anterior tooth.
6. **Cervical surface**: The surface of the tooth close to neck or cervix of the tooth.
7. **Gingival surface**: The surface of the tooth close to gingiva.

Characteristic parts of individual teeth

Crowns: It presents *three tubercles two labial and one lingual.*

Incisors: A cutting edge is formed by the fusion of labial tubercles and it joins with lingual tubercle by two lines and so *triangular space* is formed.

Canines: Lingual tubercles not prominent and a cone is formed by fusion of labial tubercles.

Premolars: Prominent lingual tubercle and one medium sized cone by fusion of two labial tubercles. So premolars are **biscuspids**.

Upper molars: Have four tubercles, 2 labial, one lingual and one additional lingual.

Lower molars: Five tubercles, two labial, two lingual and one distal tubercle.

Roots:

1. *Single root*: Incisors, canines and premolars.
2. *Bifid or double root*: First upper premolar.
3. *Two roots* (Proximal and distal): Lower molars.
4. *Three conical roots*: Two smaller labial and one larger lingual): Upper molars.
5. Roots of all teeth are flattened from proximal to distal.
6. Canines have longest roots.

Teeth of both the jaws and their occlusion

Upper incisors overbite the lower incisors, the labial borders of the occlusal surfaces of lower premolars and molars are rounded with lingual border sharp due to formation of a large curve by upper teeth than the lower teeth.

Functions:

1. **Incisors are cutting teeth** as the upper and lower incisors overlap each other like two blades of a scissor and the crown are chisel-like. Incisors cut & slice through food & make the food into pieces. Incisors support the face & lips.
2. **Canines are tearing teeth** due to rugged conical crown.
3. **Premolars are cracking teeth** (*cracking the nuts*) due to two cusps. Premolar help with aesthetics and speech.
4. **Molars are grinding teeth** with due to square crowns with five cusps. They support the checks.

Nerve supply:

1. **Upper teeth**
   a) **Molars** by posterior superior alveolar branch of maxillary nerve.
   b) **Premolars** by middle superior alveolar.
   c) **Incisors and canines**: By anterior superior alveolar nerves.
2. **Lower teeth**: Supplied by inferior alveolar branches of mandibular nerve.

APPLIED ANATOMY:

1. Teeth help in **study of ontogeny and phylogeny by providing a good data.**
2. It can be preserved as it is a most stable structure. This fact **helps in medicolegal study for identification in unrecognised dead bodies.**
3. Bad oral hygiene gives rise to pyorrhoea (*chronic discharge of pus*) from the margin of gum due to infection in between gum and teeth. This produces *foul breath.*
4. **Caries tooth** due to decalcification of enamel and dentine with softening and destruction of tooth may occur. It makes mastication painful.
5. When infection of apical part of root occurs resulting in formation of **apical abscess.**
6. **Changes in tooth are signs of some diseases** as
   a) **In scurvy** (deficiency of Vitamin C) spongy and bleeding gum + teeth.
   b) **In rickets**: Irregular dentition upper permanent incisors may be notched.
   c) In congenital syphilis: Hutchison's teeth occurs – It is also notching of permanent incisor.

DEVELOPMENT OF TEETH

Teeth arises due to interaction between oral epithelium and underlying mesoderm.

There are primary dentition (formation of deciduous teeth) and secondary dentition (formation of permanent teeth).

Primary dentition

Stages (Fig. 14.8):

1. **Dental lamina**: Ectodermal of epithelium of developing oral cavity forms a inverted 'U' shaped structure, the dental lamina, in the upper & lower jaw.
2. **Bud stage**: Dental lamina gives rise to dental buds (10 in each jaw) towards underlying mesenchyme.

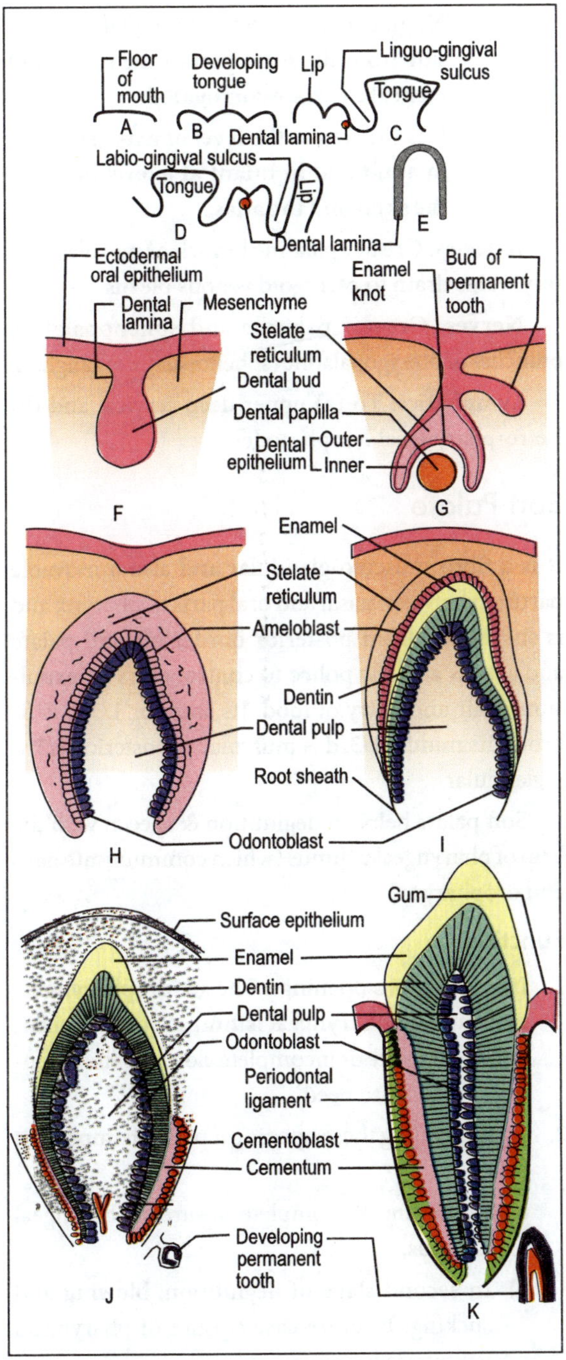

Fig. 14.8: Stages in the development of tooth; A-E. Site of development of dental lamina; F. Development of dental bud; G. Cap stage; H. Bell stage of tooth development; I. Stage of formation of dentin, enamel & root; J. Formation of cementum & root; K. Eruption of tooth

3. **Cap stage**: Mass of mesenchyme invaginates the tooth bud, resulting in cap stage. In this stage, a cap consists of:
   a) An outer layer: the **outer dental epithelium**.
   b) A inner layer: **inner dental epithelium**.
   c) Central core: Loosely arranged tissue, the stellate reticulum.

   Mesenchyme (which invaginate) originate from neural crest, forms **dental papilla**.
4. **Bell stage**: Thereafter the dental cap grows, the indentation becomes deeper, looks like bell (bell stage).
   a) **Formation of dentin**: Mesenchymal cells of the papilla near the inner dental layer differentiate into odontoblast which produce dentine. Odontoblast layer persist throughout life and produces predentine (deep to enamel).
   b) **Pulp**: Remaining cells of dental papilla form pulp of the tooth.
5. **Further development of tooth**
   a) **Formation of enamel**: During further development inner dental epithelium gives rise to ameloblast. Ameloblast produces enamel that lies over dentine.

      Some cells of inner dental epithelium form **enamel knot** which control early tooth development.

      As the enamel thickens ameloblast reticulum regress, leaving behind thin membrane on the surface of enamel. This membrane disappear after eruption of tooth.
   b) **Formation of root sheath & cementum**: Hertwig's root sheath forms by outer and inner dental epithelium. As the deposition of dentine occurs, the pulp chamber narrow and forms canal containing blood vessels & nerves of tooth.

      Mesenchymal cells (outside) in contact with root becomes **cementoblast**. Cementoblast produce cementum. Mesenchyme outside the cement layer gives rise to periodontal ligament. Periodontal ligament keep the tooth in position firmly and act as a shock absorber.

As development proceeds, crown pushed through overlying tissue layer into oral cavity, as the length of root increases.

c) **Deciduous teeth**: The eruption of deciduous or milk teeth occurs in between 6-24 months.

d) **Permanent teeth**: Buds for permanent teeth appear (in third month) on the lingual aspect of milk teeth. During 8th year, they start to grow pushing against milk teeth. As the permanent tooth grows, osteoclast remove the deciduous tooth.

PALATE

It is a structure which forms roof of mouth and floor of nasal cavity and is situated within the alveolar arches.

Different parts:

Two:

1. Hard palate (anterior two third)
2. Soft palate (posterior one third)

Hard palate

It is a bony partition between nasal cavity above and oral cavity below.

Features:

1. **Formation**: Bony palatine processes of maxillae in front and horizontal processes of palatine bone behind.
2. **Surfaces:**
   a) **Superior or upper surface** forms the floor or nasal cavity and lined by ciliated columnar epithelium.
   b) **Inferior or lower surface**
      1. Forms the roof of oral cavity
      2. Lined by stratified squamous epithelium (keratinised).
      3. Presence of mucous glands in the posterior part.
      4. Also covered by fibrous tissue and periosteum.
      5. It presents a **median raphe extending into incisive fossa** where it ends by forming a small papilla.
      6. Number of transverse folds radiate on each side from the front part of the raphe and make the surface **corrugated.**
      7. It is situated at **the level of axis vertebrae in adult** and **in infant at a level between the skull and the atlas.**

Arteries: Greater palatine branch of maxillary artery, veins drain to pterygoid venous plexus.

Nerves: Greater palatine and sphenopalatine branches of pterygopalatine (sphenopalatine) ganglion.

Lymphatics: To (a) upper deep cervical and (b) Retro-pharyngeal lymph nodes.

Soft Palate

It is a fibro musculo-glandular and also a movable partition between nasal and oral parts of pharynx and is suspended from posterior border of hard palate and acts as a traffic police to control entry or expulsion of air and entry of food. Its anterior 1/3rd is fibrous, its middle 1/3rd is muscular & posterior 1/3rd is glandular.

Soft palate helps in deglutition & speech with the help of pharyngeal isthmus (which communicate naso and oropharynx).

Function:

1. It controls two openings. The are **oropharyngeal isthmus and pharyngeal isthmus.** Control means either complete or incomplete closure of the opening according to need.
2. By controlling these opening it plays an important role.
   a) *In chewing*: By complete closure of pharyngeal isthmus.
   b) In second stage of deglutition, blowing and sucking. In every case closure of pharyngeal isthmus is necessary.
   c) In production of voice 'm n ng' partial closure of isthmus is necessary.
   d) During sneezing, partial closure of isthmus occurs so that air may also pass through mouth cavity.

e) During coughing, sputum may pass through mouth instead of narrow nasal passage which may be damaged.

Different surfaces and borders:

Surfaces: Two –

1. **Anterior or oral surface**
   a) Concave
   b) Presence of median raphe
   c) Directed downward and forward.
   d) Number of mucous glands in this surface (these glands form the main mass of the palate)
   e) Lined by stratified squamous epithelium.
2. **Posterior or nasal surface**
   a) Convex, directed backward and upward.
   b) Continuous with floor of nasal cavity
   c) Forms anterior boundary of pharyngeal isthmus
   d) Connected with tubal elevation by salpingo-palatine fold
   e) Lined by ciliated columnar epithelium except posterior part which is lined by stratified squamous.

Borders: Four

1. *Superior border* attached to posterior border of hard palate

2 & 3. *Lateral borders*: Two and continuous with pharynx.

4. *Inferior border*
   a) Free
   b) Presence of **uvula** (a conical projection) in the middle
   c) Two folds or arches: Palatoglossal (anterior) and palatopharyngeal folds (posterior). They are folds of mucous membrane containing palatoglossus and palatopharyngeal folds respectively. The space between the two folds form tonsillar fossa containing palatine tonsil.
      1. Palatoglossal fold runs downward & forward to the side sulcus terminalis of tongue in front of tonsillar fossa
      2. Palatopharyngeal fold runs downwards & backward posterior to tonsillar fossa.

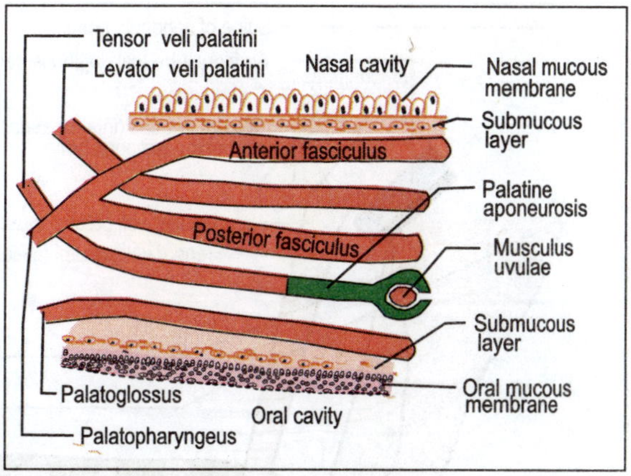

Fig. 14.9: Composition of soft palate

Composition of soft palate (Fig. 14.9)

Structurally it consists of fold of mucous membrane who contains following structures.

From above downwards:

1. *Nasal mucous membrane* (lined by mainly ciliated columnar except posterior part which is lined by stratified squamous epithelium)
2. Submucous layer containing palatine glands
3. *Anterior fasciculus of palatopharyngeus*
4. *Levator palati*
5. *Posterior fasciculus of palatopharyngeus*
6. *Tensor veli palati* ending in palatine aponeurosis which split to enclose *musculus uvulae*
7. *Palatoglossus*
8. Submucous layer containing lots of glands
9. Oral mucous membrane (lined by stratified squamous epithelium)

Palatine aponeurosis: It is the flat expanded tendon of tensor veli palati which forms the fibrous frame work of the soft palate where all the muscles of palate are attached.

Attachment:

1. *In front*: To posterior border and lower surface of hard palate up to palatine crest.
2. On each side continuous with tensor veli palati.

End: In the middle at the posterior and it splits to enclose musculus uvulae.

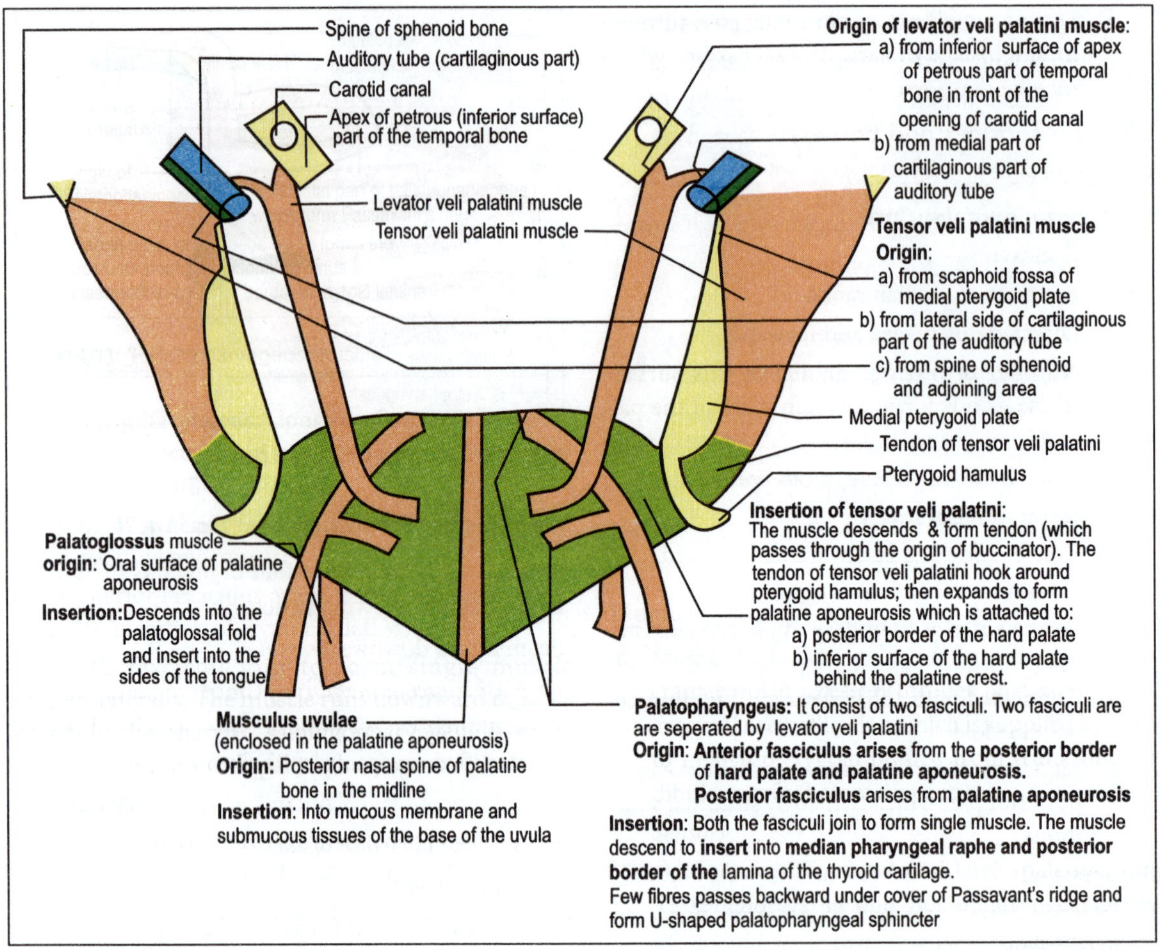

Fig. 14.10: Muscles of soft palate (origins & insertions)

MUSCLES OF SOFT PALATE (Fig. 14.10)

1. **Tensor veli palati (Fig. 14.10)**

   A. *Origin*: The muscle take origin from
      - a) Scaphoid fossa of medial pterygoid plate of sphenoid bone
      - b) Lateral aspect of cartilaginous part of pharyngotympanic tube
      - c) From spine of sphenoid, and adjoining area.

   B. *Insertion*: The tendon turns medially around pterygoid hamulus (bursa is present here in between bone & tendon) and ends in aponeurosis which is attached to hard palate.

   C. *Nerve supply*: Nerve to medial pterygoid branch of mandibular nerve before division.

   D. *Action*:
      - a) Anterior part of palate is *stretched* and depressed for closure of pharyngeal isthmus
      - b) *Dilates* pharyngo-tympanic tube and so known as dilator tubae.

2. **Levator veli palatini**

   A. **Origin**
      - a) Lower surface of apex of petrous part of temporal bone in front of the opening carotid canal.
      - b) From carotid sheath.
      - c) From cartilaginous part of pharyngo-tympanic tube [Medial lamina of cartilage].

   B. **Insertion**: The muscle descends through sinus of Morgagni (in between base of skull & superior constrictor of pharynx) into upper surface

Table 14.1: Muscles of soft palate

Muscle	Origin	Insertion	Nerve supply	Action
Tensor veli palatini – It descends	1. From scaphoid fossa of medial pterygoid plate 2. From lateral side of the cartilaginous part of auditory tube 3. From spine of sphenoid and adjoining area	With muscle of other side, forms palatine aponeurosis. It form a tendon (passes through the origin of buccinator) which hook around the pterygoid hamulus; then tendon expands to form palatine aponeurosis which is attached to— a) In the inferior surface of the hard palate behind the palatine crest b) Posterior border of the hard palate	Nerve to medial pterygoid	a) Tighten the soft palate b) Dilate the auditory tube
Levator palati – It descends	1. From the inferior surface of the apex of the petrous part of temporal bone 2. From medial part of cartilaginous part of auditory tube	Palatine aponeurosis	Pharyngeal plexus	a) Raises the soft palate to close pharyngeal isthmus b) Opens the auditory tube
Palatoglossus – It descends	Palatine aponeurosis (oral surface)	Side of tongue	Pharyngeal plexus	Pulls the root of the tongue and narrows the oropharyngeal isthmus & closes
Musculus uvulae (enclosed within palatine aponeurosis)	Posterior nasal spine of hard palate	Mucous membrane & submucous tissue of the base of the uvula	Pharyngeal plexus	Pulls up the uvula
Palatophyaryngeus (It consist two fasciculi which is separated by levator palatini)	a) Anterior fasciculi arises from the posterior border of hard palate and palatine aponeurosis b) Posterior fasciculi arises from palatine aponeurosis	Both the fasciculi join to form single muscle. The muscle descend to insert into median pharyngeal raphe and posterior border of lamina of thyroid cartilage. Few fiber passes backward under cover of Passavant's ridge and form 'U' shaped palatopharyngeal sphincter	Pharyngeal plexus	Elevate the pharynx & larynx – Closes pharyngeal isthmus

of palatine aponeurosis in between the anterior & posterior fasciculi of palatopharyngeus.

C. **Action:**

a) Elevator of soft palate and *closes* the pharyngeal isthmus

b) Opens pharyngo-tympanic tube

3. **Musculus uvulae:** A paired small muscle (enclosed by splitted palatine aponeurosis).

Origin: From posterior nasal spine of hard palate and palatine aponeurosis.

Insertion: The muscle runs backwards & downwards within tubular sheath of palatine aponeurosis & inserted into mucous membrane & submucosa of uvula.

Action: Pulls the uvula to the same side or upwards.

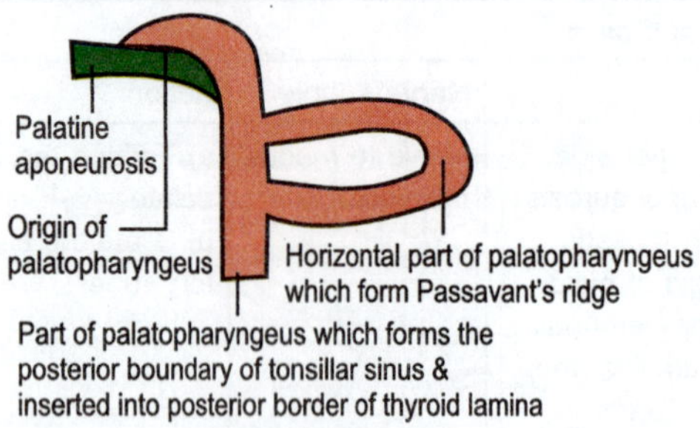

Fig. 14.11: Palatopharyngeus muscle

4. **Palatopharyngeus**: Consists of anterior and posterior fasciculus and separated from each other by levator palati.

Origin: Anterior fasciculus from hard palate and from palatine apoenurosis.

Posterior fasciculus arises from aponeurosis posterior to insertion of levator palati.

Both fasciculi join to form single muscle posterolaterally. The muscle runs downward & backward. In the pharynx, salpingopharyngeus & stylopharyngeus joins with palatopharyngeus.

Insertion:

a) Maximum fibres are inserted to posterior border of lamina of thyroid cartilage.
b) Some fibres to wall of pharynx and median raphe.
c) Some fibres of palatopharyngeus runs backward under cover of the **Passavant's ridge** and form palatopharyngeal spincter ('U'-shaped sling). (Fig. 14.11)

Action: Pulls up pharynx and larynx and helps in closure of pharyngeal isthmus.

5. **Palatoglossus**:

Origin: From lower surface of palatine aponeurosis.

Insertion: Into side of tongue.

Action: Elevator of root of the tongue to close the oro-pharyngeal isthmus.

Nerve supply of soft palate:

Motor: All the muscles of soft palate except tensor veli palati are supplied cranial root of accessory through pharyngeal plexus except the tensor veli palatini which is supplied by mandibular nerve.

Pharyngeal plexus formed by

a) *Pharyngeal branch of 9th cranial nerve.*
b) *Pharyngeal [cranial root of accessory nerve] branch of 10th.*
c) *Laryngopharyngeal branch of sympathetic.*

Arterial supply of palate

1. Greater palatine branch of 3rd part of maxillary artery
2. Ascending palatine branch of facial artery
3. Palatine branch of ascending pharyngeal arteries.

Veins: Veins drain into pterygoid and tonsillar plexuses of veins (paratonsillar vein).

Lymphatics: Drain into

a) Upper deep cervical group
b) Retropharyngeal group of lymph nodes.

Nerve supply:

1. *Motor*: All muscles of the soft palate supplied by cranial root of accessory through pharyngeal plexus except tensor veli palati which is supplied by nerve to medial pterygoid branch from trunk of mandibular nerve (before division).
2. *Sensory*:
   a) *General*: By greater and lesser palatine, long sphenopalatine and glossopharyngeal nerves.
   b) *Special sense taste*: By glossopharyngeal and lesser palatine.
3. *Secretomotor*:

   Superior salivary nucleus → Facial nerve → Greater petrosal nerve → Nerve of pterygoid canal → Relay in pterygopalatine ganglion → Postganglionic fibre passes through greater & lesser palatine nerves → Palatine glands

APPLIED ANATOMY:

In case of diptheria, soft palate may sometimes be paralysed resulting in nasal regurgitation of food and nasal tone in the voice, pulling forward of the mandible as *genioglossi is attached to genial tubercles behind symphysis menti of mandible.*

Development of palate

Palate is developed as a result of fusion of three elements (Fig. 14.12)

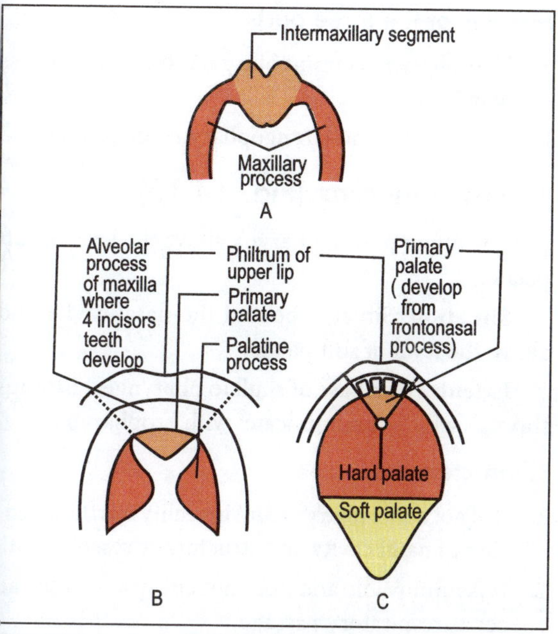

Fig. 14.12: Stages of the development of palate (A to C)

1. Premaxilla or primary palate (in relation to the incisors) develop from the frontonasal process.
2. The rest of the palate develop from two lateral palatine process of the maxillary process.

These three elements fuse from before backwards in *Y shaped manner to form definitive palate.*

Congenital anomalies: Due to failure of fusion of the three elements lead to developmental defects of the palate. This failure of fusion may be from mild degree to complete failure.

To anomalies are: (Fig. 14.13)

- Incomplete cleft palate may be only in soft or may be both in soft and hard palate
- Bifid uvula
- Complete cleft-palate (presence of Y shaped fissure).

PHARYNX (Fig. 14.14)

It is a musculomembranous tube which is functionally concerned for passage of air (in the upper and middle part) and food (in the middle and lower part).

Situation: It is situated *behind* nasal cavities, oral cavities and larynx and *in front of* cervical part of vertebral column.

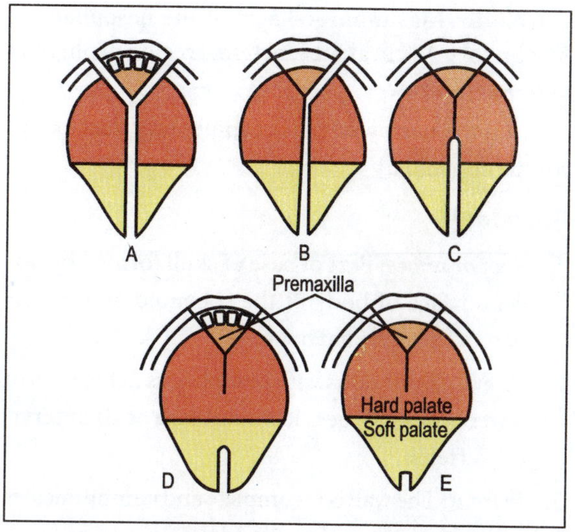

Fig. 14.13: Developmental defects of the palate. A. Complete bilateral cleft palate; B. Complete unilateral cleft palate. C. Cleft of soft palate extending into hard palate. D. Cleft soft palate. E. Bifid uvula

Extent: It extends from base of skull above to the level of sixth cervical vertebra and lower border of cricoid cartilage where it is continuous with oesophagus.

Length: 12 to 14cm.

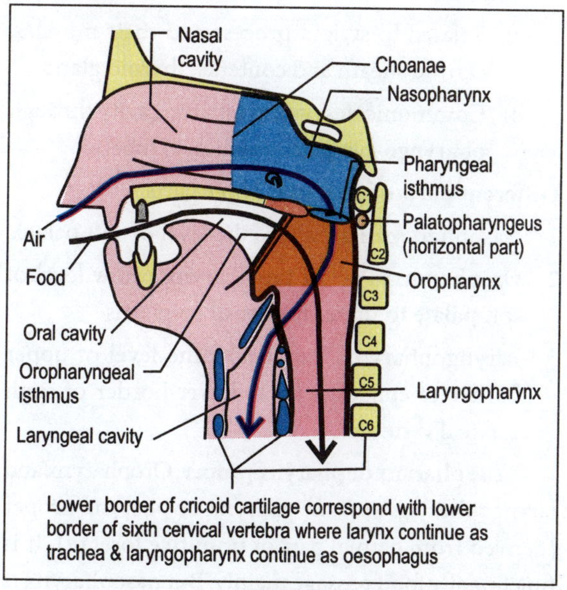

Fig. 14.14: Pathways for air (blue) and food (black) through nasal cavity & oral cavity

Width: Maximum – 3.5cm at the nasopharynx. Minimum – 1.5cm at the junctional region of pharynx and oesophagus.

[It is the narrowest part of alimentary tract except for the appendix.]

Boundary:

1. *Roof or above*: Part of base of skull formed by under surface of body of the sphenoid and basilar part of the occipital bone.
2. *Below*: Continuous with oesophagus at the level of lower border of the cricoid cartilage or sixth cervical vertebra.
3. *In front*: The wall is incomplete and communicates with (from above downwards):
   a) Nasal cavities through posterior nasal apertures (choanae or nares)
   b) Oral cavity through oropharyngeal isthmus
   c) Larynx through inlet of larynx.
4. *Behind*: Upper six cervical vertebrae with intervertebral discs, prevertebral muscles covered by prevertebral fascia and retropharyngeal space and its contents.

   Laterally:
   a) Related to styloid process and their muscles, carotid sheath and contents, thyroid gland
   b) Communicates with tympanic cavity through pharyngo-tympanic (auditory) tube.

Different parts of pharynx: Three parts

1. Nasopharynx: Part above the level of soft palate.
2. Oropharynx: Part of the pharynx below level of soft palate to upper border of epiglottis
3. Laryngopharynx: Part below the level of upper border of epiglottis up to lower border of sixth cervical vertebra.

True pharynx or pharynx proper: Oropharynx and laryngopharynx are true pharynx or pharynx proper (derived from cranial part of primitive foregut). It is functionally food passage mainly. But nasopharynx is backward extension of nasal cavity and functionally part of respiratory passage.

Mobility of the three parts:

1. Nasopharynx is immobile part (it is more or less bony)
2. Oropharynx and laryngopharynx are mobile.

1. Nasopharynx (Fig. 14.15)

It is the upper part of pharynx above the level of soft palate.

Situation: Situated behind the nasal cavity and above the level of soft palate.

Extent: From base of skull to pharyngeal isthmus through which communicates with oropharynx.

Characteristics:

1. It is not a true pharynx and in reality it is the extension of nasal cavity and structurally resembles it.
2. It is immovable and does not collapse and so can act as respiratory passage.

Features:

1. **Anterior wall**: Deficient and communicates with nasal cavity through posterior nasal apertures (Fig. 14.16)
2. **Roof and posterior wall** form a continuous slope and formed by body of sphenoid, basioccipital and anterior arch of atlas and presents
   a) *Nasopharyngeal tonsil* (adenoids): Collection of lymphoid tissue forming a conical mass at the junction of roof and posterior wall. Nasopharyngeal tonsil usually atrophies in adult. In children nasopharyngeal tonsil enlarge due to infection, known as **adenoid**; then respiration usually occurs through mouth due to obstruction of nasal respiration.
   b) *Pharyngeal bursa*: Also known as pouch of Luschka. It is a diverticulum of mucous membrane extending into nasopharyngeal tonsil. The bursa is formed due to adhesion of notochord to the dorsal wall of the pharyngeal part of the foregut.
   c) *Pharyngeal hypophysis*: Occasionally found and consists of glandular tissues similar to adenohypophysis in the roof aspect. It is formed due to backward extension of developing Rathke's pouch.

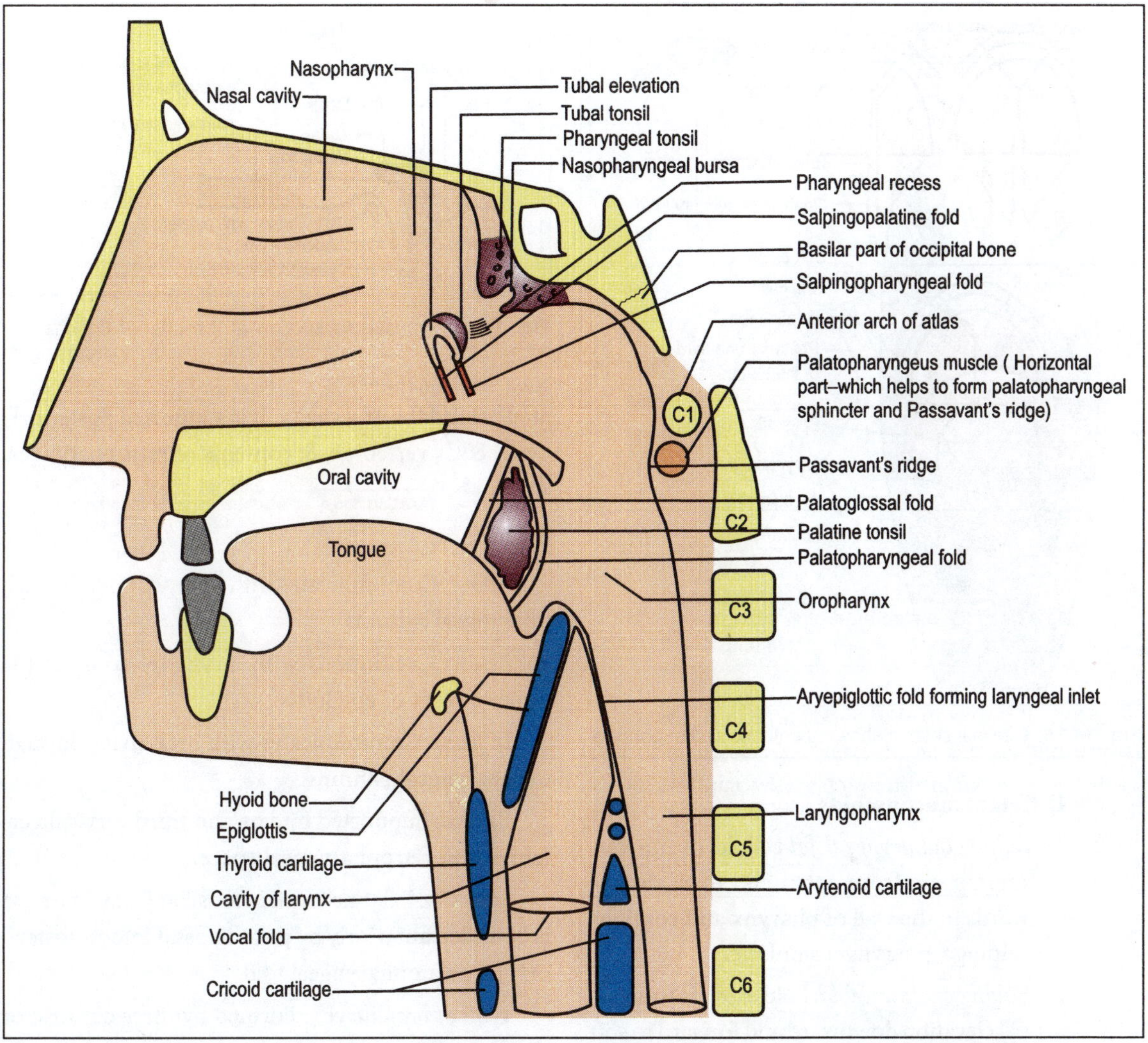

Fig. 14.15: Sagittal section through nasal cavity, nasopharynx, oral cavity, oropharynx, larynx & laryngopharynx

3. **Inferiorly or at the floor region**: Nasopharynx communicates with oropharynx through pharyngeal isthmus.

Pharyngeal isthmus:

Boundaries:

Anteriorly: Free margin of soft palate

Posteriorly: Mucous elevation of Passavant's ridge formed by palatopharyngeal sphincter.

Laterally (both side): Palatopharyngeal arch (containing the same muscle)

4. **In the lateral wall**: The features are:

a) **Pharyngeal opening of pharyngo-tympanic** (auditory) tube.

1. It is situated 1.25cm behind and little below the posterior end of inferior nasal concha.
2. Triangular in shape. The auditory tube connects the nasopharynx with tympanic cavity.

b) **Tubal elevation**: An elevation bounding above and behind the tubal opening of the tube. It is due to pharyngeal end of cartilage of auditory tube.

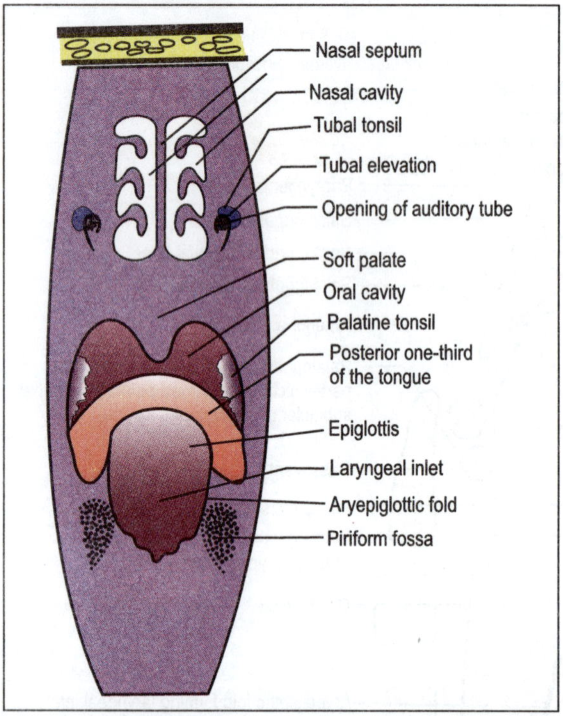

Fig. 14.16: Coronal section showing anterior wall of pharynx

c) **Different mucous folds**

1. *Salpingopharyngeal fold*: Fold of mucous membrane from tubal elevation downwards to the wall of pharynx and contains salpingo-pharyngeus muscle.
2. *Salpingopalatine fold*: Fold extends from tubal elevation downward and forward to soft palate. It contains the levator palati muscle.

d) **Tubal tonsil**: Collection of submucous lymphoid tissue posterosuperior to tubal elevation.

e) **Pharyngeal recess or fossa of Rosenmuller**: It is a deep depression behind the tubal elevation and extends between levator palati with tube and prevertebral muscles. Pharyngobasilar fascia with internal carotid artery are intimately related with it.

2. Oropharynx

It is the middle part of pharynx between soft palate above and upper border of epiglottis below and situated behind the oral cavity. It is supported posteriorly by C_2 & C_3 vertebrae, & contents of retropharyngeal space.

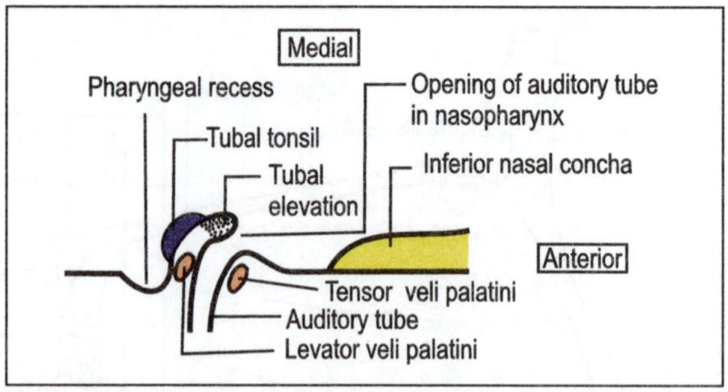

Fig. 14.17: Transverse section at the inferior concha

Boundary:

Above: Communicates with nasopharynx through pharyngeal isthmus

Below: Continuous with laryngopharynx at the upper border of epiglottis.

In front: Communicates with oral cavity through oropharyngeal isthmus

Behind: Supported by axis and third cervical vertebrae and retropharyngeal space

Laterally: Palatine tonsil in tonsillar fossa. The fossa is bounded anteriorly by palatoglossal fold & posteriorly by palatopharyngeal fold.

Wall of oropharynx: Formed by three constrictor muscles of pharynx.

3. Laryngopharynx

1. It is the lower part of pharynx below the upper border of epiglottis and lower border of cricoid cartilage and extends below up to level of cricoid cartilage and sixth cervical vertebra
2. Situated behind the larynx
3. Features are
   A. In the anterior wall
      a) Inlet of larynx (leads to laryngeal cavity)
      b) Posterior surface of cricoid and arytenoid cartilages.

B. In the posterior wall: It is supported by (from before backwards)
   a) Retropharyngeal space
   b) Prevertebral fascia
   c) Fourth cervical to sixth cervical vertebrae.

C. **In the lateral wall** (on each side): Presence of pyriform fossa – A deep depressed area lined by mucous membrane .

Important regions of pharynx

Pharyngeal isthmus: It lies between nasopharynx above and oropharynx below.

Boundary:

1. *In front*: Posterior surface and free margin of soft palate
2. *Behind*: Passavant's ridge

   [An elevation mucous membrane formed by palatopharyngeal sphincter]
3. Laterally (on each side): **Palatopharyngeal arch** containing palatopharyngeus muscle.

Physiological conditions for closure of isthmus:

1. During *sucking of milk*
2. During *second stage of deglutition*
3. During *articulation of speech of all words except m n ng (nasal tone) when partial closure is necessary.*
4. During *blowing.*

Mechanism of closure of isthmus:

1. Formation of Passavant's ridge on the posterior wall of isthmus by contraction of palatopharyngeal sphincter.
2. Simultaneous elevation of soft palate by levator palati and this posterior part of nasal surface comes in contact with Passavant's ridge and isthmus is

Inlet of larynx:

Boundaries:

Above & in front: Upper margin of the epiglottis

Below & behind: Interarytenoid fold

On each side: Aryepiglottic fold

During deglutition: Closure of inlet takes place by contraction of aryepiglotticus muscle.

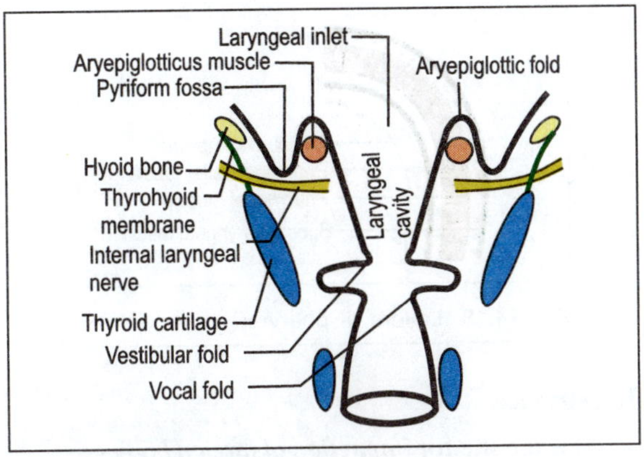

Fig. 14.18: Piriform fossa (coronal section)

Oropharyngeal isthmus

It is the opening of communication between oral cavity and the oropharynx. It lies between oral cavity and oropharynx.

Boundary:

A. *Above*: Soft palate

B. *Below*: Sulcus terminalis of the tongue

C. *On each side*: **Palatoglossal arch** containing palatoglossus muscle.

Function: It becomes closed during swallowing of food and prevents regurgitation of food from orophaynx to oral cavity.

Pyriform fossa (Fig. 14.18)

It is a deep depressed fossa lined by mucous membrane situated in the laryngopharynx and on each side of inlet of larynx.

Boundary:

Medially: Aryepiglottic fold.

Laterally: Medial surface of lamina of thyroid cartilage and membrane covered by mucous membrane.

[*Superior laryngeal vessels and internal laryngeal branch of superior laryngeal nerve pierce the thyrohyoid membrane at this site*]

Above: Piriform fossa is separated from vallecula by lateral glossoepiglottic fold.

Structures lying beneath the mucous membrane of the fossa

Superior laryngeal vessels and internal laryngeal nerve.

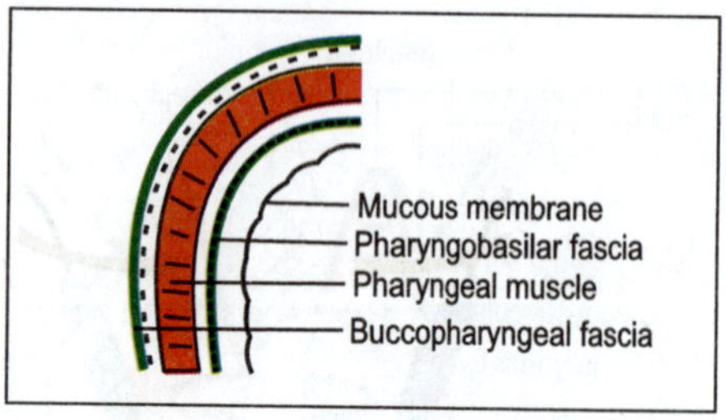

Fig. 14.19: Layers of pharynx

Importance:

1. It is the site for *impaction of foreign body.*
2. Artificially by *help of lead ball smugglers form a pouch.*

Applied anatomy: During removal of foreign body, internal laryngeal nerve lying deep to mucous membrane may be injured and cause paralysis of the supraglottic part of larynx which may result in aspiration pneumonia and ultimately may cause fatal result.

Structure of the pharyngeal wall (Fig. 14.19)

Consists of five layers from outside inwards

1. Buccopharyngeal fascia – (Loose areolar tissue): It covers the outer surface of muscles (constrictors) of pharynx. It extends over the buccinator muscle superficial to pterygomandibular raphe. It joins with the pharyngobasilar fascia at the upper border of superior constrictor of pharynx.
2. Muscular layer
   A. *Outer circular layer* consists of constrictor muscles of pharynx (superior, middle and inferior)
   B. *Inner longitudinal layer* formed by other muscles of pharynx (stylopharyngeus, salpingopharyngeus and palatopharyngeus).
   [Pharyngeal plexus of veins and nerves lie in between muscle layer and buccopharyngeal fascia].
3. *Pharyngo-basilar fascia* – Part of the submucosa forms pharyngobasilar fascia (fibrous thickening). It forms the pharyngeal raphe posteriorly.
4. *Submucous layer*
5. *Mucous membrane lined by non-keratinized stratified squamous epithelium except nasopharynx which is lined by ciliated columnar epithelium.*

Muscles of Pharynx

Constrictor muscles of pharynx: Three – Superior, middle and inferior.

General principle of constrictors

1. All the muscles arise from *front* (from ligaments, bones or cartilages) and are inserted *behind to median fibrous raphe* (extending from pharyngeal tubercle at the basilar part of occipital bone above to pharyngo-oesophageal junction below).
2. All the three muscles overlap each other form below upwards.

Superior constrictor

Origin: From above downwards (from four parts) by a continuous vertical line (Fig. 14.20).

From:

1. Posterior border of medial pterygoid plate and pterygoid hamulus
2. Posterior border of pterygomandibular raphe (from anterior border of buccinator takes origin)
3. Posterior end of mylohyoid line of mandible
4. Side of tongue (posterior part).

Insertion: Extends from pharyngeal tubercle above to median fibrous raphe up to level of vocal fold below.

a) Highest group of fibres runs upwards, backwards, & medially inserted into pharyngeal tubercle. Between base of skull & upper border of the muscle, there exist a gap which is known as **sinus of Morgagni** (which is closed by buccopharyngeal and pharyngobasilar fasciae).
b) Middle fibres runs horizontally to be inserted to fibrous raphe
c) Lowest fibres run downward, backward & medially to median raphe. Lowest fibres are covered by middle constrictor.

Nerve supply: Cranial root of accessory through pharyngeal plexus.

Middle constrictor

A fan shaped muscle.

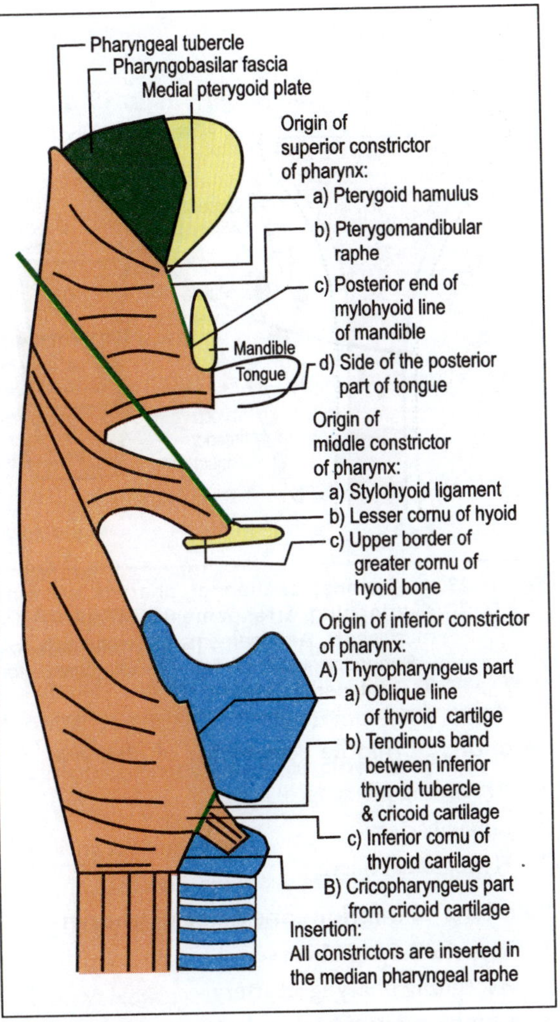

Fig. 14.20: Origin & insertion of constrictors of pharynx

Origin: From

1. Lower part of stylohyoid ligament and lesser cornu of hyoid bone
2. Upper aspect of greater cornu of hyoid bone.

Insertion: Into median fibrous raphe from pharyngeal tubercle above to more or less level of vocal fold.

a) Upper fibres cover the superior constrictor and inserted into median fibrous raphe and pharyngeal tubercle.

b) Lower fibres covered by inferior constrictor and inserted into median fibrous raphe up to vocal fold.

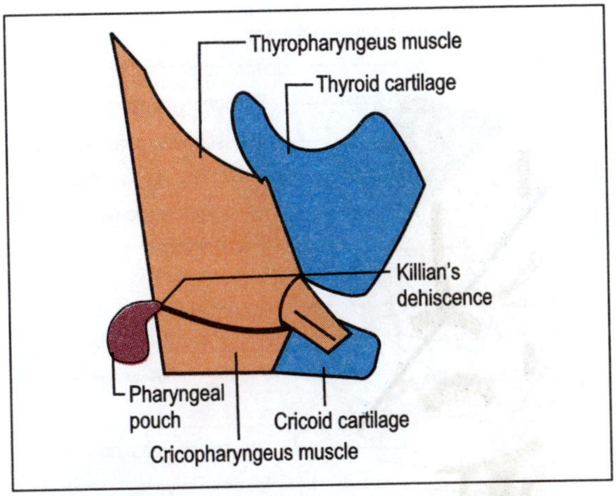

Fig. 14.21: Pharyngeal pouch

Inferior constrictor

Thickest of all the muscles and consists of two parts:

1. Thyropharyngeus
2. Cricopharyngeus

Origin:

A. **Thyropharyngeus**: From oblique line of thyroid cartilage, and from tendinous band between inferior thyroid tubercle & upper part of cricoid cartilage, and also from inferior horn of thyroid cartilage.

B. **Cricopharyngeus**: From anterior arch and side of cricoid cartilage.

Insertion: Thyropharyngeus into median raphe where as cricopharyngeus is continuous with muscle of opposite side.

a) Fibres of thyropharyngeus run upwards and backwards to median fibrous raphe.

b) Fibres of cricopharyngeus run horizontally to median fibrous raphe.

Dehiscence of Killan: It is the junctional region (posteriorly) between thyropharyngeus and cricopharyngeus. It is the weakest part.

[**Pharyngeal pouch (Zenker's diverticulum)**: Incoordination between thyropharyngeus & cricopharyngeus will lead to formation of pharyngeal pouch. When thyropharyngeous contract, if the cricopharyngeous fails to relax, the bolus of food will be pushed out through Killian dehiscence, leading to formation of pahryngeal pouch]. (Fig. 14.21)

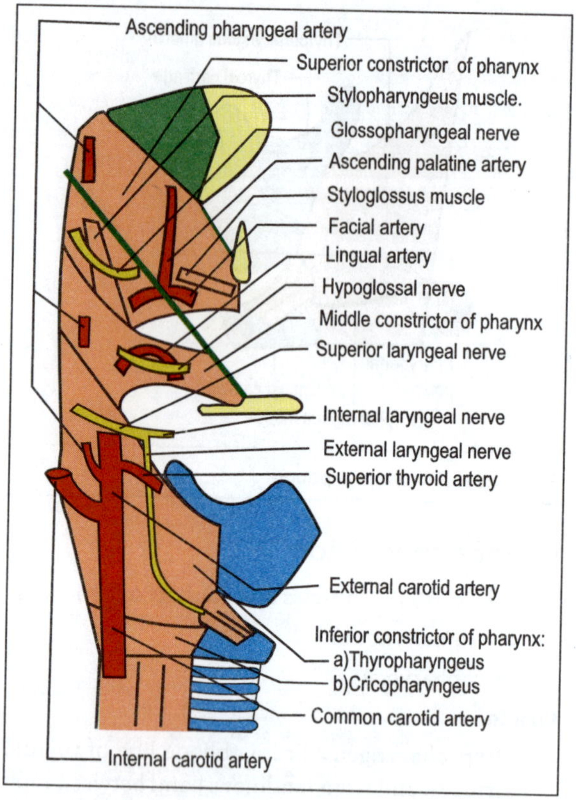

Fig. 14.22: Relations of constrictor of pharynx

Nerve supply: All the constrictors are supplied by cranial root of accessory through pharyngeal plexus.

In addition inferior constrictor is also supplied by

a) External laryngeal and
b) Recurrent laryngeal nerves

Action:

1. All constrictors help in deglutition and initiate peristalsis
2. Thyropharyngeus is propulsive in action
3. Cricopharyngeus is sphincteric. Both the muscles act alternately when one contracts other relaxes.

Relations of superior constrictor of pharynx

1. Ascending pharyngeal artery (Fig. 14.22)
2. Stylohyoid ligament
3. Stylopharyngeus muscle
4. Glossopharyngeal nerve
5. Styloglossus
6. Facial artery with **ascending palatine artery**.

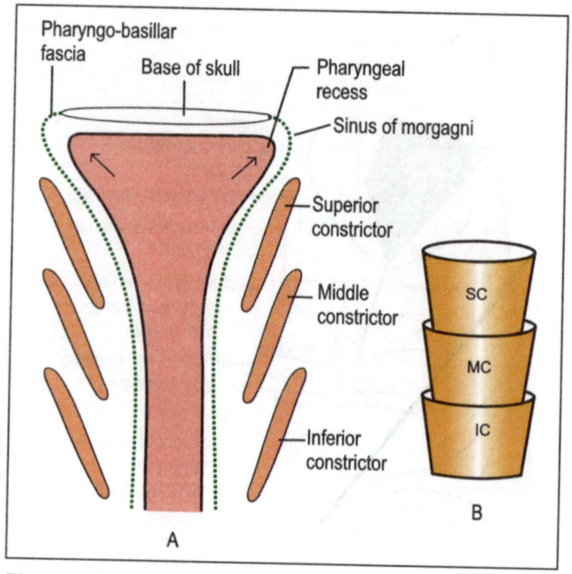

Fig. 14.23: A. Coronal section of pharynx showing overlapping arrangements of constrictor muscles; B. Arrangements of constrictors (SC – Superior constrictor; MC – Middle constrictor; IC – Inferior constrictor)

Relations of middle constrictor of pharynx

1. Ascending pharyngeal artery
2. Lingual artery
3. Hypoglossal nerve.

Relations of inferior constrictor of pharynx

1. Superior laryngeal nerve
2. Ascending pharyngeal artery
3. Common carotid artery
4. Internal carotid artery
5. External carotid artery
6. Superior thyroid artery
7. External laryngeal nerve.

Structures passing through the gaps between the constrictors

1. *Through the sinus of Morgagni i.e., space between base of skull and upper border of superior constrictor* (Figs. 14.23 & 14.24).
   a) Levator veli palati
   b) Pharyngo-tympanic tube (auditory tube)
   c) Ascending palatine artery
   d) Palatine branch of ascending pharyngeal artery.

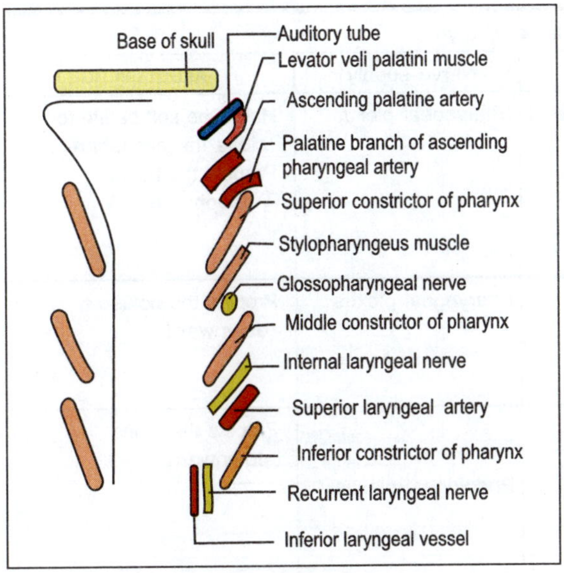

Fig. 14.24: Structures passing through the gaps in between constrictors

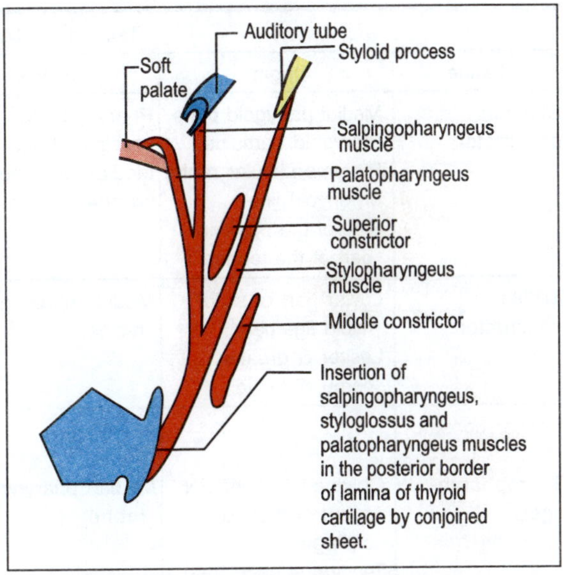

Fig. 14.25: Disposition of longitudinal muscles of pharynx

2. *Structures passing between lower border of superior and upper border of middle constrictors.*
   a) Glossopharyngeal nerve
   b) Stylopharyngeus muscle
3. *Between lower border of middle and upper border of inferior constrictors.*
   a) Superior laryngeal vessels
   b) Internal laryngeal nerve
4. *Deep to lower border of inferior constrictor*
   a) Recurrent laryngeal nerve
   b) Inferior laryngeal vessels.

Longitudinal muscles of pharynx

A. **Stylopharyngeus** (Fig. 14.25)

Origin: From medial surface of base of the styloid process of temporal bone.

Insertion: The muscle runs downward & forward (accompanied by glossopharyngeal nerve) through a gap between superior and middle constrictors, & joins with palatopharyngeus and salpingopharyngeus forms a united sheet and inserted into posterior border of lamina of the thyroid cartilage.

Nerve supply: Glossopharyngeal nerve.

B. **Palatopharyngeus:**

Origin: Two parts: Anterior fasciculus and posterior fasciculus (levator veli palatini lies between fascienti).

Both *arise* from upper surface of palatine aponeurosis after forming a single sheet.

Insertion: Into posterior border of lamina of the thyroid cartilage.

Palatopharyngeal sphincter: Few fibres of palatopharyngeus run horizontally to form 'U' shaped loop deep to mucous membrane within Passavant's ridge. Its contraction forms *Passavant's sphincter.*

C. **Salpingopharyngeus**

Origin: Lower part of tubal elevation. Fibres run vertically downward.

Insertion: Into posterior border of lamina of the thyroid cartilage.

Nerve supply: Palatopharyngeus and salpingopharyngeus are supplied by cranial root of accessory through pharyngeal plexus.

Arterial supply: By

1. Ascending pharyngeal branch of external carotid artery.

Table 14.2: Muscles of pharynx

Muscle	Origin	Incertion	Nerve supply	Action
Superior constrictor	Medial pterygoid plate Pterygoid hamulus Pterymandibular raphe Mylohyoid line Side of the posterior part of the tongue	Pharyngeal tubercle of occipital bone Median pharyngeal raphe	Pharyngeal plexus	Helps the soft palate to close the nasopharynx Propels the bolus nasopharynx
Middle constrictor	Lower part of stylo-hyoid ligament Lesser & greater cornu of hyoid	Median pharyngeal raphe	Pharyngeal plexus	Propels the bolus downwards
Inferior constric-tor:				Propels the bolus downward
Thyropharyn-geus	Oblique line & inferior cornu of thyroid catilage Tendinous band bet-ween inferior thyroid tubercle & cricoid cartilage	Median pharyngeal raphe	Pharyngeal plexus	
Cricopharyngeus	Cricoid cartilage	Median pharyngeal raphe	External laryngeal nerve	Sphincter at lower end of pharynx
Stylopharyngeus	Styloid process of temporal bone	Posterior border of thyroid cartilage	Glossopharyngeal nerve	Elevate the larynx during swallowing
Salpinogo-pharyngeus	Auditory tube	Posterior border of thyroid cartilage	Pharyngeal plexus	Elevate pharynx
Palato-pharyngeus	Palatine aponeurosis Posterior border of hard palate	Posterior border of lamina of thyroid cartilage	Pharyngeal plexus	Elevate pharynx

2. Ascending palatine and tonsillar branches of facial artery.
3. Greater palatine, pharyngeal and pterygoid branches of maxillary artery.
4. Dorsal lingual branches of lingual artery.

Veins: Veins form a plexus which also receive blood from soft palate and prevertebral region and communicate with pterygoid venous plexus above and end in internal jugular vein.

Lymphatics: Drain into retropharyngeal and deep cervical group of lymph nodes.

Nerve supply: By *pharyngeal plexus* situated on the middle constrictor muscle (*formed by pharyngeal branch of vagus containing fibres of cranial root of accessory, pharyngeal branch of glossopharyngeal and laryngopharyngeal branch of sympathetic*).

Details of nerve supply

1. **Motor**: All muscles are supplied by *cranial root of accessory through pharyngeal plexus except*:
   Stylopharyngeus which is supplied by glossopharyngeal and *inferior constrictor is also supplied by recurrent laryngeal* and *external laryngeal nerve.*
2. **Sensory**:
   A. *Nasopharynx by branch from pterygopalatine ganglion carrying fibres of maxillary nerve*
   B. *Oropharynx: By glossopharyngeal nerve*
   C. *Layngopharynx: Internal laryngeal nerve*
3. Sympathetic: Vasomotor.

SWALLOWING OR DEGLUTITION

It is a process in which food is pushed from the mouth cavity to pharynx, oesophagus and finally to stomach.

Consists of three stages

1. **First stage:** In the mouth and voluntary in character.
   a) Masticated food or bolus is imprisoned in the groove formed by heaping up of the tip and sides of tongue by contraction of superior longitudinal, vertical linguae and genioglossi and the groove being in contact with hard palate.
   b) Raising of the floor of mouth by mylohyoid and thus presses against hard palate.
      Thus the groove gradually disappears from before backwards and pushes the food into oropharynx.
   c) It is further enhanced by upward movement of hyoid bone and pushing back of the base of the tongue.
2. **Second stage:** It starts when food enters the oropharynx and it is involuntary in character, food from here may pass forwards into mouth, upwards into nasopharynx and downwards into larynx. These can be prevented by following ways.
   a) Closure of oropharyngeal isthmus is done by contraction of styloglossus and palatoglossus resulting in pulling the tongue upwards and backwards and narrowing palatoglossal arches.
   b) Pharyngeal isthmus is closed by formation of Passavant's ridge by contraction of palatopharyngeal sphincter and approximation of ridge with soft palate by elevation by levator palati and tightening by tensor veli palati.
   c) Inlet of larynx is closed by approximation of aryepiglottic folds by contraction of aryepiglotticus. It is further helpful by drawing the inlet upwards behind hyoid by thyrohyoid, stylopharyngeus and palatopharyngeus.

   So food has got no other alternative but to pass down into the laryngopharynx and further helped in this process by simultaneous contractions of superior and middle constrictors. It is involuntary in character.
3. **Third stage:** It is the contraction of inferior constrictor which helps the food to pass to oesophagus from pharynx.
   It is due to propulsive action of thyropharyngeus followed by relaxed sphincteric action of cricopharyngeus.
   Further peristaltic movements push the food down the oesophagus.

APPLIED ANATOMY:

1. Difficulty in swallowing is known as dysphagia. It may be due to any causes such as diseases of pharynx and oesophagus.
2. Removal of foreign body from the throat (pyriform fossa) may cause damage to internal laryngeal nerve which lies beneath the mucous membrane of the fossa.
3. Pressure diverticula of oesophagus or dehiscene of Killan.
   It is the formation of mucous pouch at the junction of thyropharyngeus and cricopharyngeus due to incoordination of actions of these two muscles.

Waldeyer's Ring of Lymphoid tissue (Fig. 14.26)

These are collections of lymphoid tissue situated at the different sites of pharynx ad guard the openings of gastrointestinal tract respiratory tubes and arranged in a ring like manner.

In front: Lingual tonsil

On each side: Palatine tonsil (Paired)

Posterolaterally: Tube tonsil (Paired)

Posterosuperiorly: Nasopharyngeal tonsil.

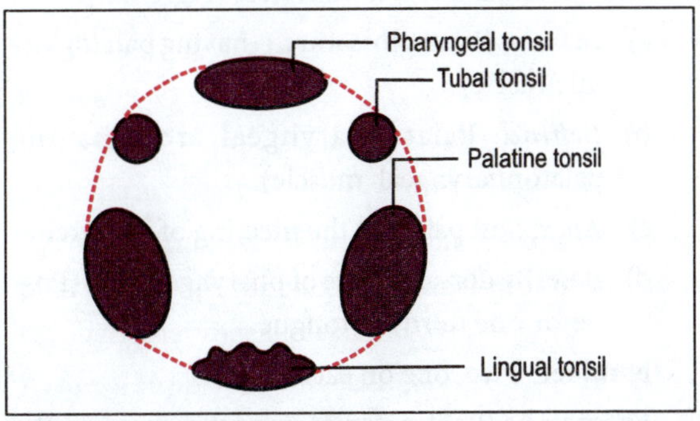

Fig. 14.26: Waldeyer's ring

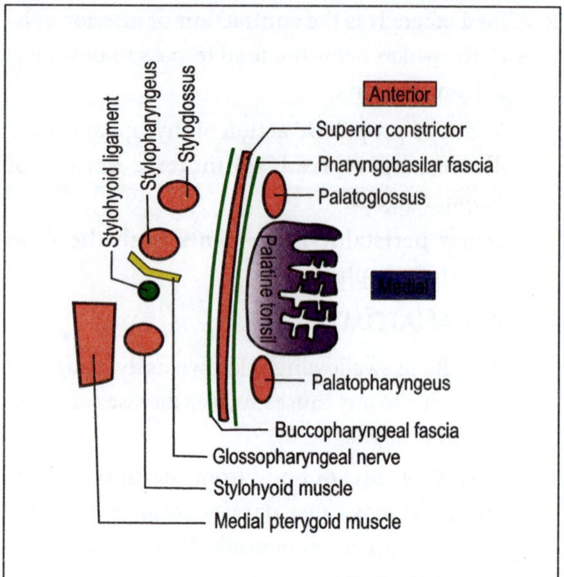

Fig. 14.27: Horizontal section of the palatine tonsil

Function: It is concerned with defensive mechanism of alimentary and respiratory systems by destruction of infecting organism at the entrance.

TONSIL

It means collections of lymphoid tissue. But usually 'Tonsil' refers to palatine tonsil.

Palatine Tonsil

It is a collection of masses of lymphoid tissue in the lateral wall of oropharynx.

Situation: Situated in the tonsillar sinus or fossa which is an angular recess bounded. (Fig. 14.27)

a) *In front*: Palatoglossal arch (having palatoglossal muscle)
b) *Behind*: Palatopharyngeal arch (having palatopharyngeal muscle)
c) *Apex*: Soft palate at the meeting of two arches
d) *Base*: By dorsal surface of pharyngeal part (Posterior one third) of tongue

Number: Two, one on each side

Extensions: Its deep surface extends beyond the tonsillar fossa or sinus.

A. *Superiorly*: Invades the soft palate
B. *Inferiorly*: Into dorsum of tongue
C. *Anteriorly*: Embedded beneath the palatoglossal arch.

Shape: Flattened or ovoid in shape.

Weight: 1.4gm

Size: In children it is enlarged but in adults it is diminished.

Capsule: Present only on lateral side and outer part is blended with palatoglossus muscle and pharyngobasilar fascia.

Other features and relations of palatine tonsil

A. **Poles**: Two
   a) Upper: Extends to soft palate and presents intratonsillar cleft
   b) Lower: Extends to dorsum of tongue.
B. **Borders**: Two
   a) Anterior: In contact with palatoglossal arch containing palatoglossus muscle.
   b) Posterior: In contact with palatopharyngeal arch containing palatopharyngeus muscle.
C. **Surface**: Two
   1. **Medial surface**
      a) Free surface
      b) Looks inwards and bound the passage from mouth to pharynx
      c) Twelve to twenty five pits leading into deep narrow recesses known as tonsillar crypts are present. They are surrounded by lymphatic follicle.
      d) Presence of two embryonic folds
         1. *Plica triangularis*: A triangular fold which extends from lower part of palatoglossal arch. Later on this fold is replaced by lymphoid tissue.
         2. *Plica semilunaris*: A fold extends from upper part of palatoglossal arch. Occasionally it is replaced by lymphoid tissue.

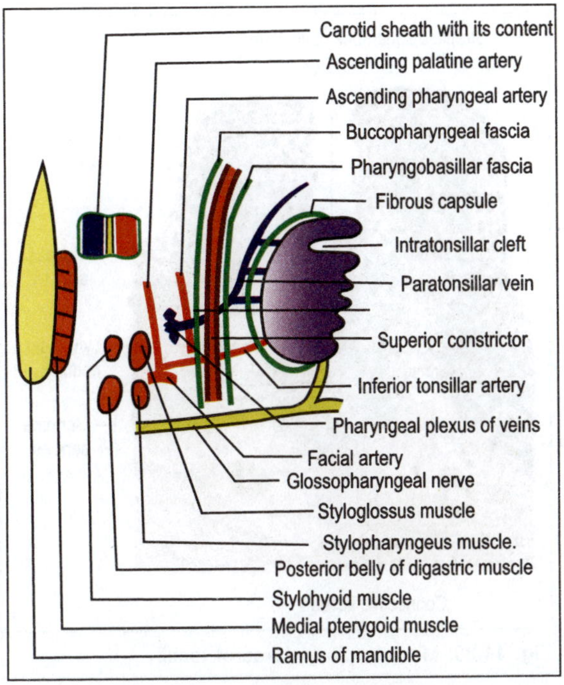

Fig. 14.28: Showing the lateral relations of palatine tonsil (coronal section)

e) *Instratonsillar cleft*: (Formerly known as supratonsillar fossa or celft).
Deep fissure in the upper part of the tonsil and represents the second pharyngeal pouch.

2. **Lateral or Deep surface**: Structures related to this surface (from deep to superficial)
   a) Capsule
   b) Loose areolar tissue with paratonsillar vein
   c) Pharyngo-basilar fascia
   d) Superior constrictor and palatopharyngeus muscle (Fig. 14.28)
   e) Buccopharyngeal fascia
   f) Styloglossus with lingual nerve
   g) Stylopharyngeus with 9th nerve
   h) Facial artery with ascending palatine and tonsillar branch
   i) Ascending pharyngeal artery
   j) Internal carotid artery
   k) Masseter
   l) Ramus of mandible

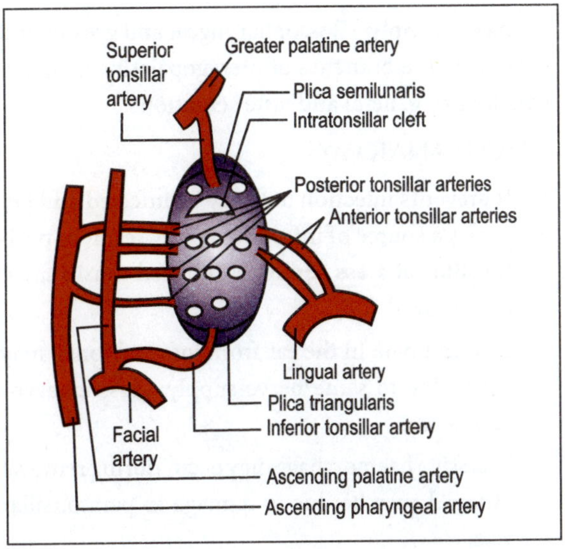

Fig. 14.29: Features of medial surface of tonsil and arterial supply of tonsil

Tonsillar Bed

The bed of the tonsil is formed by following structures:

1. Pharyngobasillar fascia
2. Superior constrictor of pharynx
3. Buccopharyngeal fascia
4. Styloglossus muscle
5. Stylopharyngeus muscle

Arterial supply: (Fig. 14.29)

1. Anterior tonsillar artery: Branch of dorsal lingual artery.
2. Superior tonsillar artery: Branch of greater palatine artery.
3. Inferior tonsillar artery: Branch of facial artery.
4. Posterior tonsillar: Branches of **ascending palatine** and **ascending pharyngeal arteries.**

Venous drainage:

Into pharyngeal venous plexus by paratonsillar vein

Lymphatics:

Drain into superior deep cervical (Jugulo-digastric) group of lymph nodes situated below and behind angle of mandible (enlarged during infection).

Nerve supply: Glossopharyngeal and greater and lesser palatine branches of pterygopalatine ganglion which carry general and taste sensations.

APPLIED ANATOMY:

1. It prevents infection but may be infected and becomes a source of infection. It may result in **peritonsillar abscess (quinsy)**. Infected tonsils must be removed.
2. Referred pain in the ear from infected tonsil may occur due to same nerve supply, glossopharyngeal nerve.
3. Excessive haemorrhage may occur during removal of tonsil may be due to damage to paratonsillar vein.
4. After removal of tonsil, taste sensation may be affected due to injury to glossopharyngeal nerve.
5. During the process of removal it is the presence or absence of capsule which will indicate whether removal is incomplete or complete.
6. Bleeding from tonsil is usually checked by removing the clots (like uterine bleeding in stopped).

Development: Developed from dorsal part of second pharyngeal pouch. It is both endodermal and mesodermal in development.

Tonsillar crypts and follicles including mucous membrane are from endoderm from second pharyngeal pouch and lymphoid tissue is mesodermal from extrapharyngeal mesoderm.

MICROSCOPIC FEATURES OF PALATINE TONSIL

Surface of the tonsil is covered by stratified squamous non-keratinized epithelium.

There are cleft-like spaces in the surface which are known as tonsillar crypts.

The maximum part of the tonsil is made up of dense collection of lymphoid nodules which are having germinal centres.

Mucous acini are present below the mucosa. (Fig. 14.30)

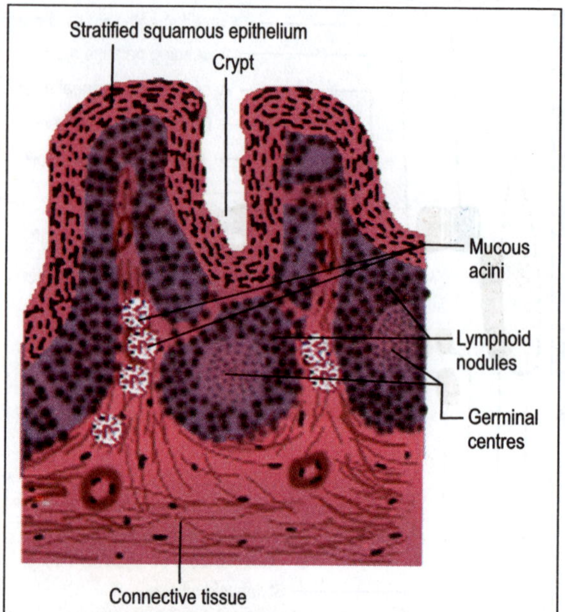

Fig. 14.30: Microscopic features of tonsil

AUDITORY TUBE (PHARYNGO-TYMPANIC TUBE OR EUSTACHIAN TUBE)

It is a channel of communication between tympanic cavity and nasopharynx and is functionally concerned for equalisation of pressure on the inner and outer aspect of tympanic membrane as air passes from pharynx to tymphanic cavity through this.

Direction:

a) It is directed *downwards, forwards* and *medially.*
b) It forms an *angle of 45° with sagittal plane* and *angle of 30° with horizontal plane.*

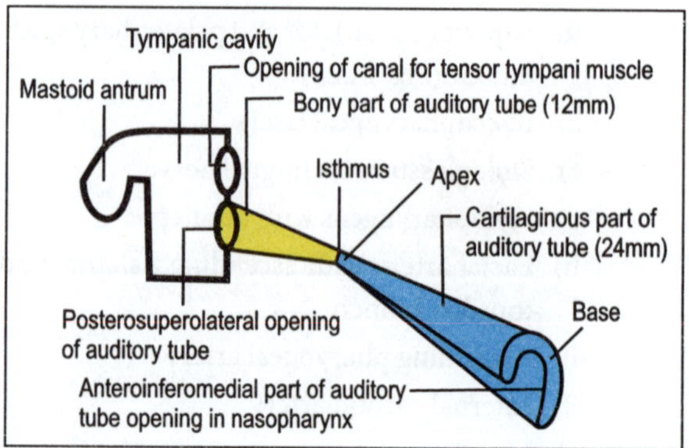

Fig. 14.31: Auditory tube

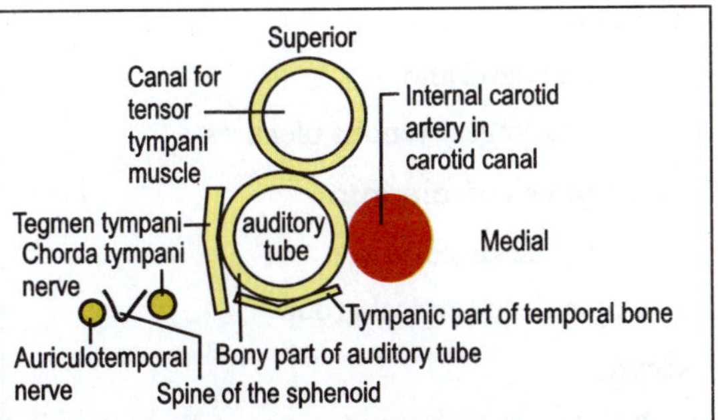

Fig. 14.32: Relations of bony part of auditory tube

Different parts: Two

I. Bony or Lateral part (Fig. 14.31)

II. Fibrocartilaginous or Medial part. (Fig. 14.32)

I. Bony part of the tube

Features:

1. It is the *posterolateral part* of the tube.
2. *Length* – 12mm
3. *Situation* – Lies within petrous part of the temporal bone.
4. *Extent* – From anterior wall of tympanic cavity to the junction between squamous and petrous part of temporal bone and on medial side of spine of sphenoid bone.
5. *Medial end* (**isthmus**) – Narrower than lateral end and presents jagged margin for the cartilaginous part.
6. *On cross-section* – Oblong i.e., greater width from side to side.
7. **Relations**:
   A. *Above* – Canal for tensor tympani muscle.
   B. *Below* – Tympanic part of temporal bone.
   C. *Laterally* – Chorda tympani nerve and spine of sphenoid bone, and auriculotemporal nerve. Temporo-mandibular joint.
   D. *Medially* – Carotid canal with internal carotid artery.

II. Fibro-cartilaginous part

Features:

1. It is the *medial part*. (Fig. 14.33)
2. *Length* – 24mm.
3. *Situation* – In the sulcus tubae (a groove between the inferior surface of petrous temporal and greater wing of sphenoid).

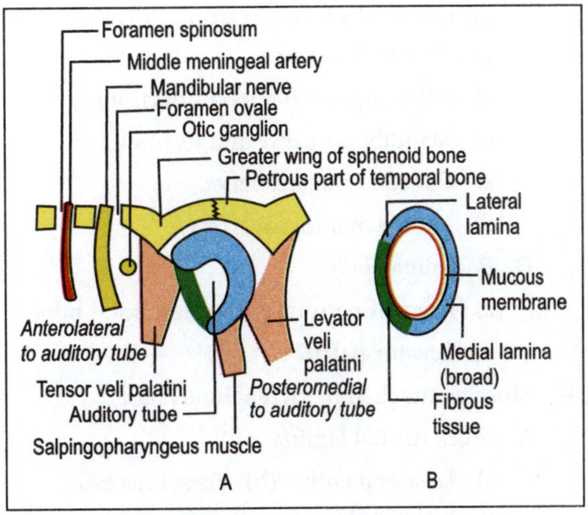

Fig. 14.33: A. Relations of cartilaginous of auditory tube; B. Section through cartilaginous part of auditory tube

4. *Direction* – *Downwards, forwards* and *medially*.
5. *Extent* – Its lateral end joins with bony part & its medial part forms an elevation (tubal elevation) in the nasopharynx (1.25cm behind the inferior nasal concha).
6. *Isthmus* – It is the *narrowest part of the tube* and is the *junctional region between bony and cartilaginous part*.
7. *Formation* – Formed by a *triangular plate of elastic fibrocartilage*.
   a) Apex – Attached to bony part.
   b) Base – Forms *tubal elevation* at the medial end.
   c) Consists of two laminae – Medial and lateral as the cartilage is bent upon itself.
   d) Floor & part of lateral lamina are deficient which is filled up by fibrous tissue.
   e) *On transverse section* – Cartilage is hook shaped i.e., *inverted 'J' shaped*.
8. *Relations:*
   A. *Above* – Sulcus tubae.
   B. *Below* – Part of tensor veli palati muscle.
   C. *Antero laterally* – Tensor veli palati muscle sepa-

rating the tube from the structures of infratemporal fossa. They are:

a) Otic ganglion and its connections.
b) Mandibular nerve and its branches.
c) Chorda tympani nerve.
d) Middle meningeal artery.

D. *Posteromedially*

a) Apex of petrous part of temporal bone.
b) Levator palati.

9. Muscles attached to cartilaginous part

A. From medial lamina

a) *Levator palati;* (b) *Tensor tympani;*
c) *Salpingopharyngeus*

B. From lateral lamina – *Tensor veli palati.*

10. It is *sandwitched between levator palati* and *tensor veli palati.*

Mucous membrane of the pharyngotympanic tube

1. It is lined by ciliated pseudostratified columnar epithelium.

Opening of the tube at the pharyngeal end

Tensor veli palatini & levator veli palatini opens the tube during deglutition.

Characteristics in children

1. As bony part is not properly developed so length is shorter and about 18nm.
2. It is more or less horizontal in disposition. [So chance of spread of infection from nasopharynx to tympanic cavity is more in case of children.]
3. Tubal elevation a the pharyngeal end is not so prominent and so passing of eustachian catheter is not so easy.

Blood supply

(a) **Arteries:**

Branches from following arteries:

1. Ascending pharyngeal
2. Middle meningeal
3. Artery of pterygoid canal.

(b) **Veins** –

1. Pterygoid and
2. Pharyngeal venous plexuses.

Lymphatics – drain into

1. Retropharyngeal and
2. Upper deep cervical group

Nerves

1. By glossopharyngeal nerve through tympanic plexus.
2. Pharyngeal branch of pterygopalatine ganglion.

APPLIED ANATOMY:

1. Introduction of Eustachian catheter. It is tubal elevation which guides the introduction of eustachian catheter into auditory tube for inflation and thereby correcting retracted tympanic membrane by equalisation of pressure and relieve all symptoms.
2. Middle ear infections are common in infants due to horizontal eustachian tube and infections from nasopharynx reach easily to middle ear.

Development – It is endodermal and mesodermal in development.

Mucous membrane is **endodermal** and from endoderm of proximal (medial) part of tubo-tympanic recess formed by the fusion of dorsal parts of first and second pharyngeal pouches.

FACTORS KEEPING THE TONSIL IN POSITION (TONSIL IS NOT SWALLOWED)

1. Situated in the deepest fossa
2. Held up by fibrous bands connecting capsule with stylo and palatoglossus muscles.
3. Attachment of capsule with pharyngobasilar fascia and superior constrictor by loose areolar tissue.
4. Perivascular stalks: Arteries supplying palatine tonsil.

chapter 15

Nose and Paranasal Air Sinuses

AT A GLANCE

- *External nose—Features, Boundaries of nostrils, Formation of skeletal framework of external nose, Bones, Cartilages, Arterial supply, Nerve supply*
- *Nasal cavity—Situation, Number, Extent; Posterior nasal apertures (Choanae); Dimensions; Boundaries–Roof, floor, medial wall (nasal septum), lateral wall, Arterial supply of septum, Venous drainage of septum, Nerve supply of septum, Development of septum, Applied anatomy of septum; Lateral wall – Formation, Features, Meatuses of nasal cavity; Arterial supply; Venous drainage; Nerve supply*
- *Paranasal air sinus—Frontal air sinus: Site, Number, Extent, Shape, Opening, Arterial supply, Veins, Nerve supply; Ethmoidal air sinus: Features, Number, Blood supply, Lymphatics, Nerve supply; Maxillary air sinus: Situation, Shape, Boundaries, Size, Opening, Relations, Blood supply, Lymphatics, Nerve supply, Development; Sphenoidal air sinus: Number, Measurement, Extent; Applied anatomy*

NOSE

It is an organ mainly for respiration but a part of it is for smell or olfaction. It consists of two parts for sake of description.

1. **External nose**
2. **Nasal cavity**

External nose (Fig. 15.1)

A pyramidal shaped projection in the midline of face below forehead and orbit and just above oral aperture (upper lip).

Features:

1. *Root*: Upper narrow part continuous with forehead
2. *Tip or Apex*: In the lower free part
3. *Nostrils or Nares (External)*: These are external piriform opening situated below and separated by nasal septum.

Boundary of the nostrils

Medially: Mobile part of nasal septum.

Laterally: Ala or nose.

4. *Dorsal nasi*: A median rounded between root and tip, and lateral surfaces meet here.

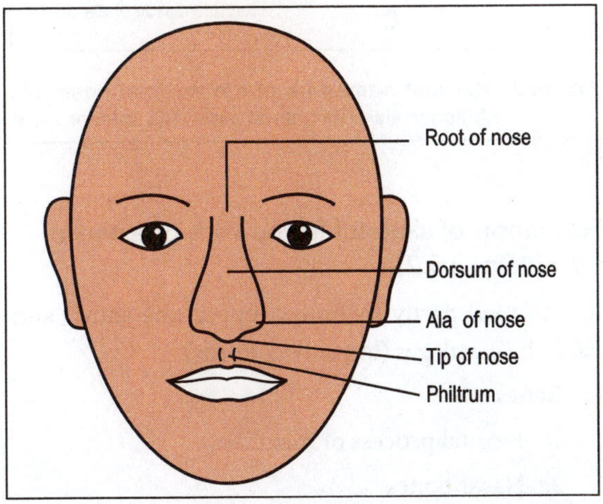

Fig. 15.1: Features of external nose

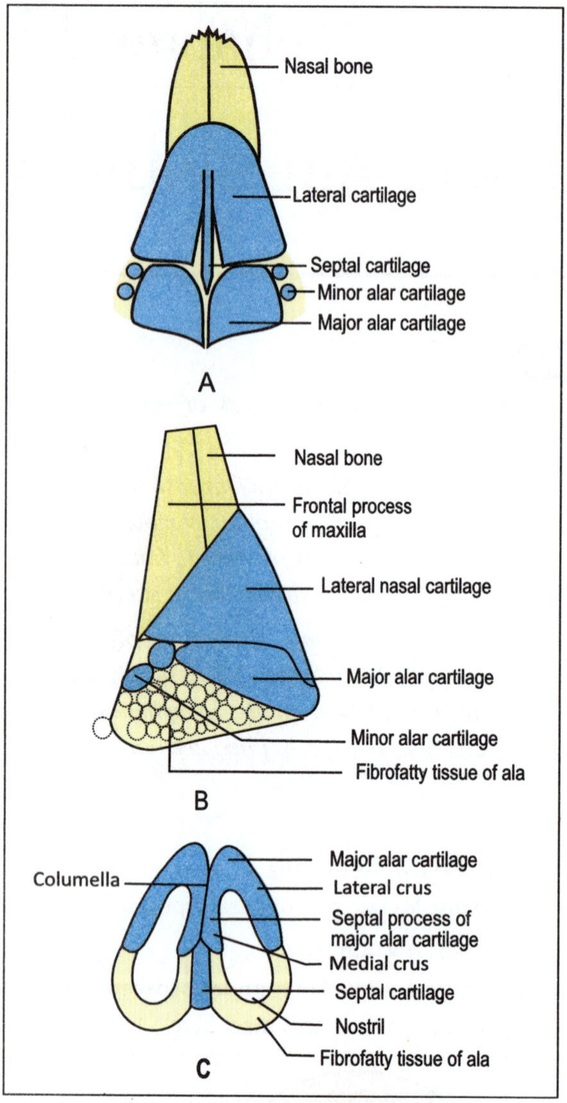

Fig. 15.2: Skeletal framework of the external nose: (A) Anterior viw; (B) Lateral view; (C) Inferior view

Formation of skeletal framework of external nose: (Fig. 15.2)

It is formed partly by bones (upper one-third) and partly by cartilages (lower two-thirds).

I. **Bones**

1. Frontal process of maxilla
2. Nasal bones
3. Nasal notch of frontal bone

II. **Cartilages**

1. **Upper lateral nasal cartilage** attached to margin of piriform aperture by fibrous tissue. The piriform aperture formed by nasal bone and frontal process of maxilla. Upper lateral nasal cartilage is continuous with septal cartilage. (Fig. 15.2A)
2. Septal cartilage is attached to anteroinferior margin of perpendicular plate. Septal cartilage not only help to form right & left nasal cavities but also provide support the dorsum of the nose.
3. Major alar cartilage is 'U' shaped having medial & lateral crus. Medial crura meet with septal cartilage. Lateral crus lie below the ala of the nose. Gap between the lateral crus and bone is filled by fibrofatty tissue.
4. Minor alar cartilage (2 or more) lie lateral to major alar cartilage.

Skin of external nose: Thin and movable over bone but thick and adherent to cartilages and fibroareolar tissue. Skin is having sebaceous gland.

Arteries of external nose

1. Dorsal nasal branch of ophthalmic artery (anastomoses with facial artery)
2. Infraorbital branch of maxillary artery (third part)
3. Alar and septal branches of facial artery.

Nerves (Sensory):

1. External nasal and
2. Infratrochlear branches of ophthalmic nerve
3. Infraorbital branch of maxillary nerve.

The muscles of external nose is supplied by facial nerve.

Applied anatomy:

Deviated nasal septum (DNS): It is common in males and usually lead to nasal obstruction which may require immediate attention. DNS may lead to sinusitis.

NASAL CAVITY

It is divided into two halves by a septum.

Boundaries of each half has medial wall, lateral wall, roof and floor.

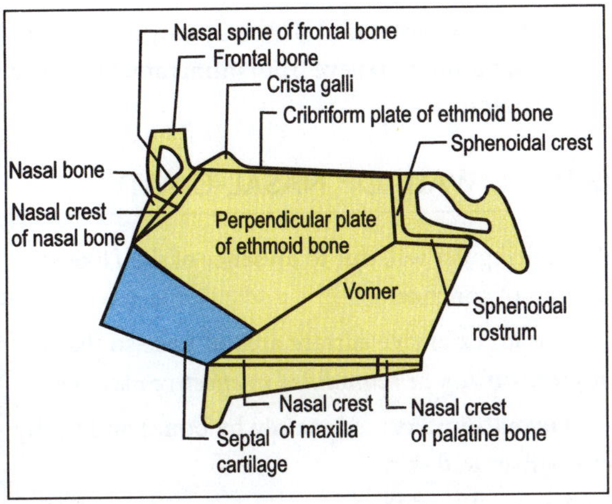

Fig. 15.3: Skeletal basis of nasal septum

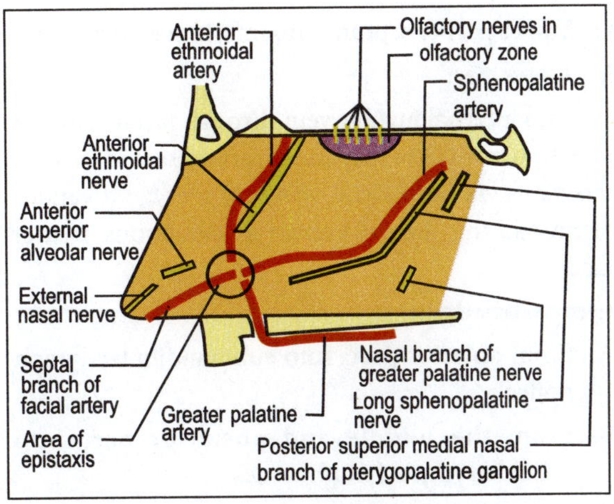

Fig. 15.4: Arterial & nerve supply of nasal septum

Medial wall or Nasal septum

It is a partition between two halves of nasal cavities and forming medial wall of the cavities.

Situation: It is usually not strictly at the median plane but usually deflected to one or other side and thereby nasal cavities become asymmetrical.

Formation: The septum is formed partly by bone and cartilage. (Fig. 15.3)

I. *Bony part*: Mainly
   1. *Perpendicular plate of ethmoid bone*: Antero-superior part of the septum.
   2. *Vomer*: Postero-inferior part of the septum.

   Other bone:

   A. *In front and above by*
      a) Nasal spine of frontal and
      b) Nasal crest formed by two nasal bones

   B. *Behind*: by sphenoidal crest & sphenoid rostrum.

   C. *Below*: by nasal crest of maxillary bones and palatine bones.

II. **Cartilaginous part**: Antero-inferior part mainly by
   1. Septal cartilage forms the major part of septum.
   2. Septal processess of two major cartilages: Both sides cartilages forms the mobile part of the septum.

   Fibrofatty tissue in the lower part & lower margin is known as **columela.**

Arterial supply:

A. Anterosuperior part is supplied by **anterior ethmoidal branch** of ophthalmic artery (Fig. 15.4)

B. Posterosuperior part is supplied by **sphenopalatine artery**: branches of third part of maxillary artery

C. Posteroinferior part is supplied by **greater palatine artery**: branch of third part of maxillary artery.

D. Anteroinferior part (vestibular region) or mobile part: **septal branch** of superior labial branch of the **facial artery.**

Little's area (Kiesselbach's plexus): It is an area in the anteroinferior [commonest area of **epistaxis (nasal bleeding)** due to trauma or ulcer] part of the septum. The following arteries anastomoses:

1. Septal branch of superior labial artery.
2. Sphenopalatine and terminal part of greater palatine arteries.
3. Anterior ethmoidal artery.

Venous drainage:

Drains from

A. Antero-superior part to superior ophthalmic vein

B. From postero-inferior part to pterygoid venous plexus.

C. Upper part of septum into inferior cerebral veins.

D. Lower part.

Into internal jugular vein through facial vein. An infection from here may cause thrombosis in cavernous sinus via deep facial vein and pterygoid venous plexus; so this area is known as dangerous area of face.

Lymphatics: drain

A. From anterior part: Into submandibular lymph nodes

B. From the middle and posterior part into retropharyngeal lymph nodes

C. From upper part: Through perineural sheaths of olfactory nerves into cerebrospinal fluid (CSF).

Nerve supply:

I. ***Olfactory region***: By olfactory nerves carrying small sensation from the upper part.

II. ***Sensory nerves***: For general sense

   A. *Anterosuperior part*: By anterior ethmoidal nerve (continuation) of nasociliary nerve.

   B. *Anteroinferior part*: Anterior superior alveolar (branch of maxillary nerve) and exteral nasal nerve (branch of anterior ethmodial nerve of nasociliary nerve of ophthalmic nerve).

   C. *Posterosuperior part*: Medial posterior superior nasal branch of the pterygopalatine ganglion.

   D. *Posteroinferior part*: By long sphenopalatine nerve of pterygopalatine ganglion nerve.

   E. *Posterior part*: Supplied by nasal branch of greater palatine nerve.

APPLIED ANATOMY:

A. Area of epistaxis or Little's area or Kiesselbach's plexus

   1. It is a commonest site for bleeding from nose (epistaxis) due to injury etc.

   2. **Deviated nasal septum** (DNS): It may be congenital or pathological. It may cause recurrent attacks of colds rhinitis usually allergic. Correction of this is necessary by submucous resection (SMR operation).

   3. Venous plexus in submucous layer may also cause profuse bleeding in patients suffering from hypertension. This is a safety mechanism of nature to relieve from intracranial vascular pressure.

LATERAL WALL OF NASAL CAVITY

It is an irregular wall due to presence of shelf like projections of conchae.

It is an extensive surface area of nose so that the *inspired air can be humidified in effective manner.*

Formation: Formed mainly by bones and partly by cartilage and skin.

I. **Bones** (Fig. 15.5)

   1. Nasal
   2. Frontal process of maxilla
   3. Lacrimal
   4. Superior and middle nasal conchae of labyrinth of ethmoid bone
   5. Inferior nasal concha
   6. Perpendicular plate of palatine
   7. Medial pterygoid plate of sphenoid
   8. Uncinate process of ethmoid bone.

II. **Cartilages**: Upper and lower nasal cartilages and

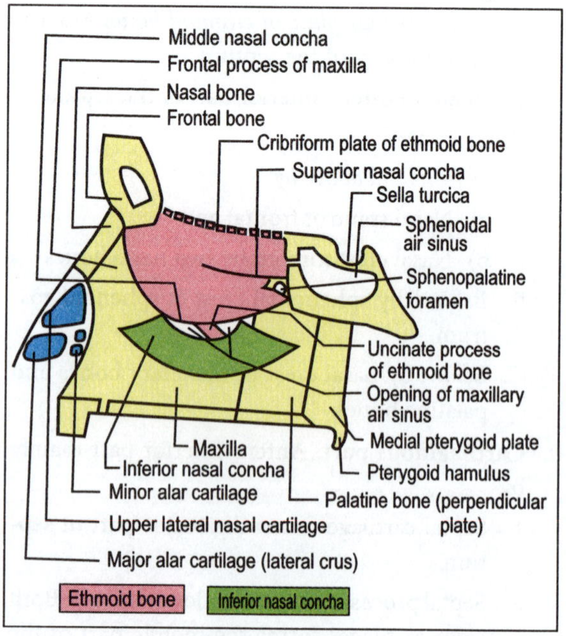

Fig. 15.5: Skeletal basis of lateral wall of nasal cavity

alar cartilage.

1. Upper lateral nasal cartilage.
2. Major alar cartilages.
3. Minor alar cartilages.

III. **Fibrofatty tissue** with covering skin in the lower part.

Features of lateral wall

I. **Nasal conchae**: Shelf like projections of curved plate of bones directed downwards and medially.

Three number: Superior concha, middle concha and inferior concha. Below and lateral to each concha is a space called meatus (Fig. 15.6).

1. ***Superior nasal concha***:
   a) It projects from the medial surface of ethmoidal labyrinth. Sphenoethmoidal recess is a depression above the superior concha and the sphenoidal air sinus opens into it.
2. ***Middle nasal concha***:
   a) A shelf like *projection from the medial surface of ethmoidal labyrinth below superior nasal concha.*
3. ***Inferior nasal concha***:
   a) It is the *lower most shelf-like projection formed by separate bone.*

II. **Meatuses of the nasal cavity**: These are spaces in the lateral wall and lie below the conchae and also named accordingly.

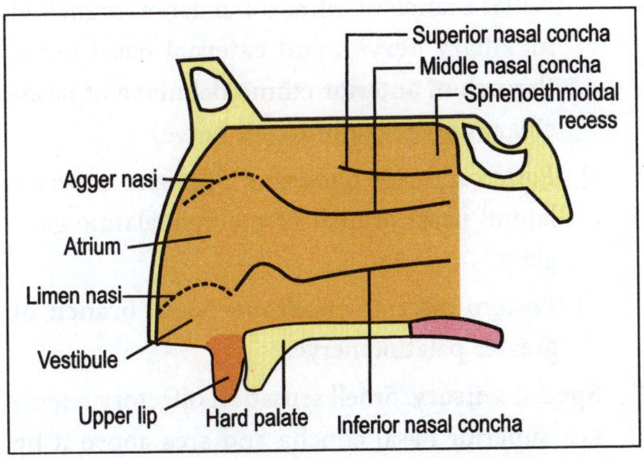

Fig. 15.6: Features of lateral wall of nasal cavity

Number: Three – superior meatus, middle meatus and inferior meatus.

Superior meatus: Shortest and shallowest of all meati and it is an area situated below and under cover of superior nasal concha.

Opening: Posterior ethmoidal sinuses opens in the superior meatus.

Middle meatus: It is the space situated below the middle nasal concha (Fig. 15.7).

Features:

1. *Bulla ethmoidalis*: a rounded bony bulging in the lateral wall due to middle ethmoidal air sinuses.
2. *Hiatus semilunaris*: It is a semilunar groove or space below the bulla ethmoidalis.
3. *Infundibulum*: The hiatus expands anteriorly (funnel shaped expansion) called infundibulum.
4. *Openings paranasal sinuses*
   a) Opening of maxillary air sinus: In the floor of hiatus semilunaris (posterior part).
   b) Opening of frontal sinus: The frontal air sinus opens into upper part of the infundibulum by frontonasal duct.

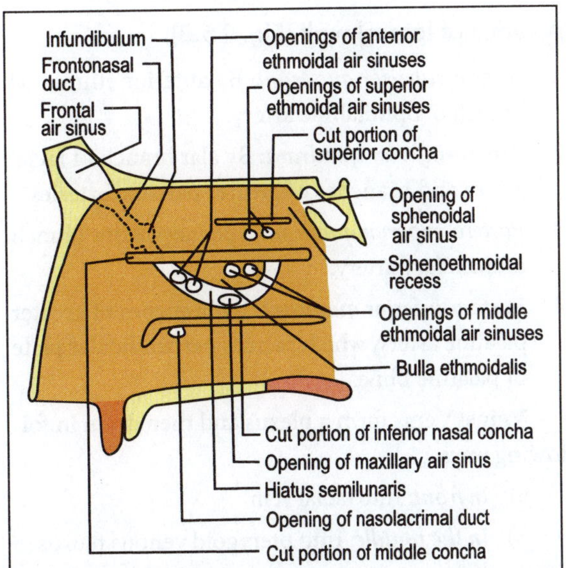

Fig. 15.7: Features of lateral wall of nasal cavity (conchae have been removed)

c) Opening of anterior ethmoidal sinus: In the middle part of hiatus.

d) Opening of middle ethmoidal air sinus: In the upper part of bulla.

5. *Atrium of middle meatus*: A depressed area situated above vestibule and is continuous with anterior part of middle meatus.
6. *Limen nasi*: A curved mucocutaneous ridge at the junction between atrium and vestibule.
7. *Agger nasi*: A mucous ridge limiting the upper part of atrium.

Inferior meatus: It is the area in the lateral wall of nasal cavity below and under cover of inferior nasal concha and largest of all meati.

Opening: Opening of nasolacrimal duct at the anterior part.

Continuity: In front with lateral wall of vestibule.

Spheno-ethmoidal recess: It is a depressed area (spheno-ethmoidal recess) above and behind superior concha.

Sphenoidal air sinus opens–

Vestibule of nose: A depressed area in the anterior and lower part of lateral wall. It is covered by skin with hairs.

Arteries of lateral wall (Fig. 15.8)

1. *Antero-superior quadrant*: By anterior ethmoidal branch of ophthalmic artery.
2. *Antero-inferior quadrant*: By alar branch of facial artery and branches of greater palatine arteries.
3. *Postero-superior quadrant*: Sphenopalatine branch of maxillary artery.
4. *Postero-inferior quadrant*: By branches of greater palatine artery, which pierces perpendicular plate of palatine bone.

Veins: Veins form a plexus and then drain in following ways

a) *In front*: Into facial vein

b) *In the middle*: Into pterygoid venous plexus

c) *Behind*: Pharyngeal venous plexus

d) *Above*: Inferior cerebral vein.

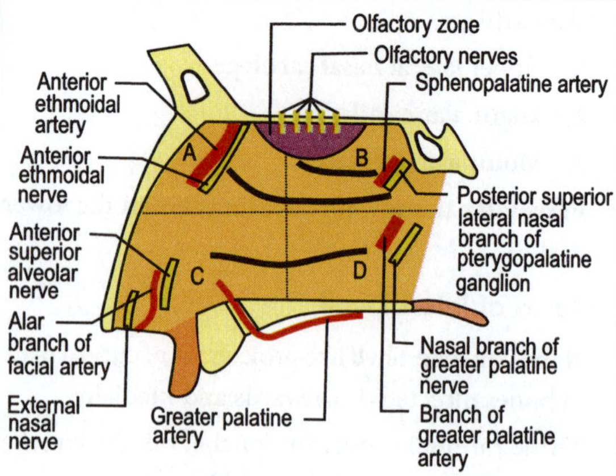

Fig. 15.8: Nerve supply & arterial supply of the lateral wall of nasal cavity. A – Anterosuperior segment; B – Posterosuperior segment; C – Anteroinferior segment; D – Posteroinferior segment

Lymphatic drainage of lateral wall of nasal cavity–

a) From the anterior half, lymph drain into submandibular group of lymph nodes.

b) From posterior half, lymph drain into retropharyngeal and upper deep cervical lymph nodes.

Nerves of lateral wall

1. **Sensory** (general sense): Supply whole of lateral wall *except the superior concha and part above it.*

   a) *Anterosuperior quadrant*: Anterior ethmoidal branch of nasociliary nerve (branch of ophthalmic nerve).

   b) *Anteroinferior quadrant*: Anterior superior alveolar branch of infraorbital nerve (branch of maxillary nerve), and external nasal nerve (branch of anterior ethmoidal nerve of nasociliary nerve of ophthalmic nerve).

   c) *Posterosuperior quadrant*: Posterior superior lateral nasal branch of pterygopalatine ganglion.

   d) *Postero-inferior quadrant*: Nasal branch of greater palatine nerve.

2. **Special sensory**: Smell sensation olfactory region i.e., superior nasal concha and area above it by olfactory nerve.

Roof:

1. Narrow transversely except posterior part.
2. Length: about 7.5cm; Width: about 1.2mm
3. *It slopes in front and behind and middle part is horizontal.*
4. **Formation:**
   A. *Anterior slope* downward and forward and is formed by nasal spine of the frontal, nasal bone and nasal cartilages.
   B. *Middle horizontal part* is formed by cribriform plate of ethmoid and it is thin and delicate. It is pierced by olfactory nerves and ethmoidal vessels. It is the highest part of roof.
   C. *Posterior part* is formed by anterior and inferior surface of body of sphenoid bone and it is less than 1cm wide and continuous with roof of nasopharynx.

Floor:

1. *Anterior-posteriorly*: Flat and almost horizontal and side to side it is concave.
2. (a) *Length* (From tip of nose to posterior border of septum): 7.5cm
   (b) *Breadth*: 1.5cm
3. *Formation*: By upper surface of hard palate (formed by palatine process of maxilla anterior three-fourth and horizontal processes of palatine bone posterior one-fourth of the hard palate).
4. A depression in the mucous membrane is present about 2cm behind the anterior end and it overlies incisive canal.

   Dimensions: Each half measures

   Height: 5cm; Length: 5-7.5cm; Width: 1.25cm near the floor and at the root only 1-2mm.

DIFFERENT SUBDIVISIONS OF NASAL CAVITY AND LINING OF EPITHELIUM OF MUCOUS MEMBRANE

Three divisions:

1. ***Vestibule***: It is the part just above the nostrils and lined by skin and coarse and stiff hairs, sebaceous & sweat glands. The hairs prevent entry of foreign particles.
2. ***Respiratory region***: Major part above vestibule and below superior nasal concha. The mucous membrane is intimately adherent to underlying bones and cartilages except the regions of inferior nasal concha. It is lined by pseudostratified ciliated columnar epithelium (respiratory epithelium).

   Goblet cells, mucous & serous glands are also present. Goblet cells secrete mucous and traps the inhaled particles & microorganisms.

   Lamina propria contains vascular spaces (the places communicates with arterioles and vessels) apart from glands. In cold, there is vasodilatation which leads to distension of vascular spaces. Few females, during menstruation, may suffer from nasal bleeding.

   Olfactory region: Roof, adjoining septal and lateral wall of nasal cavity above the superior conchae constitute the region. The mucous membrane of this region is yellowish and lined by bipolar olfactory cells, tall columnar supporting cells & basal cells.

   Bipolar cells are having peripheral process (dendrites on the surface to respond to odorous stimuli) and central process (forms the olfactory nerves – about 20 in number, pierces the cribriform plate of ethmoid bone and synapse with the mitral cells of olfactory bulb). Basal cells can regenerate to form bipolar cells.
3. ***Olfactory region***: Superior nasal concha and area above it and corresponding opposite part of nasal septum. It is lined by olfactory epithelium.

   Functions of the nasal cavity:

   a) Helps in olfaction
   b) Respiratory passage and controls the air by changing the humidity & temperature.
   c) Filters foreign particles by hairs in the vestibule.

Table 15.1: Difference between anterior and posterior nasal apertures

Anterior nasal aperture (nostril)	Posterior nasal aperture (Choanae)
1. **Cartilaginous**: Formed by alar cartilage laterally and septal cartilage medially. (Fig. 15.2B)	1. **Bony**: Formed by posterior free margin of vomer, medial pterygoid plate, body of sphenoid and posterior margin of hard palate.
2. **Mobile**	2. **Rigid**
3. Kept patent by 'U' shaped alar cartilage	3. **Fixed**
4. **Ellipsoidal** in shape	4. **Oval** in shape
5. **Controlled by** compressor and dilator muscles.	5. Does not arise
6. **Measurement**: 1.5cm-2cm antero-posteriorly 0.5cm-1cm transversely (Fig. 15.2C)	6. **Measurements**: 2.5cm vertically; 12.5cm transversely

PARANASAL AIR SINUSES (Fig. 15.9)

There are bony spaces containing air and situated around nasal cavity.

Features:

1. Situated within pneumatic bones: frontal, maxillary, sphenoid and ethmoid.
2. All the sinuses open into nasal cavity (in the lateral wall)
3. They are covered by mucous membrane which is lined by ciliated pseudostratified columnar epithelium (continuous with nasal mucous membrane).
4. They develop as mucous outgrowths of nasal cavity in the adjoining bones and are formed by dissolution of diploe substance of the bone.
5. **Growth** –
   a) At birth: rudimentary or absent.
   b) Growth starts after 2 to 3 years and grows rapidly at the age of eruption of permanent tooth i.e., at 7-8 years of age.
   c) Then during and after puberty and also in old age (due to resorption of bone).

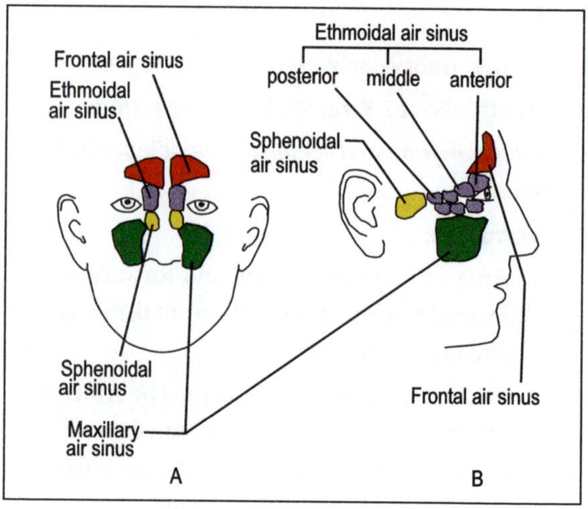

Fig. 15.9: Locations of paranasal air sinuses. A – Anterior view; B – Lateral view

So practically – Two stages of growth.
   i) During eruption of permanent teeth (7 to 8 years of age)
   ii) Post puberty age.

6. **Functions**:
   a) make the bones lighter – so the skull becomes lighter.
   b) acts as a air conditioning chamber by humidifying and warming the inspired air
   c) imparts resonance to the voice
   d) ciliated epithelium helps in drainage of mucous secretion.
7. **Applied anatomy**:
   a) As the mucous membrane of nasal cavity is continuous with the mucous membrane of the sinuses, so infection from the nose can spread easily to the sinuses and may give rise to sinusitis.
   b) When sinuses are infected the infected materials will be collected within the sinuses due to blockage of the opening into the nasal cavity and this condition may require drainage by surgical methods.
   c) During chronic sinusitis or recurrent attacks of infection the cilia of the epithelium may be lost and the result will be improper drainage as gravity also will play a least role.

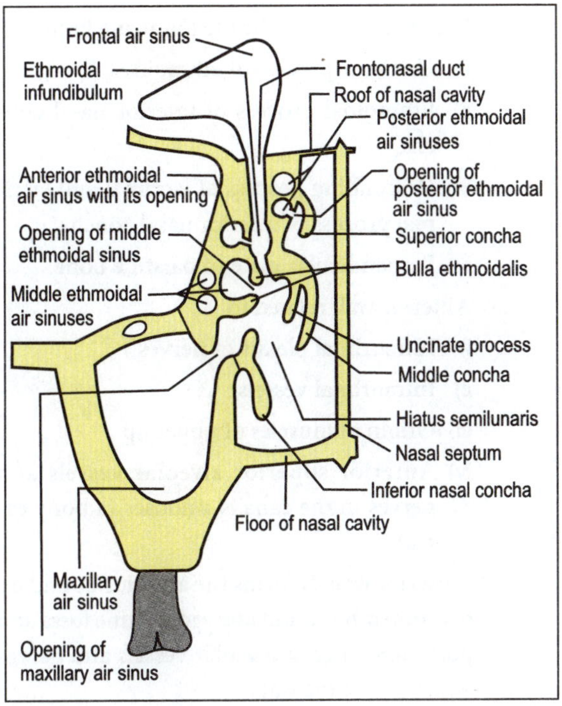

Fig. 15.10: Paranasal air sinuses

Frontal sinus:

It is a paranasal sinus in the frontal bone. (Fig. 15.10)

Site: It lies within the two tables of squamous part of frontal bone and just deep to medial part of superciliary arch.

Number: Two; one on each side.

Extent: Each sinus extends upwards above the medial end of eyebrow and behind into the medial part of roof of orbit.

Shape: More or less triangular but the two sinuses are unequal (asymmetrical).

Measurements: On average

Vertically: 3cm

Antero-posteriorly: 3cm

Transversely: 2.5cm

Opening: It opens in the anterior end of hiatus semilunaris of middle meatus through frontonasl duct. Each sinus reaches directly to infundibulum or via frontonasal duct.

Relation: Anteriorly – Superciliary arch.

Posteriorly – Frontal lobe of cerebrum.

Arterial supply: Supraorbital branch of ophthalmic artery.

Veins: Drain into junction of supraorbital and superior ophthalmic vein.

Lymphatics: Drain into submandibular lymph node.

Nerves: Supraorbital branch of frontal nerve.

Ethmoidal sinuses:

These are numerous air spaces within labyrinth of ethmoid bone on each side.

Features:

1. ***Situation***: They are situated on each side between lateral wall of nose and medial wall of orbit.
2. They are incomplete intercommunicating spaces and completed by frontal, lacrimal, maxilla, sphenoid and palatine bones.
3. ***Number***: Three to eighteen (3 to 18) but are divided into three groups – Anterior, Middle and Posterior.
   a) *Anterior group*: It consists of 3 to 7 but may be up to 1 in number. They open into middle meatus through infundibulum and hiatus semilunaris or the frontonasal duct.
   b) *Middle group*: Consists of 1 to 3 in number. It forms the bulla ethmoidalis and opens by one or two openings into the middle meatus on or above bulla.
   c) *Posterior group*: It consists of 1 to 11 in number and open mainly into superior meatus.
4. **Blood supply**: Anterior ethmoidal vessels (anterior and middle group) and posterior ethmoidal vessels (posterior group).
5. ***Lymphatics***: Into submandibular lymph node (anterior and middle group) and retropharyn-geal lymph nodes (posterior group).
6. ***Nerves***: Anterior ethmoidal nerve (anterior and middle group) and posterior ethmoidal nerve (posterior group).

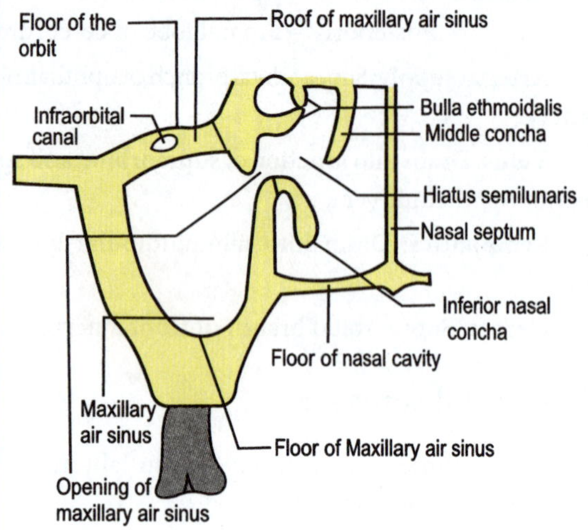

Fig. 15.11: Maxillary air sinus

Maxillary sinus: (Fig. 15.11)

It is the largest of paranasal sinuses and two in number: one on each side.

Situation: Within body of maxilla.

Shape: Pyramidal in shape, with base being directed medially towards nasal cavity and apex is directed laterally to zygomatic process of maxilla.

Size: Varies. Average measurements are:

Vertical: (Opposite first molar) – 3.5cm

Transverse: 2.5cm

Anteroposterior: 3.2cm of base

Boundaries:

a) *Apex*: Zygomatic process of maxilla.

b) *Roof*: Roof is formed by floor of the orbit. The infraorbital nerve and vessels traverse the roof in the infraorbital canal.

c) *Floor*: Alveolar process of maxilla situated 1.25cm below the level of nasal floor. It presents elevations due to roots of upper premolar and molar teeth.

d) *Base*: Nasal surface of body of maxilla which presents opening of maxillary air sinus near the roof.

Actually the opening of the maxillary air sinus is large as seen in disarticulated skull.

It is reduced in size by the following bones:

i) Uncinate process of ethmoid.

ii) Ethmoidal process of inferior nasal concha.

iii) Descending process of lacrimal and lacrimal process of inferior nasal concha.

iv) Perpendicular plate of palatine bone.

e) Anterior wall related to

i) Infraorbital plexus of nerves

ii) Infraorbital vessels

iii) Origin of muscles of upper lip

iv) Anterior superior alveolar vessels and nerves in the canalis sinuoses (a bony canal).

f) Porterior wall: It forms the anterior boundary of infratemporal and pterygopalatine fossa and posterior superior alveolar vessels and nerves which pierce the wall.

APPLIED ANATOMY:

1. Sinuses and commonly maxillary sinus are infected from nasal cavity due to continuity of nasal mucous membrane with mucous lining of the sinus and also from caries tooth.
2. Collection of infected material or pus in maxillary sinus is very common because it can be directly infected or as it is the most dependent part, so pus from infected frontal or ethmoidal sinus may collect in the maxillary sinus and besides, the drainage is very poor as the opening of this sinus lies at a higher level than the floor. Drainage is usually done by

   a) an approaching through inferior meatus (breaking the lateral wall **antral puncture**).

   b) making opening at the canine fossa.
3. **Caldwell-luc operation**: In this procedure the maxillary air sinus is approched through the incisive fossa and gingivobuccal sulcus.

Blood supply: Facial, infraorbital and greater palatine and also anterior, middle and posterior superior alveolar vessels branches of maxillary artery.

Lymphatics: Into submandibular lymph nodes.

Nerves: Infraorbital and anterior, middle and posterior superior alveolar nerves.

Sphenoidal Sinuses:

These are paranasal air sinuses situated within the body of sphenoid bone.

Number: Two, one on each side but not symmetrical and separated from each other by a septum.

Measurements: On average

Vertical: 2cm

Transverse: 1.5cm

Anteroposterior: 2cm

Extent: In front it extends up to roof of orbit and behind it extends up to margin of foramen magnum.

On each side it extends up to pterygoid canal.

Relations:

1. *Above*: Optic chiasma and pituitary gland
2. *Below*: Forms roof of pharynx (nasopharyngeal)
3. *On each side*: Cavernous sinus and internal carotid artery
4. *In front*: Spheno-ethmoidal recess
5. *Behind*: Pons and medulla separated by venous plexus (basilar).

Opening: It opens into sphenoethmoidal recess.

Blood supply: By posterior ethmoidal vessels.

Lymphatics: To retropharyngeal group of lymph nodes.

Nerve supply: Posterior ethmoidal nerve and orbital branches of pterygopalatine ganglion.

APPLIED ANATOMY:

1. Olfactory nerves may be involved during fracture of cribriform plate and result is loss of smell and discharge of cerebrospinal fluid.
2. Brain abscess in frontal lobe may result from spread of infection from frontal sinus.
3. Deviation of nasal septum usually involve cartilages & bones or cartilage only.

DEVELOPMENT OF NASAL SEPTUM

It is mesodermal in development. It is a passive phenomenon. Two nasal sacs are formed within frontonasal process (a process from roof aspect of stomodeum) and are separated from each other initially by a thick layer of mesoderm. Gradual expansion of nasal sacs results in thinning out of intervening mesoderm. The persistent thinned out intervening mesoderm between two nasal sacs from nasal septum.

DEVELOPMENT OF PARANASAL AIR SINUSES

It is the first paranasal sinus to develop. In the fourth month of foetal life a shallow groove appears in medial surface of maxilla and within six to seven years it grows rapidly an after eruption of permanent teeth it attains full size.

chapter 16

LARYNX

AT A GLANCE

- *Extent, Situation, Measurement, Relations, Structures suspending larynx from above, Functions of larynx, Framework of larynx, Skeletal framework of larynx*
- *Thyroid cartilage*
- *Epiglottis*
- *Cricoid cartilage*
- *Arytenoid cartilage*
- *Corniculate & cunaiform cartilage*
- *Developmental aspect of cartilages*
- *Joints of larynx*
- *Ligaments of larynx*
- *Quadrate membrane, crico-vocal ligament*
- *Interior of larynx*
- *Inlet of larynx, vestibula of larynx, sinus of larynx, Saccule of larynx*
- *Rima vestibuli*
- *Rima glottides*
- *Muscles of larynx*
- *Lining epithelium of larynx*
- *Arterial supply*
- *Veins*
- *Lymphatics*
- *Nerve supply of larynx*
- *Mechanism of production of larynx*
- *Applied anatomy*

Larynx is an organ of respiration and phonation (known as Sound box).

Extent: From (base of tongue) the upper border of epiglottis to the lower border of sixth cervical vertebra (lower border of cricoid cartilage). It communicate with laryngopharynx through laryngeal inlet, superiorly. Inferiorly, it continues as trachea.

Situation: Situated in the upper and front part of the neck opposite the **third cervical to sixth cervical vertebrae** in adults (male). But in children and females (also in adults) it is higher up, and laryngeal tone is high-pitched. In male, thyroid angle is more prominent (Adam's apple) and males the voice deep.

Measurement:

A. *Length*: In male: 44mm; In female: 36mm

B. *Transverse diameter*: In male: 43mm; In female: 41mm

C. *Antero-posterior diameter*: In male: 36mm; In female: 26mm

Relations:

A. *In front*: Infrahyoid muscles (thyrohyoid, sternohyoid, sternothyroid and superior belly of omohyoid). In between two groups of muscles of two sides in midline it is covered only by skin (so this part is easily approachable during laryngotomy).

B. *Lateral*: (1) Sternocleidomastoid (flanking it); (2) Lateral lobe of thyroid gland (clasping it).

C. *Behind*: Laryngopharynx.

Structures suspending the larynx (from above)

1. From hyoid bone
   a) Thyrohyoid muscle
   b) Thyrohyoid membrane
2. From base of skull
   a) Stylopharyngeus
   b) Palatopharyngeus
   c) Salpingopharyngeus

Functions of larynx

1. Acts as patent respiratory passage.
2. Sphincteric valve for prevention of entry of foreign body and specially closing the inlet during swallowing.
3. Expiratory air is utilised for production of sound
4. Also takes part in sneezing.

Frame work of larynx: It is a membranous tube lined by mucous membrane supported by cartilages which are connected with each other by membranes and ligaments and forming joints and they are moved by groups of muscles.

Skeletal framework

1. Skeleton of larynx: Formed by nine cartilages

   Cartilages are **paired** and **unpaired**

   A. **Unpaired cartilage**: (1) *Thyroid*: Haylaine type; (2) *Cricoid*: Hyaline type; (3) *Epiglottis*: Yellow elastic.

   B. **Paired**: (1) *Arytenoid*: Hyaline except apex and vocal process which are yellow elastic; (2) *Cuneiform*: Yellow elastic; (3) *Corniculate*: Yellow elastic.

All the hyaline cartilages tend to ossify by twenty fifth years of age.

THYROID CARTILAGE (Fig. 16.1)

1. It is a shield shaped unpaired cartilage situated in front part of the neck and protects larynx from front and lies opposite the level of fourth and fifth cervical vertebrae.
2. *Thyroid angle*: It consists of two laminae which fuses in front and form thyroid angle.

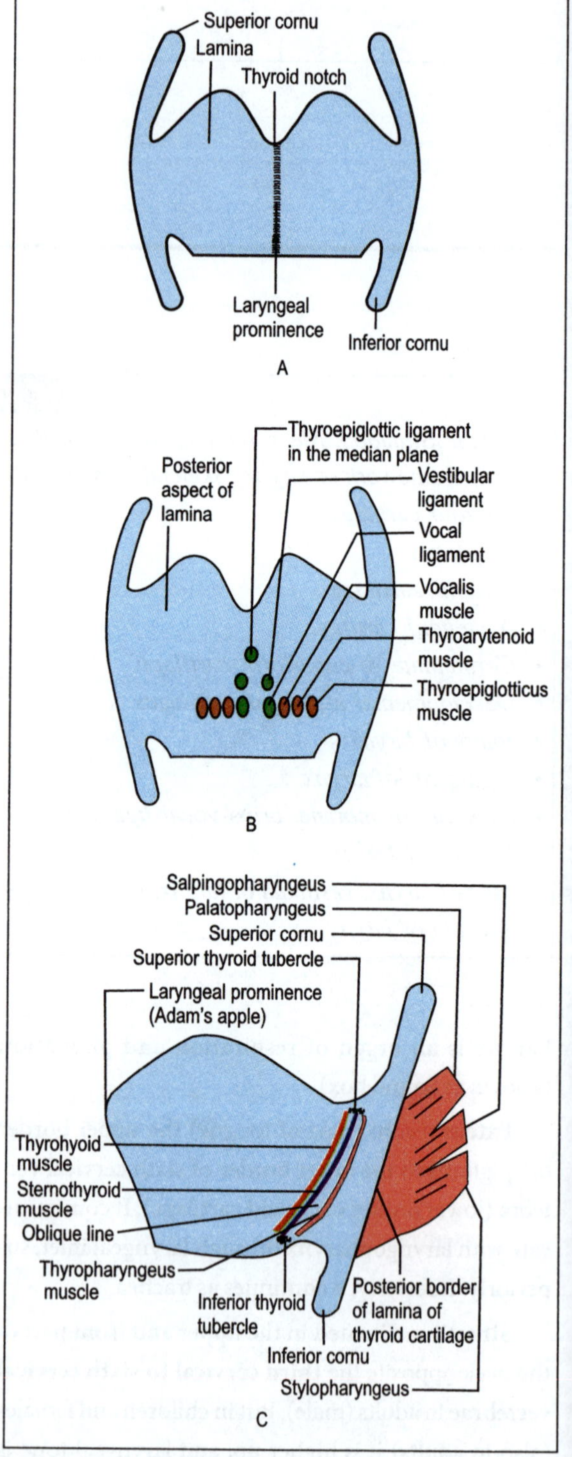

Fig. 16.1: The thyroid cartilage. A – Anterior view; B – Posterior view; C – Lateral view

In male: Thyroid angle is very **prominent** (from the time of puberty) and known as **Adam's apple.** It is about 90°.

In female and obtuse angle is 120°.

3. *Borders and surfaces of lamina of thyroid cartilage*

   Borders: Four

   A. *Upper*: Attachment of the thyrohyoid membrane
   B. *Lower*: It is straight (anteriorly) and concave (posteriorly).

      On each side: Insertion of cricothyroid muscle
   C. *Anterior*: At thyroid angle both the anterior borders meet and on posterior surface of the angle structures attached from above downwards are
      a) Thyroepiglottic ligament
      b) Paired vestibular ligament
      c) Paired vocal ligaments.

      On each side of vocal ligaments from medial to lateral.
      d) Vocalis
      e) Thyroarytenoid
      f) Thyroepiglotticus
   D. *Posterior border*: It is a free border and extends upwards and downward as superior and inferior horn
      a) Posterior border – attachment (insertion) of united tendon of three muscles – stylopharyngeus, palatopharyngeus and salpingopharyngeus.

   Surfaces: Two (Fig. 16.3)

   A. **Outer of external surface:** Oblique line extend from superior tubercle to inferior tubercle. The following muscles are attached to the oblique line:
      a) Thyrohyoid
      b) Sternothyroid
      c) Inferior constrictor muscle (thyropharyngeus). [medial to lateral]

      Upper pole of the lateral lobe of thyroid gland extends up to this ridge between sternothyroid and the inferior constrictor of pharynx.

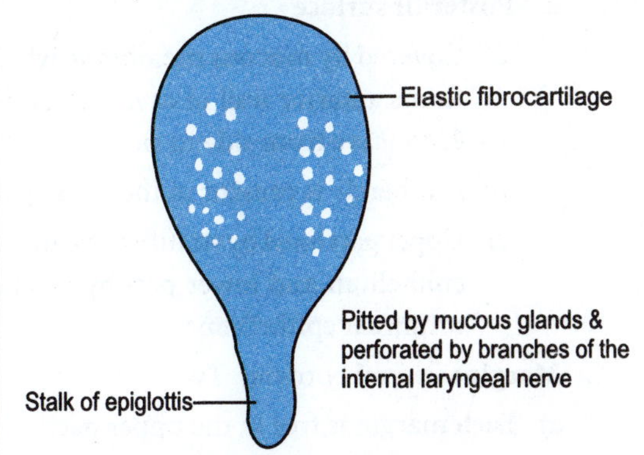

Fig. 16.2: The epiglottis (posterior aspect)

   B. **Inner surface:** Covered by mucous membrane which forms the lateral wall of the piriform fossa.

EPIGLOTTIS (Fig. 16.2)

1. It is the unpaired yellow elastic type of cartilage.
2. Situated in the upper part of anterior wall of larynx behind hyoid and base of tongue.
3. Shape: Leaf-like.
4. Ends, surfaces, and borders:

   A. Ends: Two – upper and lower
      1. *Upper end* – (also known as margin border): Free and forms anterior boundary of inlet of larynx and demarcates oropharynx and laryngopharynx.
      2. *Lower end*: Attachment of thyroepiglottic ligament (other end to posterior surface of thyroid angle)

   B. Surfaces: Two
      1. **Anterior surface:**
         a) *Upper part*: Covered with mucous membrane and one median glosso-epiglottic and two lateral glosso-epiglottic folds extend to base of tongue and enclose vallecula one on each side of median fold.
         b) *Lower part*: Attachment of hyoepiglottic ligament (other end to hyoid bone).

2. **Posterior surface**
   a) Covered by mucous membrane which forms anterior wall of cavity of larynx & concave from side to side
   b) A tubercle is present in the lower part
   c) Upper part lined by stratified squamous epithelium and lower part by ciliated columnar epithelium.

C. **Margins** (lateral borders): Two
   a) Each margin is free in the upper part
   b) Lower part – attachment of aryepiglottic folds on each side along with thyroepiglotticus and aryepiglotticus muscles.

CRICOID CARTILAGE (Fig. 16.3)

1. It is a stronger and more or less thicker cartilage forming the lower parts of anterior, lateral and major part of posterior wall of larynx.
2. **Shape**: Signet ring like.
3. **Type**: Hyaline.
4. Two parts:
   a) Narrow **anterior arch**
   b) Quadrangular **posterior lamina**.
5. **Lamina**: Quadrilateral, (posteriorly)
   A. **Borders**: Two
      a) *Upper border*: Lateral part of this border articulates with base of arytenoid cartilage.
      b) *Lower border*: Attachment of trachealis muscle.
   B. **Surfaces**: Two
      a) Anterior surface: Covered by mucous membrane of larynx.
      b) Posterior surface – present
         1. *Median ridge*: For attachment of tendon of oesophagus.
         2. *Depressed areas one on each side of ridge*: Origin of posterior cricoarytenoid muscle.
6. **Anterior arch**: Borders and surfaces of anterior arch are as follows:

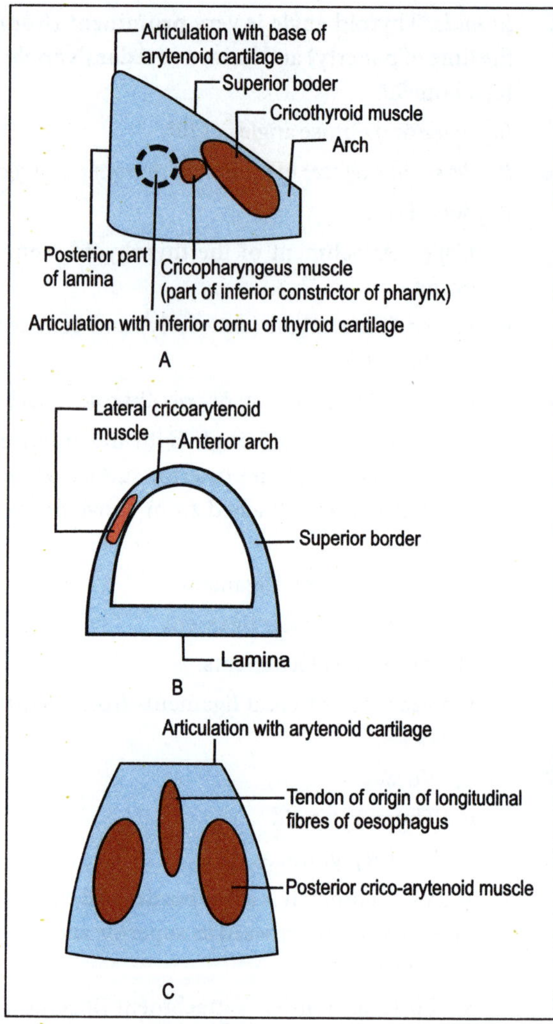

Fig. 16.3: Cricoid cartilage. A – Outer surface of arch; B – Superior view of arch; C – Posterior view of lamina

A. *Borders*: Two
   a) Upper border: It proceeds downward & forward. Origin of lateral cricoarytenoid in this border.
   b) Lower border: Attachment of cricotracheal ligament (to first ring of trachea).

B. *Surface*: Two
   a) *Outer surface*: Origin of cricothyroid in front and cricopharyngeus (part of inferior constrictor) behind.
   b) *Inner surface*: Covered by mucous membrane of the cavity of larynx.

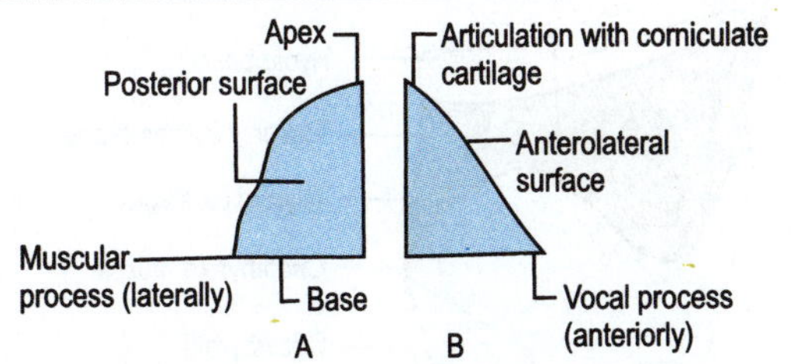

Fig. 16.4: Arytenoid cartilage. A – Posterior view; B – Antero-lateral view

ARYTENOID CARTILAGES (Fig. 16.4)

1. These are paired cartilages. Shape is pyramidal.
2. Type: Hyaline except vocal process and apex which are yellow elastic type.
3. Different parts:
   A. *Apex*: Apex is upward and medially (upper part)
      a) Articulates with corniculate cartilage and
      b) Attachment of oblique arytenoid muscle, aryepiglotticus muscle.
   B. *Base*: (Lower part) articulates with upper border of posterior lamina of cricoid forming cricoarytenoid joint (*synovial*).
   C. *Surface*: Three – Posterior, medial and antero-lateral.
      a) *Posterior*:
         1. Attachment of transverse arytenoid which extend from posterior surface of one to other (*only unpaired muscle*)
         2. Oblique arytenoids crosses each other like 'X' (attached to muscular process of one arytenoid to the apex of other arytenoid cartilage).
      b) *Medial*: Covered by mucous membrane of cavity of larynx.
      c) *Antero-lateral*: It includes vocal process and adjoining area. **Attachment below upwards are**: Vocal ligament, vocalis, vestibular ligament, thyroarytenoid muscle, and quadrate membrane.
   D. *Process*: Two – vocal and muscular.
      a) *Muscular process*: Projects laterally and insertions of lateral cricoarytenoid and posterior cricoarytenoid.
      b) *Vocal process*: Projects forward and attachment of vocal ligament at the tip and vocalis just lateral to it.

CORNICULATE AND CUNEIFORM

1. They are two paired elastic type of cartilages and are said to be detached part of arytenoid cartilages.
2. They are placed at right angles with each other.
3. Corniculate articulates with apex of arytenoid and lie in the posterior part of aryepiglottic fold.
4. Cuneiform lies in front of corniculate in the aryepiglottic folds.

Developmental aspect of cartilages – all are mesodermal in derivative.

1. *Epiglottis*: From fourth arch.
2. *Thyroid*: From fourth arches.
3. *Cricoid*: From sixth arch.
4. *Arytenoid*: From sixth arch.
5. *Corniculate and cuneiform*: Sixth arch as they are said to be detached part of arytenoid.

JOINTS OF LARYNX

Usually two –

1. Cricothyroid joint:

A pair of joints between thyroid cartilage and cricoid. (Fig. 16.5)

A. *Type*: Synovial.
B. *Bones taking part*:
   a) Inferior horn of thyroid cartilage and
   b) Facet on the side of cricoid.
C. *Ligaments*: Covered by a fibrous capsule strengthened by a fibrous band.
D. *Important relation*: Recurrent laryngeal nerve passes behind the joint to enter the larynx.

E. *Movements:*
   a) Rotation of cricoid on both the inferior horns around a transverse axis.
   b) Limited gliding movements in different directions.

2. Cricoarytenoid joints

A. These are paired joints between cricoid and arytenoid cartilages.

B. *Type*: Synovial.

C. Bones taking part are
   a) Deep grooved bases of arytenoid and
   b) Facets on the lateral part of upper border of lamina of cricoid cartilage.

D. Enclosed by a capsular ligament and presence of strong posterior cricoarytenoid ligament.

E. *Movement*:
   a) Rotation of arytenoid around an oblique axis and the effect is swinging of vocal process laterally or medially resulting in increase or decrease of rima glottidis.
   b) Gliding: It helps in approaching or receding or arytenoid from each other. These two movements combine to form lateral rotation with lateral gliding and medial rotation with medial gliding, forward movement is limited by posterior cricoarytenoid ligament.
   c) This ligament helps in slight pivotal momentum.

LIGAMENTS OF LARYNX

They are divided into two groups:

1. Extrinsic:

Those which connect amount thyroid, cricoid and epiglottis.

They are thyrohyoid membrane, hyoepiglottic and cricotracheal ligaments.

A. **Thyrohyoid membrane** with median and lateral thyrohyoid ligament (Fig. 16.5)
   a) They connect the upper border of thyroid cartilage with superior horn to upper border of hyoid bone. Subhyoid bursa lies in between posterior aspect of hyoid bone and membrane.

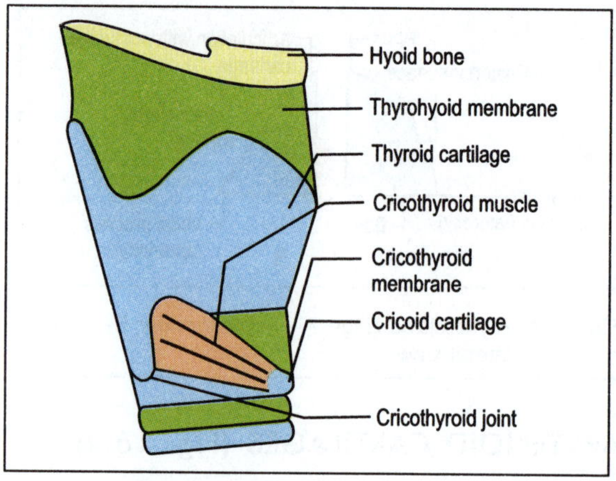

Fig. 16.5: Lateral external view of larynx

   b) **Median thyrohyoid ligament**: The median thickest part and lateral thyrohyoid ligament is the cord like structure at the posterior margin of thyrohyoid membrane. Cartilago triticea is usually present in each lateral thyrohyoid ligament.
   c) **Structures piercing thyrohyoid membrane** are superior laryngeal vessels and internal laryngeal nerve [pierce the thin part on each side of median thyroid ligament].

B. **Hyoepiglottic ligament**: Connecting epiglottis with hyoid bone.

C. **Cricotracheal ligament**: Ligament connecting lower border of cricoid cartilage with first ring of trachea.

D. Thyroepiglottic ligament is attached to posterior surface of thyroid cartilage to lower end of epiglottis.

2. Instrinsic:

These ligaments are derived from **fibroelastic membrane** of the larynx which is a broad sheet of mucous membrane in the submucous region.

This fibroelastic membrane is divided into two parts by sinus of larynx (with in cavity of larynx). (1) **Upper quadrangular**, (2) **Lower cricothyroid or Cricovocal membrane** (conus elasticus).

1. **Quadrangular or quadrate membrane (Fig. 16.6):** Quadrate membane lies in between arytenoid cartilage and epiglottis. Its lower part attached to muscular process of arytenoid cartilage (posteriorly) and to the posterior surface of thyroid cartilage (anteriorly). It lower edge (free border) forms vestibular ligament. Its upper part (aryepiglottic fold) form lateral boundary of laryngeal inlet.
2. **Crico-vocal or cricothyroid ligament (conus elasticus)**
   a) Fibroelastic sheet extends upwards and medially from the arch (upper border) of cricoid cartilage. It passes upward beneath thyroid lamina, attached to vocal process & thyroid angle.
   b) It consists of two parts:
      A. Median thicker part is known as median or anterior cricothyroid ligament.
      B. Lower lateral part is lateral cricothyroid ligament.
      C. The upper margin (free) becomes condensed to form vocal ligament.

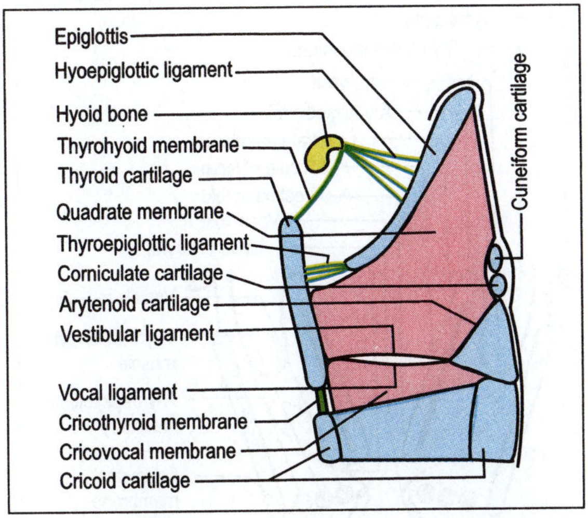

Fig. 16.6: Sagittal section of larynx showing ligaments and membranes (quadrate & cricovocal membranes)

INTERIOR OF LARYNX OR CAVITY OF LARYNX (Fig. 16.6)

Extent: It extends from inlet of larynx to lower border of cricoid cartilage.

Walls of the cavity: Anterior and posterior wall. Due to obliquity of the inlet the anterior wall is more in length than the posterior wall.

Different folds of mucous membrane within the cavity: Three pair of folds from above downward are present.

They are: (1) Aryepiglottic; (2) Vestibular; (3) vocal folds.

Fissures or spaces between the paired folds: Three spaces:

1. *Inlet of larynx*: Space between two aryepiglottic folds.
2. *Rima vestibull*: Space between two vestibular folds.
3. *Rima glottidis*: Space between two vocal folds.

Different subdivisions:

Cavity of larynx is divided into three parts by two pair of folds – vestibular and vocal folds.

1. *Vestibule or upper part*: Part above the vestibular folds (from aryepiglottic fold [laryngeal inlet] to vestibular fold).
2. *Intermediate part of sinus of larynx (also known as ventricle)*: Part between vestibular folds above and vocal folds below.
3. *Infraglottic or lower part*: Below the vocal folds. It is featureless but lined by loose mucous membrane.

Inlet of larynx

1. It is the opening of entrance of larynx through which larynx opens into the laryngopharynx.
2. **Boundary**:
   A. *In front*: Upper border of epiglottis.
   B. *Behind*: Inter arytenoid folds (mucous folds)
   C. *On each side*: Aryepiglottic folds (contains aryepiglotticus and thyroepiglotticus muscles).
3. **Slope of inlet**: Downwards and backwards.
   A. Closure – due to contraction of aryepiglotticus.
   B. Opening: By thyroepiglotticus.

Vestibule of larynx

1. It is the upper part of larynx between inlet of larynx above and vestibular folds below.

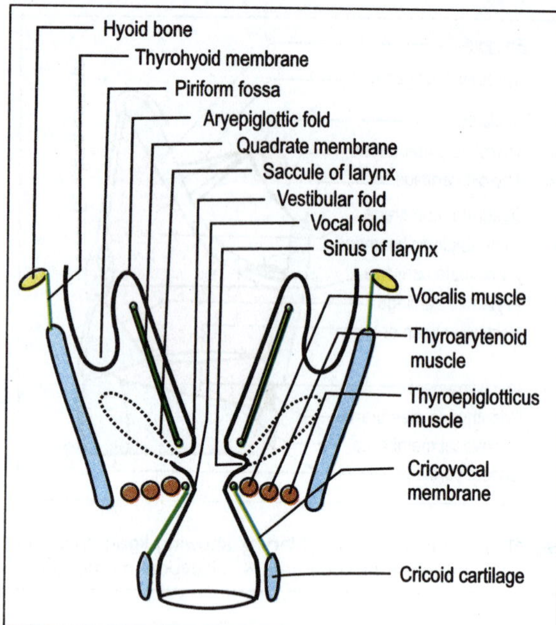

Fig. 16.7: Coronal section through larynx

2. **Boundary**
   A. *Anterior wall*: Posterior surface of epiglottis.
   B. *Posterior wall*: Interarytenoid mucous membrane above vestibular folds.
3. It acts as a resonating chamber.

Ventricle or sinus of larynx

1. It is the middle part of cavity of larynx and is the smallest of three divisions and the part between rima vestibuli above and rima glottidis below.
2. It presents a deep mucous recess extending to lamina of thyroid cartilage.
3. Opening of saccule is present on anterior part of each side.

Saccule of larynx (Fig. 16.7)

1. A mucous diverticulum arises from anterior part and on each side of sinus of larynx.
2. It extends blindly upwards between the vestibular fold and lamina of thyroid cartilage.
3. The wall is studded with 60-70 mucous glands. Secretions of thee glands lubricate the vocal fold particularly during production of voice. So it is called "oil can" for "vocal fold".

Rima vestibuli:

It is a space or fissure between two vestibular folds

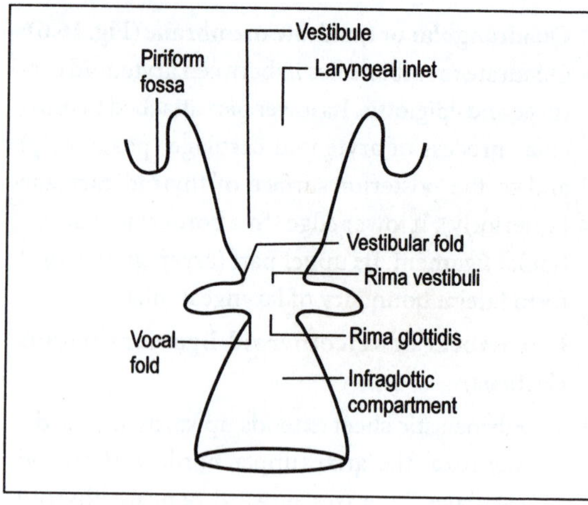

Fig. 16.8: Coronal view of vestibule, rima vestibuli and rima glottidis

which are folds of mucous membrane containing vestibular ligaments (lower condensed part of quadrate membrane) (Fig. 16.8).

Action:

1. It acts as exit valve so that it allows entry of air during inspiration but prevents exit of air during expiration.

VESTIBULAR FOLDS: (Also known as ventricular fold or false vocal cord)

1. **Formation**: Each is a fold of mucous membrane containing vestibular ligament which is lower condensed and thickened free lower margin of quadrate membrane.

Arterial supply:

By superior laryngeal branch of superior thyroid branch of external carotid artery.

Nerve supply:

Internal laryngeal branch of superior laryngeal (branch of vagus).

VOCAL FOLDS (known as vocal cords)

a) They are paired folds of mucous membrane containing vocal ligament (upper condensed and thickened free margin of cricovocal membrane).
b) **In living condition**: It appears white as it is least vascular.

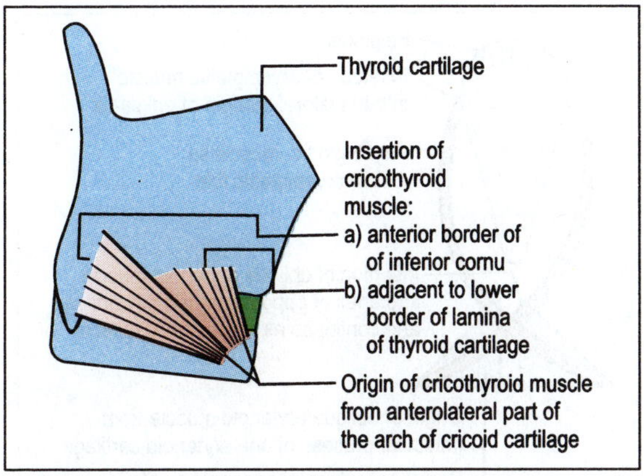

Fig. 16.9: Cricothyroid muscle

c) It is lined by stratified squamous epithelium without any submucous tissue and so mucous membrane is more or less intimately adherent to underlying ligament.

d) It is lubricated by mucus from glands of saccule.

e) *Vocal fold is least vascular and submucous tissue is absent.* So during inflammation there will be lesser oedema larynx and chance of suffocation is least. Besides, due to phonation vocal folds vibrate and due to less amount of blood supply there will be least chance of bleeding.

INTRINSIC MUSCLES OF LARYNX

1. **Cricothyroid (Fig. 16.9 & Fig. 16.10)**

   Origin: From lateral surface of arch of cricoid cartilage.

   Insertion: (a) Anterior border of inferior cornu and (b) Adjacent part of inferior border of lamina of the thyroid cartilage.

   Action: Tensor of the vocal cords.

2. **Posterior cricoarytenoid (Fig. 16.11)**

   Origin: From posterior surface of the cricoid lamina.

   Insertion: Muscular process of arytenoid.

   Action: Abductor of the vocal cord.

3. **Lateral cricoarytenoid (Fig. 16.12)**

   Origin: From lateral aspect of upper margin of anterior arch of cricoid.

   Insertion: Into muscular process of arytenoid.

   Action: Adductor of vocal cord.

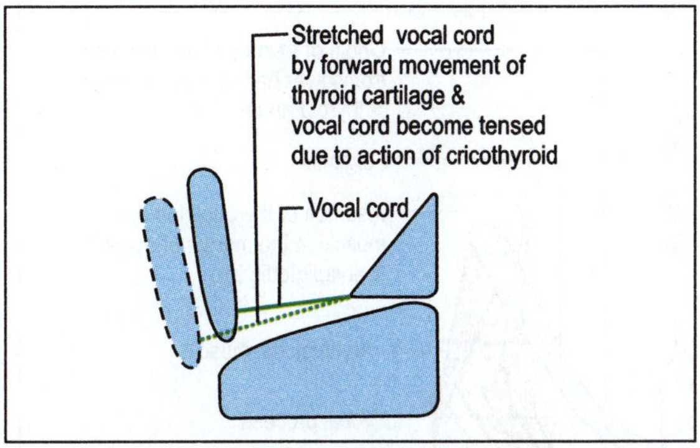

Fig. 16.10: Action of the cricothyroid

4. **Transverse arytenoid**

   Origin: From posterior surface of arytenoid of one side

   Insertion: To posterior surface of arytenoid of other side.

   Action: Adductor of vocal cord.

5. **Oblique arytenoid (Fig. 16.13)**

   Origin: From muscular process of one arytenoid.

   Insertion: To apex of other arytenoid.

   Action: Closing the inlet of larynx.

6. **Aryepiglotticus**

   Origin: Few fibres of oblique arytenoid continues from the apex of arytenoid continue as aryepiglotticus (below aryepiglottic fold).

   Insertion: To margin of epiglottis and known as aryepiglotticus.

   Action: Closing inlet of larynx.

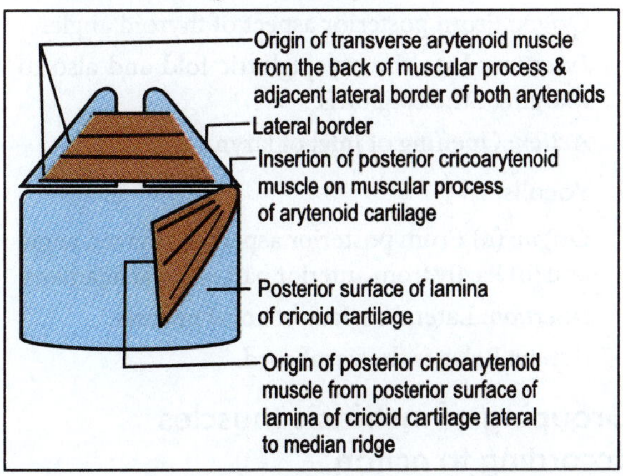

Fig. 16.11: Transverse arytenoid and posterior cricoarytenoid muscles

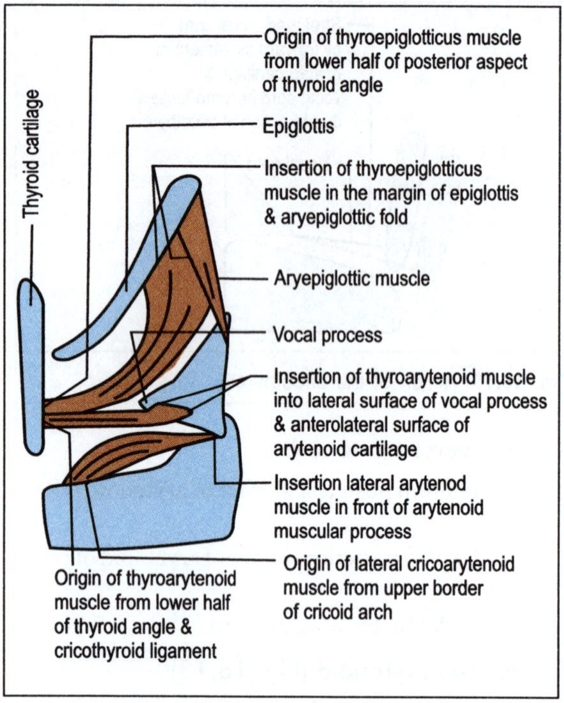

Fig. 16.12: Aryepiglottic, thyroepiglottic, thyroarytenoid and lateral cricoarytenoid muscle

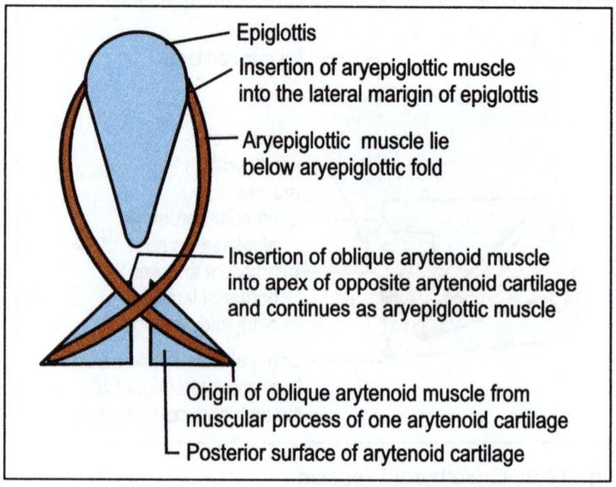

Fig. 16.13: Oblique arytenoid and aryepiglottic muscles

7. **Thyroarytenoid (Fig. 16.14)**

   Origin: From posterior aspect thyroid angle and cricothyroid ligament.

   Insertion: Into anterolateral surface of arytenoid cartilage.

   Action: Relaxation of vocal cord.

8. **Thyroepiglotticus**

   Origin: From posterior aspect of thyroid angle.

   Insertion: Into the aryepiglottic fold and also to margin of the epiglottis.

   Action: Opening of inlet of larynx.

9. **Vocalis**

   Origin: (a) From posterior aspect of thyroid angle and (b) Partly from anterior part of vocal ligament.

   Insertion: Lateral surface of vocal process.

   Action: Relaxes the vocal cord.

Grouping of instrinsic muscles according to action

1. **Acting on inlet of larynx**

   A. *Closing*: a) Oblique arytenoid; b) Aryepiglotticus.

   B. *Opening*: Thyro-epiglotticus.

2. **Acting on vocal cords and on rima glottidis**

   A. *Abductor of vocal cord and thus opening of glottis*

   Posterior cricoarytenoid: Only abductor (safety muscle of larynx).

   B. *Adductors of vocal cord and closure of glottis*

   (a) Lateral cricoarytenoids; (b) Transverse arytenoids; (c) Oblique arytenoid

   C. *Tensor of vocal cord*: Cricothyroids

   D. Relaxing vocal cord

   a) Thyroarytenoid; b) Vocalis

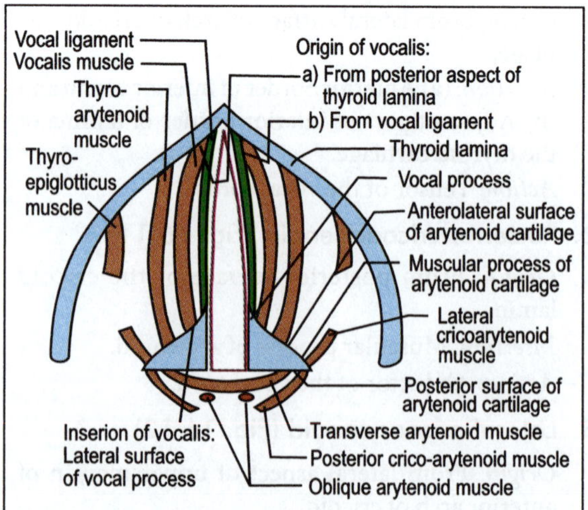

Fig. 16.14: Intrinsic muscles of larynx in transverse section at rima glottidis

Table 16.1: Actions of intrinsic muscles of larynx

Movements	Muscles
1. Closing inlet of larynx	1. Oblique arytenoid Aryepiglotticus
2. Opening inlet of larynx	2. Thyroepiglotticus
3. Abductor of vocal cord	3. Posterior cricoarytenoid
4. Adductor of vocal cord	4. Lateral cricoarytenoid Transverse arytenoid Oblique arytenoid
5. Tensor of vocal cord	5. Cricothyroid
6. Relaxing vocal cord	6. Vocalis Thyroarytenoid

Rima glottidis (Glottis):

Broadly it is a space between two vocal folds.

Features:

1. It is the narrowest part of the larynx.
2. It is a fissure antero-posteriorly.
3. It is longer in male than female.
   In male: 23mm
   In female: 17mm
4. **Boundary**
   A. *In front*: Angle of the thyroid cartilage.
   B. *Behind*: Mucous fold between two arytenoid cartilages.
   C. *Laterally*: Vocal fold in front and vocal processes behind.

Table 16.2: Intrinsic muscles of larynx

Muscle	Origin	Insertion	Action
1. Cricothyroid pass backward and upwards	Anterolateral part of arch of cricoid cartilage	a) Inferior cornu and b) Adjacent part of inferior border of lamina of the thyroid cartilage	Tensor of vocal cord
2. Transverse arytenoid Rectangular shpaped Unparied muscle	Posterior surface of one arytenoid	Posterior surface of another arytenoid	Adductor of vocal
3. Oblique arytenoid	Muscular process of one arytenoid cartilage	Apex of opposite arytenoid	Closing of inlet of larynx Adductor of vocal cord
4. Aryepiglotticus – Oblique arytenoid continue as aryepiglotticus	Originate from the apex of arytenoid and continues below the aryepiglottic fold	Margin of epiglottis	Closing of inlet of larynx
5. Lateral cricoarytenoid passes upwards and backwards – a triangular muscle	Lateral part of upper border of cricoid arch	Muscular process of arytenoid cartilage	Adductor of vocal cord
6. Posterior cricoarytenoid passes upwards laterally – a triangular shaped	From posterior surface of lamina of the cricoid cartilage lateral to median ridge	Muscular process of arytenoid cartilage	Abductor of vocal cord
7. Thyroarytenoid passes backwards & upwards	From posterior aspect of thyroid angle	Anterolateral surface of arytenoid cartilage	Relaxation of vocal cord
8. Thyroepiglotticus passes upwards into aryepiglottic fold	Posterior aspect of thyroid angle	Into aryepiglottic fold & margin of epiglottis	Opening of inlet of larynx
9. Vocalis passes backwards	a) From posterior aspect of thyroid angle; b) partly from vocal ligament	Lateral surface of vocal process	Relax the vocal cord

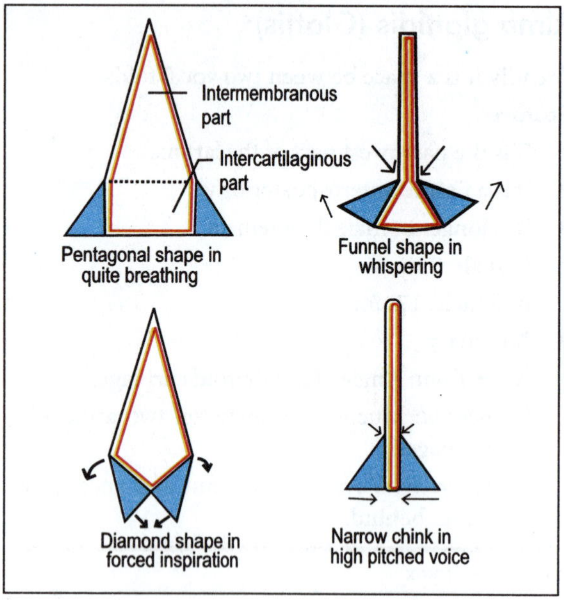

Fig. 16.15: Different shape of rima glottidis in different condition

5. *Different parts*: Two –
   A. *Intermembranous part*: Anterior 3/5th of the space and between two vocal folds.
   B. *Intercartilaginous part*: Posterior 2/5th of the space between vocal processes of arytenoid cartilages.

Shape and appearance of rima glottidis: It depends upon type of breathing and phonation. (Fig. 16.15)

1. **During quiet breathing** and **at rest**, intermembranous part is triangular and the intercartilaginous part is quadrangular between the medial surfaces of arytenoid cartilage. Rima glottidis becomes pentagonal. (Fig. 16.15A)
2. **During forced inspiration**: Rima glottidis is diamond shaped due to abduction of vocal cord (Fig. 16.15C).
3. **During phonation and production of high pitched sound** rima glottidis becomes a narrow chink as vocal folds adducted. (Fig. 16.15D).
4. **During whispering**: Intermembranous part becomes closed but intercartilaginous remains open triangular gap. Rima glottidis looks like inverted funnel.

ARTERIAL SUPPLY OF LARYNX

A. Above the vocal fold: Superior laryngeal branch of superior thyroid artery.
B. Below the vocal fold: Inferior laryngeal artery branch of inferior thyroid artery.
C. Vocal fold: Both the above arteries.

VENOUS DRAINAGE OF LARYNX

The veins draining the larynx accompany the arteries supplying the larynx.

The veins are:

a) Superior laryngeal vein drains to superior thyroid vein.
b) Inferior laryngeal vein drains to inferior thyroid vein.

LYMPHATICS DRAINAGE

A. *Above the vocal fold*: Drains into prelaryngeal and jugulo-digastric lymph node.
B. *Below the vocal fold*: Drain into pre and paratracheal group of lymph nodes, then drain into lower deep cervical lymph nodes.
C. *At the vocal fold*: Lymphatics drain into both the above ways and acts as water shed line.

NERVE SUPPLY OF LARYNX

Motor:

1. Except cricothyroid all muscles are supplied by recurrent laryngeal nerve.
2. Cricothyroid: By external laryngeal branch of superior laryngeal branch of vagus.
3. Transverse arytenoid has double nerve supply. By both recurrent laryngeal and internal laryngeal branch of superior laryngeal nerve.

Sensory: Mucous membrane above the vocal fold by internal recurrent laryngeal nerve and below the vocal fold by recurrent laryngeal nerve. Vocal fold by both the nerves.

Secretomotor: Laryngeal glands by recurrent laryngeal nerve mainly.

APPLIED ANATOMY:

1. Paralysis of recurrent laryngeal nerve and effects on larynx.
   A. When nerve of one side is involved (during partial thyroidectomy). The affected vocal fold is paramedian in position and the unaffected vocal fold moves freely to the opposite vocal fold.
      a) Voice: hoarse
      b) Respiration: No difficulty.
   B. In case of paralysis of both the recurrent laryngeal nerves. Both the folds are more or less fixed in paramedian in position.
      The person complains of:
      a) Difficulty in respiration
      b) Difficulty in production of vice
      To relieve tracheostomy will be the choice of treatment.
   C. If recurrent laryngeal and external laryngeal nerves are involved – the vocal folds are in cadaveric position (further abducted and fixed).
   D. **Semon's Law**: It is manifested in chronic type of paralysis of recurrent laryngeal nerves i.e., slowly growing tumour pressing upon the nerve.
      According to this law: Abductors are involved first and other muscles follow.
      During recovery abductor recovers last.
      It is probably due to thickly myelinated fibres supply the abductors and these nerve fibres are affected by oxygen lack as a result of pressure.
2. *Foreign body* may be lodged due to narrowness (narrowest part of respiratory tract) but if passes it will pass through trachea and bronchi easily and may be caught in a narrow bronchiole.
3. *Laryngeal oedema* may be allergic or infective due to inflammation and may cause pain, dyspnoea with inspiratory stridor and fatal result may occur due to asphyxia.
4. Posterior cricoarytenoid is called safety muscle of larynx. It is the only abductor muscle of larynx.
   If this becomes paralysed, the adductor muscles will close the glottis and the person may be subjected to death due to suffocation.
   So posterior cricoarytenoid muscle due to its action of abduction is saver of life and so called safety muscle of larynx.

Development:

Mucous membrane is endodermal and from cranial part of laryngotracheal diverticulum which arises from ventral aspect of pharyngeal part of foregut.

MUCOUS MEMBRANE AND LINING EPITHELIUM OF LARYNX

A. *Epithelium*: The whole of mucous membrane of larynx is lined by *pseudo-stratified ciliated columnar epithelium*. The areas below lined by *stratified squamous epithelium:*
   a) Aryepiglottic fold
   b) Upper part of posterior surface of epiglottis
   c) Vocal fold
B. Taste buds in the epithelium – present in aryepiglottic fold and in epiglottis.
C. Mucous glands can be seen all over the mucous lining. They are numerous on the posterior surface of the epiglottis, aryepiglottic fold and in the saccules. There are no mucous glands in vocal folds.

MECHANISM OF PRODUCTION OF VOICE (PHONATION)

Four process produce the voice

1. **Expired air** from the lungs initiate and also responsible for intensity and loudness.
2. **Vibration** of vocal folds by the expired air – responsible for pitch of voice.
3. **Resonation** by column of air from lip and nostrils to vocal fold responsible for quality and vowels.
4. **Articulation** by lips, tongue, teeth and palate. Mainly consonants are produced.

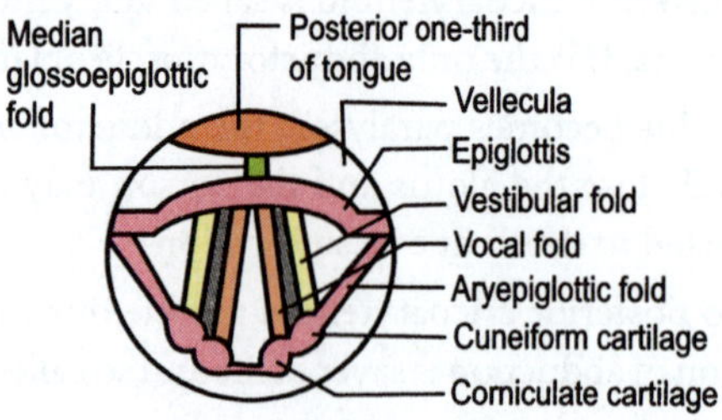

Fig. 16.16: Laryngoscopic view of laryngeal cavity showing laryngeal inlet and rima glottidis

Clinical note:

Vocal nodules or singer's nodule

- Individuals who often use vocal cords, they develop inflammatory nodules.

  Those nodules are bilateral.

VOCAL FOLD AS VALVE

It allows exit of air during *expiration but prevents entrance of air during inspiration.*

This valve action is due to upward and medial direction of vocal fold.

This is required for holding the breath at the end of expiration in order to have free movements of arm by inspiratory muscles as serratus anterior and pectoralis major.

STRUCTURES SEEN BY LARYNGOSCOPE

The following structures can be seen by laryngoscope: (Fig. 16.16)

1. Posterior Brd of tongue.
2. Epiglottis
3. Aryepiglottic fold
4. Vestibular fold
5. Vocal fold
6. Sinus of the larynx
7. Velleculae
8. Piriform fossa.

chapter 17

TONGUE

AT A GLANCE

- *Parts of tongue*
- *Dorsum of tongue*
- *Different types of papillae*
- *Features of posterior one third or pharyngeal part of tongue*
- *Inferior surface of tongue*
- *Taste buds*
- *Muscles of tongue: Extrinsic (Genioglossus, Styloglossus, Hyoglossus & Palatoglossus); Intrinsic muscles (Superior longitudinal, Inferior longitudinal, Transverse & Vertical)*
- *Arterial supply of tongue*
- *Veins*
- *Lymphatic drainage*
- *Nerve supply*
- *Development*
- *Microscopic anatomy of tongue*
- *Applied anatomy*

TONGUE

The tongue is a mobile organ which forms floor of oral cavity (anterior $\frac{2}{3}$rd) and anterior wall of oropharynx (posterior $\frac{1}{3}$rd). (Fig. 17.1)

The parts of tongue

A. Broadly two parts according to situation:

1. **Oral part** (Part in the mouth)
2. **Pharyngeal part** (Part in the oral part of pharynx)

Two parts are demarcated in the dorsum by 'V' shaped sulcus known as sulcus terminalis.

B. It has four parts:

1. **Tip or apex**: Free anterior end which usually lies behind incisor teeth.
2. **Root**: That part of the tongue attached to mandible in the floor of mouth and extends from symphysis menti to hyoid bone and formed by genioglossus muscles (lower fibres) and related to mylohyoid and geniohyoid muscles.
3. **Body**: It has two surfaces: [(a) Dorsal or upper convex; (b) Lower or inferior surface], and two lateral margins.
4. **Base**: Formed by posterior one third directed backwards towards the oropharynx.

Dorsum or dorsal surface of body of tongue (Fig. 17.2)

It is convex in all directions and pink and moist in appearance. It is divided into two parts by **sulcus terminalis** (a sulcus) into

1. *Anterior two third* (part in front of the sulcus) or oral part and
2. *Posterior one third* (part behind the sulcus) or pharyngeal part.

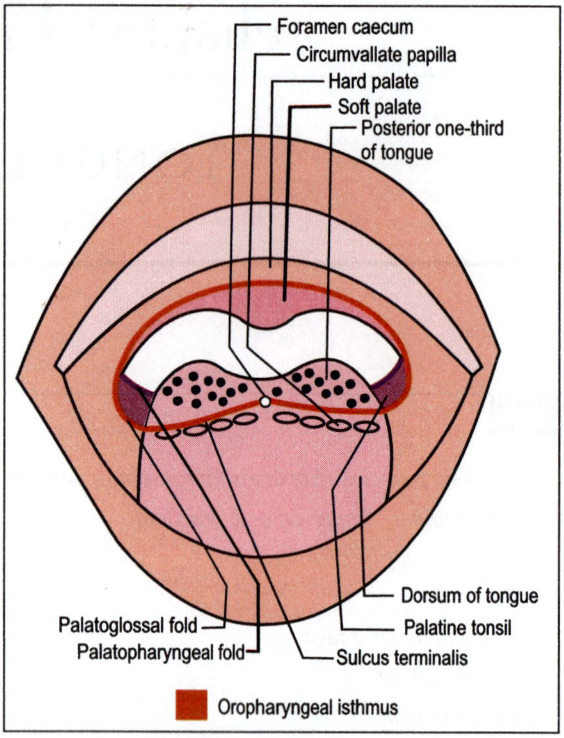

Fig. 17.1: Oral cavity and oropharynx. (Red line indicate oropharyngeal isthmus)

Sulcus terminalis: A 'V' shaped sulcus demarcating two parts of tongue extends forwards and laterally from a central median pit known as foramen caecum. Foramen caecum represents upper end of median thyroid diverticulum.

Features of anterior two third or oral part of tongue (Dorsal surface)

1. It is velvety in appearance due to absence of submucous coat and mucous membrane being adherent to underlying musculature.
2. Situation: In the floor and within oral cavity.
3. Margins: Free.
4. Mobility: Freely mobile.
5. Papillae foliate (Foliate papillae): Three or four vertical ridges of mucous membrane situated at the margin of tongue on each side and in front of sulcus terminalis. They contain taste buds.
6. The surface presents:
   a) Median furrow

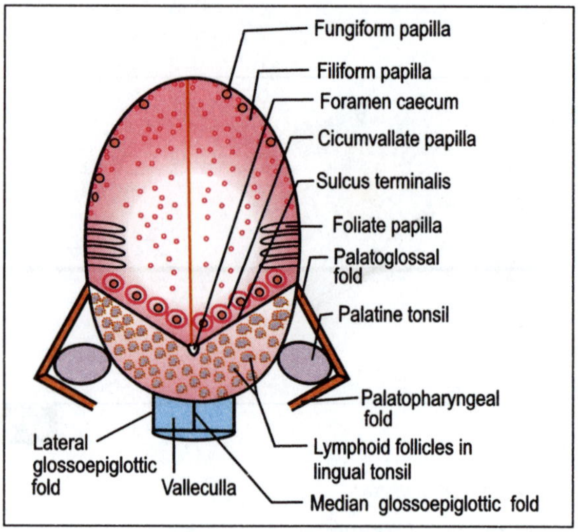

Fig. 17.2: Features of dorsum of tongue

   b) Rough in appearance due to presence of different types of papillae.
7. *Papillae of tongue*: These are projections of lamina propria covered by mucous membrane producing roughness of the surface.

Different varieties or types of papillae

Three types:

1. **Vallate papillae**:
   a) Larger papillae, 8-12 in numbers
   b) Situated in front and parallel to sulcus terminalis
   c) Shape: truncated conical (cylindrical) projection with broad base directed towards dorsal surface of tongue and surrounded by a circular sulcus. The outer wall of the sulcus id known as vallum. Taste buds are present in the walls of sulcus. Sulcus also receives openings of ducts of serous glands.
2. **Fungiform papillae**: Large rounded bright elevations with narrower pedicle and situated near the margins and tip of tongue. Usually numerous and contain taste buds.
3. **Filiform papillae**: Smallest of the three types and more or less scattered all over the dorsum of anterior two third of tongue. They are numerous small conical projections. They do not contain taste buds. They give this part of tongue a velvety appearance. Tips of papillae are keratinized which helps the food to stay for while.

Features of posterior one third or pharyngeal part of tongue

1. It is the part behind sulcus terminalis.
2. It differs from anterior two third of tongue so that it has no papillae but presence of submucous coat separating the muscles from mucous membrane.
3. Mucous membrane is thick and movable.
4. Presence of **lingual tonsil** in the submucous coat and they are collections of encapsulated lymphatic follicles. Follicles consist of collection of lymphocytes. So mucous membrane is nodular in appearance.
5. Presence of mucous and serous glands.

Posterior most part of tongue presents

a) **Median glosso-epiglottic fold**: Single fold of mucous membrane extending from tongue to epiglottis in the median plane.

b) **Lateral glossoepiglottic fold**: A pair of folds of mucous membrane on each side extending to pharynx.

c) **Vallecula**: A pair of shallow depressions on each side of median glosso-epiglottic fold.

Inferior or under surface of tongue

Features:

1. No papillae are present. (Fig. 17.3)
2. *Frenulum linguae*: A median fold of mucous membrane extending from tongue to floor of mouth.
3. *Sublingual papillae and openings of submandibular ducts*: Paired elevations on each side of base of frenulum and in which the openings of submandibular ducts are present.
4. *Profunda or deep lingual veins*: One on each side are present on each side of frenulum linguae and medial to plica fimbriate. Lingual nerve & artery lie medial to deep lingual vein.
5. Plica fimbriate: A pair or fringed fold of mucous membrane situated lateral to profunda lingual vein and extends forwards and medially towards the tip.

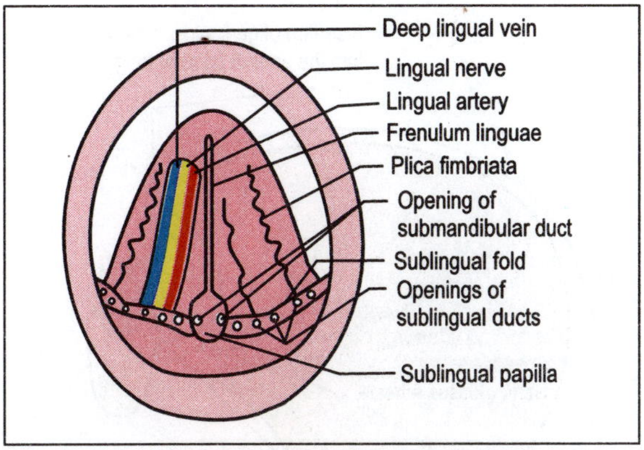

Fig. 17.3: Inferior surface of tongue and parts of floor of mouth

Lateral margins: Two:

1. Covered with mucous membrane.
2. At the junction of anterior two third and posterior one-third each margin gives attachment to palatoglossal arch.

MUSCLES OF TONGUE

Its **two groups**: (A) **Extrinsic**; (B) **Intrinsic**. Both the group of muscles are present in each half (right and left half) of tongue divided by a midline fibrous septum.

A. **Extrinsic muscles** are muscles which connect tongue to other structures such as mandible, hyoid, styloid process and the palate and they alter position of tongue.

   They are five pairs of muscles:

1. **Genioglossus**: (Fig. 17.4)

   Origin: From upper genial tubercle and proceed in fan shaped manner. It forms main part of tongue.

   Insertion:

   - Upper fibres inserted into tongue from the root to apex.
   - Middle fibres (lie deep to hyoglossus) are continuous with middle constrictor of pharynx.
   - Lower fibres are inserted to body of hyoid.

   Action: Upper fibers retract the lip and the middle fibres depress and it is the lower fibre which help in protrusion of tip of tongue.

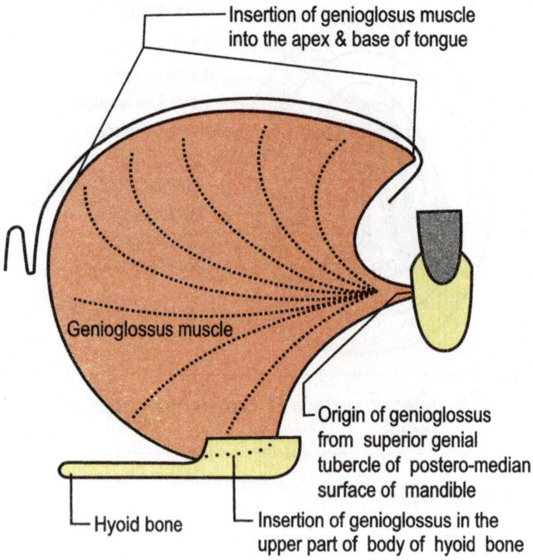

Fig. 17.4: Genioglossus muscle

It is called safety muscle of tongue because it prevents falling back of tongue and thus protecting from suffocation due to obstruction of respiration.

2. **Hyoglossus**: (Fig. 17.5)

Origin: From upper surface of greater cornu and partly from body of hyoid bone.

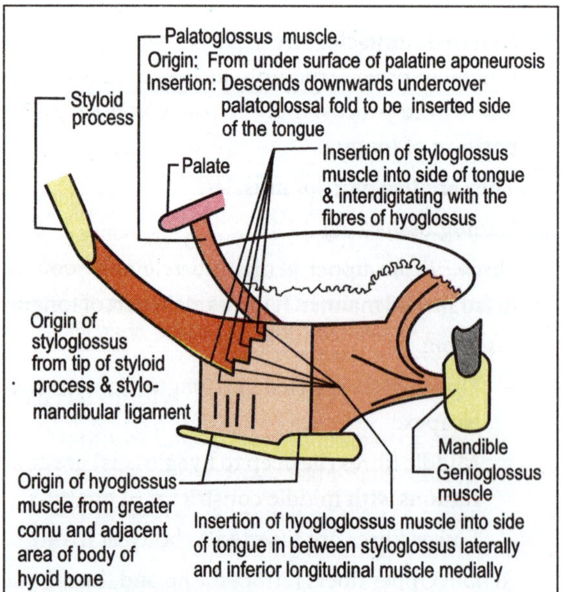

Fig. 17.5: Extrinsic muscles of tongue

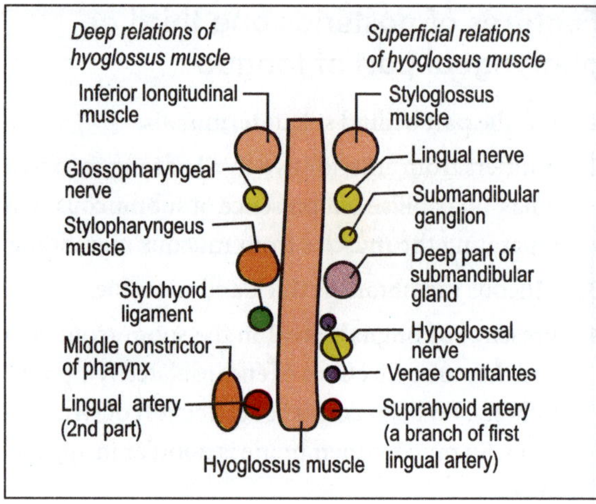

Fig. 17.6: Relations of hyoglossus

Insertion: Into side of tongue (posterior half) in between styloglossus (laterally) and inferior longitudinal muscles (medially).

Action: Depression of the sides of tongue and makes dorsal surface convex.

Relations: (Fig. 17.6)

a) *Superficial: From above downwards.*
   1. Styloglossus.
   2. Lingual nerve with submandibular ganglion suspended from the nerve.
   3. Deep part of submandibular gland with duct.
   4. Hypoglossal nerve, with a pair of veins.
   5. Suprahyoid branch of lingula artery.

   All the above structures are covered by mylohyoid muscle.

b) *Deep*: Inferior longitudinal muscle of tongue middle constrictor, stylopharyngeus, glossopharyngeal nerve, stylohyoid ligament and lingual artery (2nd part).

3. **Styloglossus**:

Origin: From tip of styloid process and stylomandibular ligament.

Insertion: To side of tongue, interdigitate with the hyoglossus.

Action: Retraction of tongue backward and upward.

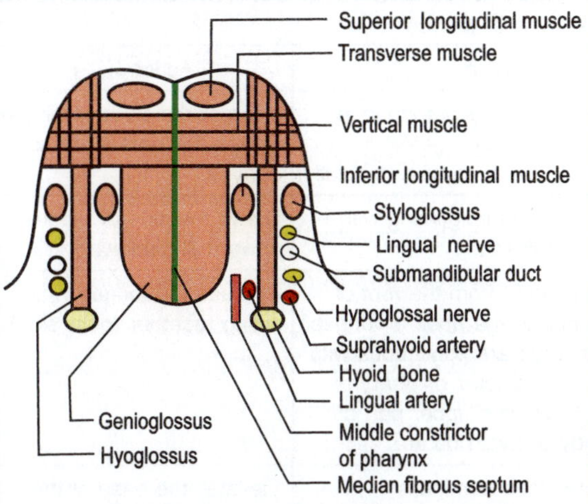

Fig. 17.7: Coronal section of the tongue showing intrinsic & extrinsic muscle of tongue

4. **Chondroglossus**: It is detached part of hyoglossus.

   Origin: Lesser cornu and part of body of hyoid bone.

   Insertion: To side of tongue.

   Action: Depression of side of tongue.

5. **Palatoglossus**: The muscle lie below the palatoglossal fold.

   Origin: From lower surface of palatine aponeurosis.

   Insertion: Into side of tongue, in front of sulcus terminalis.

   Action: Elevator of base of tongue and narrowing the oropharyngeal isthmus.

B. **Intrinsic muscles**: These are muscles attached to submucous fibrous layer and median septum and also alter the size and shape of tongue (Fig. 17.7). They are four pairs of muscles:

1. **Superior longitudinal**: Situated deep to mucous membrane of the dorsum of tongue.

   Origin: They arise from median septum.

   Insertion: Are inserted into side of tongue.

   Action: Reduces of the length of tongue and making the dorsal surface concave from side to side.

2. **Inferior longitudinal**: Situated deep to mucous membrane of the inferior surface of tongue.

   Origin: Arising from posterior part of side of tongue both the muscle.

   Insertion: Into front part of median septum.

   Action: Shortening the tongue and making its dorsal surface convex.

3. **Verticalis linguae**: Each is situated at the borders of front part of tongue.

   Origin: Arising from deep to mucous membrane of dorsum each.

   Insertion: Into sides of tongue.

   Action: makes the tongue broad & flatter, in the process the dorsal surface becomes concave from side to side.

4. **Transverse linguae**: Situated on each side from margin to median septum.

   Origin: Arises from median septum.

   Insertion: Into the sides of tongue.

   Action: Narrowing and elongation of tongue.

In summing up the muscles of tongue

Extrinsic: which alter the position of tongue.

1. Genioglossus
2. Hyoglossus
3. Styloglossus
4. Chondroglossus
5. Palatoglossus

Intrinsic: which alter the size and shape of tongue.

1. Superior longitudinal
2. Interior longitudinal
3. Vertical linguae
4. Transverse linguae

Action of muscles of tongue

1. Protrusion of tongue: Genioglossus.
2. Retraction of tongue: Styloglossus backward.
3. Depression of the tongue: Hyoglossus and chondroglossus.
4. Elevation of the tongue: Palatoglossus.
5. Dorsal surface of the tongue is made convex: Hyoglossus and inferior longitudinal.
6. Dorsal surface of the tongue is made concave: Genioglossus, styloglossus, superior longitudinal and vertical linguae muscles.
7. Elongation of the tongue: Transverse linguae.
8. Shortening and widening of the tongue: Superior and inferior longitudinal, vertical linguae muscles.

Table 17.1: Extrinsic muscles of tongue

Muscles	Origin	Insertion	Action
1. Hyoglossus – Quadrilateral muscle	Upper surface of greater cornu and adjacent part of body of hyoid bone	Posterior half of side of tongue in between styloglossus (laterally) & inferior longitudinal muscle (medially)	Depress the sides of tongue. Makes the dorsal surface convex.
2. Styloglossus	Tip of the styloid process & adjacent stylohyoid ligament	Side of tongue interdigitating with fibers of hyoglossus	Draws the side of tongue upward & backward
3. Genioglossus (fan shaped)	Superior genial tubercle of the posteromedian surface of the mandible	a) Upper fibers – from the root of the tongue to the apex of tongue b) Middle fibres are continuous with middle, constrictor of pharynx c) Lower fibers into upper part of the body of hyoid bone	Protrude the tongue while acting together (both side)
4. Palatoglossus – It lies below the palatoglossal fold	From oral surface of palatine aponeurosis	In front of sulcus terminalis (side of the tongue)	Elevates the base of the tongue Narrows the oropharyngeal isthmus

Table 17.2: Intrinsic muscles of tongue

Muscles	Location	Action
1. Superior longitudinal muscles	Below the mucous membrane	Reduce the length of tongue Make the dorsum of tongue concave
2. Inferior longitudinal muscles	Near the inferior surface of tongue (between genioglossus & hyoglossus)	Shorten the length of the tongue Make the dorsum convex
3. Transverse	Median septum to side of tongue	Make the tongue narrow Increases the length of tongue
4. Vertical	In the lateral part of dorsum of tongue	Makes the dorsum broad & concave from side to side.

Table 17.3: Movements of tongue and muscles involved

Movement of tongue	Muscles
1. Protrusion	1. Genioglossal of both side
2. Retraction	2. Styloglossus & hyoglossus
3. Depression	3. Hyoglossus
4. Elevation	4. Palatoglossus (both side)
5. Changes in shape	5. Intrinsic muscles

Arterial supply:

1. Mainly by lingual artery branch of external carotid (Pharyngeal part by dorsal lingual and rest of the part by profunda linguae artery).
2. Tonsillar and ascending palatine branch of facial artery (tip of tongue).
3. Ascending pharyngeal branch of external carotid artery.

Venous drainage

1. Venae comitantes accompanying hypoglossal nerve.
2. Deep vein (Main vein): Deep vein accompany lingual artery. All veins unite to form lingual vein and end in internal jugular or common facial vein.

Nerve supply: (Fig. 17.8)

Motor: All extrinsic and intrinsic muscles except palatoglossus are supplied by hypoglossal nerve. Palatoglossus is supplied by cranial root of accessory through pharyngeal plexus.

Sensory: From anterior two-third of tongue–

1. a) *Lingual nerve*: General sensory of anterior two third of tongue.
   b) *Chorda tympani nerve*: Special sense taste of anterior two third except vallate papillae.

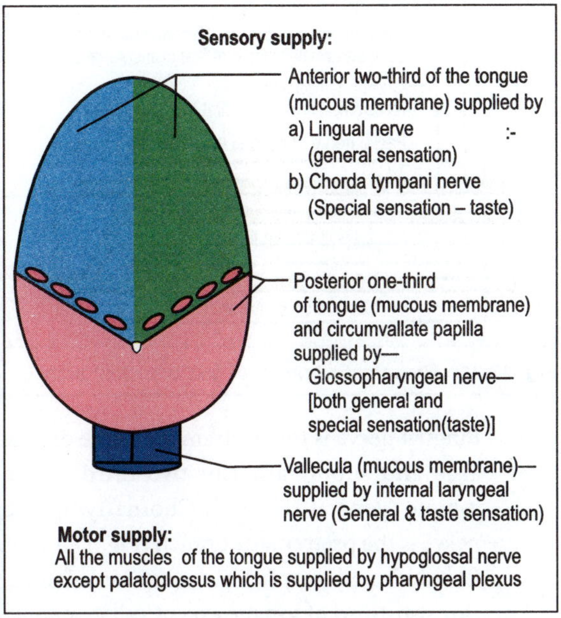

Fig. 17.8: Nerve supply of the tongue

2. **Glossopharyngeal:** Both general sensory and special sense taste of posterior one third of tongue including vallate papillae.
3. **Internal laryngeal nerve** (branch of vagus): Sensory supply (general sensory & taste) of vallecula (posterior most part of tongue).

LYMPHATIC DRAINAGE (Fig. 17.9)

1. **Apical set:** Lymph drainage from tip and inferior surface of tongue into submental lymph nodes after piercing mylohyoid muscle. The efferents from submental lymph nodes drain to submandibular lymph nodes, jugulo-omohyoid lymph nodes and jugulo-diagastric lymph nodes.
2. **Marginal set:** Lymph from marginal portion of anterior two-thirds of tongue (in front of sulcus terminalis) drain to submandibular lymph nodes, jugulo-digastric lymph nodes and jugulo-omohyoid lymph nodes.
3. **Central sets:** Lymph from central portion of anterior two-thirds of tongue drain bilaterally drain into jugulo-omohyoid & jugulo-digastic lymph nodes. A few lymph vessels ends in submandibular lymph nodes after piercing mylohyoid muscle.

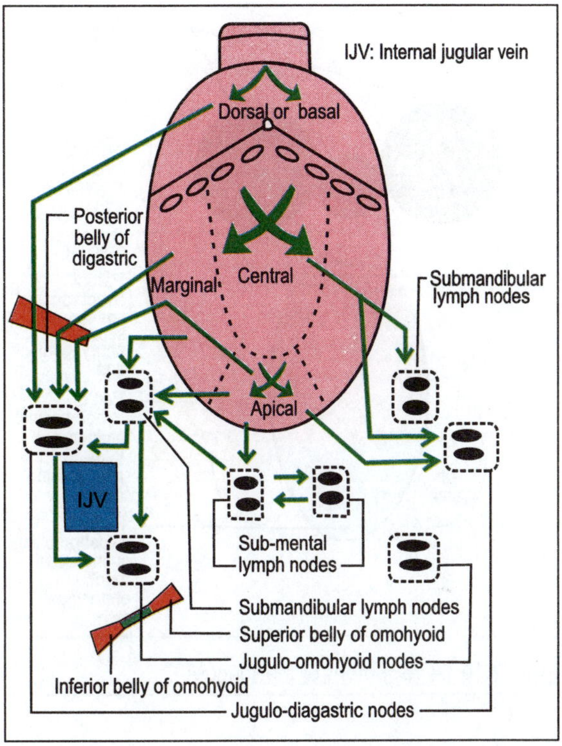

Fig. 17.9: Lymphatic drainage of the tongue

4. **Basal (or dorsal) set:** Lymph from root of the tongue and posterior one-third of the tongue drain bilaterally into jugulo-digastric lymph nodes (after piercing) pharyngeal wall, & some lymph vessels end in jugulo-omohyoid lymph nodes (after piercing thyrohyoid membrane).

Speciality of lymphatics:

1. Lymphatics do not accompany the blood vessels.
2. Richest lymph drainage occur from the tip of the tongue. Lymph from this area drain into all cervical lymph nodes.

DEVELOPMENT OF TONGUE

Tongue is composite in development and developed from three sources.

A. **Mucous membrane:**

1. **Anterior two third** – developed from two lingual swellings and tuberculum impar of first branchial arch. (Fig. 17.10)

   Therefore, mucous membrane of anterior two-

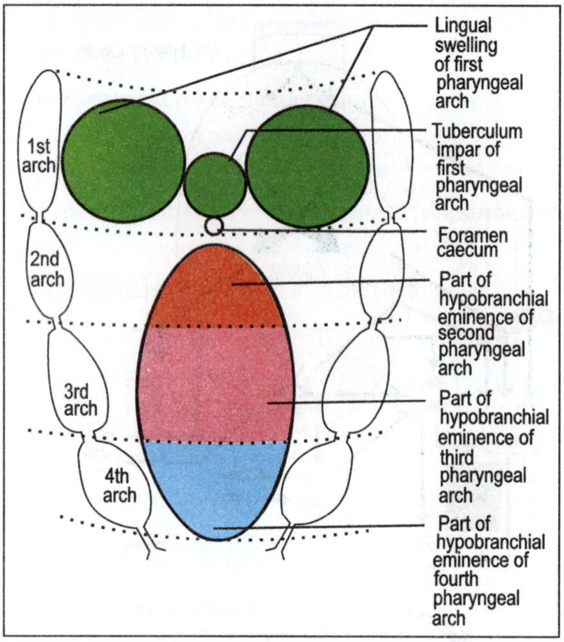

Fig. 17.10: Development of the tongue

third is supplied by lingual nerve (posttrematic branch) of 1st arch and chorda tympani nerve (pre-trematic branch) of 1st branchial arch.

2. **Posterior one third of tongue**: Developed from third arch element of hypobranchial eminence. Therefore, posterior 1/3rd of tongue is supplied by glossopharyngeal nerve (both general & taste sensation) which is nerve of IIIrd branchial arch.
3. **Vallecula**: Developed from the fourth arch element of hypobranchial eminence. Therefore vallecula is supplied by internal laryngeal nerve (nerve of IV pharyngeal arch).

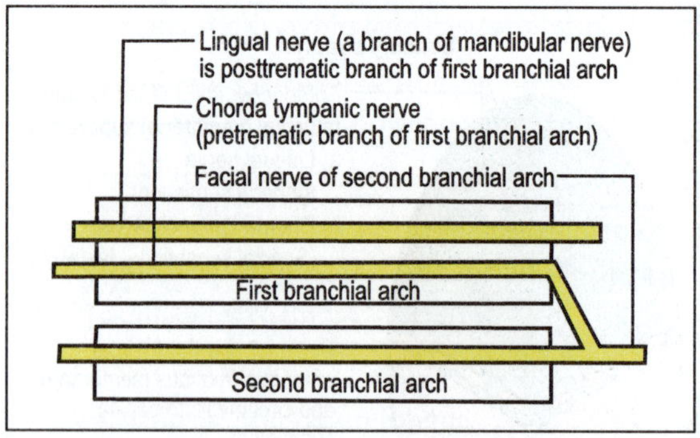

Fig. 17.11: Pretrematic branch of first branchial arch

Lingual nerve is the postrematic nerve of first arch and supply anterior two-third of the tongue (general sensory). Chorda tympanic nerve is the pretrematic branch (Fig. 17.11) of first arch and supply taste sensation of anterior two-third of tongue except vallate papilla (Fig. 17.11). Glossopharyngeal nerve is nerve of third pharyngeal arch. Glossopharyngeal nerve supply both general & taste sensation to posterior one-third of tongue along with vallate papilla. Internal laryngeal nerve supply valleculae & it is the nerve of fourth pharyngeal arch which is concerned with general & taste sensation.

B. **Muscles**: The muscles of tongue develop from the occipital mytome which is supplied by segmental nerves. Afterwards the muscles migrate anteriorly superficial to carotid arteries, thereby hypoglossal nerve (formed by segmental nerves) lie superficial to both carotid arteries.

Anomalies:

1. Tongue tie or ankyloglossia (short frenulum)
2. Macroglossia (large tongue)

Table 17.4: Developmental explanation of innervation of tongue

Structures	Source of development	Nerve supply
Mucous membrane		
Anterior 2/3rd of tongue	First branchial arch	Lingual nerve (post-trematic nerve of 1st arch) Chorda tympani nerve (pre-trematic nerve of 1st arch)
Posterior 1/3rd of tongue	Third branchial arch	Glossopharyngeal nerve (nerve of IIIrd arch)
Vallecula	Fourth branchial arch	Internal laryngeal nerve (nerve of IV arch)
Muscles	Occipital myotome	Hypoglossal nerve

3. Microglossia (small tongue)
4. Aglossia (absence of tongue)
5. Hemiglossia (Half of anterior two-third tongue absent)
6. Lingual thyroid (failure of formation of median thyroid diverticulae)
7. Bifid tongue.

MICROSCOPIC ANATOMY OF TONGUE

1. **Mucosa** of the tongue consists of outer epithelial layer and underlying lamina propria (connective tissue layer)
2. Covered by mucous membrane lined by stratified squamous epithelium.

   Mucous membrane (in front of sulcus terminalis) bears numerous projections or papillae. Each papilla consists of lining epithelium and core of connective tissue. The epithelium over the papillae is partly keratinized.

   The papillae are of various types as follows:

   - **Circumvallate papillae** (8-12 in number) are arranged single row (V-shaped) in front and parallel to sulcus terminalis. The wall in the groove present taste buds. Bottom of the groove receives the ducts of serous glands.
   - **Fungiform papillae** are broad rounded elevations and narrower base. They bear taste buds. (Fig. 17.12)
   - **Filiform papillae** are most numerous on entire two thirds of the tongue. Tips of the papillae are keratinized, which makes the surface rough. They donot have taste buds.
3. Serous glands is surrounded by skeletal muscles of tongue.
4. Submucous layer absent in the dorsal surface of anterior two-third of tongue and present in posterior one-third of tongue.

   Lymphoid follicles are present in posterior one-third of tongue.

   On the inferior surface, it is thin.

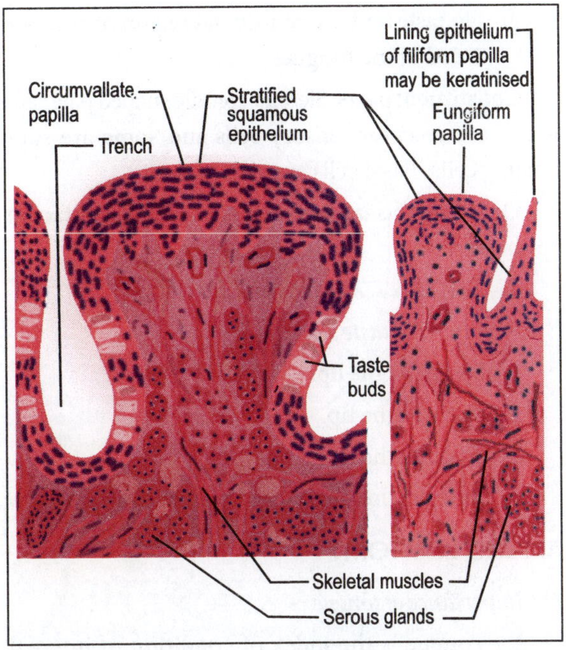

Fig. 17.12: Microscopic features of circumvallate, fungiform & filiform papillae

Taste buds

These are spherical modified epithelial cells (Fig. 17.13).

Sites: Within the epithelium of

a) Mucous membrane of tongue
b) Inferior surface of soft-palate
c) Posterior surface of epiglottis
d) Posterior wall of oropharynx
e) On the sides of vallate, fungiform papillae, and foliate
f) Posterior one-third of the tongue.

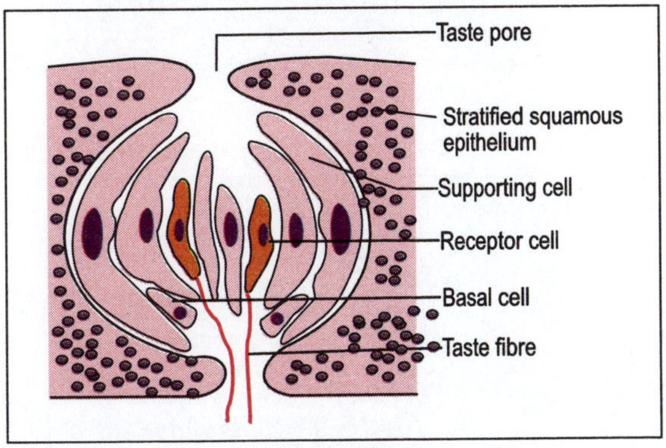

Fig. 17.13: Cells in the taste bud

g) No taste bud on mid-dorsal region of anterior 2/3rd of the tongue.

Constituent parts: Slender spindle shaped pale cells which are receptor sensory cells and some are supporting cells. Basal cells are also present.

Opening: *Gustatory pores situated* at the surface of epithelium.

Types of taste sensations and sites of tongue.

Four types of taste sensation:

1. Sweet: At the lip.
2. Salty: At the tip.
3. Sour: At the margins.
4. Bitter at the pharyngeal part of tongue.

APPLIED ANATOMY

A. *Importance of tongue*

1. Tongue is the index of condition of internal organs and also mirror of gastrointestinal tract.

   Coated: In gastrointestinal condition such as non-movement of bowel or any pathological condition.

   Macroglossia: Pituitary tumour.

   Raw beef tongue: In some metabolic diseases as diabetes mellitus.

   Fissured tongue: Vitamin deficiency.
2. Cyanosis: Marked in tongue.
3. In jaundice: Yellow tinge in under surface of tongue.
4. Movement of tongue in relation to deglutition.

   It plays its role in first stage (voluntary stage).

   a) In the beginning – formation of a groove on the dorsum by contraction of vertical intrinsic muscles.

chapter 18

EAR

AT A GLANCE

- *External Ear: Auricle – Surface; Structure, Skin, Cartilages, Ligaments muscles, Nerve supply, Blood supply, Lymphatic drainage, Development; External acoustic meatus – Extent, Shape, Parts (Cartilaginous, Bony), Constrictions, Relations, Blood supply, Nerve supply, Applied anatomy; Tympanic membrane – Colour, Shape, Disposition or attitude; Dimensions, Circumference of membrane; Different parts; Structure; Blood supply, Lymphatic drainage; Nerve supply; Development; Applied anatomy*
- *Middle Ear: Different part; Boundaries & Features of different walls of middle ear – Roof, Floor, Lateral wall, Medial wall, Anterior wall, Posterior wall; Contents of middle ear; Ear ossicles – Malleus, Incus, Stapes; Mastoid antrum; Mastoid air cells (Types); Blood supply, Lymphatics, Nerve supply; Development; Applied anatomy of middle ear*
- *Internal Ear: Bony labyrinth, Membranous labyrinth, Cochlea; Spiral lamina, Vestibule, Semicircular canals; Membranous labyrinth, Cochlear duct; Spiral organ of corti, Applied anatomy*

It is an organ of hearing and balance. It consist of three parts: (1) External ear, (2) Middle ear and (3) Internal ear

EXTERNAL EAR

It is concerned for collection & transmission of sound wave to tympanic membrane. It consists of two parts: (1) Pinna or auricle and (2) External acoustic (auditory) meatus

1. **Auricle or pinna**: It is a shell-like projection from the side of head and collects sound vibrations. Features: Two surfaces – Lateral and cranial.
   a) **Lateral surface**: It is irregular and presents elevations and depressions. (Fig. 18.1)

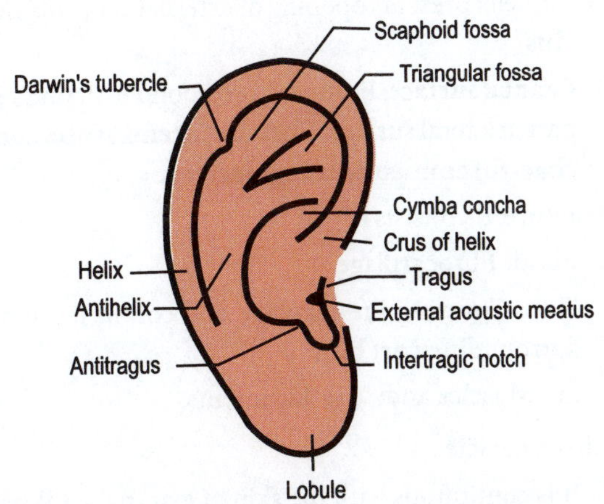

Fig. 18.1: Features of lateral surface of right auricle

They are

1. *Helix*: It is the prominent outer rim and consists of two limbs. The anterior limb ends as crus of helix which divides concha into upper smaller and lower larger part.

   Posterior limb presents and elevation (occasionally) known as **Darwin's tubercle.**

2. *Antihelix*: It is another prominent margin situated in front and parallel to posterior part of helix and encircling concha (deep depressed area). In the upper end it divides into two crura and enclose area deep (depression) known as triangular fossa.
3. *Scaphoid fossa*: Narrow area between helix and antihelix.
4. *Tragus*: An elevated part (triangular part of cartilage) guarding the depression of concha.
5. *Antitragus*: Triangular elevation opposite the tragus and separated from it by inter-tragic notch.
6. *Cymba conchae*: Small part of concha above crus of the helix.

   [It corresponds to *suprameatal triangle and tympanic antrum lies just deep to it*]

Lobule of ear: Part below the antitragus, skin covering fibro fatty tissue.

Outer opening of external auditory (acoustic) meatus: Larger part of the concha below the crus of the helix presents opening of external acoustic meatus.

b) **Cranial surface**: Features correspond to depressed part of lateral surface. They are (a) **eminentia conchae,** (b) **eminentia trangularis** etc.

Structure: It consists of

1. Elastic fibrocartilage
2. Skin: Covering the cartilage and connected with surrounding part by

   (a) Muscles and; (b) Ligaments

Skin of auricle

1. It is continuous with the skin of external auditory meatus.
2. Intimately adherent to cartilage.
3. Fine hairs with sebaceous glands are present in concha and scaphoid fossa, coarse hairs may be some times present in tragus, antitragus and intertragic notch of the elderly persons.

   [Hairy pinna is genetic characteristic of 'Y' linked genes]

Cartilage of auricle

1. A single piece in each auricle continuous with cartilage of external acoustic meatus.
2. **Type**: Yellow elastic cartilage.
3. It is absent or deficient in lobule, tragus and crus helix.
4. It present elevations and depressions and they are known as spine of helix in front, tail of helix below, eminentia concha etc.

Muscles of auricle: Two group –

1. **Extrinsic**: Auricularis anterior, superior and posterior.
   a) *Auricularis anterior*: Smallest and arises from lateral margin of epicranial aponeurosis and inserted into spine of helix.
   b) *Auricularis superior*: Largest muscular arises from epicranial aponeurosis and inserted into upper part of cranial surface of auricle.
   c) *Auricularis posterior*: Arises from mastoid part of temporal bone and inserted into eminentia conchae.

   Nerve supply: Auricularis anterior and superior by temporal branches of facial and posterior by posterior auricular branch of facial nerve.

2. **Intrinsic muscles** are in between cartilages.

   Action: They modify shape of ear.

   Nerve supply: Muscles on lateral surface by temporal branches and on cranial surface by posterior auricular branch of facial nerve. (Fig. 18.2)

Ligaments of auricle: Consists of two group

1. **Extrinsic**: Those ligaments which connect auricle with temporal bone. They are anterior and posterior.
2. **Intrinsic**: They connect various parts of cartilage. The main ligaments are:
   a) A fibrous band between tragus and crus helix

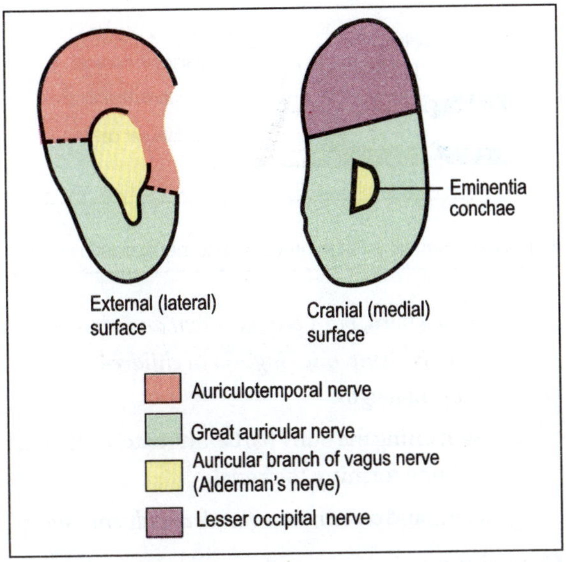

Fig. 18.2: Nerve supply of auricle

and completes the meatus anteriorly and forms part of concha.

b) Another band between antihelix and tail of helix.

Arterial supply of auricle:

1. *Posterior auricular branch of external carotid*: Cranial surface and posterior part of lateral surface.
2. *Anterior auricular branch of superficial temporal*: Anterior part of lateral surface.
3. *Branch from occipital artery – upper part of cranial surface.*

Veins: Correspond to arteries and drain *superficial temporal and external jugular veins.*

Arterio – venous anastomoses are numerous in auricle.

Lymphatics: Drain into

1. Parotid
2. Upper deep cervical
3. Mastoid lymph nodes

Sensory nerves of auricle:

1. Great auricular: Supplies most of cranial (medial) surface and posterior part of lateral surface (helix, antihelix and lobule)
2. *Lesser occipital*: Supplies upper part of cranial (medial) surface.
3. *Auricular branch of vagus*: Supplies concha and eminentia conchae (posterior part).
4. *Auriculo-temporal*: Supplies part of lateral surface (tragus, crus of the helix and its adjacent part of the helix).

Development: It is ectodermal in development and formed around the first branchial cleft.

External acoustic (auditory) meatus

It is a canal and part of external ear and conducts sound waves from concha to tympanic membrane.

Extent: From bottom of concha to tympanic membrane.

Shape: 'S' shaped and according to direction it is divided into three parts:

1. Par externa: Medially, forwards and upwards
2. Par intermedia: Medially, backwards and upwards
3. Par internal: Medially, forwards and downwards. (Fig. 18.3).

[So during examination it may be straightened by pulling the ear upwards, backwards and slight lateral wards].

On section: Oval

Length: 24mm

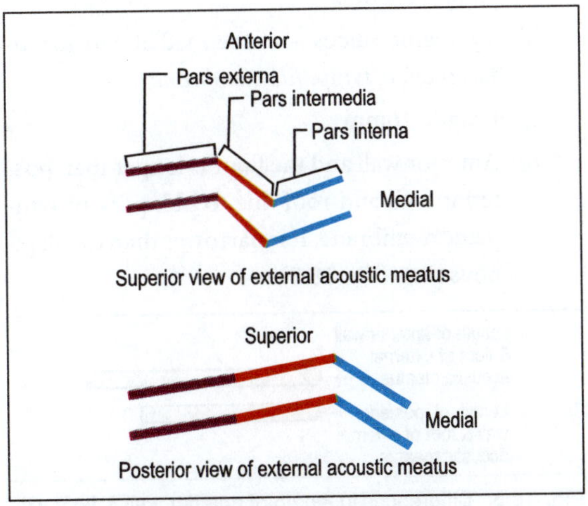

Fig. 18.3: Parts of external acoustic meatus

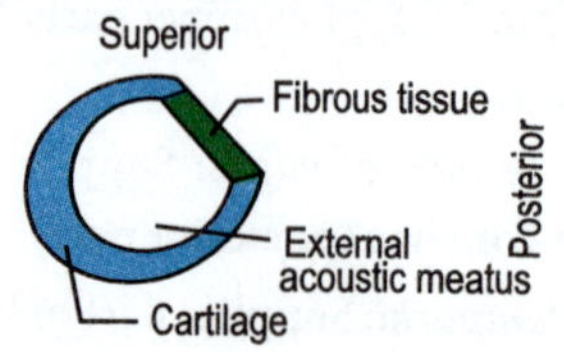

Fig. 18.4: Transverse section through the cartilage of external acoustic meatus

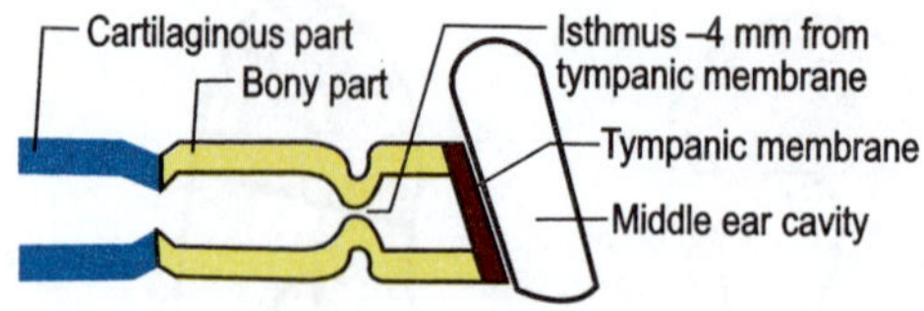

Fig. 18.6: Showing the isthmus of external acoustic meatus

Different parts:

1. **Cartilaginous part**: Lateral one third (8mm).
2. **Bony part**: Medial two third (16mm).

1. **Cartilaginous part**: (Fig. 18.4)
   a) Cartilage is continuous with cartilage of auricle
   b) Posterosuperior part of the canal is *deficient* and *replaced by fibrous tissue*
   c) Length: 8mm
   d) Lining skin is *intimately adherent* to underlying cartilage.
   e) *Ceruminous glands (modified sweat glands)* and hair follicles are *limited to cartilaginous part only*. [Secretion of ceruminous glands are *cerumen or earwax*].
2. **Bony part**
   a) It is formed mainly (anterior inferior, part of posterior) by tympanic part of temporal and posterosuperior part by squamous part of temporal bone
   b) Tympanic sulcus – at the medial end for *attachment of tympanic membrane*
   c) Length: 16mm
   d) Anterior wall and the floor is longer than posterior wall and roof due to obliquity of tympanic membrane. It is narrower than cartilaginous part. (Fig. 18.5)

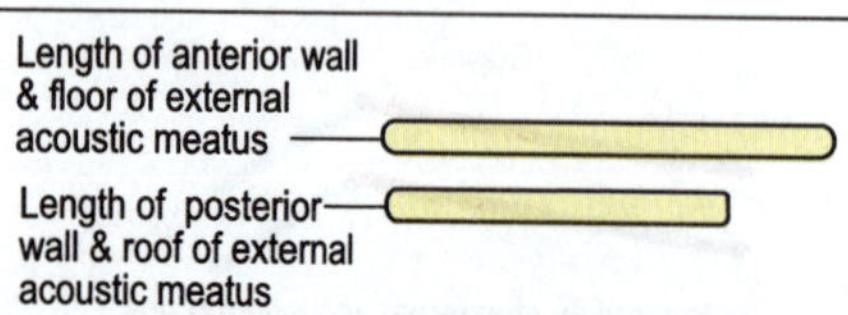

Fig. 18.5: Differences in length of anterior wall & floor with roof & posterior wall of external acoustic meatus

   e) In *newborn, bony part is absent and represented by only 'tympanic ring'. So in children it is very short in length.*
   f) Skin lining the bony part is intimately adherent to bone forming the canal.
   g) Hairs and *ceruminous glands are absent usually.*

Constrictions:

Two constrictions:

1. One at the junction between bony and cartilaginous part. The clearance of this constriction is important while removing foreign body.
2. **Isthmus**: In the bony part and situated at about 2cm deep from the bottom of concha. (Fig. 18.6)

Arteries:

1. Anterior auricular branch of superficial temporal arteries.
2. Posterior auricular branch of external carotid.
3. Deep auricular branch of maxillary artery.

Veins:

Drain into

a) External jugular vein
b) Maxillary veins and
c) Pterygoid venous plexus

Lymphatics:

Drain into preauricular, post auricular and superficial cervical lymph nodes.

Nerve supply:

1. Auriculo temporal nerve – roof and anterior wall.
2. Auricular branch of vagus: A floor and posterior wall. (Fig. 18.7)

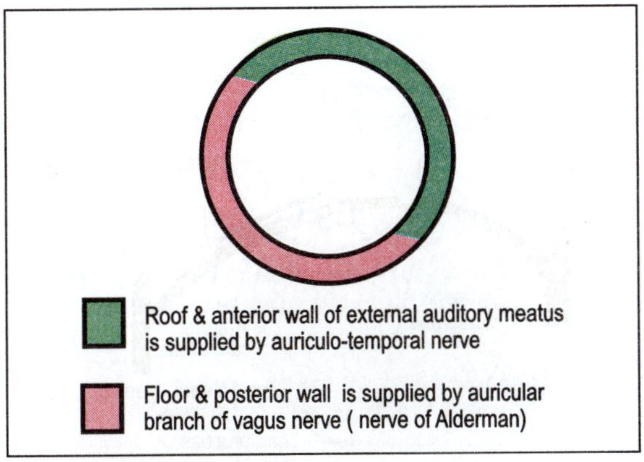

Fig. 18.7: Nerve supply of external acoustic meatus

APPLIED ANATOMY:

1. Examination of meatus by *aural speculum*
   a) In adult: As the meatus is 'S' shaped, so ti must be drawn upwards, backwards and slightly laterally to make it straight.
   b) In children: Meatus is short as *bony part is not developed* and so *tympanic membrane is directed downwards* and *downwards and backwards* and *special care should be taken in introducing the speculum* and *short length of the meatus must be kept in mind* so that *tympanic membrane may not be damaged.*
2. Any infection in the meatus is very much *painful* as skin is *intimately adherent to underlying cartilage and bone.*
3. Cerumen or ear wax serves many useful purposes.
   a) *prevent injury to lining epithelium by water*
   b) *prevents entrance of insects*
   c) *keeps the temperature warm and humid* within the meatus so that vibrations of sound waves may pass smoothly.
4. Foreign body may be lodged in *two regions at the isthmus (2cm from bottom of concha) or at the junctional region of bony and cartilagious part.* These are two regions of constrictions.
5. Syringing of the ear for removal ear wax or removal of foreign body may cause *irritation of auricular branch of vagus.* This *results in persistent cough and death due to sudden stoppage of heart by vagal stimulation.*

   Slight irritation will cause increase of appetite reflexly.
6. Referred pain in the ear from caries tooth or cancer tongue may occur *due to distribution of mandibular nerve.*

Development:

1. The *cuticular layer is ectodermal from first branchial cleft and meatal plate arising from the cleft* which *undergoes canalisation.*
2. Rest of the wall is mesodermal from extrapharyngeal mesoderm.

TYMPANIC MEMBRANE

It is cuticulo-muco-fibrous sheet interposed between external auditory meatus and middle ear cavity.

Colour: Pearly grey, semitransparent but may present yellowish tinge depending on tis vascularity.

Shape: Nearly oval more or less elliptical.

Disposition or attitude: It makes an angle of 55° with the floor of the meatus and the tympanic membrane faces downwards, forwards and laterally.

Dimensions: Greatest 9 to 10mm downwards and forwards. (Fig. 18.8)

Shortest: 8 to 9mm.

Circumference of membrane: The greater part of the circumference is thickened which is lodged in the tympanic sulcus of the medial end of external acoustic meatus.

The sulcus is deficient above. Here lies the notch. From the margins of the notch, two bands, anterior & posterior malleolar folds are attached to the lateral process of the malleus.

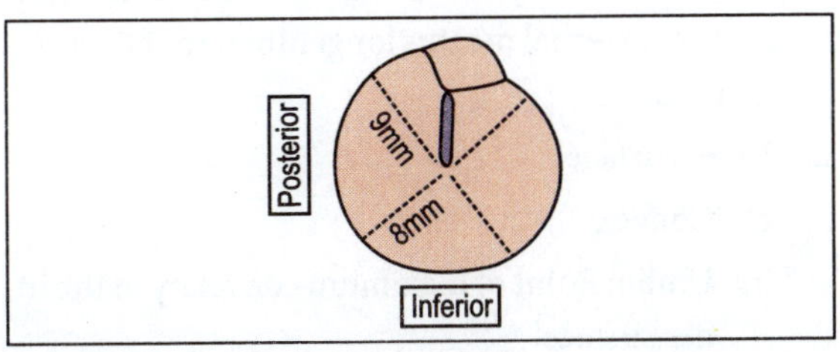

Fig. 18.8: Measurements of tympanic membrane

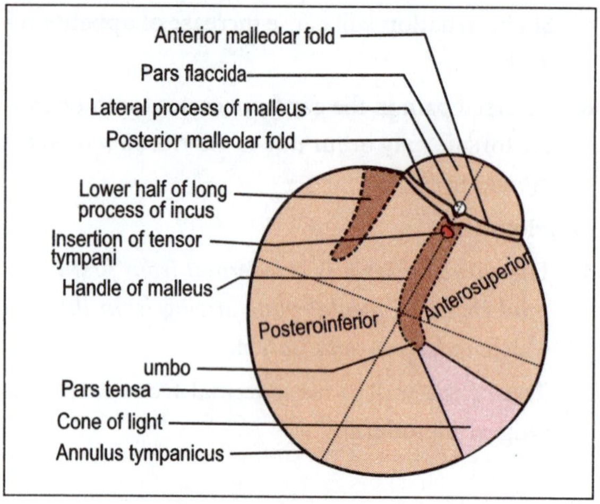

Fig. 18.9: External surface of tympanic membrane as seen through otoscope

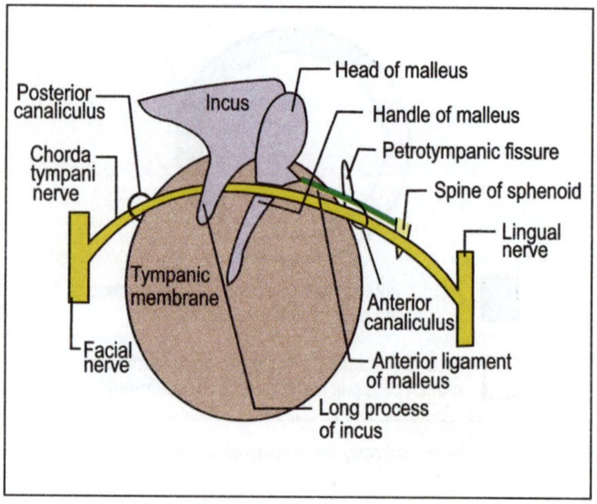

Fig. 18.10: Chorda tympanic nerve in relation to tympanic membrane

Different parts: Malleolar folds divide the tympanic membrane into two parts: (Fig. 18.9)

1. **Par flaccida**
   a) It is the part above the malleolar folds. It is triangular.
   b) It is lax and thin and sometimes perforated.
   c) Intermediate fibrous tissue is absent so thin and lax. It is replaced by loose areolar tissue.
2. **Par tensa**:
   a) Remaining part below the malleolar folds is tense and thick by the attachment of handle of malleus and radiating fibres of intermediate layer from the handle is being disposed.
   b) It presents all the three layers including the intermediate fibrous tissue.

Different surfaces: Two –

1. Outer surface: Concave, directed downwards, forwards, & laterally; due to which the anterior wall & floor of external meatus longer than roof & posterior wall.
2. Inner surface:
   a) Convex
   b) **Umbo**: Point of maximum convexity in the inner surface
   c) Two important features
      i) *Attachment of handle of malleus between mucous and fibrous layers* extending up to the centre of the membrane.
      ii) *Crossing medial to handle of malleus by chorda tympani nerve in between mucous and fibrous layer* at the junction of par flaccida and par tensa. (Fig. 18.10)

Cone of light: During otoscopic examinations highly refractive area is the antero-inferior quadrant of the membrane and known as cone of light.

Structure: It is 1mm thick and consists of three strata.

1. ***Outer cuticular layer***: It is continuous with the skin of external auditory meatus and lined by stratified squamous epithelium.
2. ***Intermediate fibrous layer***: It consists of two sets of fibres
   a) *Superficial radiating fibres* which diverge from the centre.
   b) *Deeper circular fibres:* They are plenty at the periphery. It is scanty in the centre.
3. *Inner mucous layer* is lined by *ciliated columnar epithelium.* (Fig. 18.11)

Arteries: Arteries descend from above to supply the membrane. They are –

a) Deep auricular branch of maxillary artery (cuticular layer — outer surface)

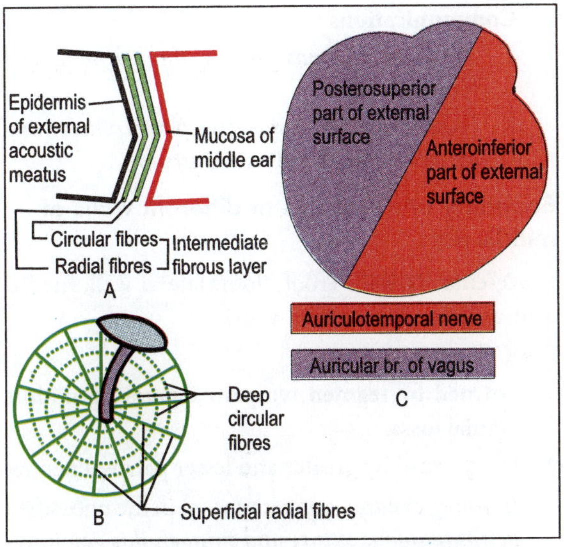

Fig. 18.11: A – Structure of tympanic membrane; B – Intermediate fibers; C – Nerve supply of external surface of tympanic membrane

b) Posterior tympanic branch, a branch from stylomastoid artery (a branch of posterior auricular artery) supplies mucous surface.

c) Anterior tympanic branch of maxillary artery (mucous surface).

Veins:

1. Superficial veins from outer surface to external jugular vein
2. Deep veins from inner surface to
   a) Transverse sinus
   b) Veins of duramater
   c) Plexus of veins on auditory tube and pterygoid venous plexus

Lymphatic drainage: Into preauricular and retropharyngeal lymph nodes.

Nerve supply:

1. Outer surface:
   a) Anteroinferior surface is supplied by auriculotemporal nerve.
   b) Posterosuperior surface is supplied by auricular branch of vagus nerve.
2. *Tympanic plexus (formed by tympanic branch of glossopharyngeal) – mucous layer.*

Development: It is tridermal in formation i.e., developed from three sources (three germinal layers).

a) **Outer cuticular layer** is developed from ectoderm.

b) **Intermediate fibrous tissue** is developed from mesoderm.

c) **Inner mucous layer:** It is developed from endoderm.

Clinical subdivisions of the membrane: It is divided into four quardrants by means of two imaginary lines through the umbo. One is drawn along the handle of malleus and the other at right angle to it through umbo.

Paracentesis of tympanic membrane: It is done in acute otitis media (acute infection of middle ear forming pus). The pus is drained by giving incision at the postero-inferior quadrant (Myringotomy). If it is not done automatic rupture of membrane occurs resulting in chronic discharge of pus (chronic otitis).

The **postero-inferior quadrant is chosen for incision because**

a) *Arteries* which supply the membrane descend from above

b) *Chorda tympani nerve crosses the membrane in the upper part*

c) It is the *most dependent part*

d) The *lower part is vascular* and *heals quickly.*

MIDDLE EAR

It is an irregular laterally compressed space with petrous part of temporal bone and functionally concerned with the transmissions of vibrations of tympanic membrane to medial wall and to internal ear by the movement of ossicles contained within the cavity.

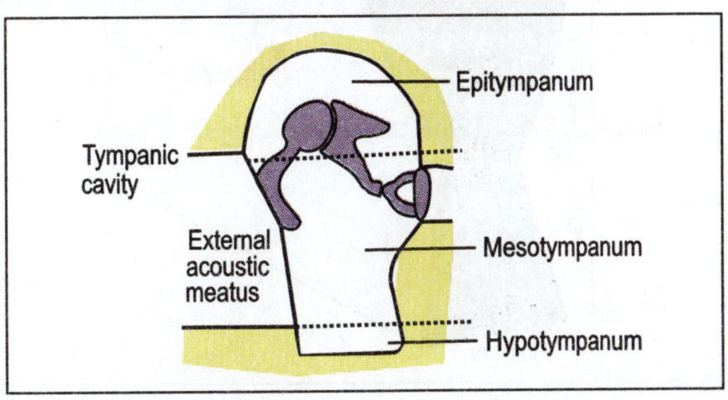

Fig. 18.12: Subdivisions of the tympanic cavity or middle ear

Different parts:

Usually three:

1. **Tympanic cavity proper (Mesotympanum)**: Part opposite the tympanic membrane and it is the narrowest part containing handle of malleus, long process of incus and stapes. (Fig. 18.12)
2. **Epitympanic (attic)**: Part above the level of tympanic membrane containing head of malleus, body and short process of incus.
3. **Hypotympanum** part below the level of tympanic membrane.

Shape and size: Middle ear is sandwiched between external & internal ears, in coronal section, it looks like biconcave disc. Outside the mucous membrane, middle ear contains following strucutres:

1. Three ossicles: Malleus, incus & stapes.
2. Two muscles: Tensor tympanic, stapedius.
3. Blood vessels & nerves.

Measurement are:

Vertical: 15mm (Fig. 18.13)

Anteroposterior: 15mm

Transverse diameter: At the roof – 6mm

Opposite the centre of tympanic membrane: 2mm

At the floor: 4mm

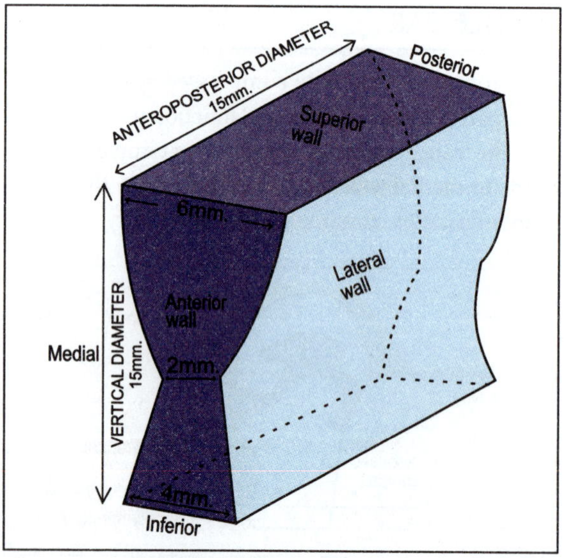

Fig. 18.13: Diameters of different parts of the middle ear cavity

Communications:

1. *Anteriorly* with *nasopharynx through pharyngo-tympanic tube.*
2. *Posteriorly* with *mastoid (tympanic) antrum and air cells through aditus to antrum.*

Boundary and features of different walls of middle ear:

It presents six walls (roof, floor, lateral wall, medial wall, anterior & posterior walls).

Roof: (Fig. 18.14)

1. Formed by tegmen tympani separating middle cranial fossa.
2. It is pierced by greater and lesser petrosal nerves.
3. *In young children* a gap is present in the unossified *petrosquamous suture and through this gap infection may spread from tympanic cavity to meninges.*
4. The tegmen tympani also form roof of the canal for tensor tympani.

Floor:

1. Formed by a convex plate of bone (Jugular fossa) separating superior bulb of internal jugular vein.
2. Sometimes bony partition may be deficient and so tympanic cavity and vein will be separated from each other by mucous membrane and fibrous tissue.
3. Opening for tympanic branch of glossopharyngeal nerve is present on the antero-medial aspect of floor.

Lateral wall: (Fig. 18.15)

1. Mainly formed by the mucous covering the medial surface of the *tympanic membrane* (which presents maximum convexity towards the tympanic cavity; **umbo** is the maximum point of convexity) lodged in a tympanic sulcus (which is deficient above). Handle of malleus extend up to umbo. Par tensa of tympanic membrane is attached to handle of malleus. Chorda tympanic nerve lies medial to malleus.
2. Posterior canaliculus for chorda tympani nerve: Situated at the junction of posterior and lateral walls behind tympanic membrane. Chorda tympani nerve enters the tympanic cavity through it. Chorda tympani nerve leaves the middle ear through anterior canaliculus.

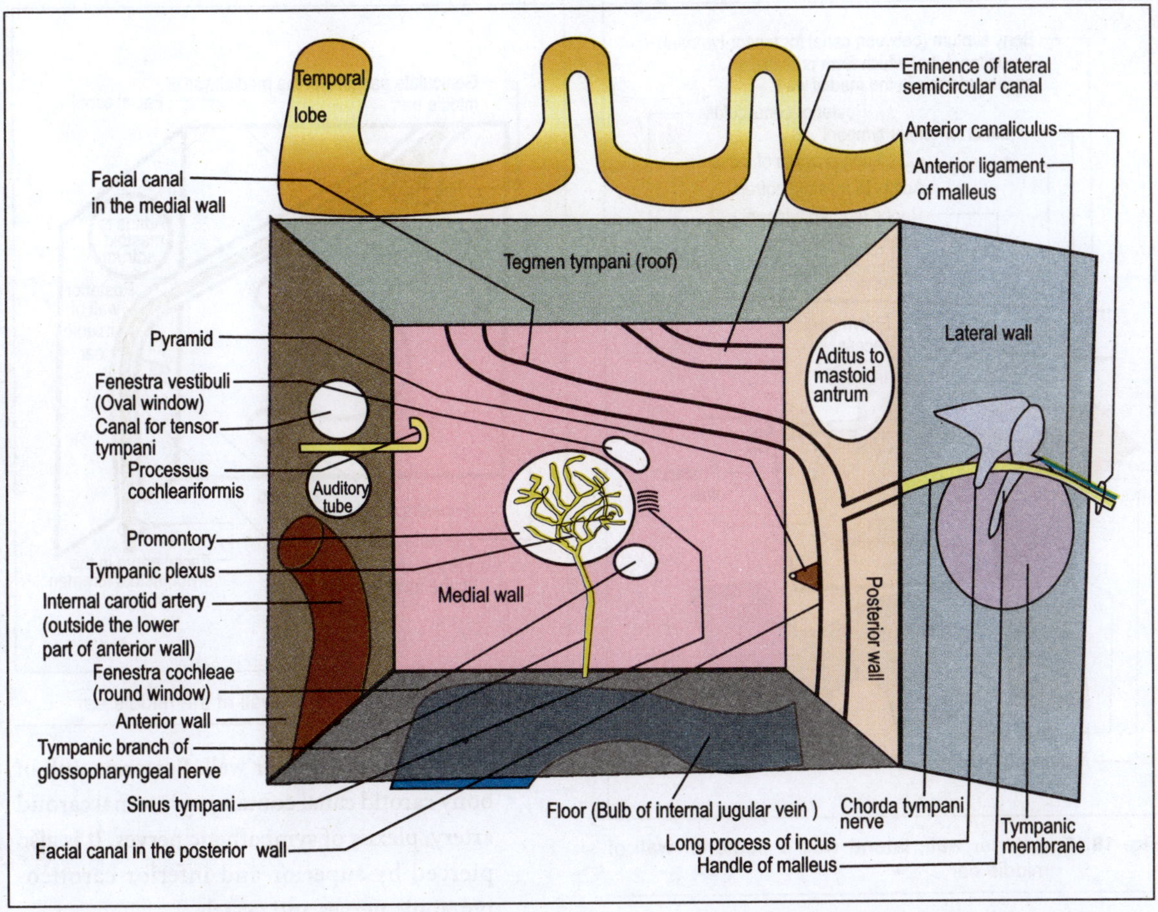

Fig. 18.14: Boundaries & relations of the middle ear

3. *Petrotympanic fissure*: Situated near the anterior margin of tympanic membrane. Transmitting tympanic branch of maxillary artery, chorda tympanic nerve & anterior ligament of malleus. Anterior canaliculus for chorda tympanic nerve either present with in fissure or in front of fissure.
4. *Epitympanic or upper part*: Formed by squamous part of temporal bone and contains
   a) Head of *malleus*
   b) Body of *incus.*

Medial wall:

Formed by bony labyrinth of internal ear and it separates middle ear from internal ear.

The features are: (Fig. 18.16)

1. ***Promontory***: A rounded elevation caused due to underlying first turn of cochlea. It presents tympanic plexus which is formed by tympanic branch of glossopharyngeal nerve.
2. ***Fenestra vestibuli***: A kidney shaped opening situated behind and above promontory. It is closed by base of stapes and annular ligament.
3. ***Fenestra cochleae***: A round opening below and behind promontory and is closed by secondary tympanic membrane.

   It separates the tympanic cavity from scala tympani of internal ear.
4. *Prominence of facial nerve canal*: Extends backwards and downwards, above promontory and fenestra vestibuli to reach below the aditus, and continue as vertical part of canal along the posterior wall of tympanic cavity.

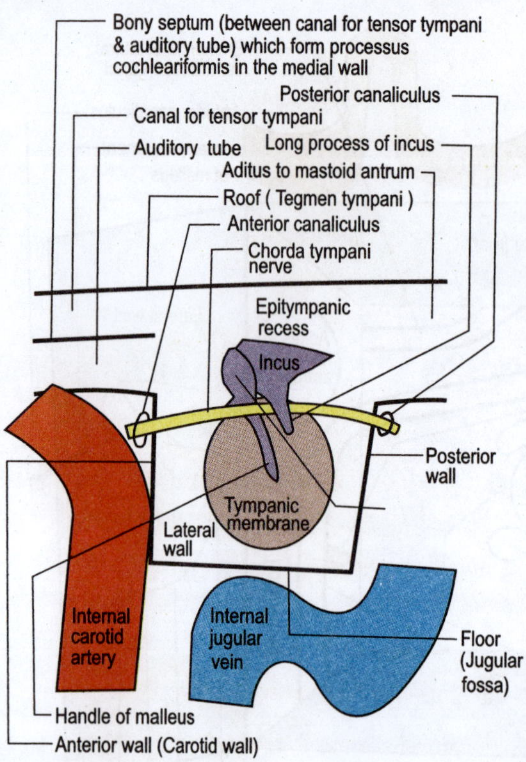

Fig. 18.15: Anterior wall, lateral wall & posterior wall of middle ear

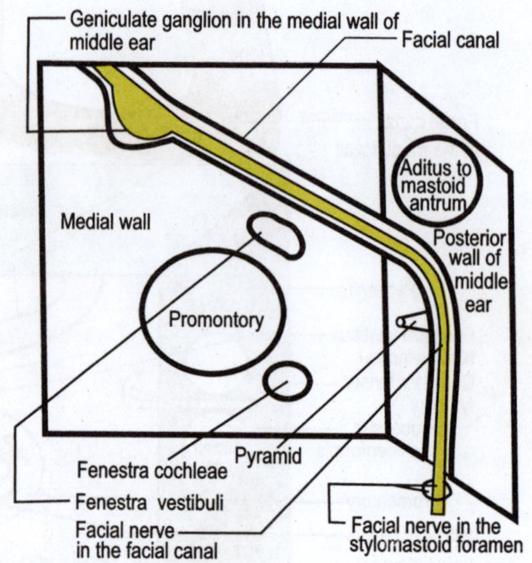

Fig. 18.16: Medial & posterior wall of the middle ear

5. *Sinus tympani*: A depression (between fenestra vestibuli and fenestra cochleae) behind the promontory indicating the position of ampulla of posterior semicircular canal.
6. *Processus cochleariformis*: A curved process above promontory forming a pulley by the septum (between auditory tube and canal for tensor tympani muscle).
7. *Eminence of lateral semicircular canal*: It lies in above the facial canal.

Anterior wall

1. Formed by meeting of roof, medial and later walls.
2. Three important features from above downwards are
   a) Upper canal for tensor tympani muscle
   b) Lower opening of canal for bony part of pharyngo-tympanic (auditory) tube.
   c) Lower part of anterior wall: Posterior wall of bony carotid canal containing internal carotid artery, plexus of sympathetic nerves. It is also pierced by superior and inferior carotico-tymapnic nerves and vessels.
   d) A bony septum between the two canals (for tensor tympani and auditory tube) is extended to the medial wall as curved lamina known as processus cochleariformis.

Posterior wall:

It is wider above and presents following features from above downwards

1. ***Aditus to the mastoid antrum***: A large *aperture communicate epitympanic recess with the mastoid antrum.*
2. ***Fossa incudis***: *A depression which lodges* short process of incus.
3. ***Pyramid***: *A conical elevation in front of vertical part of facial nerve canal and it contains stapedius muscle* and communicates with vertical part of facial nerve canal and through that a branch from 7th nerve passes to supply the muscle. At the apex

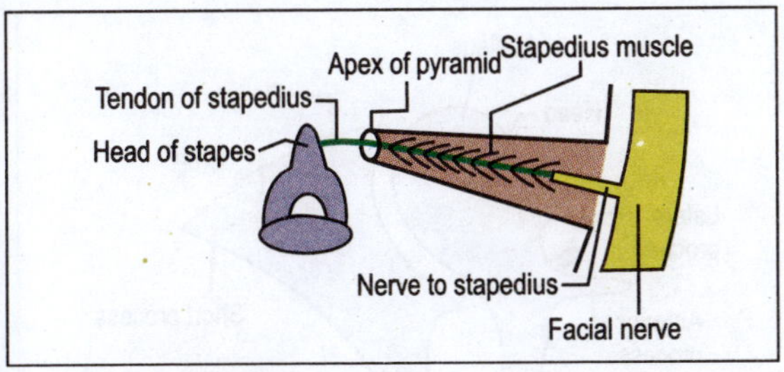

Fig. 18.17: Stapedius

of pyramid, the tendon of stapedius comes out, through a pinpoint opening. (Fig. 18.17)

4. ***Vertical part of facial nerve canal***: Situated below the aditus to mastoid antrum in the lower part of posterior wall and facial nerve runs downwards through it up to stylomastoid foramen.
5. ***Posterior canaliculus for chorda tympani***: *Situated lateral to pyramid.*

Contents of middle ear:
1. 'Air' only
2. Three ossicles: Malleus, incus and stapes and ligaments connecting them

Arterial supply: Six sets of arteries: (Fig. 18.18)
a) Stylomastoid branch of posterior auricular artery.
b) Anterior tympanic branch of maxillary artery (through petrotympanic fissure).
c) Petrosal branch of middle meningeal artery through fissure for greater petrosal nerve.
d) Superior tympanic branch of middle meningeal artery (through canal for tensor tympanic muscle).
e) A branch from ascending pharyngeal artery and a branch from artery of pterygoid canal (along pharyngo-tympanic tube).
f) Tympanic branch from internal carotid artery.

Venous drainage: The veins of tympanic cavity drains into
1. Superior petrosal sinus.
2. Pterygoid venous plexus.

Nerve supply:
1. Tympanic branch of glossopharyngeal nerve: It enters the tympanic cavity through tympanic canaliculus. It forms tympanic plexus on the promontory. It is sensory in nature.
2. Superior and inferior carotico-tympanic nerves from the sympathetic plexus around the internal carotid arteries.
3. Chorda tympanic nerve is closely related to tympanic membrane.
4. Facial nerve runs in facial canal which is related to medial and posterior wall of middle ear.

Lymphatic drainage: The lymphatics of tympanic cavity drains into
1. Deep cervical lymph nodes.
2. Retropharyngeal lymph nodes.

APPLIED ANATOMY OF MIDDLE EAR:

1. Otitis media (infection of middle ear) with or without discharge of pus is due to spread of infection from nasopharynx through auditory tube.
2. Otitis media is very common in children because length of auditory tube is very short 19mm and disposed horizontally and not obliquely downwards and medially as in adult.
3. Different course of spread of infection in otitis media will be any of the following:
   a) If tympanic membrane is ruptured pus will be discharged through external ear.
   b) The infection may spread upwards through the roof and may cause meningitis and brain abscess.

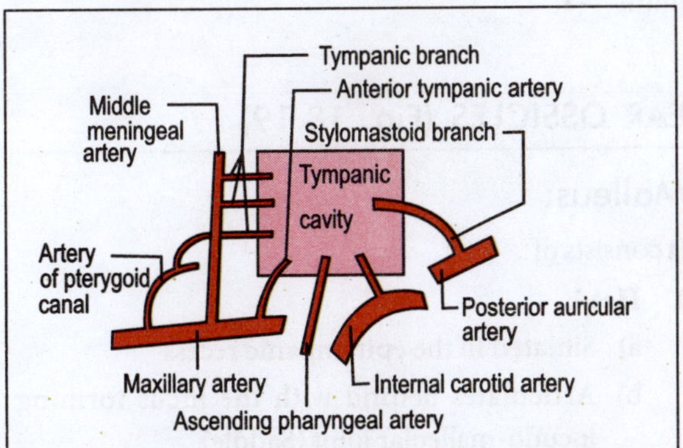

Fig. 18.18: Arterial supply of middle ear

c) If infection spreads downwards and may cause thrombosis of internal jugular vein.

d) It may spread backwards and may cause mastoiditis and mastoid abscess and thrombosis of sigmoid sinus.

4. Chronic discharge of pus through the ear indicates perforated tympanic membrane from acute otitis media (infection of middle ear) or mastoid abscess.
5. In case of acute otitis media pus likes drained by myringotomy (i.e., by giving incision to the tympanic membrane). The site of choice of incision should be postero-inferior quadrant so that
   a) Chorda tympani nerve and blood vessels supplying the membrane may not be injured, the nerve crosses in the upper part and blood vessels supply from above downwards.
   b) Lower part being vascular heals quickly.
6. Bleeding through ear and discharge of C.S.F. through ear occurs due to breaking the roof of the middle ear in case of fracture of middle cranial fossa.

MUCOUS MEMBRANE MIDDLE EAR OR TYMPANIC CAVITY

The cavity is lined by ciliated columnar epithelium except the posterior wall, posterior part of medial wall and ossicles which are non-ciliated flattened epithelium.

EAR OSSICLES (Fig. 18.19)

Malleus:

It consists of

1. **Head:**
   a) Situated in the epitympanic recess
   b) Articulates behind with the incus forming incudo-malleolar joint (Saddle)
   c) Superior and lateral ligaments are attached to it.

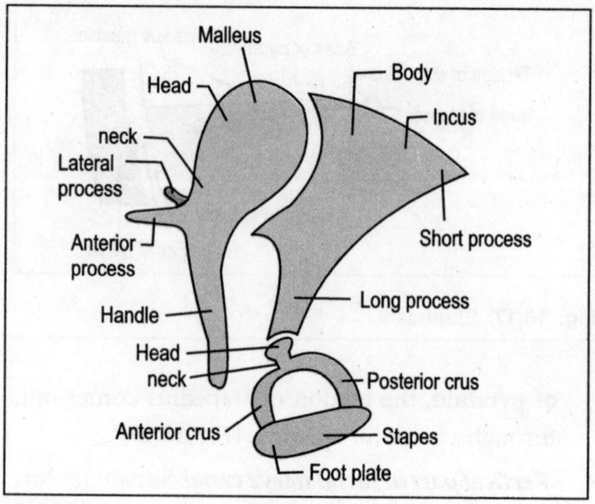

Fig. 18.19: Ossicles of middle ear

2. **Neck:**
   a) Situated in the par flaccida part of tympanic membrane
   b) Related medially to chorda tympani nerve
3. **Processes**
   a) *Handle*: Attached to medial surface of tympanic membrane and directed downward and backward.
   b) *Anterior process*: Connected to spine of sphenoid bone by anterior ligament (passes through petrotympanic fissure).
   c) *Lateral process*: Anterior and posterior malleolar folds are attached to it.
   d) It is a *derivative of Meckel's cartilage (Skeletal element of first branchial arch).*
   e) Tensor tympani muscle is attached in the medial surface in the upper end.

Incus:

It looks like premolar tooth and consists of

a) *Body:* Large, articulate with the head of the malleus.

b) *Short process*: Directed backwards and fixed to fossa incudis by posterior ligament of incus in the posteroinferior part of epitympanic recess.

c) *Long process*: Directed downwards and parallel to handle of malleus and its tip articulates with head of stapes and forms incudo-stapedial joint (*ball and socket*).

d) It is a *derivative of Meckel's cartilage (Skeletal element of first branchial arch).*

Stapes:

1. It is stirrup shaped and consists of
   a) *Head*: Forms cup shaped facet for articulation with lentiform nodule of tip of long process of incus and forms incudostapedial joint (*ball and socket*)
   b) *Neck*: Narrow and posteriorly stapedius is inserted.
   c) *Two limbs*: Anterior and posterior diverge from each other and is attached to foot plate or base (reniform).
   d) *Foot plate or base*: It fits to fenestra vestibuli by an annular ligament.
2. *Derived from Reichert's cartilage (Skeletal element of second branchial arch)*

Joints of the ossicles:

All the joints are synovial joints. Joint between incus & malleus is saddle joint. Joint between incus & stapedius is a ball & socket joint. They conduct sound vibrations from tympanic membrane to oval window and subsequently to perilymph to endolymph of inner ear.

Otosclerosis: *It is a condition characterised by abnormal ossification between base of stapes and fenestra vestibuli and this results in loss of mobility of stapes causing deafness (conductive).*

Muscle of ossicles (middle ear): Two: (1) Tensor tympani; (2) Stapedius.

1. **Tensor tympani**

Origin: From the wall of auditory tube and sulcus tubae.

Insertion: Into medial surface of root (upper part) of handle of malleus, after turning at processus cochleariformis.

Nerve supply: Nerve to medial pterygoid from trunk of mandibular nerve.

Action: It draws the handle of malleus medially and makes the tympanic membrane more tense (tightened).

Development: It is derived from myotome of first branchial arch.

2. **Stapedius**

Origin: From pyramid (elevation on the posterior wall). Exit through apex of pyramid.

Insertion: Into the posterior surface of the neck of stapes.

Nerve supply: Facial nerve.

Action: Drawing the stapes laterally.

Both *tensor and stapedius produce dumping effect on the sound vibrations* resulting in preventing production of loud sounds (*paralysis of stapedius – causes hyperacusis*).

Development: Derived from second arch myotome.

Mastoid Antrum

It is an air sinus in the basal part of petrous part of temporal bone developmentally but in adult it is within mastoid part. (Fig. 18.20)

Features:

1. It is formed as a backward extension of tympanic cavity.

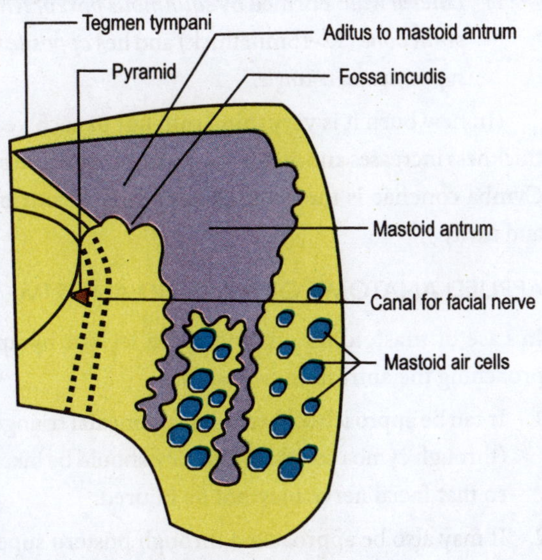

Fig. 18.20: Mastoid antrum

2. It is very well developed (full adult size) in the new born and very little development takes place after birth.
3. Dimension: Vertical – 10mm; Transverse – 10mm; Anteroposterior – 10mm.
4. Capacity = 1ml
5. Lined by non-ciliated columnar epithelium.
6. **Boundary**:
   a) *Roof*: Thin plate of bone (*tegmen tympani*) separating it from middle cranial fossa containing temporal lobe.
   b) *Floor*: Present perforations communicating mastoid air cells lined by mucoperiosteum.
   c) *Anterior wall*: In the upper part is the *aditus to tympanic antrum* (opening of communication between epitympanic part of tympanic cavity and antrum).

      In the lower part: *Vertical part of facial nerve canal.*
   d) *Posterior wall*: Formed by thin plate or bone separating from sigmoid sinus and mastoid air cells may be present.
   e) *Medial wall*: Petrous temporal bone.
   f) *Lateral wall*: Formed by *squamous part of temporal bone* (12-15mm thick) and lies *opposite to suprameatal triangle.*

(In new born it is very thin 1mm but in each year thickness increases and attains its maximum thickness. Cymba conchae is the route of approach to antrum and cavity.)

APPLIED ANATOMY OF MASTOID ANTRUM:

In case of mastoiditis – pus may be let out by approaching the antrum in two ways.

1. It can be approached through suprameatal triangle (through cymba conchae) and care should be taken so that facial nerve may not be injured.
2. It may also be approached through postero superior aspect of external acoustic meatus close to tympanic membrane. (Transmeatal approach)

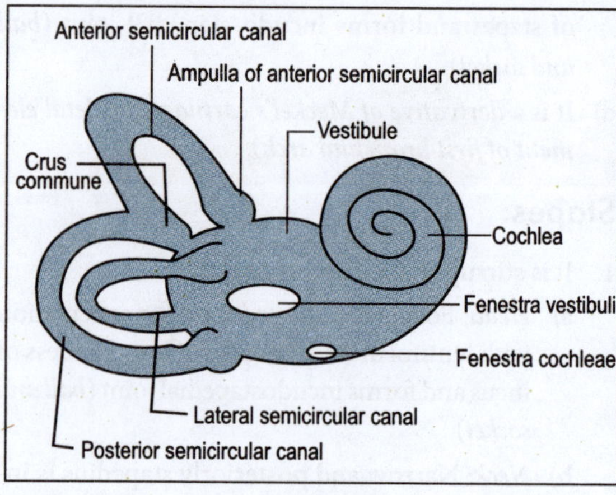

Fig. 18.21: Bony labyrinth of inner ear

INTERNAL EAR

It consists broadly two parts:

A. Outer bony labyrinth
B. Inner membranous labyrinth

A. Bony Labyrinth (Fig. 18.21)

1. Situation within petrous part of temporal bone.
2. Consists of three bony parts which inter communicate with each other.
3. The constituent parts from before backwards are
   a) Cochlea
   b) Vestibule, semicircular cannals
4. Each part is filled with perilymph.
5. Bony labyrinth contains membranous labyrinth within them.
6. Total length of bony labyrinth – 18mm.

Cochlea:

1. It is one of the constituent of bony part of labyrinth.
2. *Shape*: Conical and resembles the shell of a snail.
3. *Extent*: Apex (known as copula) directed towards tympanic cavity and base lies at the internal acoustic meatus.
4. *Measurement*: From apex to base – 5mm; at the base – 9mm.

5. Different parts: Two–
   A. *Modiolus* – a central pillar or axis
      a) Conical in shape
      b) Base towards internal acoustic meatus
      c) Length in 5mm long
      d) Tractus spiralis foraminosus is present at the base and through this cochlear nerve passes.
   B. *Cochlear canal*
      a) Canal arranged spirally around the modiolus.
      b) *Length*: 35mm long.
      c) Consists of *two and three fourth turns.*
      d) *Apical turn begins at the cupola* and basal turn produces **promontory** at the medial wall of middle ear.
      e) *Divisions*: Cochlear canal is partially divided by osseous spiral lamina. They are scala vestibuli above and scala tympani below. They are continuous with each other at the apex by an opening known as ***helicotrema***.
      f) At the base, **scala tympani** presents *fenestra cochleae closed by secondary tympanic membrane* and *aqueduct of cochlea (a narrow channel)* which *communicates perilymph with CSF of subarachnoid space through* ***cochlear canaliculus***.
      g) Content: *Perilymph*.

Osseous spiral lamina

1. A spiral ridge of bone projecting from the modiolus like a cork-screw into the cochlear canal.
2. The free margin of the lamina splits into two lips *by a sulcus*.
3. The **vestibular membrane** is attached to upper lip while basilar membrane is attached to lower lip. They contain cochlear duct (scala media) which divides scala vestibuli and scala tympani. Scala vestibuli and scala tympani is continuous with each other through small opening (helicotrema) at the apex of cochlea.

Vestibule:

1. It is the central part of bony labyrinth situated medial to tympanic cavity and lies *between cochleae in front* and *semicircular canals behind*.
2. *Shape*: Bilaterally compressed ovoid body.
3. *Dimensions*
   a) Anteroposterior and
   b) Vertical: 5mm
   c) Width: 3mm
4. *Content*: Membranous saccule and utricle.
5. Communications and features of different walls.
   A. *In the lateral wall*: **Fenestra vestibuli** is present and closed by foot plate of stapes, and annular ligament. Facial nerve passes laterally above (roof) the vestibule.
   B. *In the posterior wall*: Five openings of three semicircular canals.
   C. *In the medial wall*: The wall is divided by vestibular crest (*an oblique ridge*) into.
      a) *Spherical recess (in front)*: Saccule is lodged in this recess and this recess presents *foramina for transmission of lower divisions of vestibular nerve to saccule.*
      b) *An elliptical recess* (behind) contains *utricle*. The floor of this recess presents *foramina for upper division of vestibular nerve* and *ampullae of superior and lateral semicircular ducts.* Just below the elliptical recess, opening of **aqueduct of vestibule** is present. Tubular prolongation of saccus and ductus endolymphaticus passes through aqueduct of vestibule. Aqueduct of vestibule is a bony canal.

      Another recess, *cochlear recess* is present in between two splitted parts of vestibular crest at its lower part.
   D. *Anterior wall of the vestibule is having one opening which communicate with scala vestibuli of the cochlear canal.*

   Relations:

   a) *Above*: Facial nerve runs from medial to lateral.

b) *Medially*: Internal acoustic meatus.

c) *Laterally*: Tympanic cavity.

Semicircular canals

Features:

1. These are three bony canals situated behind vestibular part of bony labyrinth.
2. The three canals are superior or anterior, lateral and posterior.
3. Each canal is set at right angles to each other and forms two third of a circle.
4. They are 15-20mm long.
5. *Opening*: They open by five openings as upper end of posterior and medial end of anterior canal unite to form crus commune which opens at the medial wall of the vestibule.
6. Each end before opening expands to form *ampulla*.
7. a) *Anterior canal*: Lies in vertical plane with convexity upwards and forms ***arcuate eminence*** in the anterior surface of petrous part. It ampulla lies anterolaterally and posterior end unites with upper end of posterior canal and forms ***crus commune***, which opens into medial wall of vestibule.

   b) *Posterior canal*: Lies parallel to the long axis of petrous part of temporal bone. Its convexity is directed backward and ampullated end lies below (communicates with vestibule and supplied by branch of vestibular nerve which passes through foramen singulare in the internal acoustic meatus) and the upper end forms *crus commune*. It lies in vertical plane.

   c) *Lateral canal:* It lies in horizontal plane with convexity posterolaterally.
8. *Lateral semicircular canals* of two sides lie in same plane. Two openings in vestibuli.

B. Membranous Labyrinth

I. Consists of closed membranous sacs and ducts intercommunicating with each other and lie within bony labyrinth and contain endolymph.

II. Constituent parts of membranous labyrinth are:

1. *Cochlear duct* lying within bony cochlea. (Fig. 18.22)
2. *Saccule and utricle* lying within vestibule.
3. *Three semicircular ducts* lie with respective bony canal.

Functionally: The membranous labyrinth consist of two components: (Fig. 18.23)

A. Cochlear duct: for hearing;

B. Saccule, utricle are concerned with static balance & linear acceleration.

Semicircular ducts are concerned with kinetic balance and angular acceleration.

Semicircular ducts open into utricle which joins with saccule by 'Y' shaped **utriculosaccular duct** and saccule communicates with cochlear duct by ductus reunions.

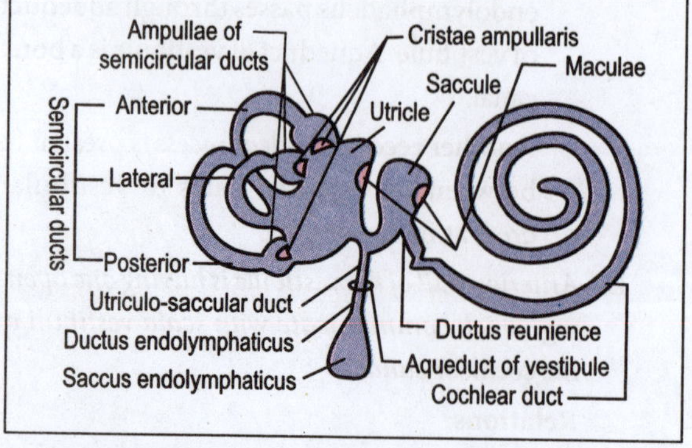

Fig. 18.22: Membranous part of internal ear

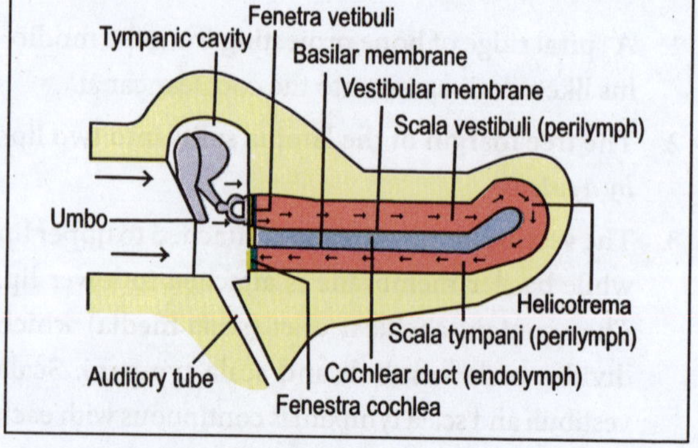

Fig. 18.23: Propagation of sound waves

Cochlear duct (also known as Scala Media)

Situation: Situated at the outer wall of bony cochlear canal between scala vestibuli and scala tympani.

Disposition: It consists of spiral course of two and three fourth turns.

Boundary:

a) *Medially or roof*: Vestibular membrane (Reissner's).

b) *Laterally*: Stria vascularis.

c) *Below or floor*: Osseous spiral lamina and basilar membrane. Basilar membrane is divided into:

1. Lateral part: Zona pectinate.
2. Medial part: Zona arcuata; organ of corti rest on it.

On cross section: Triangular.

Stria vascularis: Consist of stratified epithelium (specialised) with rich plexus of capillaries. It secretes endolymph.

Vestibular lip gives attachment to membrana tectoria & vestibular membrane.

Spiral organ of corti:

It is the peripheral organ of hearing and is the content of cochlear duct and rests on **basilar membrane.** (Fig. 18.24)

Constituent parts: It consists of:

1. **Membrana tectoria**: *Gelatinous structure which is attached to vestibular lip of osseous spiral lamina and covers the inner and outer hair cells. The hair cells are stimulated by the shearing force between the hair cells and tectorial membrane.*
2. Supporting *Deiter's and Hensen's cell.* The Deiter's cells are situated below the outer hair cells. The Hensen's cells lie outside the hair cells.
3. *Tunnel of corti* containing cortilymph: It is the triangular *interval between inner and outer rod cells.*
4. Hair cells and cochlear nerve.

   Inner hair cells: Afferent fibres of cochlear nerve make direct synapse. Inner hair cells are supplied numerous cochlear nerve fibers.

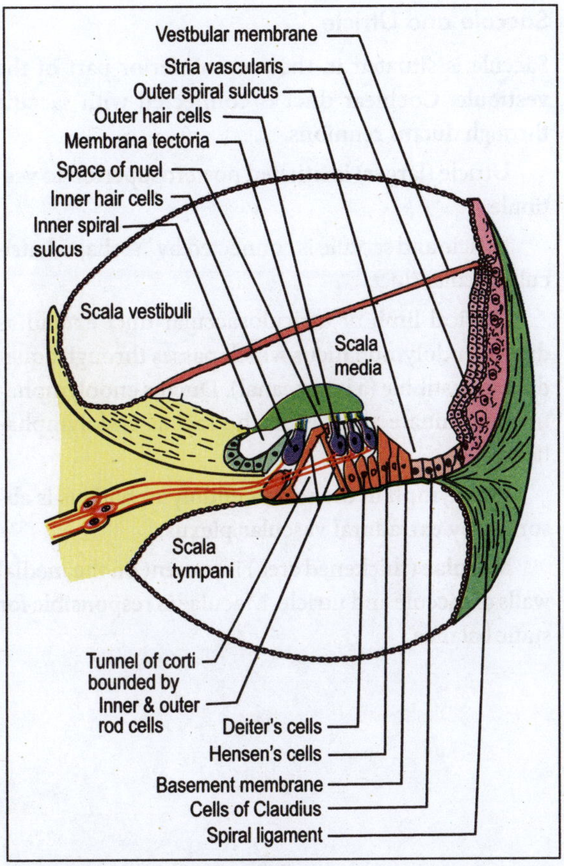

Fig. 18.24: Structure of organ of corti

   Outer hair cells: Receive direct synapse with afferent and efferent fibres of cochlear nerve. Outer hair cells modulate the function of inner hair cells.

5. *Outer tunnel and space of Nuel*: In addition to tunnel of corti there are two more spaces.

Ten ganglion of cochlear nerve are connected to each inner hair cells and concerned with discrimination of sound waves. Each ganglion cell are connected with ten outer hair cells and allow us to hear very quiet sounds.

Basal turn of cochlea is concerned with high pitched sound and apical turn of spiral organ is concerned with low pitched sound.

Noise or loud sound damage hair cells & kill the hair cells, since cochlear hair cells cannot grow back, this manifest as permanent hearing loss.

Saccule and Utricle

Saccule is situated in the anteroinferior part of the vestibule. Cochlear duct is connected with saccule through ductus reunions.

Utricle (larger) is situated posterosuperior to vestibule.

Utricle and saccule is connected by 'Y' shaped utriculosaccular duct.

Vertical limb of utriculosaccular duct extend as ductus endolymphaticus which passes through aqueduct of vestibule (a bony canal). Ductus endolymphaticus terminate as dilation the saccus endolymphaticus.

Endolymph in the saccus endolymphaticus is absorbed by extradural vascular plexus.

Maculae (thickened area) is present on the medial walls of saccule and utricle. Maculae is responsible for static balance.

Semicircular duct

Semicircular canals contain semicircular ducts. Semicircular ducts open in the utricle through five openings.

Ampulla is dilated part of each duct which contains receptors called **crista ampullaris**. These receptors are responsible for kinetic balance.

APPLIED ANATOMY OF INTERNAL EAR

1. Tinnitus: Peripheral cochlear disease followed by deafness.
2. **Vertigo**: Due to excessive stimulation of semicircular ducts.
3. Meniere's disease: Due to attacks of vertigo, tinnitus and hearing impairment (progressive). There may be distension of cochlear duct. Reducing sodium intake may relieve the symptoms.

chapter 19

EYEBALL

AT A GLANCE

- *Development of optic nerve and retina, iris & choroid cornea & sclera*
- *Sclera*
- *Choroid*
- *Ciliary body*
- *Iris*
- *Retina*
- *Aqueous humour*
- *Lens*
- *Vitreous body*
- *Suspensory ligament of lens*

EYEBALL

Location: The eyeball is located anterior one-third of the orbital cavity. It is enclosed by a membranous envelop called fascial bulbi or Tenon's capsule which separate the eyeball from fat.

Each of the anteroposterior, transverse and vertical diameters of normal eyeball measures about 24mm.

Coats or Tunics or the eyeball

The eyeball consists of three layers:

1. An outer fibrous coat consisting of sclera and cornea.
2. A middle vascular coat consists of choroid, ciliary body and iris.
3. An inner nervous coat consist of the retina.

Outer fibrous tissue

SCLERA

It is outer protective fibrous coal and forms posterior five-sixth of the eyeball. Sclera's dense connective tissue maintain the shape of eyeball.

White of eye: The part of the sclera is opaque so known as 'white of eye', (as this part is covered by conjunctiva).

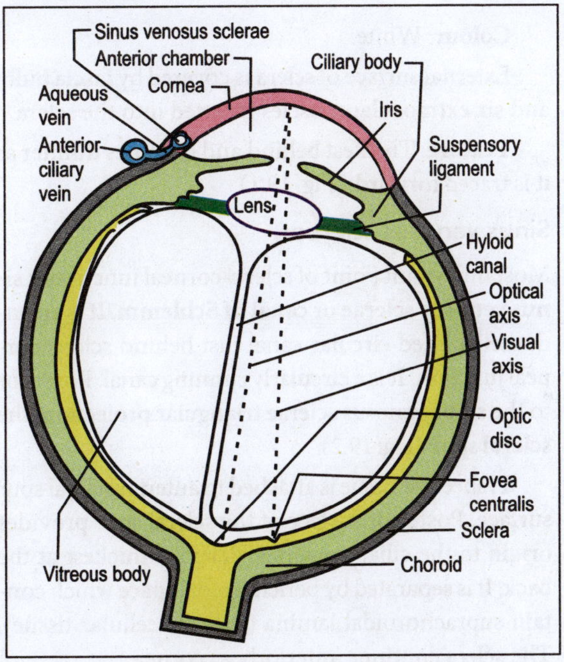

Fig. 19.1: Horizontal section of right eyeball

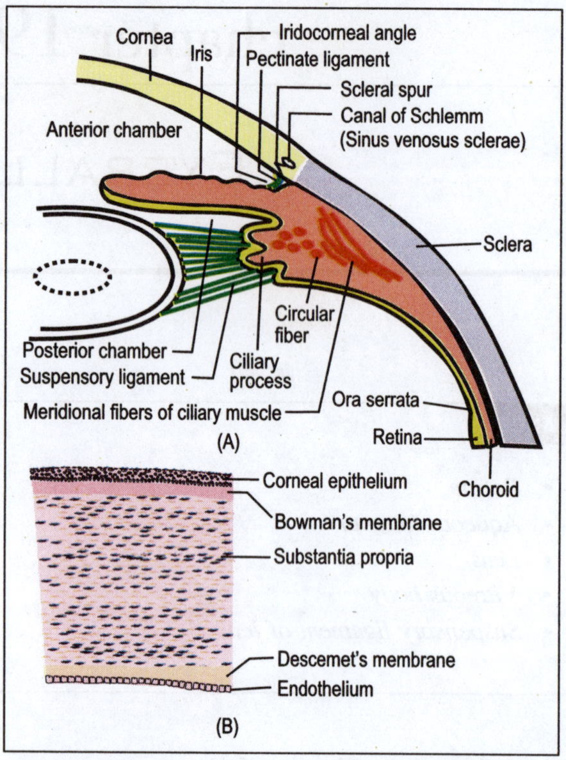

Fig. 19.2: (A) Features of ciliary body & cornea-sclearal juction (limbus); (B) Microscopic features of cornea

Colour: White.

External surface of sclera is covered by fascia bulbi and six extraocular muscles inserted into the sclera.

Texture: Thickest behind and becomes thinner as it is traced forward. (Fig. 19.1)

Sinus venosus sclerae:

Most important point of sclero-corneal junction is **sinus venosus sclerae** or **canal of Schlemm.** It is an endothelial lined circular canal just behind sclero-corneal junction. It is a circularly running canal. Posterior to the sinus venosus sclerae triangular projection, the **scleral spur** (Fig. 19.2).

Trabecular tissue is attached to anterior scleral spur surface. Posterior surface of the scleral spur provides origin to the ciliary muscles. Sclera is thickest at the back. It is separated by perichoroidal space which contain suprachoroidal lamina (delicate cellular tissue). The sclera continue anteriorly as cornea.

The sclera joins with dural sheath of optic nerve.

Function of sclera:

1. It protects & maintain the shape of eyeball, provide attachment of extraocular muscles.
2. Maintains the optimal intraocular pressure 15-20mm of Hg. Venous pressure should be maintained more than 20mm of Hg.
3. Eyeball moves within fascia bulbi (in episcleral space).

Structure of sclera:

Consists of fibrous tissue, elastic fibres and pigments.

These fibrous tissue are arranged longitudinally and coronally and determined by intraocular tensions, pull of muscles and stress and strain. Different parts of sclera perform different functions due to different orientations of fibres.

Structure piercing the sclera:

1. Optic nerve pierces the sclera 3mm inferomedial to posterior pole of the eyeball. The site is known as **lamina cribrosa** due to perforation by optic nerve fibres (make the area sieve-like—weakest part).
2. Anteriorly: Anterior ciliary vessel close to corneoscleral junction.
3. *Middle set*: 4mm behind the equator of eye for exit of venae vorticosae (choroid veins).
4. *Posterior set*: Around the entrance of optic nerves for long and short ciliary nerves and vessels.

Blood and Nerve supply: Almost *avascular except* the area *where bulbar conjunctiva* is *attached* to sclera by episclera (loose connective tissue).

It is *vascular* by *conjunctival blood vessels.*

Blood supply by ciliary vessels and *nerves by ciliary nerves.*

CORNEA

It is anterior 1/6the of the outer fibrous tunic.

Function: Transparent avascular and projecting part and responsible for major part of refraction of rays of light (it forms one of the refractive media of eyeball).

Shape: Almost circular broader transversely than vertical.

Texture: Thickness – 1mm at periphery & 0.5mm in the centre.

Limbus or sulcus sclerae is the junctional part between sclera and cornea. Most of refraction occur at surface of cornea.

Surface:

A. *Anterior*: Convex anteriorly and covered by conjunctiva.
B. *Posterior*: Perfectly circular and exceeds anterior surface in diameter. This surface presents sulcus circularis cornea. It is a furrow on the inner surface of cornea between sclero-corneal junction and attachment of iris and bounded by *trabecular tissue*.

Microscopic features of cornea (Fig. 19.2)

From outside inwards

1. *Corneal epithelium*: It is lined by non-keratinized stratified squamous epithelium.
2. *Anterior elastic lamina (Bowman's membrane)*: Structureless homogeneous mass without any elastic fibres.
3. *Substantia propria*: Composed of 200-250 lamella (flattened). Each lamella contain bundles of parallel fine collages fibrils. All fibrils are embedded in ground substance (rich in chondroitin sulphate) which makes the cornea transparent.
4. *Posterior elastic lamina (Descemet's membrane): Structureless homogeneous mass with elastic fibres.*
5. *Endothelium or posterior epithelium:* Cuboidal cells which covers the posterior surface of the cornea.

Vascular supply: It is nonvascular, capillaries from conjunctival and scleral vessels from loops at its circumference and by diffusion supply nutrition to periphery also gets nutrition from aqueous humour, and tears (lacrimal secretion) spread over the anterior surface of cornea.

Nerve supply: Numerous by short ciliary (branches from ciliary ganglion) and long ciliary nerves. (Branches of nasociliary nerves).

APPLIED ANATOMY:

1. **Corneal graft**: Cornea is avascular and lack of antigen; for those reasons cornea is usually grafted from one person to other.
2. **Corneal opacity**: Injury may cause corneal opacity.

MIDDLE VASCULAR COAT

It consist of three parts: Choroid, ciliary body and iris.

CHOROID

It is the posterior part of vascular tunic of eyeball and consists of thin highly vascular pigmented layer lining the inner surface of posterior part of sclera and outer surface of retina.

Extent: It extends anteriorly up to ora serrata where it is continuous with ciliary body.

Colour: Brown or chocolate colour.

Texture: Thicker posteriorly and thinner anteriorly.

Surfaces:

1. *External*: Loosely connected with sclera by lamina fusca or suprachoroid lamina, which is transversed by ciliary vessels and nerves.
2. *Internal*: Intimately adherent with retina.

   Structures piercing it: Optic nerve pierces it posteriorly with which it is firmly adherent and also attached with sclera firmly in this part.

Arteries: They are derived from **long & short ciliary arteries.**

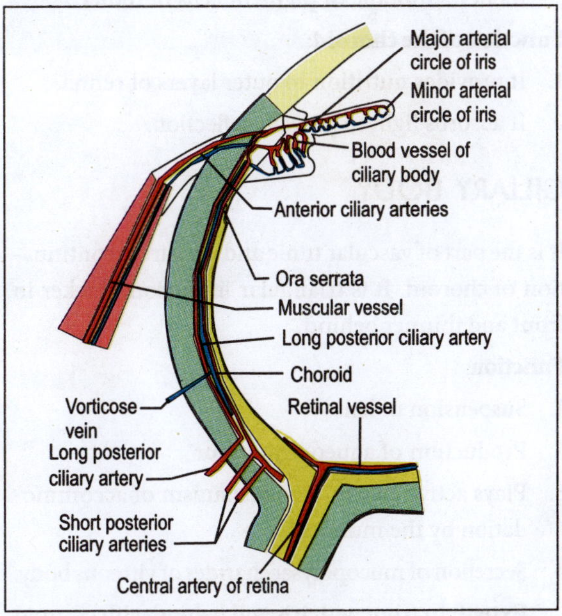

Fig. 19.3: Vessels of the eyeball

Venae vorticosae formed by converging veins & pierces the sclera near the equator to end in the ophthalmic veins.

Structure: Structurally it forms two layers from outside inwards:

1. **Suprachoroid lamina**: Delicate nonvascular lamellae consisting of network of fine collagen, elastic fibres and branched cells containing dark brown pigments. This space is transversed by long posterior ciliary vessels and nerves.
2. *Vascular lamina*: This layer is divided on the basis of calibre of vessels.

   The inner layer contains arterioles and layer of longer vessels are arteries (short posterior ciliary) and veins which converge in whorls to form 4 to 5 *vorticose veins*. These vorticose veins pass through sclera to open in ophthalmic veins. (Fig. 19.3)
3. *Intermediate choroido-capillary lamina*: This lamina consists of capillaries packed closely together. It nourishes the outer part of retina by diffusion. This layer ends at *ora serrata*.
4. *Inner based lamina or membrane of Bruch*: A thin *structureless transparent lamina* is united to basement membrane of pigment cells of retina.

Function of the choroid:

1. It provides nutrition to outer layers of retina
2. It absorbs light to prevent reflection.

CILIARY BODY

It is the part of vascular tunic and the direct continuation of choroid. It is triangular in section, thicker in front and thinner behind.

Function:

1. Suspension of lens
2. Production of aqueous humour
3. Plays active role in the mechanism of accommodation by the muscles
4. Secretion of mucopolysaccharides of vitreous body.

Extent: In front with iris and behind with choroid (at the ora serrata of retina)

On cross section: Triangular being thick in front and thin behind.

Different parts: It consist of:

1. Ciliary ring.
2. Ciliary processes
3. Ciliary muscles.

1. **Ciliary ring**: Also known as pars plana (an outer fibrous ring). The peripheral rim of it is ora serrata where nervous part of retina ends. Choroid continue as ciliary ring.
2. **Ciliary process**: Also known as corona ciliaris or pars plicata. It is the anterior one-third ridged part of ciliary body. It consists 70 to 80 ridges (ciliary process) formed by inward foldings of ciliary body.

   The grooves between the ciliary process provides attachment to the fibre of suspensory ligament.

   Inner end of ciliary process is in the posterior chamber of eye and secrete aqueous humour deeper layer of ciliary epithelium is pigmented.
3. **Ciliary muscles**: (*No chorio-capillary lamina*). A ring of unstriped muscles consisting of three parts. All muscle (meridional, radial and circular) fibres arise from posterior surface of the scleral spur.

   Contraction of fibres (particularly radial and circular) are responsible *for focussing lens for near vision i.e., accommodation* (lens become round).

   As the ciliaris muscle relax, elastic recoil of suprachoroid lamina causes the tension of suspensory ligament resulting in flattening of lens for distant vision.

Nerve supply: Short ciliary nerves from ciliary ganglion & preganglionic parasympathetic fibres coming from Edingeer Westphal nucleus through third nerve, & relay in ciliary ganglion.

Structure of ciliary body: It consist of bilaminar epithelium, ciliary stroma and ciliary muscles.

1. **Bilaminar**: i.e., 2 layered ciliary epithelium superficial.

   Deep: Cuboidal loaded with pigments.
2. Ciliary stroma consist of loose collagen fibres which supports ciliary vessels, nerves & muscles. Arteries are from long posterior ciliary arteries, which

form capillary plexus in ciliary process. They also form arterial circle at the periphery of iris. Veins join vorticose veins.

3. Ciliary muscles.

IRIS

It is a circular contractile coloured curtain and forms the anterior part of the vascular tunic of eyeball. Its peripheral margin is attached to the anterior surface of ciliary body.

Situation: Suspended in the aqueous humour between cornea in front and lens behind.

Pupil: Central aperture in the iris which controls the amount of light which enters into the eye. So by pupil, iris acts like an adjustable diaphragm.

Division of the space between cornea and lens.

It divides the space into two chambers: Anterior and posterior.

They communicate with each other through *pupil*

Attachment: Attached peripherally to the middle of anterior surface of ciliary body and to posterior elastic lamina of cornea by *pectinate ligament* but separated from cornea by *iridocorneal angle*.

Central free margin forms the pupil and rests against lens.

Colour: Depends upon the number of pigment cells and vary from individual to individual.

Structure: From outside inwards

1. No distinct endothelial layer; its anterior surface presents crypts. Anterior border or this surface is formed by fibroblast & melanocyte & blends with pectinate ligament (derived from Descement's membrane of cornea).
2. Stroma of connective tissue cell: It contains collagen fibres, fibroblast, melanocytes, vessels, nerves & muscles. Consists of involuntary muscles two types:
   A. Circular muscle fibres forming sphincter pupillae lying behind at the margin of pupil. (Fig. 19.4)

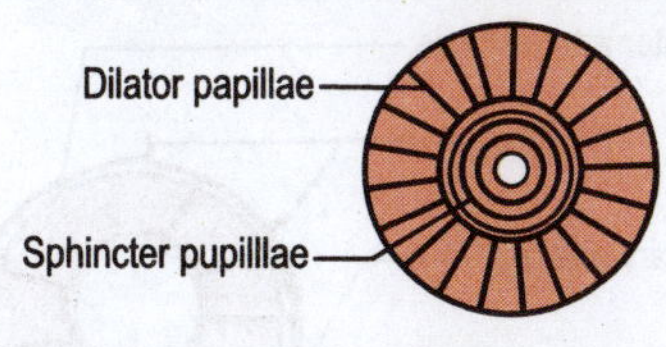

Fig. 19.4: Muscles of iris

(This muscle *constricts the pupil and supplied by parasympathetic nerve fibres which carry post ganglionic fibres from ciliary ganglion*).
The preganglionic fibres will come from Edinger-Westphal nucleus.
When light reaches the retina, iris contracts (pupillary light reflex), iris also contract during adjustment of eye for near vision (accommodation reflex) Atropine drops causes dilatation of pupil, actions of sphincter pupillae and ciliaris muscles are blocked by blocking the action acetyl choline. The muscles are covered by collagen fibers.

   B. Radiating fibres forming **dilator pupillae**. These fibres are ill defined sheet of radial fibres situated near the posterior surface of iris. It is supplied by sympathetic fibres. (Postganglionic from superior cervical sympathetic ganglion and coming via long ciliary branches of nasociliary).

3. Two layers of pigmented epithelial cells are continuous with ciliary part of retina.
   The colour of iris depends upon type of pigment.
   The colour of iris may be brown, blue, or pink (due to blood) or black.

Arterial supply:

Long posterior ciliary arteries and **anterior ciliary arteries.**

Both are branches of ophthalmic arteries.

They form two arterial circles in the iris.

1. Major arterial circle of iris: Arterial circle formed by the joining of above two sets of arteries at the periphery of iris. (Fig. 19.5)

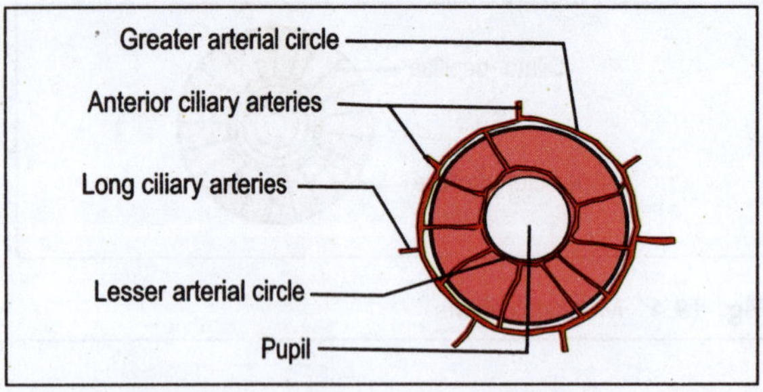

Fig. 19.5: Arteries of iris

2. Minor arterial circle of iris: It is an arterial circle at the margin of the pupil and formed by the vessels which pass from the major circle in the iris radially towards the margins of pupil.

Nerve supply:

1. Sympathetic nerve supply dilator pupillae and blood vessels. Long ciliary nerve convey sensory fibres.
2. Parasympathetic fibres supply the sphincter pupillae.

INNER NERVOUS COAT

RETINA

It is the innermost, neural and sensory tunic of the eyeball and forms reception area for visual impression.

Surface:

1. External: Attached to choroid.
2. Internal: In contact with hyaloid membrane of the vitreous body.

Texture: Very thin and delicate and varies from 0.56mm near the optic disc to 0.1mm near the equator.

Continuity: Posteriorly it is continuous with optic nerve and anteriorly ora serrata, where nervous part ends and from here it (non nervous pigmented layer with deeper epithelium) is continuous with back of the ciliary processes and iris. Thus retina forms three different parts:

1. **Optic part**: Nervous part and is sensitive to light. This part lies behind ora serrata and extends from optic disc behind to ora serrata in front.
2. **Ciliary part**: The part of retina (*non nervous part*) *behind to back of the ciliary processes.*
3. **Iridial part**: It is also *non-nervous part behind to iris in front.*

Both *ciliary and iridial part of retina are non-nervous and so insensitive to light.*

Ora serrata: It is the junctional region between nervous and nonnervous part of retina.

Colour: Purple tint due to rhodopsin or visual purple but become bleached when exposed to light and becomes clouded and opaque.

Structure of retina

Structurally it consists of ten layers from outside inwards–

1. **Pigmented epithelium**: It consist of single layer of cuboidal cells, resting on basal lamina of choroid. Cytoplasm contain melanin pigments. Cytoplasmic infoldings are there in basal region & microvilli are present in the apical area towards rods & cones outer segment. (Fig. 19.6)

   Functions:

   a) Absorbs light & prevent reflection.

   b) Provide nutrition to avascular outer zone of retina (3-4 layer) by diffusion.

2. **Layer of light receptors i.e., rods and cones:**

   Rods and cones:

   a) Rods & cones are photoreceptor.

   b) Rods response to dim light & cones response to bright light.

3. **External limiting membrane**: It is a membrane perforated by central processes of rods and cones.
4. **Outer nuclear layer**: Contains nuclei and central processes of rods and cones.
5. **Outer plexiform**: Here rod spherules and cone pedicles synapse with bipolar & horizontal cells.
6. **Inner nuclear layer:** Contain cell bodies of bipolar cells which from the first neurone of visual pathway. It also contain cell bodies horizontal cells, amacrine cells & Muller's cells.

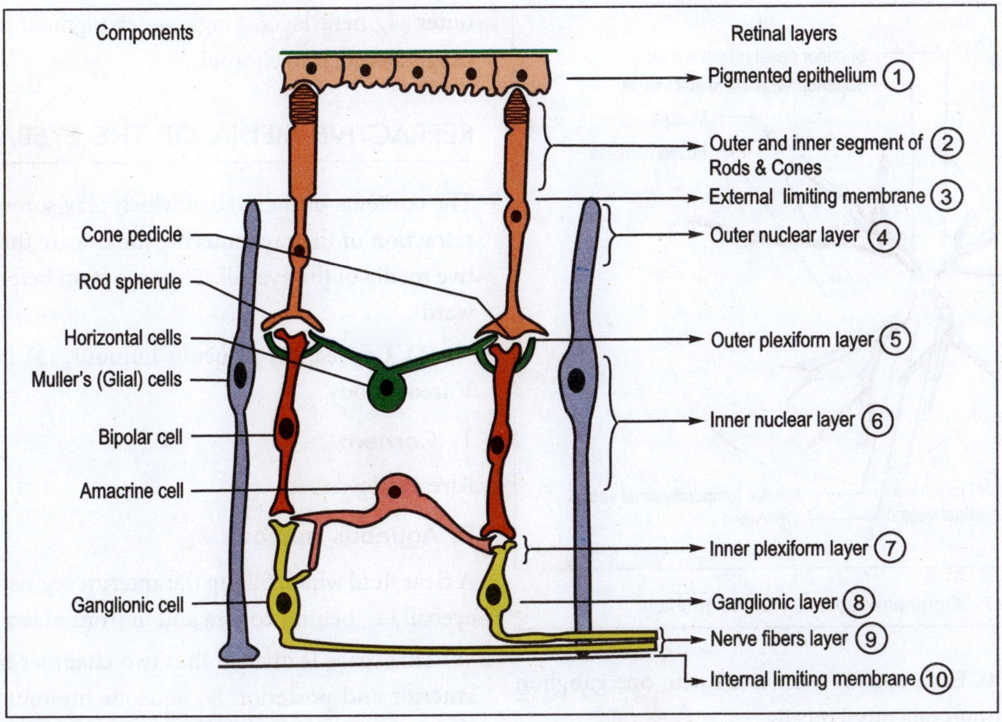

Fig. 19.6: Retinal layers

7. **Inner plexiform**: An acellular layer and zone of arborisation of bipolar and ganglion cells. In this layer, synapse among the bipolar, amacrine and ganglion cells can be seen.
8. **Ganglion cell layer**: Contain cell bodies of ganglion which form second order neurones of visual path.
9. **Stratum opticum**: Consists of nerve fibres which are the axons of ganglion cells and form optic nerve.
10. **Internal limiting membrane**: It is formed by junctional complexes of inner ends of Muller's cells (in between retina and vitreous body).

Functionally three sets of neurons in longitudinal column (from outside inwards):

a) Rods & cones and their process occupy 2nd to 5th layer.

b) Bipolar cells with denarites and axons occupy 5th to 7th layers.

c) Ganglion cells and their axons are placed in 8th & 9th layer.

Integration of these cells with horizontal cells & amacrine cells.

Muller's cells support all the neurons.

Structures seen through an ophthalmoscope (Fig. 19.7)

1. **Macula lutea**: An oval yellowish area in the centre of posterior part of retina (posterior pole). It is free of blood vessels. It is about 3mm lateral to optic disc yellow colour is due to presence of xanthophyll pigment. Measurement: Horizontally – 2mm; Vertically – 1mm.
2. **Fovea centralis**: Central depressed region of macula lutea. It is the thinner part of retina and area for acute vision. Rods are absent and only cones are present in this area. It is about 0.4mm in diameter. Bottom of fovea centralis is known as foveola. Number of cones in this area is about

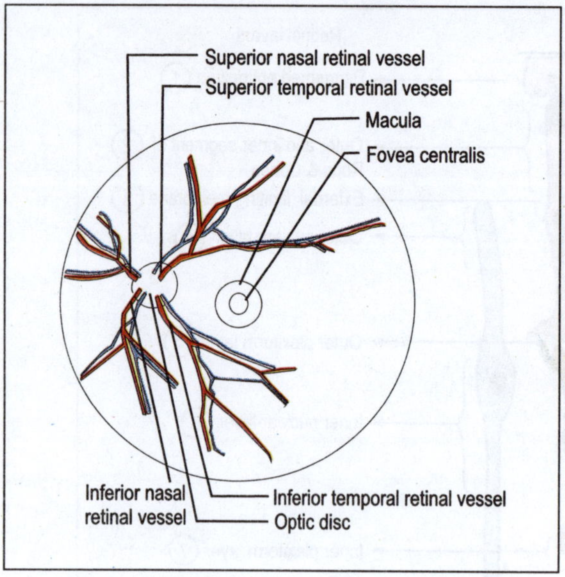

Fig. 19.7: Ophthalmoscopic view of retina

4000. Each cone is connected with one ganglion through one bipolar cells.

3. **Optic disc**: It is the area of retina which lies 3mm *to the nasal side of macula lutea* (posterior pole) and where *optic nerve pierces* the retina.

   Diameter is 1.5mm. The circumference of the area is raised and the central part is depressed and produces "*physiological cup*". It is *pierced by central artery and vein of retina*. It is *insensitive to light* due to *absence of rods and cones*. So it is also known as **blind spot**.

Blood supply of retina

Retina is interposed between two sets of arteries and veins.

These two sets are:

1. Ciliary vessels of choroid.
2. Central artery and vein of retina.

Lymphatics: Exist but is doubtful about their emergence.

APPLIED ANATOMY:

Detachment of retina – A condition in which inner nine nervous layer of retina is separated from single outer pigment layer. Single outer pigment layer remains attached to choroid.

REFRACTIVE MEDIA OF THE EYEBALL

The contents of the eyeball which play some part in refraction of the rays entering the eye are the refractive media of the eyeball. They are from before backwards.

(1) Cornea, (2) Aqueous humour, (3) Lens, (4) Vitreous body.

1. Cornea:

Already described.

2. Aqueous humour:

A clear fluid which fills up the anterior segment of the eyeball i.e., behind cornea and in front of lens.

This space is divided into two chamber by iris—anterior and posterior. So aqueous humour fills up both anterior and posterior chambers which communicate with each other through pupil.

Quantity: Small.

Formation: By active transport and diffusion from the capillaries of the ciliary processes.

Circulation: After being formed by ciliary processes it at first fills up the posterior chamber from there is passes to anterior chamber through the pupil. Then form the iridocorneal angle of anterior chamber it passes through the spaces of the angle (i.e., spaces of fontana between the fibres of ligamentum pectinatum) and the canal of Schlemm (sinus venosus sclerae), and finally drains into the anterior ciliary veins. (Fig. 19.8)

Composition: (1) Ascorbic acid (high concentration, (2) Glucose, (3) Amino acid.

Conclusions:

1. It *nourishes the avascular tissue like lens and cornea.*
2. *Maintains intraocular pressure* and thereby *maintains constancy of the optical dimensions of the eyeball.*

Normal intraocular pressure: 15 to 20mm Hg.

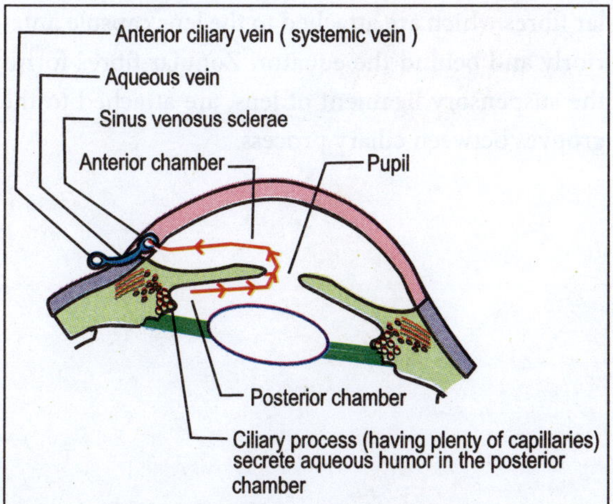

Fig. 19.8: Red line indicate the pathway of aqueous humour

APPLIED ANATOMY

Glaucoma: Due to increased intraocular tension by interference in the drainage of aqueous humour into the canal of Schlemm. This condition will produce cupping of the optic disc and followed by pressure atrophy of retina which will result in blindness.

The interference in the drainage may be due to adhesion between iris and lens. In that case iridectomy may reestablish flow of aqueous humour from posterior chamber to the anterior chamber.

3. Lens

It is a transparent, biconvex structure which lies in between iris & vitreous body. The average diameter of the lens is above 1cm.

1. It presents anterior & posterior surfaces. Equator is the marginal circumference. Anterior surface is flattened & posterior surface is convex.
2. Central point of both surfaces are the poles.

   Axis of the lens passes through poles.

Structure: It consists of capsule, anterior epithelium and lens fibres.

1. **Lens capsule:** It is transparent elastic membrane.
2. **Anterior epithelium**: Beneath the capsule the anterior surface of the lens is lined by a single layer of cuboidal cells.
3. Amorphous substance
4. **Lens fibres:**
   a) Fibres of outer laminae are nucleated and equatorially form a nuclear layer (recently formed). Deeper fibres are nonnucleated (old) and serrated.
   b) Total number of fibres (cells) is estimated to be about 2000 in adult.
   c) They contain crystallins (semistiff transparent proteins).

Clinical notes: The lens plays a big role in accommodation & absorb ultraviolet rays. As age advances power of accommodation decreases, the condition called presbyopia.

Opacity of the lens is known as cataract.

Suspensory ligaments of lens: The ligament extend from the ciliary process to the anterior surface & periphery of the lens. Ligament keep the lens in position, and ligament also keep the lens flattened. Ligaments are also attached to the lens behind the equator. (Fig. 19.9)

4. Vitreous body:

It is a transparent, jelly like mass occupying posterior 4/5th of eyeball. It is having 99% of water, some salts, collagen fibrils, and hyaluronic acid. A narrow hyaloid canal from optic disc through the body to the posterior surface of the lens. The vitreous body is covered by delicate and transparent hyaloid membrane.

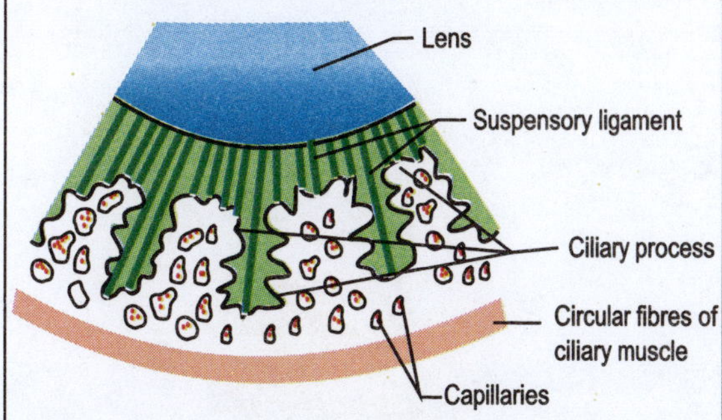

Fig. 19.9: Schematic diagram showing suspensory ligament

Anteriorly the membrane forms a depression, hyaloid fossa, upon which lens rest. In this region the membrane is having series of furrows into which ciliary processes can be seen. Anterior layer form zonular fibres which are attached to the lens capsule anteriorly and behind the equator. Zonular fibres forms the suspensory ligament of lens, are attached to the grooves between ciliary process.

chapter 20

CRANIAL NERVES

AT A GLANCE

- *Olfactory nerve*
- *Optic nerve*
- *Oculomotor nerve*
- *Trochlear nerve*
- *Trigeminal nerve*
  – *Maxillary nerve*
  – *Mandibular nerve*
  – *Ophthalmic nerve*
- *Abducent nerve*
- *Facial nerve*
- *Vestibulo cochlear nerve*
- *Glossopharyngeal nerve*
- *Vagus nerve*
- *Accessory nerve*
- *Hypoglossal nerve*
- *Glossopharyngeal nerve*
- *Vagus nerve*
- *Accessory nerve*
- *Hypoglossal nerve*

OLFACTORY NERVE

Definition: It is the first cranial nerve and nerve of smell and form first order neuron of olfactory pathway.

Type: Special sensory type.

Functional component: *Special somatic afferent (SSA)* fibres: The fibres carry sensation of smell from olfactory region of nasal cavity.

Origin: From olfactory epithelium in (Fig. 20.1) olfactory region of nasal cavity (superior nasal concha and opposed part of nasal septum).

[Olfactory epithelium consists of bipolar (Fig. 20.2) cells supported by sustentacular cells periphery processes from olfactory hairs which are stimulated by volatile smell sensations dissolved by mucus. Central processes or axons of the cells form olfactory nerves].

So olfactory nerves consists of 15 to 20 bundles on each side and formed from the axons or central processes of olfactory cells.

Course: After origin they pass through the cribriform plate of the ethmoid bone and within the cranial cavity they end.

Termination: They terminate by forming synaptic glomeruli with mitral cells of olfactory bulb where second neuron starts.

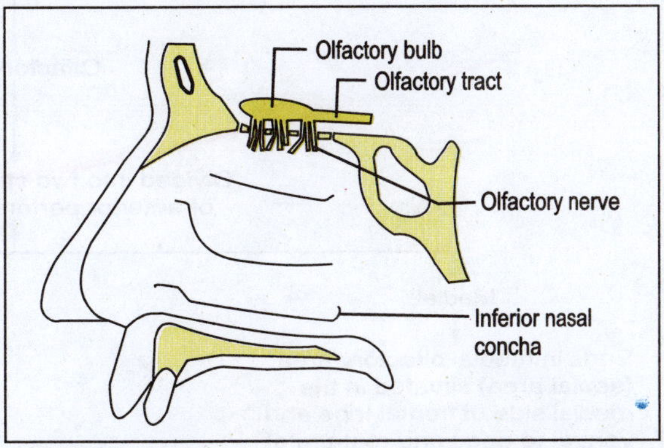

Fig. 20.1: Olfactory nerves in the lateral wall of nasal cavity

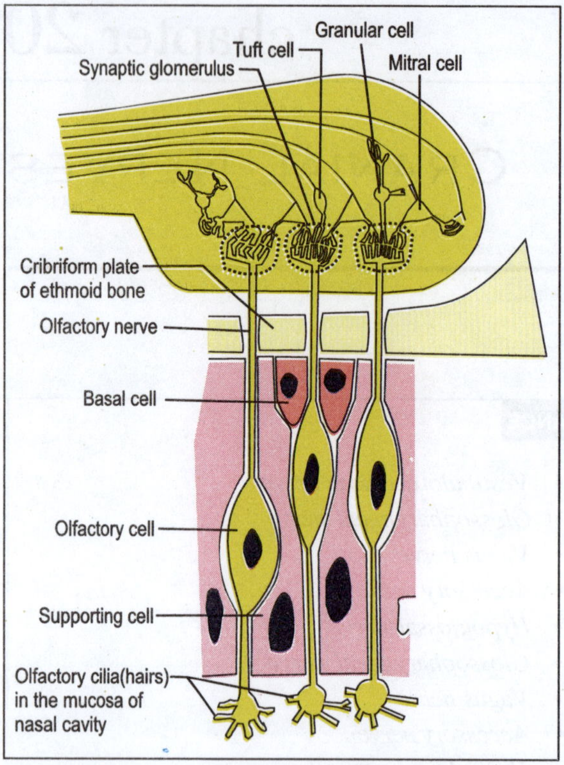

Fig. 20.2: Olfactory cell in olfactory bulb

Characteristic: These nerves are provided with meningeal sheaths (Dura, arachnoid and pia mater).

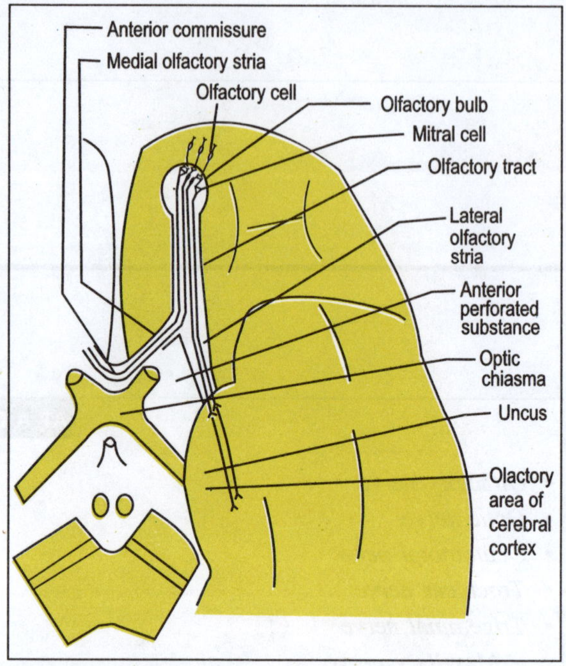

Fig. 20.3: Olfactory pathway

Olfactory Pathway

Olfactory pathway consists of olfactory nerves, olfactory bulbs, olfactory tracts and striae ending in septal area in paraterminal gyrus and pyriform area.

Bipolar olfactory nerve cells

↓

Olfactory nerves (axons of the cells)

↓ **(Passes through cribriform plate of ethmoid bone)**

Olfactory bulb

↓ **(Neurons end and form synaptic glomeruli with mitral cells)**

Olfactory tract

↓ **(Anterior olfactory nucleus – collection of cells along the tract and axons contribute in forming the tract. It receives axons from mitral cells)**

Divided into two striae in the region of anterior perforated substance

↓

Medial

↓

Ends in medial olfactory area (septal area) situated in the medial side of frontal lobe and ventral to genu and rostrum of corpus callosum. It is the par olfactory area and contain septal nuclei.

Lateral

↓

Ends in pyriform area (lobe), which consists of uncus, Limen insulae and entorhinal area. It is also known as primary olfactory cortex (Fig. 20.3) function is perception of smell.

APPLIED ANATOMY:

Anosmia: Due to several reasons (atrophic rhinitis etc.) there may be loss of sensa of smell.

OPTIC NERVE

It is the second cranial and is nerve of vision.

Type: Special sensory type.

Functional components:

1. **Special somatic afferent** (SSA)
2. Afferents for visual reflex
3. Few afferents.

Characteristics: It is not a true peripheral nerve. Because:

1. It is an outgrowth of brain.
2. It is covered by three layers of meninges and subarachnoid space is prolonged into it.
3. It gets rich blood supply as vascular pial sheath gives numerous septa into the substance of the nerve.

Measurements:

Total length: 4cm

Intraorbital part: 25mm

Part within optic canal: 5mm

Intracranial part: 10mm.

Origin: Its fibres origin from ganglionic layer of retina and form optic nerve.

Emergence: Fibres after being originated, converge in the optic disc, and pierce the choroid and sclera of eyeball about 3mm towards the nasal side from fovea centralis.

Course: After emerging out of the eyeball it passes through the orbit for a short course and enters the cranial cavity by passing through the optic canal.

End: It ends by uniting with the fellow of the opposite side and forming optic chiasma.

Different parts: So its course can be divided into **three parts**:

1. On the orbital cavity: Intraorbital part, (25mm)
2. Within optic canal
3. In the cranial cavity: Intracranial part.

1. **Intraorbital part**: The part of optic nerve lying within the orbit and extends from posterior pole of eyeball to **optic canal**. Length – 25mm.
2. In the optic canal

   Length : 5mm

   Here,

   a) Ophthalmic artery lies below and lateral to nerve.

   b) Nerve is separated from sphenoidal and posterior ethmoidal air sinus by a thin plate of bone.
3. **Intracranial part**: It runs backwards and medially from the optic canal to optic chiasma.

   Length: about 10mm

The fibres in optic nerve are arranged in the same positions as they took origin from four quadrants of retina.

Optic Chiasma

It is a flattened bundle of nerve fibres.

Situation: Above the body of sphenoid bone at the junction of anterior wall & floor of third ventricle.

Shape: Quadrilateral

Continuity: Anterolaterally with optic nerve & posterolaterally with optic tracts.

Relations:

1. Above: Third ventricle, lamina terminalis, optic recess & crossed by anterior communicating artery.
2. Below: Diaphragm sellae near optic groove.
3. Posteriorly: Tuber cinerium & infundibulum.
4. Laterally: Internal carotid artery & anterior perforated substance.
5. Postero-inferior: Pituitary gland.
6. Anterior: Lamina terminalis, anterior communicating artery.

Components:

1. Fibres from nasal half of each retina including nasal half of macula lutea cross the median plane and enter the optic tract of opposite side.
2. Fibres from temporal half of retina do not cross but pass backwards in the optic tract laterally and above.

Arterial supply: Optic chiasma is supplied by

branches of anterior cerebral, internal carotid, middle cerebral arteries, and posterior communicating artery.

Optic Tract

Origin: From the posterolateral end of optic chiasma.

Components: Ipsilateral temporal fibres & contralateral nasal fibres.

Course: It passes backwards along the anterolateral boundary of the interpeduncular fossa and crosses the cerebral peduncle to end in lateral geniculate body, & few fibres end in superior colliculus through superior brachium.

Arterial supply: Optic tract is supplied by branches of anterior choroidal, middle cerebral & posterior communicating arteries.

Lateral geniculate body (LGB)

It is ovoid (collection of grey matter) postero-inferior to pulvinar part of thalamus. The grey matter of LGB is having six layers from ventral to dorsal side. Neurons in the layers 1, 4 & 6 receives contralateral nasal fibres, where as neurons of layers 2, 3 & 5 receives ipsilateral temporal fibers. A few fibers retinotectal fibers passes through LGB without relaying to pretactal nucleus and superior colliculi through superior brachium.

The axons of neurons in LGB form optic radiation to terminate in visual cortex.

Arterial supply: Lateral geniculate body is supplied by branches of posterior cerebral and posterior chovoidal artery.

Optic radiation

Origin: From lateral geniculate body.

Termination: Visual cortex of occipital lobe.

Course: Passes through retrolenticular part of internal capsule.

Upper fibres (carrying information from upper halves of both retinae) terminate in upper anterior part of calcarine sulcus.

Lower fibres (carrying information from lower halves of both retinae) terminate below the calcarine sulcus. The fibres lies in relation to roof of the inferior horn of lateral ventricle. The fibres form a loop (Meyer's loop) anteriorly in temporal lobe.

Macular fibres (located in the centre of optic radiation) terminate in posterior most part of visual cortex.

Arterial supply: Optic radiation is supplied by branches of anterior choroidal artery, middle & posterior cerebral arteries.

Visual cortex

Visual cortex or striate cortex (area 17 of Broadmann) is in depths of calcarine sulcus. Upper lip of calcarine sulcus receive information from upper quadrant of retina & lower lip of calcarine sulcus receives information from lower quadrant of retina. Occipital pole receives from macular fibres.

Arterial supply: Visual cortex is supplied by branches of posterior & middle cerebral arteries.

Visual pathway

It is functionally concerned for receptions, transmission and perception of visual impulses. It consists of

1. **Retina**: Three layers of cells concerned for initiation and transmission of visual impulses. They are
   a) Rods (for dim vision at the periphery) and cones (for acuity of vision);
   b) Bipolar cells.
   c) Ganglion cells.
2. **Optic nerve**: (Formed by axons of ganglion cells).
   ↓
3. **Optic chiasma**
   ↓
4. **Optic tract**
   ↓
5. **Lateral geniculate body**
   ↓
6. **Optic radiation.** (Fig. 20.4)
   ↓
7. **Visual cortex in occipital lobe (area 17 - striate area)** (Fig. 20.5): Here size, shape, colour etc., are received. **Parastriate and peristriate** (visual association areas are 18, 19) will interpret the impressions received in the light of past experience.

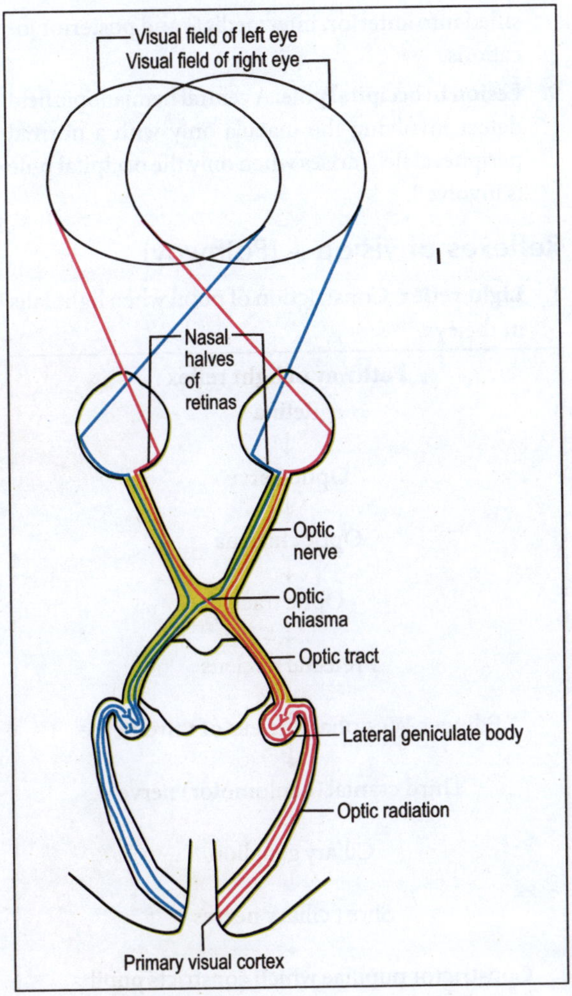

Fig. 20.4: Optic pathway

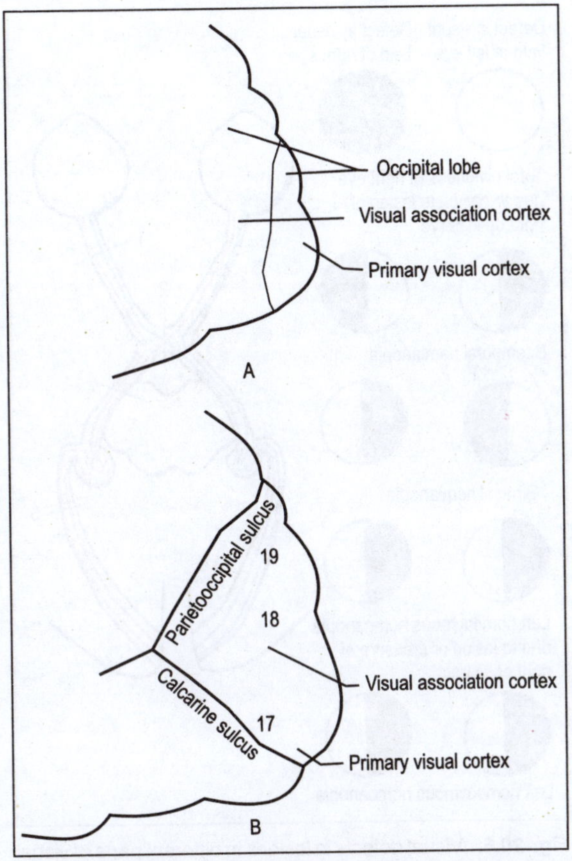

Fig. 20.5: (A) Lateral aspect of occipital lobe; (B) Medial aspect of occipital lobe

Lesion of different parts of pathways and effects

1. **Retina**: Scotoma (blind spots in certain parts)
2. **Optic nerve**: Due to injury and effect is blindness. Tumour of the base of the frontal lobe may involve the optic nerve with following manifestations:
   a) Atrophy of optic nerve on the effected side.
   b) Optic disc may be involved on the normal side due to increased pressure in cerebrospinal fluid.
   c) Central scotoma in the ipsilateral eye
   d) Anosmia ipsilaterally

   The condition is known as **Foster Kennedy Syndrome**, which is due to optic nerve compression, olfactory nerve compression. There may be memory loss and emotional lability (i.e. frontal lobe signs).
3. **Optic chiasma**:
   a) **Central part**: Bitemporal hemianopia (due to pressure on optic chiasma in the midline by tumour of pituitary gland)
   b) **Peripheral part (both side)**: Binasal hemianopia.

   (Hemianopia is loss of vision in one half of field of vision)
4. Complete injury to optic tract, geniculate body, optic radiation and visual cortex of one side loss of field of vision of opposite side such as if lesion is on left side then it will result in right homonymous hemianopia.

   Hemianopia means loss in one half of field vision (right or left). (Fig. 20.6)

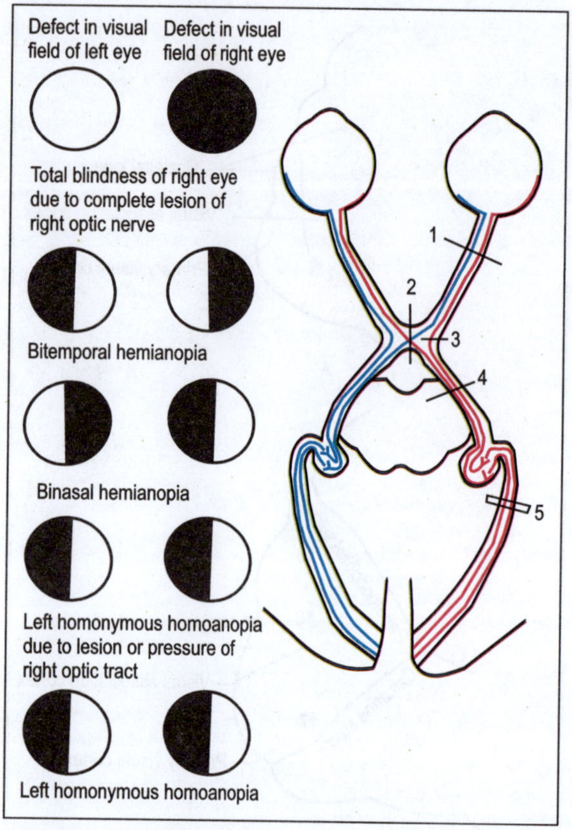

Fig. 20.6: Visual defects in lesions in different parts of visual pathway

Homonymous when same half of field of vision of both the eyes are affected.

Heteronymous when different halves of field of vision are affected.

5. **Lesion in optic tract**: Lesion of left optic tract leads to right homonymous hemianopia. Pupillary reflex absent.
6. **Lesion of lateral geniculate body**: Leads to contralateral homonymous hemianopia.
7. **Lesion of optic radiation**: Upper fibers of optic radiation involvement lead to contralateral inferior quadrantic hemianopia.
   Lower fibers (including Meyer's loop) involvement leads to contralateral superior quadrantic hemianopia.
8. **Lesion of visual cortex**: Involvement of posterior cerebral artery leads to contralateral homonymous hemianopia. Lesions of striate cortex can be classified into anterior, intermediate and posterior locations.
9. **Lesion in occipital pole**: A central hemianopic field defect involving the macula only with a normal peripheral field arises when only the occipital pole is involved.

Reflexes of vision – (Pathway)

1. **Light reflex**: Constriction of pupil when light falls in the eye.

Pathway of light reflex

Retina
↓
Optic nerve
↓
Optic chiasma
↓
Optic tract
↓
Pretectal nucleus
↓
Edinger Westphal nucleus of third nerve
↓
Third cranial (oculomotor) nerve
↓
Ciliary ganglion
↓
Short ciliary nerves
↓
Constrictor pupillae which constricts pupil

[Consensual reflex: It is constriction of both the pupil and due to bilateral connection of the pretectal nucleus with both the Edinger Westphal nuclei of the third nerve.]

2. **Accommodation reflex**: Accommodation is adjustment of optical apparatus for near vision and it is a convergent reaction.

   It consists of three actions: (a) Convergence of eye, (b) Constriction of pupil, (c) Lens becomes more convex anteriorly.

Pathway of accommodation

Retina
↓
Optic nerve
↓

Contd........

Optic chiasma
↓
Optic tract
↓
Lateral geniculate body
↓
Optic radiation
↓
Visual area in occipital lobe
↓
Superior longitudinal fasciculus
↓
Superior colliculus, frontal eye filed, Edinger Westphal nucleus of third nerve
↓
For Medial rectus muscle, (Convergence for constriction of pupil) Ciliary ganglion and Sphincter pupillae and Ciliaris muscle for increasing curvature of lens

Argyll Robertson Pupil: It is a condition where light reflex is lost and accommodation reflex is present. It is due to affection on light reflex pathway syphilis.

(**To remember**: A.R.P. – Accommodation Reflex Present).

OCULOMOTOR NERVE

It is the third cranial nerve supplying all the muscles of the eyeball except lateral rectus and superior oblique and also supplies sphincter pupillae and ciliaris muscle.

Functional components & nuclei of origin:

1. **General Somatic Efferent (GSE) fibers**: The fibers arise from main nucleus of **oculomotor nucleus** to supply all the extraocular muscles except lateral rectus (supplied by VIth cranial nerve) and superior oblique (supplied by IVth cranial nerve).
2. **General Visceral Efferent (GVE) fibers**: The fibers arise from Edinger-Westphal nucleus (parasympathetic component) to relay in ciliary ganglion to supply sphincter pupillae and ciliaris muscles.

Origin: (Deep origin or nucleus of origin) Nucleus of the third nerve lies in the grey matter of upper part of cerebral aqueduct of midbrain at the level of superior colliculi.

Course: Divided into two:

A. **Intraneural (part within brain)**;

B. **Extraneural part (outside the brain)**.

A. **Intraneural part**: From the nucleus of origin the fibres pass through the tegmentum, red nucleus and medial part of substantia nigra in a curved manner and finally emerges out of the brain from the medial side of the crus crebri through oculomotor sulcus.

B. **Course outside the brain**: (Fig. 20.7)

1. The fibres of the oculomotor nerve after emerging out of the brain through oculomotor sulcus passes through the pia mater and runs in the subarachnoid space.
2. **In the interpeduncular cistern**: It at first lies between posterior cerebral and superior cerebellar arteries and in the interpeduncular cistern and on the lateral side of posterior communicating artery. While emerging from interpeduncular cistern, it pierces the arachnoid mater.
3. Then the nerve lies in the interval between free and attached margins of terntorium cerebelli.
4. After that it passes lateral to posterior clinoid process and pierces the meningeal dura mater.
5. Then it transverses the lateral wall of the cavernous sinus.

   In the lateral wall of cavernous sinus: Here from above downwards, the structures are:

   a) Oculomotor nerve,
   b) Trochlear nerve
   c) Ophthalmic division of trigeminal nerve.
6. At the anterior part of the cavernous sinus oculomotor nerve divides into superior and inferior division.
7. Finally these two divisions enter the orbit by passing through **superior orbital fissure within common tendinous ring**. In between the two divisions, nasociliary nerve lies and abducent nerve lies lateral to inferior division.
8. **Within orbit**:

   a) The superior division of the oculomotor nerve ascends on the lateral side of optic nerve and lies below the superior rectus. Here it supplies superior rectus muscle and levator palpebrae superioris muscles.

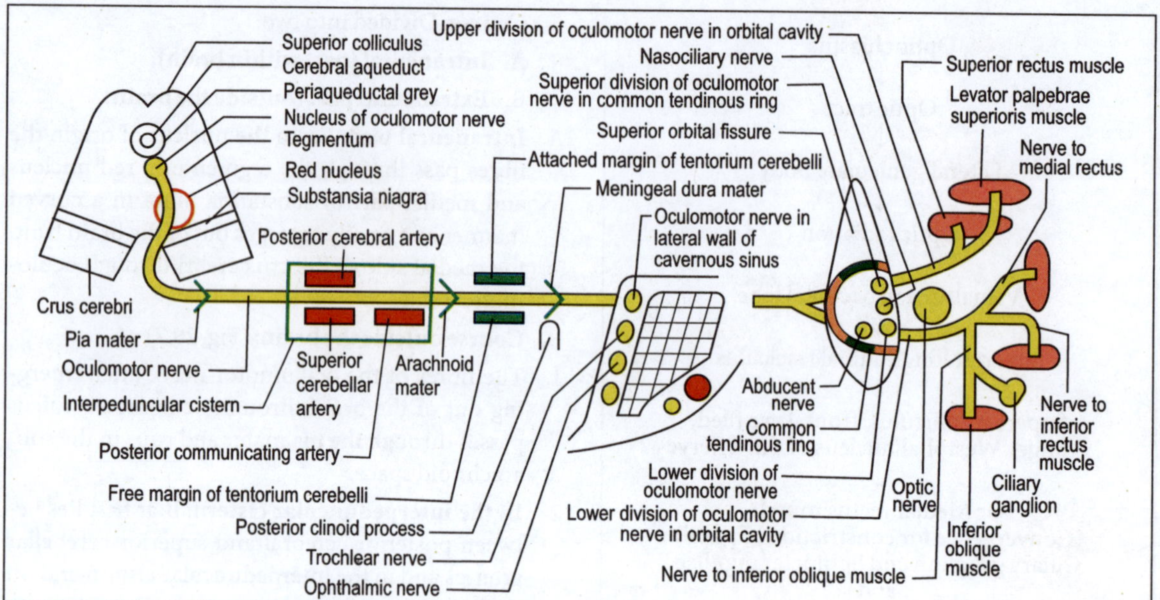

Fig. 20.7: Course, relations & branches of the oculomotor nerve

b) The inferior division lies below the optic nerve and divides into three branches: medial, central & lateral. Medial branch supply medial rectus. Central branch supply inferior rectus. Lateral branch before supplying inferior oblique send a twig to ciliary ganglion.

The twig to the ciliary ganglion carries parasympathetic component for the ciliary ganglion.

APPLIED ANATOMY

Paralysis or injury of oculomotor nerve:

Effects are:

1. **Ptosis**: Drooping of upper eyelid due to paralysis of levator palpebrae superioris.
2. Lateral strabismus (squint) due to unopposed action of lateral rectus (due to paralysis of medial rectus).
3. **Dilatation of pupil** due to paralysis of sphincter pupillae muscle.
4. Loss of accommodation due to paralysis of ciliaris muscle.
5. Slight prominence of eyeball owing to most of the muscles of eyeball being relaxed.
6. Diplopia.
7. **Weber's syndrome.** (Ipsilateral oculomotor nerve palsy & contralateral upper motor neuron paralysis of body due to involvement of corticospinal tract.

The third nerve is usually affected due to syphilitic periarteritis of posterior cerebral and superior cerebellar arteries as the nerve passes between them.

Ciliary ganglion

It is one of the parasympathetic ganglion. It is functionally connected with oculomotor nerve and topographically with nasociliary nerve. **Refer chapter 9 for details.**

TROCHLEAR NERVE

It is the fourth cranial nerve which supplies superior oblique muscle of eyeball.

Type: Motor

Functional components & nuclei of origin:

1. **General Somatic Efferent (GSE)**: The fibers arises from trochlear nucleus in the midbrain (at the level of inferior colliculus) & supply superior oblique muscle.

2. **General Somatic Afferent (GSA)**: The fibers carries propriocaptive fibers from the superior oblique to the mesencephalic nucleus of trigeminal nerve.

Characteristics:

1. Most slender of all cranial nerves.
2. Only cranial nerve which emerges from the dorsal aspect of brain stem.
3. Only cranial nerve which crosses the nerve of the opposite side before emergence from the brain stem.
4. A nerve which supplies only one muscle superior oblique muscle (like abducent nerve supplying later rectus).

Origin (Deep or Nucleus of origin): Nucleus of the trochlear nerve lies in the anterior grey matter part of the cerebral aqueduct at the level of inferior colliculi.

Course:

Intraneural (part within the brain): From the nucleus of origin the nerve runs backwards and laterally in the tegmentum and then turns backwards around the central grey matter towards the dorsal aspect of the brain stem. Here the two nerves cross each other before emergence.

It emerges out below inferior colliculus and on surface of superior medullary velum and on each side of frenulum veli.

Intracranial part: After emerging from the brain it crosses superior medullary velum, superior cerebellar peduncle and winds round crus cerebri and temporal lobe and reaches the ventral aspect. Here it pierces the pia mater. Then the nerve lies in the interpeduncular cistern and passes between posterior cerebral & superior cerebellar arteries. After emerging out of interpeduncular cistern, the nerve pierces arachnoid mater and appears between free and attached margins of tentorium cerebelli. It then pierces duramater on the lateral side of posterior clinoid process.

After that it runs forward in the lateral wall of the cavernous sinus below oculomotor nerve and above ophthalmic and maxillary nerve. Then it enters the orbit by passing through lateral part of superior orbital fissure outside common tendinous ring.

In the orbit it terminates.

Termination: In the orbit it terminates by supplying orbital surface of superior oblique muscle.

APPLIED ANATOMY:

If the nerve is injured, downward and lateral movement of eyeball will not be possible and no difficulty so long the patient looks above the horizontal level. Double vision will occur if he looks downward and the patient has a pathetic look and so this nerve is known as pathetic nerve.

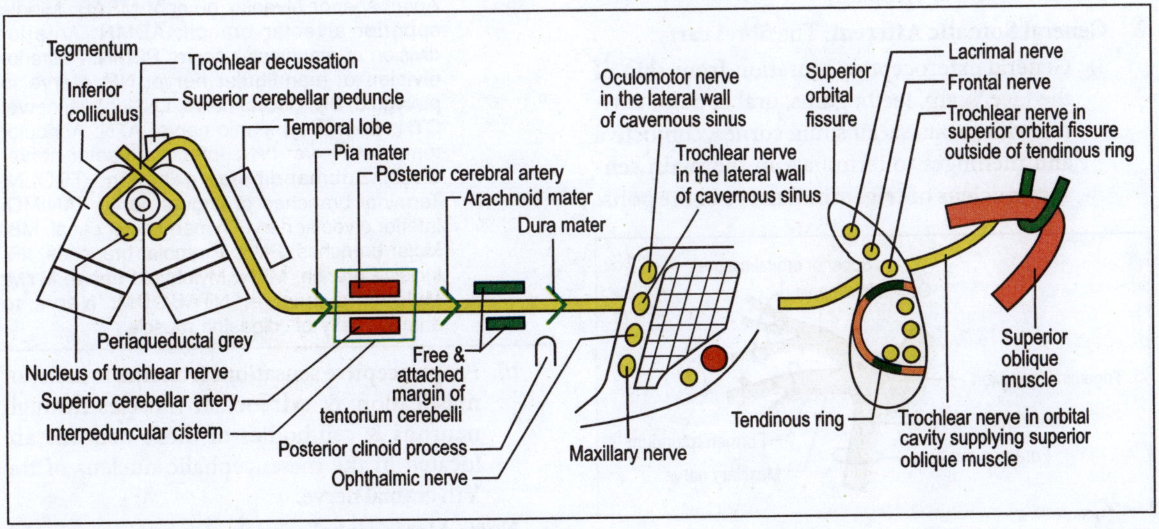

Fig. 20.8: Course, relations & supply of the trochlear nerve

TRIGEMINAL NERVE

The trigeminal nerve is the cranial nerve. It is the fifth cranial nerve.

Functional roots:

1. Large sensory root.
2. Small motor root.

It is having one sensory ganglion (trigeminal ganglion).

Three subdivisions:

1. Ophthalmic nerve (sensory)
2. Maxillary nerve (sensory)
3. Mandibular nerve (mixed)

(**Note**: All the parasympathetic ganglia are linked (Fig. 20.9) with the branches of trigeminal nerve:

a) Ciliary ganglion: Nasociliary branch of ophthalmic nerve)

b) Pherygopalatine ganglion: Maxillary nerve.

c) Otic ganglion: Mandibular nerve.

d) Submandibular ganglion: Lingual branch of mandibular nerve.

Functional components & nuclei of origin:

1. **Special Visceral Efferent (SVE)**: The fibres arises from **motor nucleus** which is situated in the pons and this motor nucleus represent special visceral efferent column. The fibre supply muscles derived from 1st pharyngeal arch (muscles of mastication, mylohyoid anterior belly of digastric, tensor veli palatine & tensor tympani).
2. **General Somatic Afferent**: The fibres carry:
   a) General exteroceptive sensation from skin of the face, scalp, teeth, gums, oral & nasal cavities with paranasal air sinus, cornea, conjuctiva and meninges to terminate in the **main sensory nucleus of trigeminal nerve** in the pons.

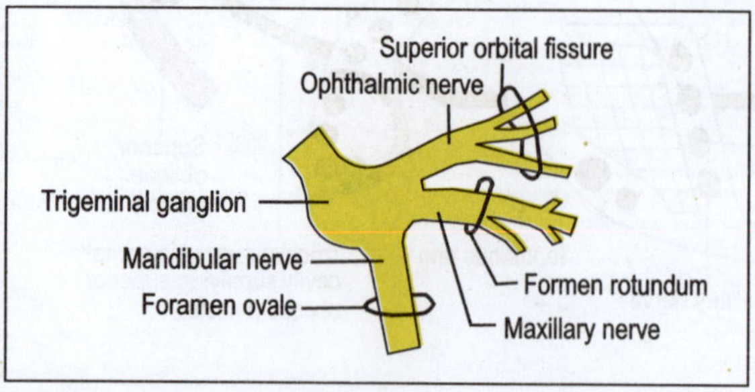

Fig. 20.9: Trigeminal ganglion & branches

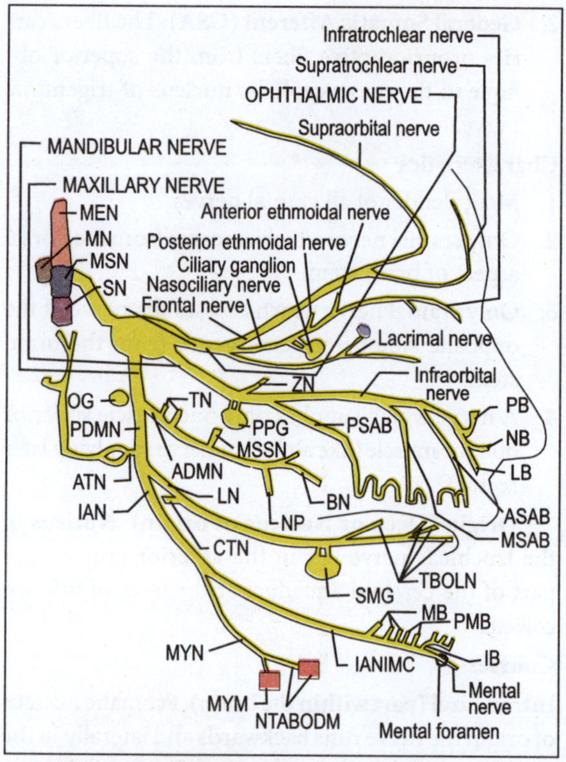

Fig. 20.10: Trigeminal nerve with its branches, MEN: Mesencehalic nucleus in midbrain & pon; MN: Motor nucleus of pons; MSN: Main sensory nucleus pons; SN: Spinal nucleus; OG: Otic ganglion; ZN: Zygomatic nerve; TN: Temporal branches; MSSN: Masseteric nerve; PPG: Pterygopalating ganglion; PSAB: Posterior superior alvelolar nerve; PB: Palpebral branch; NB: Nasal branch; LB: Labial branch; ASAB: Anterosperior alveolar branch; MSAB: Middle superior alveolar branch; ADMN: Anterior division of mandibular nerve; PDMN: Posterior division of mandibular nerve; NP: Nerve to pterygoid, BN: Buccal nerve; LN: Lingual nerve; CTN: Chorda tympanic nerve; ATN: Auriculotemporal nerve; IVN: Inferior alveolar nerve; SMG: Submandibular ganglion; TBOLN: Terminal branches of lingual nerve; IANIMC: Inferior alveolar nerve in mandibular canal; MB: Molar branches; PMB: Premolar branches, IIB: Incisive branch, MYN: Mylohyoid nerve; MYM: Mylohyoid muscle; NTABODM: Nerve to anterior belly of digastric muscle

   b) Proprioceptive sensations from the muscles of mastication, & extraocular muscles through neurons & cell bodies of those neurons are located in the mesencephalic nucleus of the Vth cranial nerve.

Note: Mesencephalic nucleus contains unipolar neuron.

Course, relations & distributions

The nerve emerges from the junction of middle cerebellar peduncle with pons.

When the Vth nerve lies on petrous (apex) temporal bone, the nerve is having ovale enlargement (trigeminal ganglion). The trigeminal ganglion lies on trigeminal fossa.

The ganglion gives origin to ophthalmic, maxillary & mandibular nerve: (Fig. 20.10)

1. The **ophthalmic nerve** (sensory) at once enter the lateral wall of cavernous sinus & then the nerve divides into three branches—lacrimal, frontal & nasociliary. Those three branches enter the orbit through the superior orbital fissure.

   The ophthalmic nerve supplies cornea, conjunctiva, upper eyelid, scalp (anterior part) and nose. **Refer chapter 9.**

2. **Maxillary nerve** (sensory) passes forward in the

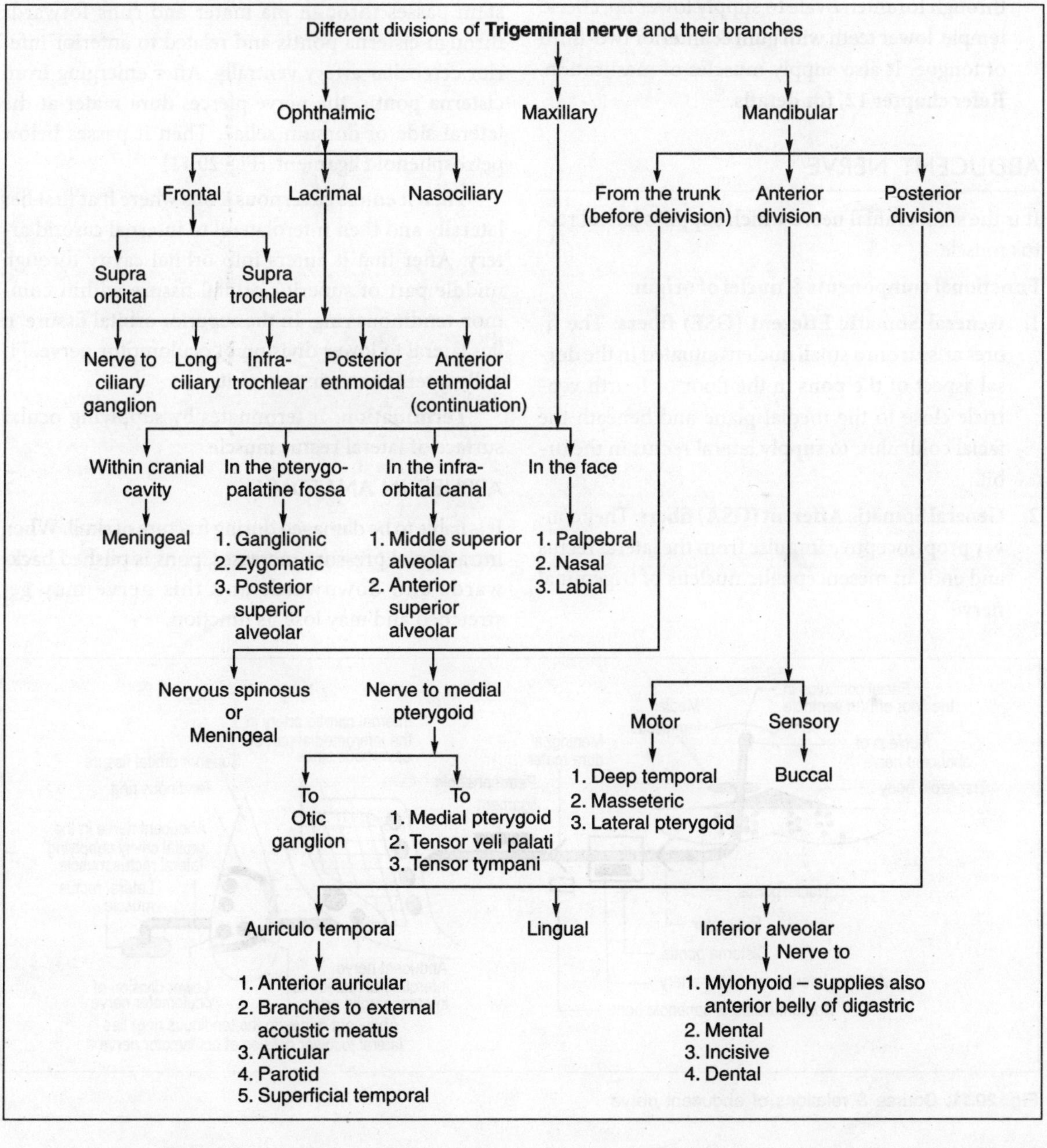

lateral wall of cavernous sinus to the foramen rotundum to enter the pterygopalatine fossa. Then the nerve passes through the infraorbital fissure, infraorbital groove and infraorbital canal to emerge through infraorbital foramen. **Refer chapter 12.**

The maxillary nerve supplies skin of cheek, nose, upper lip, upper teeth & gum and maxilla.

3. **Mandibular nerve** (mixed): The nerve passes through foramen ovale to supply lower lip, cheek, temple, lower teeth with gum & anterior two-third of tongue. It also supply muscles of mastication. **Refer chapter 12, for details.**

ABDUCENT NERVE

It is the sixth cranial nerve which supplies lateral rectus muscle.

Functional components & nuclei of origin:

1. **General Somatic Efferent (GSE) fibers**: The fibres arise from a small nucleus situated in the dorsal aspect of the pons in the floor or fourth ventricle close to the medial plane and beneath the facial colliculus, to supply lateral rectus in the orbit.
2. **General Somatic Afferent (GSA) fibers**: They convey proprioceptive impulse from the lateral rectus and ends in mesencephalic nucleus of trigeminal nerve.

Facial colliculus: An elevation in the floor of fourth ventricle due to hooking of seventh cranial nerve underlying **nucleus of abducent nerve.**

Course within brain and superficial origin: The fibres after arising from the nucleus passes through medial lemniscus, trapezoid body and nuclei pontis and emerge at the furrow between lower border of pons and pyramid of medulla oblongata.

Course: The abducent nerve after leaving the brain stem passes through pia mater and runs forwards through cisterna pontis and related to anterior inferior cerebellar artery ventrally. After emerging from cisterna pontis, the nerve pierces dura mater at the lateral side of dorsum sellae. Then it passes below petrosphenoid ligament. (Fig. 20.11)

Then it enters cavernous sinus where it at first lies laterally and then inferolateral to internal carotid artery. After that it enters into orbital cavity through middle part of superior orbital fissure within common tendinous ring. In the superior orbital fissure, it lies lateral to lower division of oculomotor nerve. Finally it terminates in the orbit.

Termination: It terminates by supplying ocular surface of lateral rectus muscle.

APPLIED IN ANATOMY:

It is liable to be damaged during fracture of skull. When intracranial pressure increases, pons is pushed backwards and downwards and this nerve may get stretched and may lose its function.

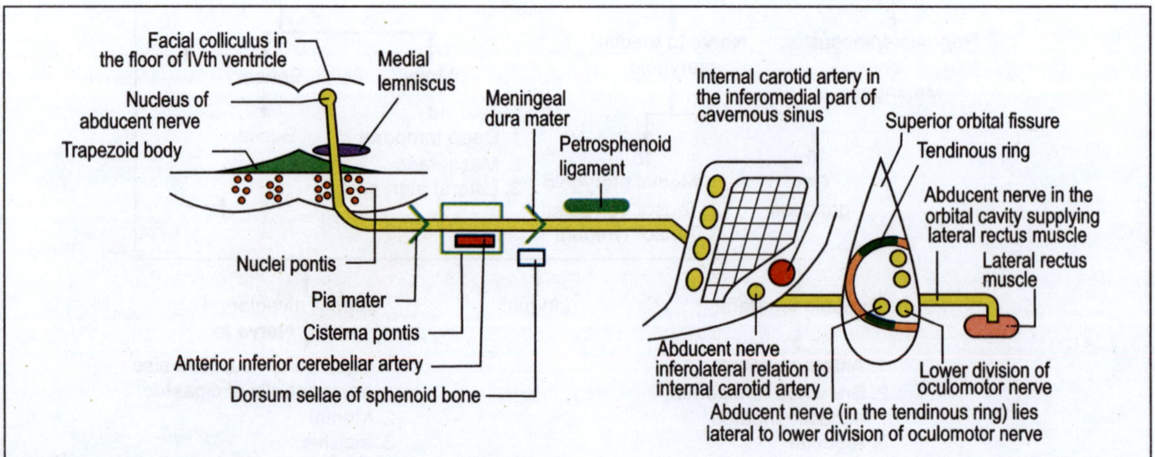

Fig. 20.11: Course & relations of abducent nerve

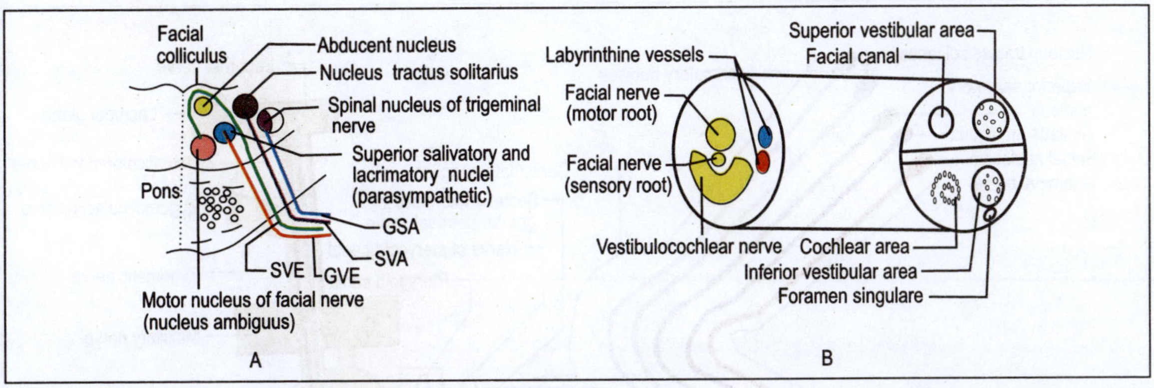

Fig. 20.12: A – Functional components and nuclei of origin of facial nerve; B – Facial nerve in internal acoustic meatus

Effects of paralysis:

1. Convergent squint due to unopposed action of medial rectus.
2. Often diplopia with convergent squint will be present.

FACIAL NERVE

The facial nerve (VII cranial nerve) consist of motor & sensory root (nervus intermedius).

Functional components & nuclei of origin:

1. **Special Visceral Efferent (SVE)** or **Branchial Efferent (BE) fibres**: It arises from **nucleus ambiguus** & supply the muscles of facial expression which are developed from second branchial apparatus.
2. **General Visceral Efferent (GVE)** fibres: They (preganglionic fibres) arise from **lacrimatory nucleus** & **superior salivatory nucleus** to supply secretomotor fibers to lacrimal gland, submandibular gland and sublingual glands. (Fig. 20.12)
3. **Special Visceral Afferent (SVA)** fibres: They carry taste sensations from the anterior two-thirds of tongue (except vallate papillae) and soft palate to **nucleus tractus solitaries.**
4. **General Somatic Afferent (GSA)** fibres: The fibres carry general sensation from skin of the auricle to the spinal nucleus of trigeminal nerve. (Fig. 20.13)

Course & relations:

Intraneural course

The motor fibres from the motor nucleus run posteromedially to abducent nucleus & then posterior to abducent nucleus occupying the facial colliculus of the floor of the fourth ventricle. Then the fibres run lateral to abducent nucleus. The fibres emerge at the junction of pontomedullary junction between olive & inferior cerebellar peduncle. At the same site sensory fibres emerge.

Course in the posterior cranial cavity

It emerges from brainstem. It proceeds towards internal acoustic meatus. Facial nerve with its two roots lie on the groove of vestibulocochlear nerve. Motor root is large and sensory root is smaller. Sensory root lie in between motor root & vestibulocochlear nerve in the internal acoustic meatus. Labyrinthin vessels also accompany them. At the lateral end of internal acoustic meatus two roots unit to form trunk of facial nerve.

Intracranial – intrapetrous part:

At the bottom of the meatus (internal) both roots (motor & sensory) unite to form trunk of facial nerve which passes through facial canal.

The course in the facial canal is divided into three segments:

1. **First part or vestibular or labyrinthine segment**: The facial canal lies in the anterior part of roof of vestibule of inner ear to reach the medial wall of the middle ear. (Fig. 20.14)
2. **Second or tympanic segment**: Here the facial canal takes sharp turn posteriorly. At the site of sharp turn the facial nerve bears geniculate ganglion. The facial nerve passes posteriorly & downwards above

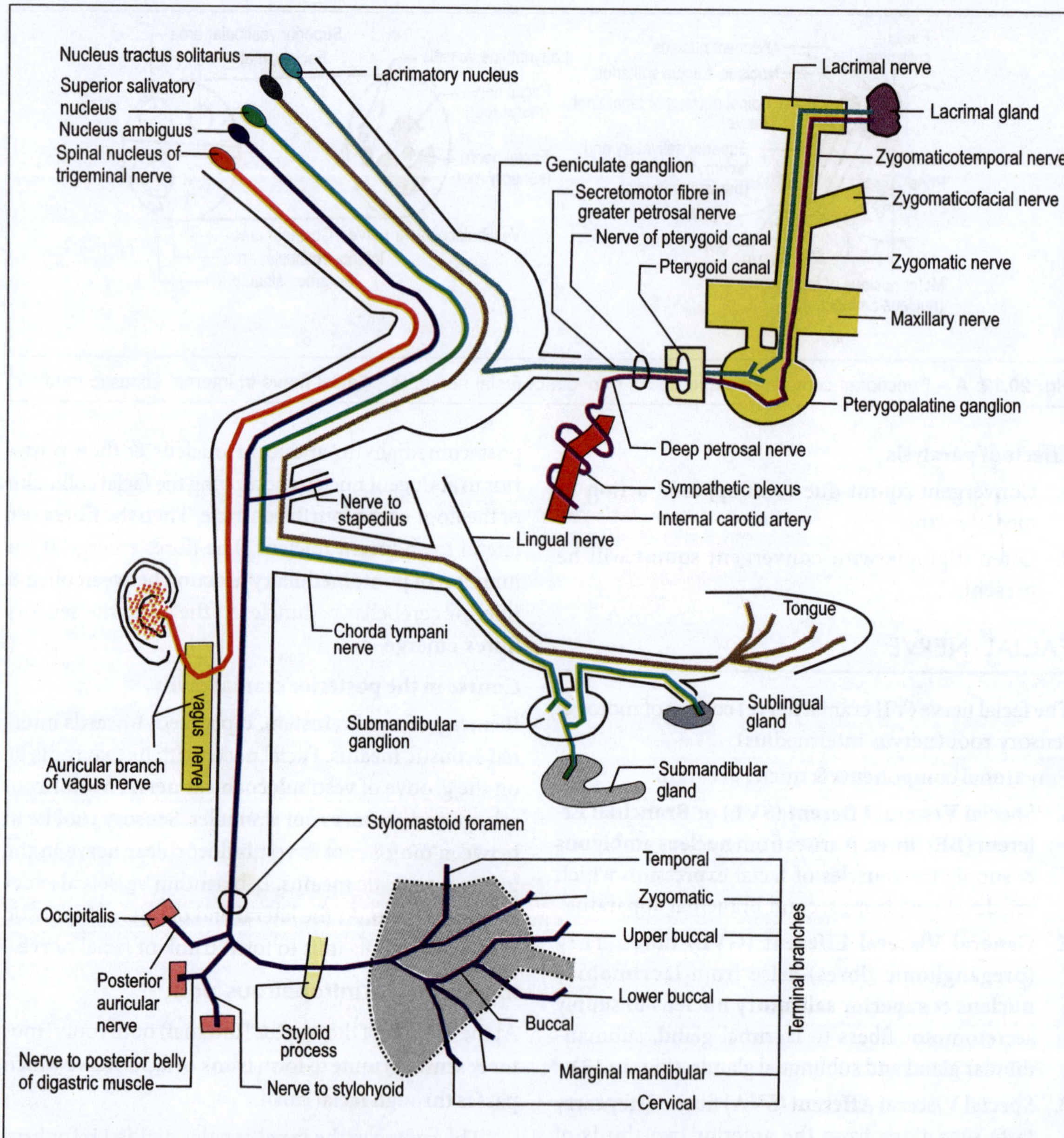

Fig. 20.13: Nuclei of origin & branches of facial nerve

the promontory & fenestra vestibuli to reach the posterior wall of middle ear.

3. **Third or mastoid part (vertical part)**: In the posterior wall of middle ear the facial nerve lies below the aditus to mastoid antrum. Then the facial nerve passes vertically downwards to reach the stylomastoid foramen at the base of skull.

Extracranial course: After exiting from the stylomastoid foramen the facial nerve runs forwards superficial to styloid process and passes through the parotid gland. The nerve gives five terminal branches.

Branches of facial nerve

1. Within the facial canal – a) Greater petrosal nerve;

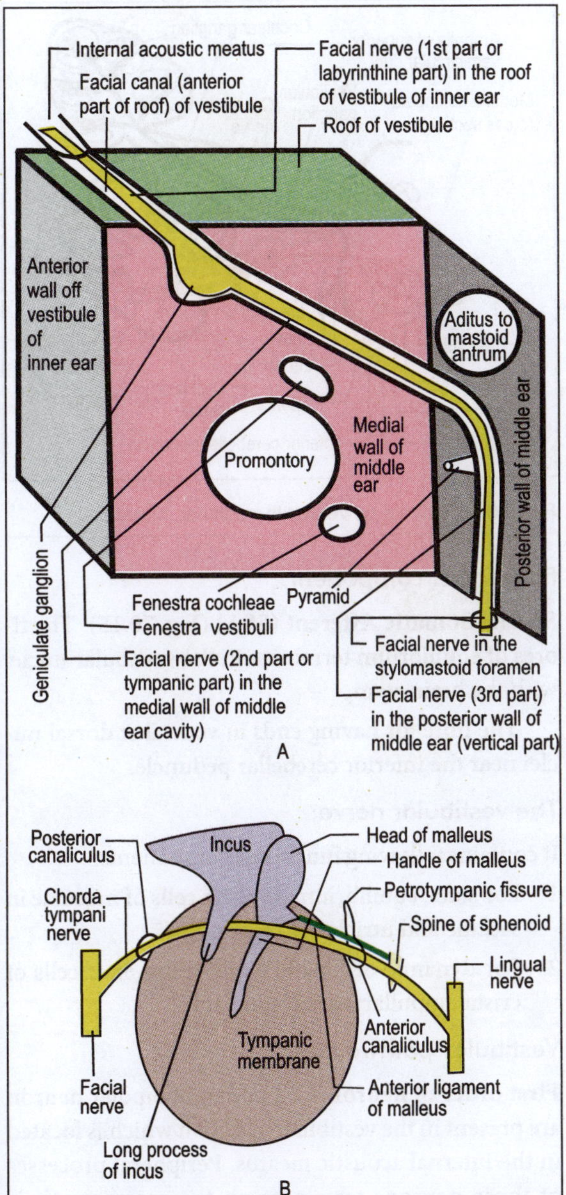

Fig. 20.14: A – Facial nerve in relation to internal & middle ear; B – Chorda tympani nerve

b) The nerve to the stapedius; c) The chorda tympani; d) Communicating branch to auricular branch of vagus.

2. After the exit from stylomastoid foramen

   a) Posterior auricular nerve; b) Digastric; c) Stylohyoid.

3. Terminal branches within parotid gland

   a) Temporal; b) Zygomatic; c) Buccal (upper & lower); d) Marginal mandibular; e) Cervical.

Distributions of branches of facial nerve

1. **From the geniculate ganglion: Greater petrosal nerve** arises from geniculate ganglion. It carries secretomotor fibres (after relaying in pterygopalatine ganglion) to supply lacrimal gland and glands of palate & nose. The greater petrosal nerve is joined by **deep petrosal nerve** to form the nerve of the pterygoid canal. The nerve of pterygoid canal joins with pterygopalatine ganglion.

   The taste fibre for soft palate, passes through greater petrosal nerve, nerve of pterygoid canal, pterygopalatine ganglion (without relaying) & lesser palatine nerve to supply soft palate.

2. **Nerve to stapedius**: It arise from the facial nerve opposite to pyramidal eminence & supplies the stapedius. Injury to this nerve produces hyperacusis.

3. **Chorda tympani nerve**: It arises from facial nerve in the facial canal in the posterior wall of the middle ear. The nerve enters the middle ear cavity through posterior canaliculus & runs forward in the medial surface of the tympanic membrane at the junction of pars tensa & pars flaccida.

   Chorda tympani nerve leaves the middle ear through anterior canaliculus (which lies in the medial part of petrotympanic fissure). In the infratemporal fossa, chorda tympani nerve joins with lingual nerve. It carries taste fibers for anterior 2/3rd tongue except vallate papillae and preganglionic secretomotor fibers for submandibular and sublingual gland.

4. **Communicating branch to auricular branch** of vagus.

5. **Posterior auricular branch** supply occipitalis muscle of occipitofrontalis. It also supply auricularis posterior muscle.

   Muscular branches to posterior belly of digastric & stylohyoid .

6. **Terminal branches**: Refer chapter 2.

APPLIED ANATOMY

Supranuclear paralysis: It involves the upper motor neuron and results in impairment or loss of movements of lower half of face of opposite side. In some individual emotional movements like jokes or distress are lost. Volitional movements are more affected in the affected side.

Nuclear involvement: An injury in the pons near facial colliculus results in lower motor neuron paralysis. It leads to loss of movements in all facial muscles and associated internal strabismus due to involvement of lateral rectus muscle of the eyeball.

Sometimes pontine lesion lead to Millard-Gublar syndrome which results in contralateral hemiplagia & ipsilateral facial palsy.

Infranuclear paralysis: Sings & symptoms of infranuclear lesions depends on the site of the lesions:

1. **Lesions in the internal acoustic meatus**: Lesion at this site produces Bell's palsy (lower motor neuron paralysis of all facial muscles on the affected side) and deafness (due to involvement of vestibulo-cochlear nerve).
2. **Lesion at genu**: Lesion produces diminished lacrimation & salivation from submandibular gland & sublingual gland, reduced taste sensation of anterior two-third of tongue, hyperacusis due to involvement of nerve to stapedius and signs of Bell's palsy.

   During recovery some of the regeneratng salivary fibres may be misdirected & supply as secretomotor fibres to lacrimal gland. In such case there may be paroxysmal lacrimation during eating and this condition is known as **crocodile tear syndrome**.
3. Lesion of facial nerve between genu and pyramidal eminence produce all signs & symptoms as mentioned in (2), except problem of lacrimation & taste sensation from soft palate.
4. An injury of facial nerve

VESTIBULO-COCHLEAR NERVE

It is the VIIth cranial nerve. The vestibulo-cochlear nerve consist of two components—the vestibular nerve for balance and the cochlear nerve for hearing.

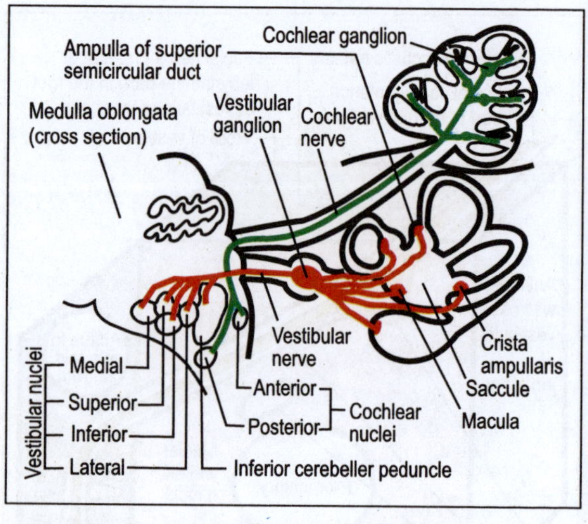

Fig. 20.15: Nuclei of vestibulo-cochlear nerve

Functional component:

Special Somatic Afferent (SSA) (Fig. 20.15): The fibres of equilibrium terminate in the vestibular nuclei with the brain stem.

The fibre for having ends in ventral & dorsal nuclei near the inferior cerebellar peduncle.

The vestibular nerve:

It contains following functional components:

1. For static equilibrium, the hair cells of maculae in saccule and utricle are responsible.
2. For dynamic or kinetic equilibrium, hair cells of crista ampullaris are responsible.

Vestibular pathway:

First order of neuron: Cell bodies of bipolar neuron are present in the vestibular ganglion which is located in the internal acoustic meatus. Peripheral processes of those neurons terminate on the receptors (hair cells) in the maculae (Fig. 20.16) and crista ampullaris (Fig. 20.17) central processes of those neurons form vestibular nerve. Vestibular nerve end in vestibular nuclei (Fig. 20.18). Some fibres of central processes directly end flocculo-nodular lobe.

Second order of neuron starts in the vestibular nuclei and terminate in postero ventral nucleus of thalamus. Some fibres joins with medial longitudinal fasciculus (MLF) to join with 3rd, 4th, 6th & 11th cranial nerve. (Fig. 20.18)

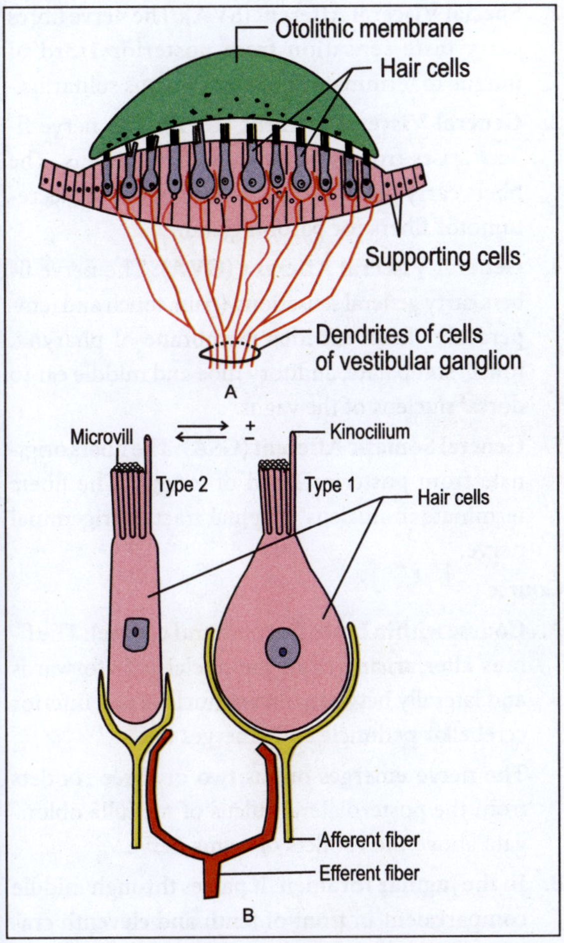

Fig. 20.16: A – Structure of macula; B – Magnified hair cells

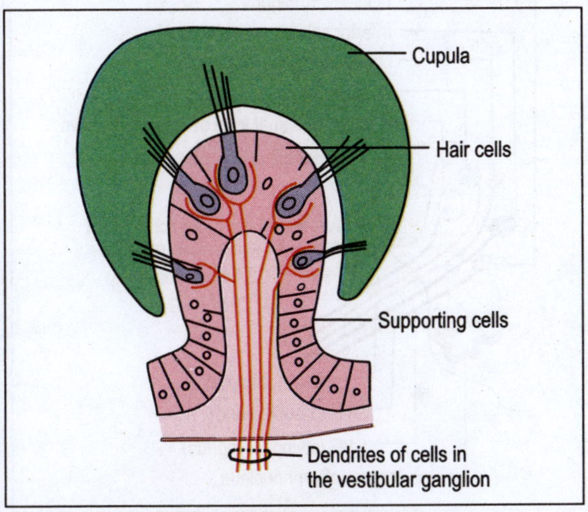

Fig. 20.17: Structure of crista ampullaris

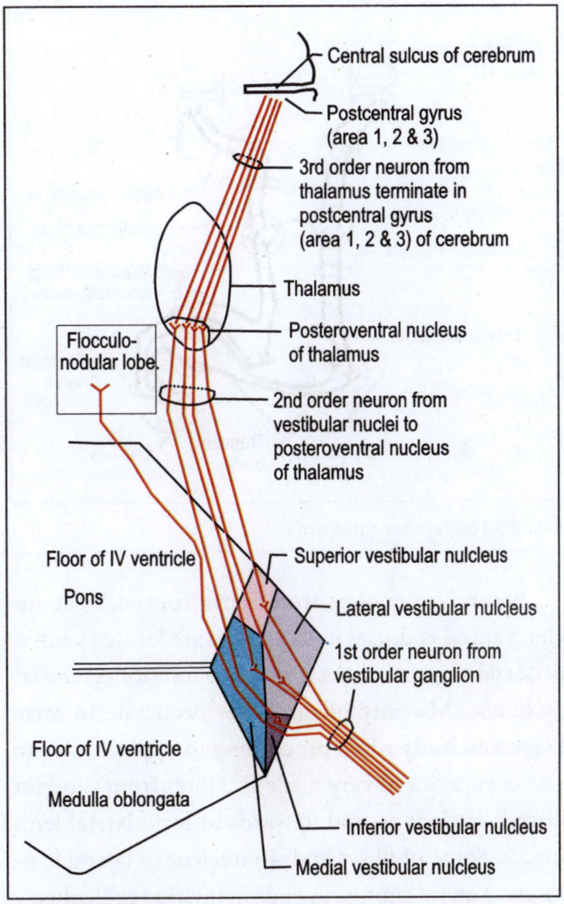

Fig. 20.18: Vestibular pathway

Third order of neuron starts from thalamus to terminate in posterior central gyrus (areas 3, 1 & 2).

APPLIED ANATOMY:

Involvement of this pathway will lead to vertigo, nystagmus.

The cochlear nerve

It contains about 23,000 fibres.

Auditory pathway

First order of neuron: Cell bodies of these neurons (bipolar) lies within spiral ganglion. The spiral ganglion is located in the modiolus of the cochlear. Peripheral processes of the bipolar neuron terminate in the hair cells in the spiral organ of corti. Central processes form the cochlear nerve. The fibres in the cochlear nerve terminate in cochlear nuclei (Fig. 20.19).

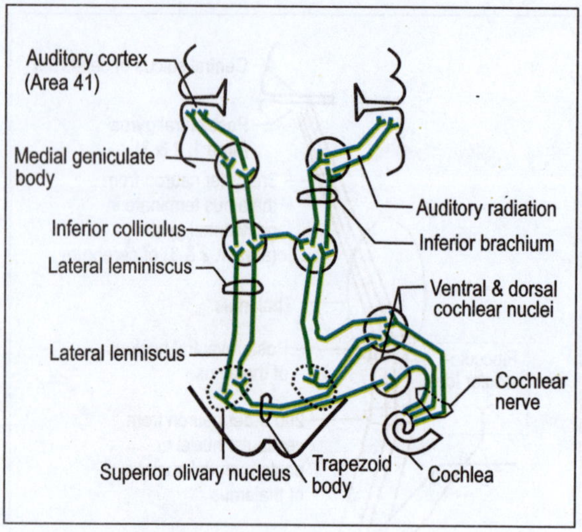

Fig. 20.19: Auditory pathway

Second order of neuron: Starts from cochlear nuclei (ventral & dorsal nuclei which are located ventral & dorsal respectively in relation to inferior cerebellar peduncle. Majority of the fibres decussate to form **trapezoid body** while proceeding to opposite side to end in superior olivary nucleus. Fibres from superior olivary nucleus ascend upwards to form lateral lemniscus. Some of fibres ends in nucleus of lateral lemniscus. Lateral lemniscus ends in inferior colliculus.

Third order of neuron: It starts from inferior collicus to end in medial geniculate body. The fibers form inferior brachium.

Fourth order of neuron: It starts from medial geniculate body to terminate in auditory cortex (area 41). The fibers from **auditory radiation.**

GLOSSOPHARYNGEAL NERVE

It is nine cranial nerve which supplies only one stylopharyngeus.

Type: Mixed nerve consisting of motor and sensory fibres.

Functional components & nuclei of origin:

1. **Branchial Efferent or Special Visceral Efferent (SVE)**: The nerve fibers arises from nucleus ambiguus to supply stylopharyngeus.
2. **Special Visceral Afferent (SVA)**: The nerve fibres carry taste sensation from posterior 1/3rd of tongue to terminate in nucleus tractus solitarius.
3. **General Visceral Efferent (GVE)**: The nerve fibers arises from inferior salivatory nucleus. The fibers carry preganglionic parasympathetic secretomotor fibers for parotid gland.
4. **General Visceral Afferent (GVA)**: The nerve fibers carry general sensations (pain, touch and temperature) from mucous membrane of pharynx, tonsil, soft palate, auditory tube and middle ear to dorsal nucleus of the vagus.
5. **General Somatic Afferent (GSA)**: The fibers originate from posterior 1/3rd of tongue. The fibers terminate in nucleus of spinal tract of trigeminal nerve.

Course

A. **Course within brain (intraneural course)**: The fibres after arising from the nuclei pass forwards and laterally between olivary nucleus and inferior cerebellar peduncle and emerges out.

The nerve emerges out as two or three rootlets from the posterolateral sulcus of medulla oblongata above the rootlets of vagus nerve.

B. **In the jugular foramen**: It passes through middle compartment in front of tenth and eleventh cranial nerves in a separate sheath. (Fig. 20.21)

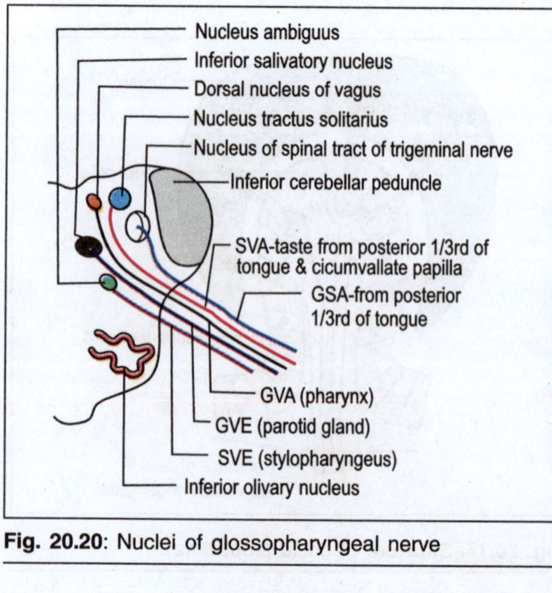

Fig. 20.20: Nuclei of glossopharyngeal nerve

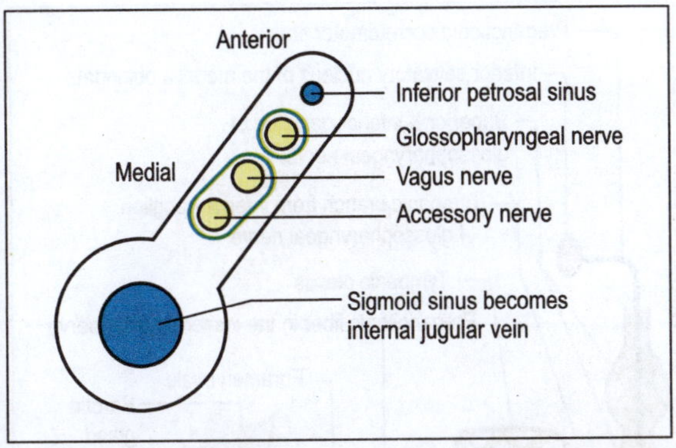

Fig. 20.21: Structures passing through jugular foramen

C. **Extracranial part**: After exit from jugular foramen, it passes downwards in between internal jugular and internal carotid artery and afterwards passes between internal and external carotid arteries and pass deep to styloid process and muscles attached to it (Fig. 20.22). Subsequently, it reaches the posterior border of stylopharyngeus and lies upon the muscle and passes deep to stylohyoid ligament and next passes through the gap between superior and middle constrictor muscles of pharynx. Finally, it passes deep to posterior border of hyoglossus and terminate. (Fig. 20.23)

Termination: It terminates by dividing into branches of distribution to tongue, tonsil and palate.

Ganglion of the nerve: Two ganglia:

1. **Superior ganglion**: Situated in the nerve trunk just above the jugular foramen. It is very small and is a detached part of inferior ganglion. It has no branches.
2. **Inferior ganglion**: Relatively larger and situated on the inferior surface of petrous part of temporal bone.

Its peripheral branches carry taste and general sense from posterior one third of tongue including vallate papillae and also general sense from tonsil, pharynx and sift palate.

Branches - from the ganglion

1. Distributing branch – Tympanic branch

Branches of glossopharyngeal nerve

A. **Branches of distribution**

1. **Tympanic branch**: It arises from inferior ganglion

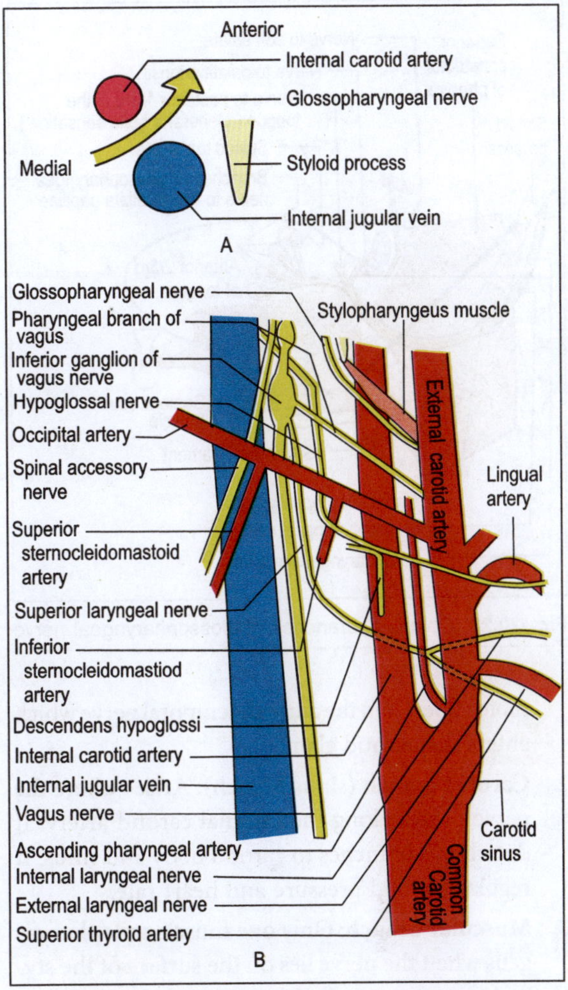

Fig. 20.22: A – Glossopharyngeal nerve at the base of the skull; B – Last four cranial nerves

and carries prepanglionic secretomotor parasympathetic fibres for parotid gland. (Fig. 20.24)

After origin it enters the tympanic cavity through tympanic canaliculus and forms tympanic plexus on the medial wall (promontory) of the tympanic cavity.

The main important nerve which is formed from tympanic plexus is lesser petrosal nerve.

Lesser petrosal nerve passes out of the tympanic cavity through a hiatus in the anterior surface of petrous part of temporal bone and then enters the infratemporal fossa through foramen ovale and relay in otic ganglion. Postganglionic secreto-

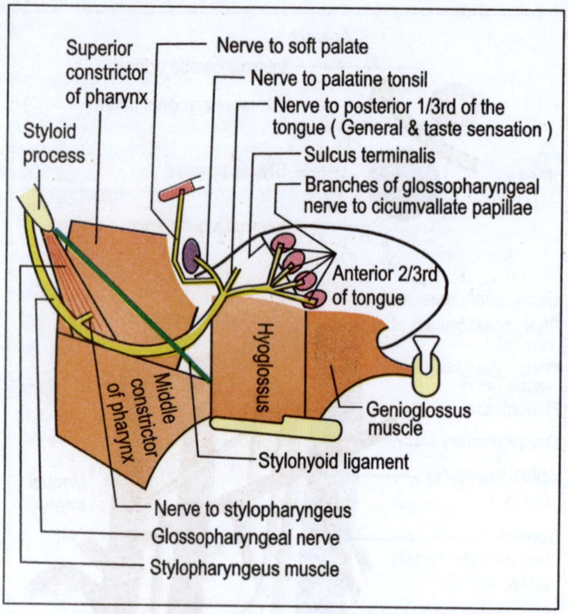

Fig. 20.23: Course & branches of glossopharyngeal nerve

motor fibers join the auriculotemporal nerve which enters the parotid gland.

2. **Carotid branch** (sinus branch): Arises where the nerve passes along the internal carotid artery. It distributes branches to carotid body and sinus. It regulates blood pressure and heart rate.
3. **Muscular branch**: Only one muscle stylopharyngeus when the nerve lies on the surface of the stylopharyngeus. (Stylopharyngeus is derived from third arch myotome).
4. **Pharyngeal**: These branches arise when the nerve passes through the gap between superior and middle constrictor muscles.

   They form pharyngeal plexus with pharyngeal branch of vagus and laryngo pharyngeal branch of sympathetic. This plexus supply sensory branches to mucous membrane of pharynx. Pharyngeal plexus lies on middle constrictor of pharynx.
5. **Tonsillar branch**: Supply (sensory) palatine tonsil and soft palate.
6. **Lingual branches**: Arise from glossopharyngeal nerve and distribute to posterior one third of tongue including vallate papillae and carry general and taste sensation.

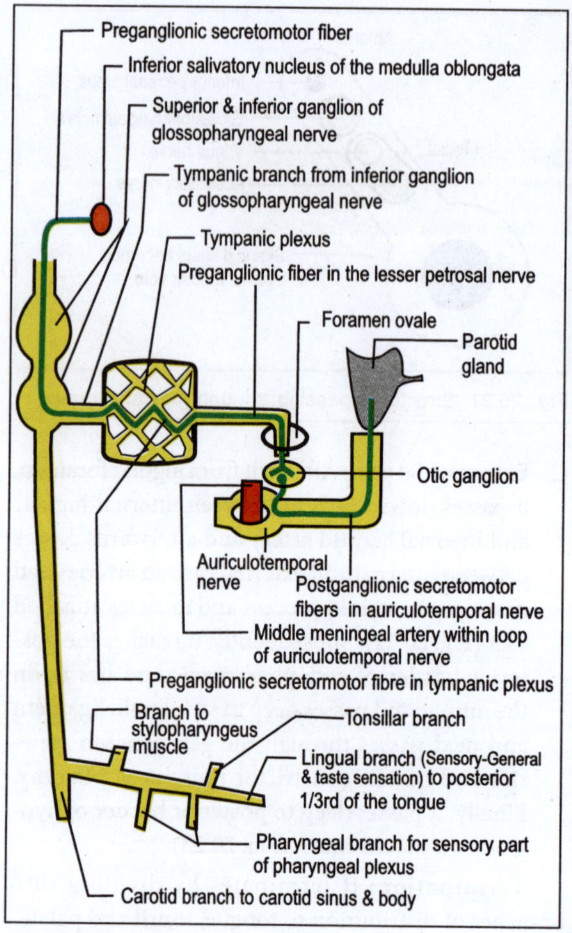

Fig. 20.24: Branches of glossopharyngeal nerve with elaboration of tympanic branch

APPLIED ANATOMY:

Glossopharyngeal nerve is not involved separately usually, it may be injured along with tenth nerve.

1. Acute pharyngitis may cause referred pain in the ear but inflammation of pharyngotympanic tube must be excluded.
2. Reflex contraction of muscles of throat if posterior wall of pharynx is stimulated and 9th nerve can be tested in this way.
3. Taste sensation of posterior one-third of tongue will be lost in case of involvement of 9th nerve.
4. After series of coughing carotid sinus may be subjected to pressure and results in syncope or cardiac arrest. This is due to stimulation of cardioinhibitory centre reflexly by sinus nerve.

VAGUS NERVE

It is the tenth cranial nerve.

Type: Mixed nerve.

Functional components & nuclei of origin

1. **Branchiomotor or Special Visceral Efferent (SVE)**: The nerve fibers arises from nucleus ambiguus to supply muscles of palate, larynx & pharynx.
2. **General Visceral Efferent (GVE)**: The nerve fibers originate from dorsal nucleus of vagus to supply (parasympathetic part) heart, bronchial tree, pharynx (lower part) foregut, mid gut (up to right 2/3rd of transverse colon), liver & pancreas.
3. **Special Visceral Afferent (SVA)**: The nerve fibers taste sensation from valleculla and upper anterior pat of epiglottis to terminate in nucleus tractus solitarius.
4. **General Visceral Afferent (GVA)**: The fibres carry general sensation from mucous membrane of digestive and respiratory tracts, to end dorsal nucleus of vagus.
5. **General Somatic Afferent (GSA)**: The fibers carry general sensation from skin, of auricle, external acoustic meatus, tympanic membrane (outer surface) to end in nucleus of spinal tract of the trigeminal nerve.

Course

A. **Intraneural course**: Fibres from the nuclei unit to form several (about 10) rootlets and passes laterally and forwards between olivary nucleus and inferior cerebellar peduncle. (Fig. 20.25)

   It emerges out from the postero lateral sulcus of medulla between olive and inferior cerebellar peduncle below the 9th nerve and under cover of flocculus.

B. **Extracranial course**: The nerve comes out of cranial cavity by passing through middle compartment of jugular foramen behind the 9th nerve. Within jugular foramen vagus nerve & 11th nerve enclosed in common dural sheath. (Fig. 20.21)

   Within the jugular foramen the nerve is having superior ganglion, where as inferior ganglion is below the foramen. Superior ganglion is having cell bodies of neurons which are concerned with GSA fibres, where as cell bodies in inferior ganglion are concerned with GVA fibres. Cranial root of accessory nerve joins with inferior ganglion.

   In the neck: The nerve runs vertically downwards within the carotid sheath up to root to neck. Within the carotid sheath the nerve lies between internal jugular vein laterally and internal carotid artery medially up to upper border of thyroid cartilage and below it common carotid artery medially. But the nerve lies in a more posterior plane between them. (Fig. 20.26)

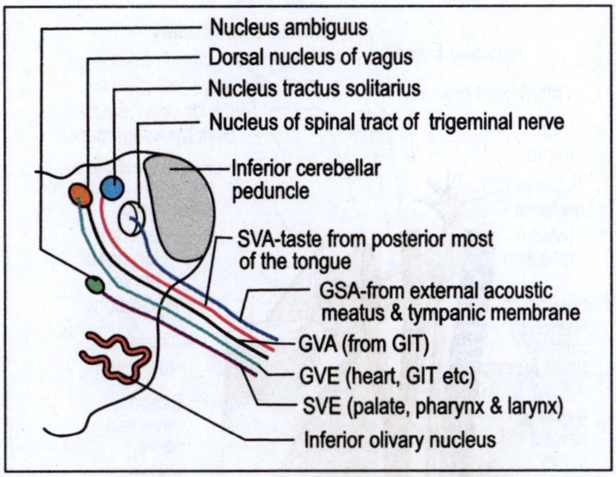

Fig. 20.25: Functional components & nuclei of origin of vagus nerve

Branches of Vagus Nerve

A. Branches from superior ganglion
   1. Meningeal
   2. Auricular branch

B. Branches from inferior ganglion
   1. Pharyngeal nerve
   2. Branches to carotid body
   3. Superior laryngeal nerve
   4. Cardiac branches: superior and inferior cervical
   5. Right recurrent laryngeal (Right vagus)

A. Branches from superior ganglion

1. **Meningeal branch**: It supplies the meninges of posterior cranial fossa.

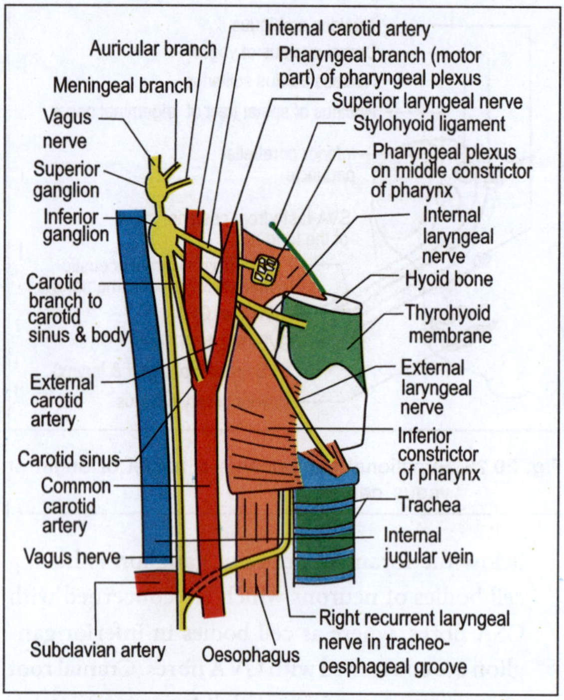

Fig. 20.26: Course of cervical part of vagus nerve with its branches

2. **Auricular branch**: Also known as **Alderman's nerve.** This nerve after origin from superior ganglion of vagus runs upward and backwards and pass through mastoid canaliculi and tympanomastoid fissure and finally ends by supplying branches to
   a) Skin of cranial surface of auricle (pinna)
   b) Floor and posterior wall of external acoustic meatus and
   c) Adjoining part of tympanic membrane.

B. Branches from inferior ganglion

1. **Pharyngeal branches**: They are actually the fibres of cranial root of accessory. They form pharyngeal plexus along with pharyngeal branch of glossopharyngeal, laryngopharyngeal branch of sympathetic. The plexus lies on middle constrictor. The fibres of cranial root of accessory through it supply muscles of soft palate and pharynx. Sensory fibres are responsible for reflex (deglutition). (Fig. 20.26)
2. **Branches of carotid body.**
3. **Superior laryngeal nerve**: It arises from inferior ganglion and nerve of fourth arch. It runs downwards and forwards and pass medial to internal carotid artery and divide into internal and external laryngeal nerve. Cranial part of accessory nerve fibres are not present in this nerve.

   A. **Internal laryngeal**: It pierces the thyrohyoid membrane along with superior laryngeal artery (branch of superior thyroid which is a branch of external carotid artery).

   It lies beneath the mucous membrane of pyriform fossa. It supplies:
   a) Vallecula, mucous membrane of pyriform fossa and larynx up to vocal fold.
   b) Transverse arytenoid muscle.

   B. **External laryngeal nerve**: It is purely a motor nerve and accompanies superior thyroid artery and leaves the artery distal to upper pole of lateral lobe runs deep to the upper pole and supplies:
   a) Cricothyroid muscle.
   b) Inferior onstrictor.

   (Which is also supplied by recurrent laryngeal and cranial rot of accessory through pharyngeal plexus).
4. **Cardiac branches**: Arise from the trunk in the neck. They are superior and inferior. All the cardiac branches of both the vagi except the inferior cervical cardiac branch join to form deep cardiac plexus. The inferior cervical cardiac branch take part in the formation of superficial cardiac plexus.
5. **Recurrent laryngeal nerves** – Two: right and left. Cranial part of accessory nerve fibres are present in this nerve.

Right recurrent nerve arises from right vagus at the root of the neck and loops below the first part of right subclavian artery and runs upwards behind the right common carotid artery reaches in the groove on the right side between trachea and oesophagus and runs upwards and finally supply all the muscles of larynx except cricothyroid (supplied by external laryngeal), inferior constrictor muscle of pharynx and mucous membrane of larynx below vocal folds. (Fig. 20.27)

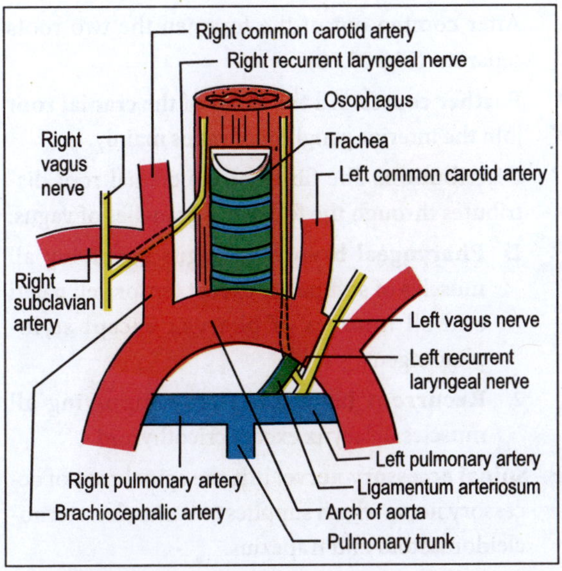

Fig. 20.27: Recurrent laryngeal nerve

Left recurrent laryngeal nerve: It is the branch of left vagus nerve in the thorax.

Origin: It arises from the left vagus when the vagus nerve crosses the left and anterior aspect of arch of aorta.

Course: After origin it hooks round the ligamentum anteriosum below the arch of aorta and runs upward in the groove in the left side between trachea and oesophagus. It enter the neck lying in the groove. Then passes deep to lower boarder of inferior constrictor muscle of pharynx. Finally, it passes behind cricoarytenoid joint and enters the larynx and terminates.

Termination: By dividing into branches.

Branches:

a) **Cardiac branches** – forming deep cardiac plexus.

b) **Muscular branches** – to all intrinsic muscles of larynx except cricothyroid and also a branch to inferior constrictor.

c) Branches to trachea and oesophagus for supplying muscles, glands and mucous membrane.

d) Sensory branches to mucous membrane of larynx below vocal fold and receive fibres from internal laryngeal nerve.

APPLIED IMPORTANCE OF VAGUS NERVE:

1. Auricular branch of vagus if irritated by scratching, or by earwax or syringing the ear with warm water. This irritation may cause reflex vomiting and also stoppage of heart by reflex irritation of vagus.

   This nerve is called Alderman's nerve because mild irritation of this nerve by soft cotton with rectified spirit may reflexly stimulate vagus nerve and result in increase of gastric movements and thus increase of appetite and this is done by British Alderman before dinner.

2. Recurrent laryngeal nerve may be injured during operation on thyroid and application of ligature of inferior thyroid artery. It may also be compressed during enlargement of thyroid, specially a growth. Its affection causes hoarseness of voice.

3. Vagotomy i.e., section of anterior and posterior vagal trunks are sometimes done in treatment of peptic ulcer.

4. Enlarged bronchial lymph nodes in children compress recurrent laryngeal nerve and produces persistent cough.

5. If vagus nerve nuclei in medulla is damaged or nerve trunk in its intracranial course is involved, then its functions are interfered and produces palpitation, increased pulse rate, constant vomiting, slowing of respiratory rate and sense of suffocation.

ACCESSORY NERVE

It is the eleventh cranial nerve and consists of two roots: (A) Cranial; (B) Spinal.

A. **Cranial root**: It is said to be detached part of vagus and so accessory to vagus. It distributes its fibres though the vagus.

   Type: Purely motor nerve.

B. **Spinal root** is known as spinal accessory.

Functional component & nuclei of origin:

1. **Special Visceral Efferent (SVE)**: The fibers arises from nucleus ambiguus to supply all the muscles

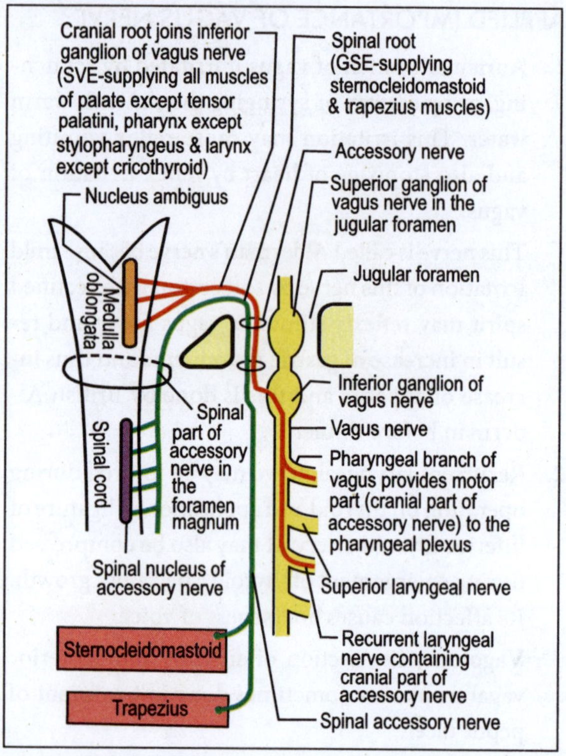

Fig. 20.28: Functional component & nuclei of origin of accessory nerve

of palate except tensor veli palatini, pharynx except stylopharyngeus & larynx except cricothyroid muscles.

2. **General Somatic Efferent (GSE)**: The fibers arises from spinal nucleus (in the anterior horn) of accessory nerve to supply sternocleidomastoid & trapezius.

A. **Cranial root**:

Deep origin or nuclei of origin: From lower part of nucleus ambiguus in medulla and possibly from dorsal nucleus of vagus.

It emerges out from posterolateral sulcus of medulla oblongata just below just below the vagus nerve.

Course: After emergence the rootlets unite and pass laterally to jugular foramen where it unite with the spinal root and form the trunk of accessory nerve. Then it passes through middle compartment of jugular foramen within a common sheath with vagus.

After coming out of the foramen the two roots separate. (Fig. 20.28)

Further course: All the fibres of the **cranial root** join the inferior ganglion of vagus mainly.

Distribution: The fibres of the cranial root distributes through the following branches of vagus:

1. **Pharyngeal branch of vagus** supplying all muscles of soft palate except tensor veli palati and all muscles of pharynx except stylopharyngeus.
2. **Recurrent laryngeal nerve** supplying all muscles of larynx except cricothyroid.

B. **Spinal accessory nerve**: It is the spinal root of accessory nerve which supplies two muscles: sternocleidomastoid and trapezius.

Type: Purely motor.

Functional component: Somatic efferent for trapezius & sternocleidomastoid.

Deep origin or nucleus of origin: From an elongated motor nucleus situated in the lateral part of anterior grey column of spinal cord extending from first cervical to fifth cervical segments (upper five cervical segments) of spinal cord.

Course:

I. **In the vertebral canal**: The nerve fibres after emerging from lateral aspect of spinal cord ascend. During the process of ascent the rootless unite to form single trunk.

II. **In the cranial cavity**: The nerve enters the cranial cavity by passing through foramen magnum. The nerve then runs to the jugular foramen. Here it joins with the cranial root and form the trunk of accessory nerve.

In the jugular foramen: It passes through middle compartment of jugular foramen along with ninth, tenth cranial nerves. The accessory nerve passes in a common dural sheath along with vagus nerve and comes out of cranial cavity. (Fig. 20.21)

Extracranial part:

1. After coming out of jugular foramen both the roots (cranial and spinal) are separated (the cranial root joins inferior ganglion of vagus nerve).

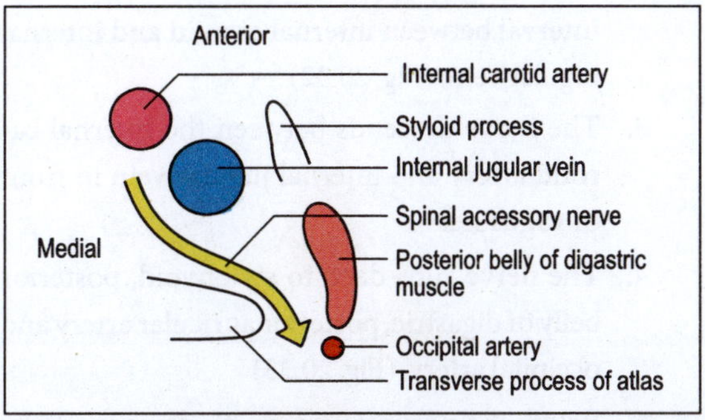

Fig. 20.29: Course & relations of spinal accessory nerve at the base of the skull

2. Then the nerve (spinal accessory) passes backwards and laterally behind internal jugular vein (in 66% cases) or in front of vein (33%). Here it passes in front of tip of atlas but itself is crossed by occipital artery. (Fig. 20.29)
3. Then the nerve runs downwards obliquely deep to styloid process, stylohyoid and posterior belly of digastrics.
4. It reaches the upper part of carotid triangle and accompanied by superior sternocleidomastoid branch of occipital artery.
5. It disappears by passing deep to a point of junction of upper one third and lower two thirds of anterior border of sternocleidomastoid muscle.
6. **In the posterior triangle**: The nerve emerges from posterior border of sternocleidomastoid muscle.
7. Then the nerve crosses the triangle superficially lying upon levator scapulae muscle.
8. Here it is also intimately related with cervical lymph nodes and $C_{3,4}$ nerves. Finally, it again disappears about 5cm above the clavicle by passing deep to anterior border of trapezius. (Fig. 20.30)
9. **Termination**: It terminates on the deep to trapezius by uniting with third and fourth cervical nerves and forming subtrapezoid plexus.

Branches of distribution:

1. It supplies sternocleidomastoid along with C_2 and C_3.
2. It also supplies trapezius along with C_3 and C_4 forming subtrapezoid plexus.

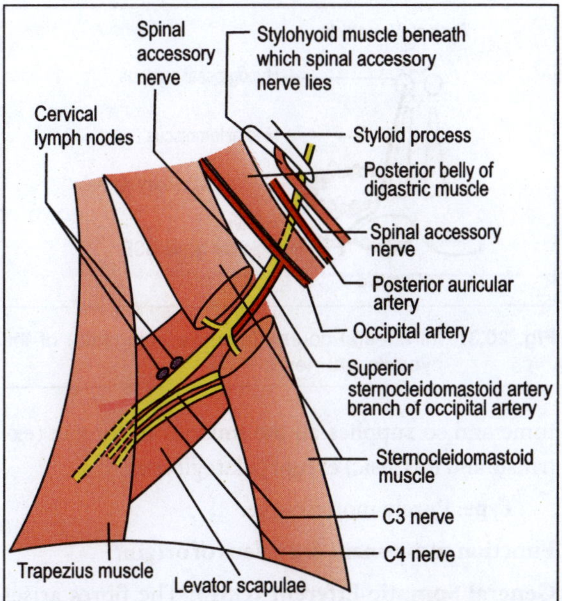

Fig. 20.30: Extracranial course & relations of spinal accessory nerve

APPLIED ANATOMY:

1. Spasmodic torticollis may result from central irritation of spinal accessory due to clonic spasm of sternocleidomastoid.
2. The nerve may be injured during removal of enlarged tubercular lymph node in the posterior triangle or incision of any inflammatory abscess at the posterior border of sternocleidomastoid. So incision should be given across the muscle and not at the posterior border.
3. If the nerve is injured in the posterior border of sternocleidomastoid – only trapezius will be involved producing:
   a) Slight winging of scapula
   b) Difficulty to raise the hand above had after being abducted by deltoid.
4. If injured in the anterior triangle both sternocleidomastoid and trapezius will be involved.

HYPOGLOSSAL NERVE

It is the 12th cranial nerve and nerve of occipital myo-

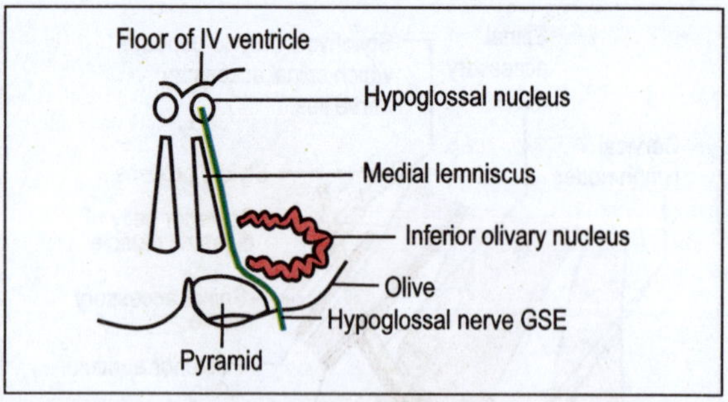

Fig. 20.31: Intraneural course (medulla oblongata) of the hypoglossal nerve

tome and so supplies all the muscles of tongue (extrinsic and intrinsic) except palatoglossus.

Type: Purely motor nerve.

Function component & nucleus of origin:

General Somatic Efferent (GSE): The fibres arises from **hypoglossal nucleus** which is present near the hypoglossal triangle of floor of IVth ventricle. Hypoglossal nucleus lies in the open part of medulla oblongata. It supplies all muscles of the tongue except palatoglossus which is supplied by pharyngeal plexus.

Course:

a) **Intraneural course**: The fibres after arising from the hypoglossal nucleus passes lateral to medial lemniscus and pyramidal tract. The fibres passes medial to inferior olivary nucleus. (Fig. 20.31)

It emerges at the anterolateral sulcus of medulla oblongata between pyramid and olive.

b) **Intracranial course**: After coming out of medulla the rootlets pass behind the vertebral artery and run laterally and form two roots. Then they pierce the duramater and pass through the anterior condylar canal and comes out of cranial cavity. In the canal the two roots unite to form a single trunk.

c) **Extracranial part**:

1. After coming out of the anterior condylar canal the nerve lies in a deeper plane than internal carotid artery, 9th, 10th and 11th cranial nerves and internal jugular vein.
2. Then it passes downwards and laterally behind the internal carotid artery and lies in the interval between internal carotid and internal jugular vein. (Fig. 20.32)
3. The nerve descends between the internal carotid artery and internal jugular vein in front of vagus nerve.
4. The nerve runs deep to stylohyoid, posterior belly of digastric, posterior auricular artery and occipital artery. (Fig. 20.33)
5. Below the occipital artery it curves medially round lower sternocleidomastoid branch of occipital artery.
6. It crosses the internal and external carotid artery, and crosses the loop of first part of lingual artery and reaches the posterior border of hyoglossus muscle.
7. Then the nerve lies on hyoglossus.
8. The nerve passes deep to tendon of posterior belly of digastric and stylohyoid muscle. Then it runs on the superficial surface of hyoglossus.
9. As it lies on the hyoglossus it is related above to lingual nerve, submandibular ganglion, deep part of submandibular gland with duct.
10. At the anterior border of hypoglossus it lies on the surface of genioglossus and runs forward and upwards up to tip of tongue and terminates.

Termination: It terminates by distributing branches to muscles of tongue except palatoglossus.

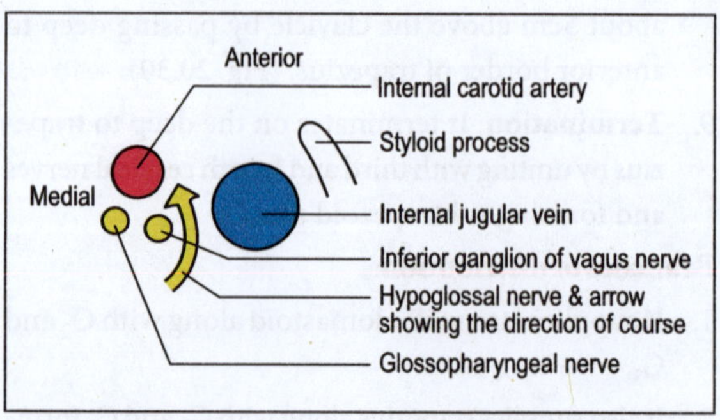

Fig. 20.32: Hypoglossal nerve at the base of the skull

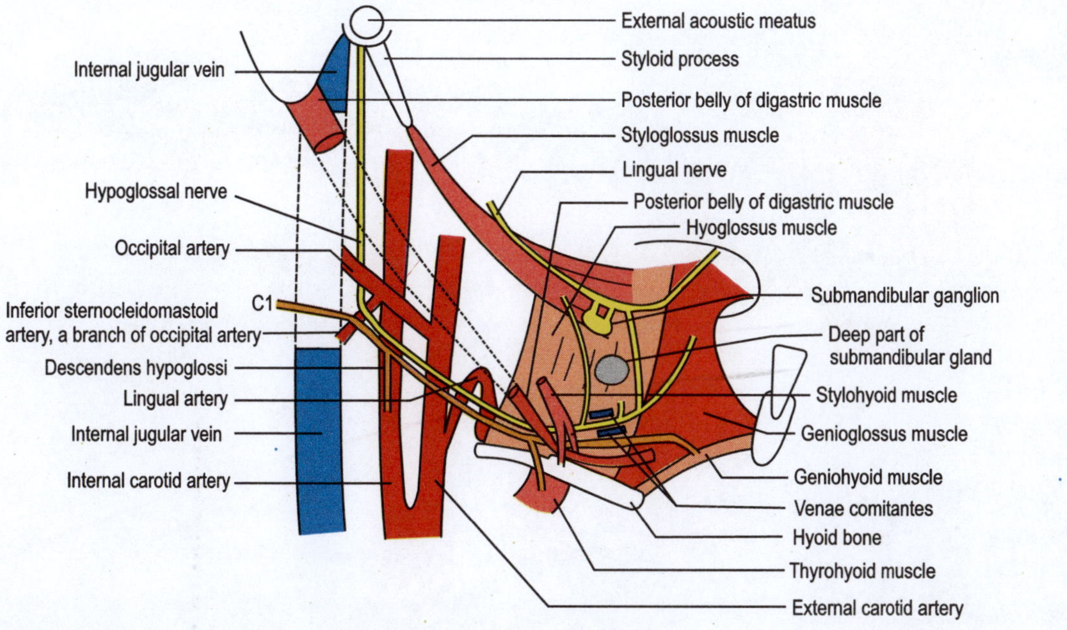

Fig. 20.33: Extracranial course, relations & branches of the hypoglossal nerve

A. **Branches containing fibres first cervical nerve**
   1. Meningeal
   2. Descendens hypoglossi
   3. Thyrophyoid
   4. Geniohyoid

B. **Branches of the hypoglossal nerve proper**: All muscles of tongue except palatoglossus (which is supplied by cranial root of accessory through pharyngeal plexus) (Fig. 20.34).

APPLIED ANATOMY:

Paralysis of tongue muscles with geniohyoid, thyrohyoid and muscles supplied by ansa may be paralysed.

If one side: Tongue will be deviated to same side due to paralysis of genioglossus.

CHARACTERISTICS:

1. The nerve passed deep to posterior belly of digastric twice.
2. The lower sternocleidomastoid branch of occipital artery prevents the ascent of hypoglossal nerve.

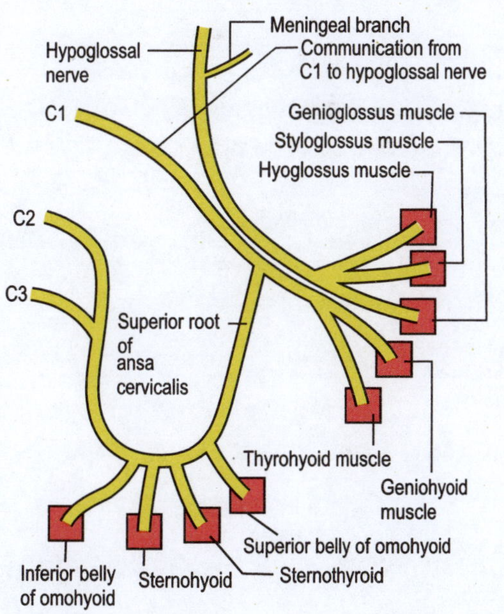

Fig. 20.34: Distribution of hypoglossal nerve

chapter 21

SURFACE AND RADIOLOGICAL ANATOMY (HEAD & NECK)

AT A GLANCE

- *Surface landmarks and bony points*
- *Arteries, Veins and Nerves of Head and neck region*
- *Different glands, air sinuses and other structures of Head and neck region*
- *Radiological anatomy of head & neck*

SURFACE LANDMARKS AND BONY PROMINENCE (MAINLY POINTS)

1. **External occipital protuberance and Inion (felt only in adults)**: A point on the occipital bone (back of head – a knob-like feeling) and is on the upper end of the furrow of the back of neck. Central point is the Inion.
2. **Superior nuchal line**: A transversely arched line over the ridge on each side of external occipital protuberance (prominence at the upper end of nuchal furrow of the back of neck) towards the mastoid process.
3. **Nasion**: A point on the depression at the root of nose (overlies the fronto-nasal suture and actually meeting of internasal and frontonasal suture).
4. **Pterion (Sylvian point)**: A point 3.5cm behind frontozygomatic suture (felt as a depression in the upper part of lateral orbital margin) and 3.8cm above zygomatic arch (midpoint) or 1.5cm above the frontozygomatic suture.

Importance:

a) *Meeting point of 4 bones*: Frontal, squamous part of temporal, parietal (anteroinferior angle) and greater wing of sphenoid.

b) *Important landmark* (for surgery) because deep to it lies anterior branch of middle meningeal artery.

c) It also overlies anterior pole of insula, middle cerebral artery and point of division of lateral sulcus of brain into 3 rami.

d) It is also site of anterolateral fontanelle in foetal skull.

e) Site for trephining the skull in case of surgery.

5. **Asterion**: A point 3.5cm behind the external acoustic meatus and 1.2cm above the line joining the meatus and inion (most median prominent point on the external protuberance which is felt in the upper end of nuchal furrow of the back).

Importance:

a) It is the meeting point of 3 bones: Parietal

(posteroinferior angle), occipital and mastoid part of temporal.

b) On the inner surface a groove is present for lodgement of transverse sinus and beginning of sigmoid sinus.

c) Site for posterolateral fontanelle in foetal skull.

6. **Bregma**: A point of junction of midline of scalp and the line drawn from the preauricular point (just in front of auricle) vertically upwards which will cut up to midline of scalp. (It is the junctional region of coronal and sagittal suture and it is the site of anterior fontanelle of foetal skull and is important in foetus for dehydration or increased pressure of CSF).

7. **Lambda**: A point about 6.5cm above Inion (central prominence of external occipital protuberance). [It is the meeting of sagittal and lambdoid suture and site for posterior fontanelle in foetal skull.]

8. **Glabella**: It is median elevation between two superciliary arches and just above nasion, (superciliary arches are elevations on each side above the upper margin of medial part of upper margin of orbit and nasion is the depression on the upper part of root of nose).

9. **Supraorbital margin**: A line on the upper margin of eyebrow. (Fig. 21.1)

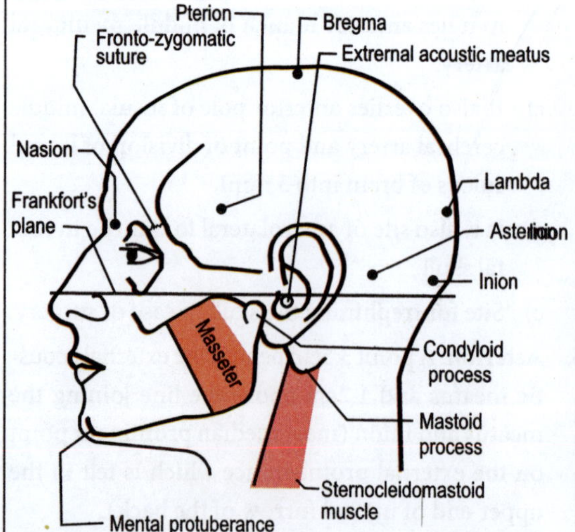

Fig. 21.1: Important points in the head

10. **Supraorbital notch**: A point on the junction of medial $\frac{2}{3}$rd and lateral $\frac{1}{2}$rd of supraorbital margin (upper margin of eyebrow).

11. **Superciliary arch**: A curved line on the respective side (on slightly) above the medial part of orbit and on rounded elevation. (It lies between supraorbital margin below and frontal eminence above, which is superolateral rounded elevation of forehead).

12. **Infraorbital foramen**: A point 1cm (slightly) below the infraorbital margin and on the vertical line joining the supraorbital notch (a point of junction of medial of $\frac{1}{3}$rd and laterally $\frac{2}{3}$rd of supraorbital margin) to base of mandible.

13. **Mental foramen**: A point on the midway between the upper and lower border of mandible and on the vertical line joining supraorbital notch to base of mandible. (It lies vertically below the interval between two premolar teeth).

14. **Frontal eminence**: A point on each side on the superolateral rounded elevation on the forehead and above superciliary arch.

15. **Parietal eminence**: A point on each side is to be given on the most prominent part of the lateral aspect of head (maximum convex part) and it will be far above and little behind the auricle.

16. **Head of mandible**: Condyloid process of mandible. A point in front of tragus (a projection in the anterior part of *Pinna or auricle*). It can be felt at the time of movement of lower jaw.

17. **Frontozygomatic suture**: A point on the slightly depressed area at the upper and outer border of orbital cavity.

18. **Zygomatic arch**: A line at the region of meeting of temple and cheek and in front of ear and the posterior end will be just above *tragus*. (It can be felt).

19. **Mastoid process**: A point on the process situated behind lower part of the auricle and directed downwards and forwards.

20. **Supramastoid crest**: A curved line about 2.5cm long is to be drawn above the external acoustic meatus and curves upwards and backwards (can be felt above the posterior part of root of the auricle).

21. **Suprameatal triangle (Macewan's)**: A point behind external acoustic meatus and in front of vertical line drawn upwards from posterior margin of the meatus. (Point may be placed in the depression above and behind the meatus covered by Helix).

    [*Mastoid antrum* lies 1.25cm deep to it and in child it is superficial].

    The point can also be placed in *Cymba conchae*, which is the conchal area above crus helix (anterior end of helix). It overlies suprameatal triangle.
22. **Preauricular point**: A point in front of upper part of tragus (a projection of auricle or pinna in front of concha which is the beginning of external acoustic meatus).
23. **Auricular point**: a point at the centre of the external acoustic meatus.
24. **Reid's base line**: 2 points
    a) 1st: A point at the lower border of orbit.
    b) 2nd: A point at the centre or external acoustic meatus (auricular point). The line joining these two points will be drawn.

    Importance: In trephining the skull, this line is a guide to the surgeon to measure the points above the lesion according to site of lesion.
25. **Frankfort's plane**: A line drawn through lower margin of orbit and upper margin of external acoustic meatus.
26. **Philtrum**: A point in the median vertical groove above upper lip.
27. **Lobule**: A point on the lower small part of auricle.
28. **Angle of mouth**: A point in front of 1st premolar tooth.
29. **Angle of mandible**: A point (can be felt) just below and in front of lobule of ear.
30. **Sternoclavicular joint**: A point on the medial end of clavicle when arm is abducted.
31. **Spine of 7th-cervical vertebra or vertebra prominence**: A point is to be placed on the visible prominence at the lower end of median nuchal furrow at the back of the neck and the head is being flexed (bowed down).
32. **Transverse process of Atlas**: A point is to be given in the midway between tip of mastoid process (behind lower part of auricle) and angle of mandible (in front and below lobule of ear).
33. **Carotid tubercle**: (prominence of anterior tubercle of transverse process of 6th cervical vertebra) – A point is to be given after feeling on the anterior border of Sternocleidomastoid muscle at the level of cricoid cartilage (about 3cm from median plane).
34. **Laryngeal prominence or Adam's apple (Thyroid eminence)**: A point on the easily felt median eminence in front of the neck just below the hyoid (which lies below mandible) (not prominent in women).
35. **Hyoid bone**: A point or line on bony eminence below mandible and above thyroid eminence.
36. **Arch of Cricoid cartilage**: A line on the prominence below the thyroid eminence in the median plane.
37. **Bifurcation of common carotid artery**: a point is placed on the anterior border of Sternocleidomastoid at the level of upper border of thyroid cartilage.
38. **Beginning of facial artery in face**: a point on the base of mandible at the anterior border of masseter (Masseter should be contracted after clenching the teeth).

Venous sinuses

1. *Superior sagittal sinus*: 2 points
   a) 1st: A point on the glabella (median elevation between 2 superciliary arches).
   b) 2nd: A point on the Inion (central point of external occipital protuberance – an eminence on the upper end of nuchal furrow).

   A line joining these two points will be drawn in such a way that it will be gradually broader from before backwards. Lines should be 1.25cm apart.
2. *Transverse sinus*: 2 points
   a) 1st: A point on Inion.
   b) 2nd: A point on the Asterion (a point 3.5cm behind external acoustic meatus and 1.2cm above the line joining the meatus and inion).

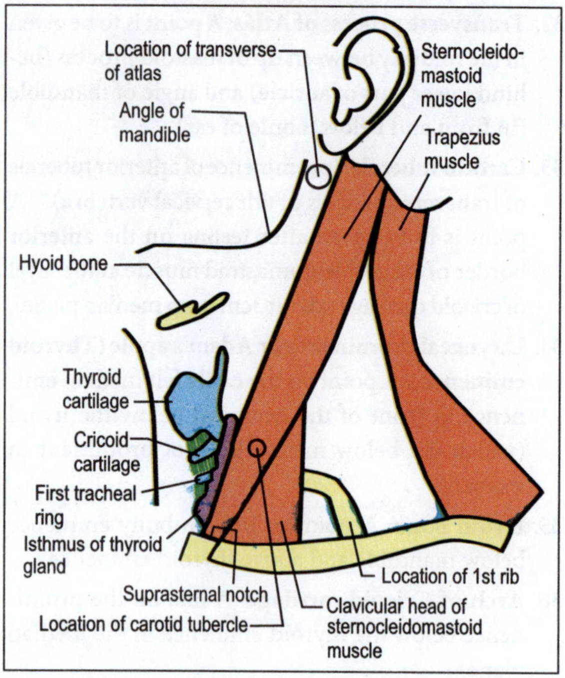

Fig. 21.2: Important points in the neck

A broad line joining the two points should be drawn with slight convexity upwards (1.25cm above).

3. *Sigmoid sinus*: 2 points.
   a) 1st: A point on the asterion [2(a)] (Fig. 21.2)
   b) 2nd: A point about 1.2cm above the tip of mastoid process (point behind lower part of the auricle).

   A broad line joining these two points is to be drawn.

   Two parallel lines, 1.2cm apart should be drawn from inion to 1.2cm above the tip of mastoid process.

OTHER IMPORTANT SURFACE MAKINGS IN CONNECTION WITH BRAIN

1. *Middle meningeal artery* (Fig. 21.4)

   A. *Trunk*: 2 points
      a) 1st: A point middle (above) of the zygoma
      b) 2nd: A point 2cm above the first point (a).

   The line joining these two points should be drawn upwards and forwards. The artery divides deep to second point (b).

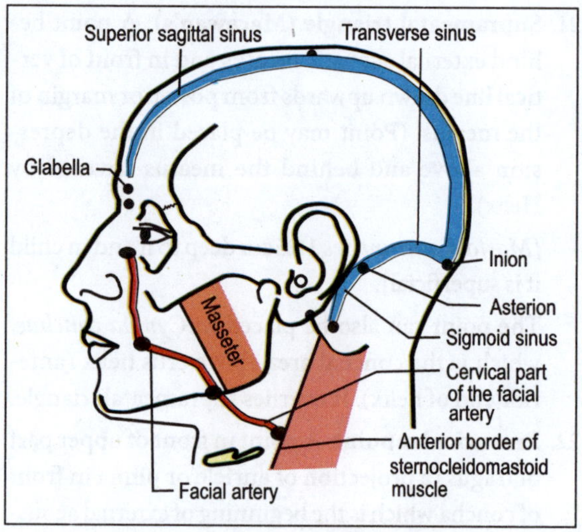

Fig. 21.3: Surface anatomy of superior sagittal, transverse & sigmoid sinuse and facial nerve & artery

   B. *Anterior divisions (branch)*: 2 points
      a) 1st: A point at the pterion (Sylvian point).
      b) 2nd: A point on the midway between inion and nasion.

   The line joining points A(b), B(a) & B(b) represents anterior division.

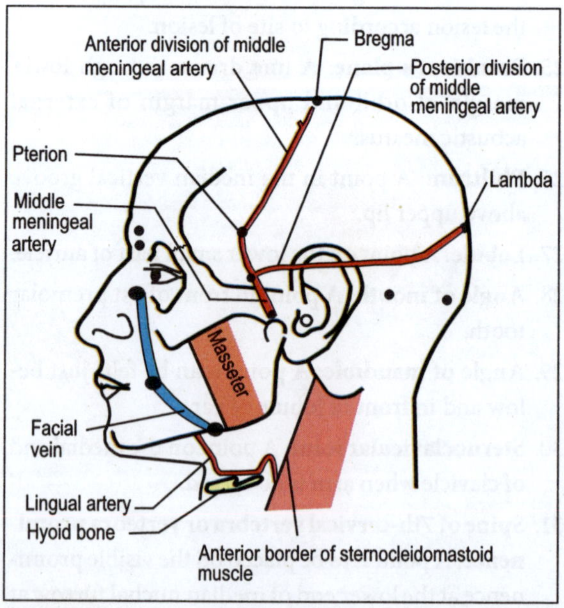

Fig. 21.4: Surface anatomy of middle meningeal & lingual arteries and facial vein

C. *Posterior division (branch)*: 4 points

a) 1st: A point at the *lambda*. (7cm above the external occipital protuberance).

The line joining points A(b) and C(a) represents posterior division.

Trigeminal ganglion: A point on the lateral aspect of head just in front of preauricular point which is a point in front of tragus. (The ganglion lines 5cm deep to this point).

Arteries of Head and Neck (Lines) (Fig. 21.5)

1. *Right common carotid artery*: 2 points

a) 1st: A point on the right sternoclavicular joint.

b) 2nd: A point on the anterior border of sternocleidomastoid muscle at the level of the upper border of thyroid cartilage.

The line joining these two points is to be drawn.

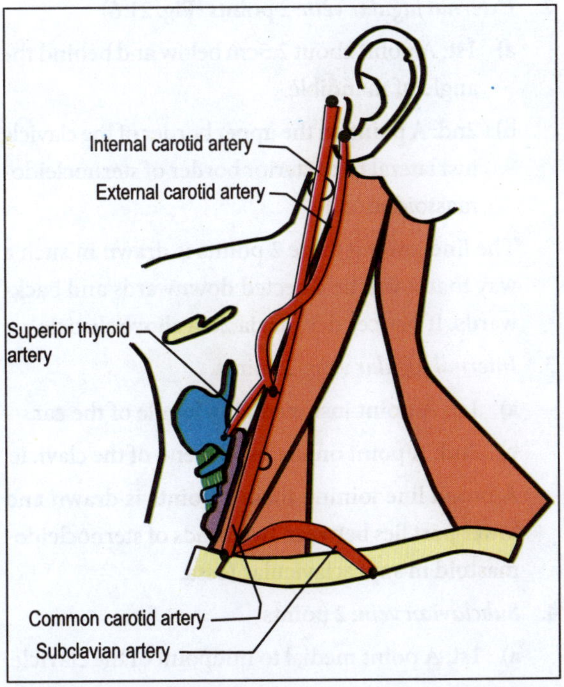

Fig. 21.5: Surface anatomy of common, internal & external carotid arteries along with superior thyroid & subclavian arteries

2. *Left common carotid artery*: 3 points

a) 1st: A point little left of the centre of the manubrium sterni.

b) 2nd: A point on the left sternoclavicular joint.

c) 3rd: A point on the anterior border of left Sternocleidomastoid muscle at the level of upper border of thyroid cartilage.

A broad line joining these three points is to be drawn (The part between (b) and (c) artery in the neck) and part (a) and (b) is artery in the thorax).

3. *External carotid artery*: 2 points

a) 1st: A point on the anterior border of the sternocleidomastoid at the level of the upper border of thyroid cartilage.

b) 2nd: A point on the posterior border of neck of mandible.

The line joining these two points will be drawn in such a manner so that lower half will be convex forwards and the upper half is gradually concave forwards.

4. *Internal carotid artery*: 2 points

a) 1st: A point on the anterior border of sternocleidomastoid at the level of upper border of thyroid cartilage.

b) 2nd: A point at the posterior border of condyle of mandible.

The line joining these two points is to be drawn.

5. *Superior thyroid artery*: 2 points

a) 1st: A point just above 4(a) at the lines of upper border of thyroid cartilage.

b) 2nd: A point on the 2cm front of the anterior border of sternocleidomastoid at the level of arch of cricoid cartilage.

The line joining these two points is to be drawn in such a way that it will be directed downwards and medially.

6. *Facial artery*: 4 points

a) A point on the anterior border of sternocleidomastoid muscle just above the tip of greater cornu of the hyoid bone.

b) 2nd: A point on the mandible at the antero-inferior (lower part of anterior border) part of masseter muscle.

c) 3rd: A point about 1.2cm lateral to angle of mouth.

d) 4th: A point at the medial angle of the eye.

The line joining these points is to be drawn in such a way that the part (a) and (b) (part in the neck) will be straight and curves round the mandible and the rest of the part will be tortuous. (part in the face).

7. *Transverse facial artery*: A transverse line just below the zygomatic arch is to be drawn.

8. *Lingual artery*: A line is to be drawn from tip of greater cornu up to whole greater cornu and vertically upwards up to floor of mouth. The beginning will be a loop.

9. *Subclavian artery*: 2 points

a) 1st: A point on sternoclavicular joint.

b) 2nd: A point on middle of lower border of the clavicle.

The line joining the 2 points is to be drawn in such a way that it will form an arch 2cm above the clavicle.

On the left side: Another point just left of centre of manubrium sterni is to be taken and this point is to be joined with (a) by a vertical line.

Veins of Head and Neck

1. *Facial vein*: 3 points

a) 1st: A point at medial angle of the eye.

b) 2nd: A point just below and in front of angle of mouth.

c) 3rd: A point anteroinferior part of masseter muscle.

The line joining these 2 points should be drawn in such a manner that from (a) it will run downwards and backwards for a small distance and then vertically downwards across the cheek.

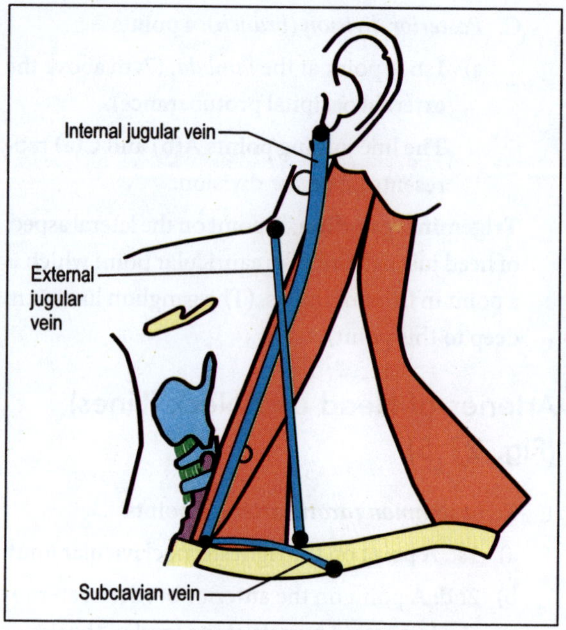

Fig. 21.6: Surface anatomy of external & internal jugular vein along with subclavian vein

2. *External jugular vein*: 2 points (Fig. 21.6)

a) 1st: A point about 2.5cm below and behind the angle of mandible.

b) 2nd: A point on the upper border of the clavicle just lateral to posterior border of sternocleidomastoid muscle.

The line joining these 2 points is drawn in such a way that it will be directed downwards and backwards. It pierces deep facia 2cm above clavicle.

3. *Internal jugular vein*: 2 points

a) 1st: A point just medial to lobule of the ear.

b) 2nd: A point on the medial end of the clavicle.

A broad line joining these 2 points is drawn and lower part lies between two heads of sternocleidomastoid in supraclavicular fossa.

4. *Subclavian vein*: 2 points

a) 1st: A point medial to midpoint of the clavicle.

b) 2nd: A point on the medial end of the clavicle.

A broad line joining these two points should be drawn along the clavicle.

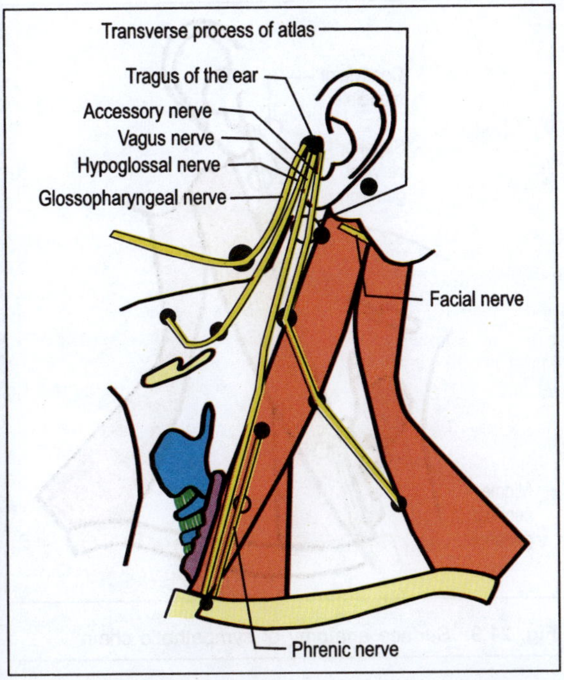

Fig. 21.7: Surface anatomy of vagus, spinal accessory, hypoglossal, phrenic nerves and glossopharyngeal nerves

Nerves of Head and Neck

1. *Vagus nerve in the neck*: 2 points (Fig. 21.7)
   a) 1st: A point below preauricular point.
   b) 2nd: A point medial to medial end of clavicle.

   The line joining these 2 points should be drawn vertically downwards.
2. *Spinal accessory nerve in the neck*: 5 points
   a) 1st: A point little below the preauricular point.
   b) 2nd: A point on the tip of transverse process of atlas (midpoint between angle of mandible and tip of mastoid process of temporal bone).
   c) 3rd: A point on the junction of upper 1/3rd and lower 2/3rd of anterior border of sternocleidomastoid muscle.
   d) 4th: A point on the middle of posterior border of sternocleidomastoid muscle.
   e) A point about 6cm above the clavicle on the anterior border of trapezius.

   The line joining these 5 points is to be drawn.
3. *Hypoglossal nerve*: 3 points
   a) 1st: A point little below the preauricular point.
   b) 2nd: A point just above behind greater cornu of hyoid.
   c) 3rd: A point on the midway between angle of mandible and symphysis menti.

   The line joining these 3 points should be drawn in a curved manner with concavity upward. (Head of the person should be extended i.e., bent backward).
4. *Facial nerve*: 2 point
   a) 1st: A point on the middle of anterior border of mastoid process..
   b) 2nd: A point behind the neck of mandible.

   A short horizontal line joining these 2 points is drawn across the lobule of ear. (Fig. 21.3)
5. *Mandibular nerve*: 3 point
   a) 1st: A point on centre of zygomatic arch.
   b) 2nd: A point front of head of mandible on the posterior part of mandibular notch.
   c) 3rd: A point at the line of 2nd molar tooth midway between upper and lower borders of body of the mandible.

   The line joining these 3 points is to be drawn vertically downwards.
6. *Auriculotemporal nerve*: 2 point (Fig. 21.8)
   a) 1st: A point in front of head of mandible.
   b) 2nd: Preauricular point.

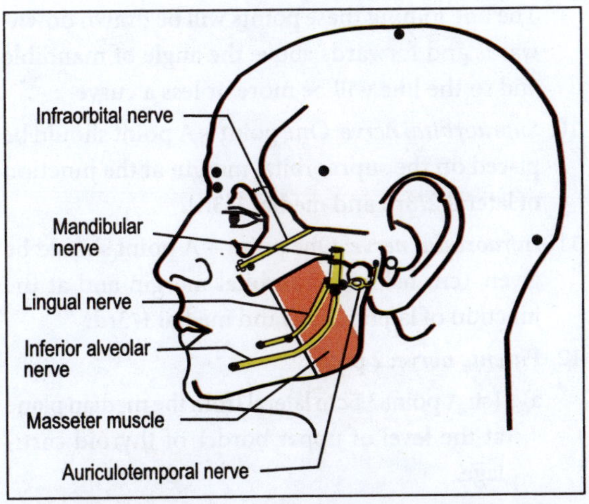

Fig. 21.8: Surface anatomy of infraorbital, lingual, inferior alveolar and auriculotemporal nerve

A line from (a) should be drawn backwards crossing the neck of mandible and then upwards to (b) and the line should extend beyond (b).

7. *Lingual nerve*: 3 point (Fig. 21.8)
   a) 1st: A point in the posterior part of mandibular notch in front of head of mandible.
   b) 2nd: A point little below and behind last lower molar tooth.
   c) 3rd: A point opposite the 1st lower molar tooth.

   The line joining these 3 points should be drawn in such a way that the concavity will be between (b) and (c) and will be directed upwards.
8. *Inferior alveolar nerve*: 2 point
   a) 1st: A point on the midway between anterior and posterior borders of the ramus of the mandible just below the level of last lower molar tooth.
   b) 2nd: A point just opposite the lower 2nd premolar tooth midway between upper and lower borders of the body of mandible.

   The line joining these 2 points will be directed downwards and forwards.
9. *Glossopharyngeal*: 2 point
   a) 1st: A point on the anterio-inferior part of tragus (more or less preauricular point).
   b) 2nd: A point on the body of mandible, anterosuperior to the angle of mandible.

   The line joining these points will be drawn downwards and forwards above the angle of mandible and so the line will be more or less a curve.
10. *Supraorbital nerve*: One point – A point should be placed on the supraorbital margin at the junction of lateral 2/3rd and medial 1/3rd.
11. *Infraorbital nerve*: One point – A point should be given 1cm below infraorbital margin and at the junction of lateral 2/3rd and medial 1/3rd.
12. *Phrenic nerve*: 2 point
    a) 1st: A point 3.5cm lateral from the median plane at the level of upper border of thyroid cartilage.
    b) 2nd: A point on the sternoclavicular joints.

    The line joining these 2 points will be drawn.

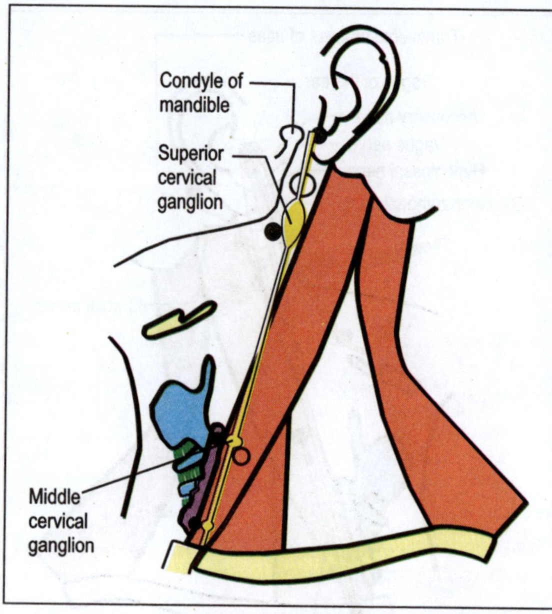

Fig. 21.9: Surface anatomy of sympathetic chain

13. *Cervical sympathetic trunk*: 2 points with ganglia.
    a) 1st: A point at the posterior border of condyle of mandible.
    b) 2nd: A point at the sternoclavicular joint.

    The line joining these 2 points is to be drawn.

    Ganglia will be marked by three points in the following way: (Fig. 21.9)

    Superior cervical ganglion: It will be marked from transverse process of atlas to tip of greater cornu of hyoid.

    Middle cervical ganglion: It will be marked at the level of arch of cricoid cartilage.

    Inferior cervical ganglion: To be marked about 3cm above sternoclavicular joint.
14. *Brachial plexus*: 2 points
    a) 1st: A point midway between anterior and posterior borders of Sternocleidomastoid at the level of cricoid cartilage.
    b) 2nd: A point just lateral to midpoint of the clavicle.

    The line joining these two points will be drawn and it is the upper limit of trunk.

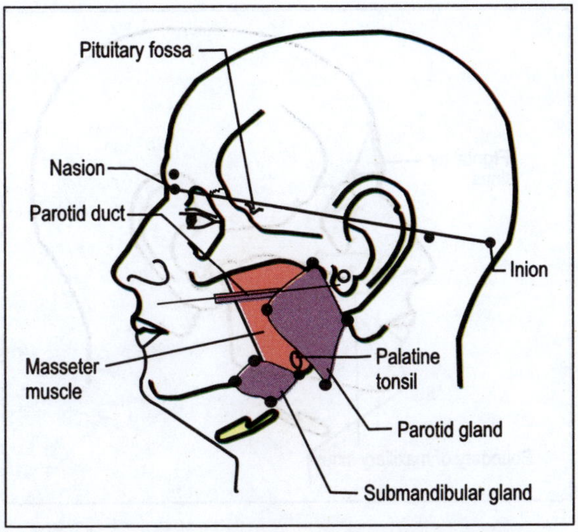

Fig. 21.10: Surface anatomy of glands, parotid duct, palatine tonsil with pituitary gland

GLANDS OF HEAD AND NECK, AIR SINUSES AND OTHER STRUCTURES

1. *Parotid gland*: 4 points (Fig. 21.10)
   a) 1st: A point on the upper border of the condyle of mandible.
   b) 2nd: A point just above the centre of Masseter muscle (which will be contracted by clenching teeth).
   c) 3rd: A point 2cm below and behind the angle of mandible.
   d) 4th: A point on the upper part of the anterior border of mastoid process.

   The line should be drawn in such a way that the three borders of the gland will be drawn by joining the points in the following way:

   A. *Anterior border*: The line joining (a) and (b) will be directed downwards and forwards and (b) and (c) are joined in downward and backward direction.
   B. *Superior border*: It should be drawn by joining (a) and (d) in a curved manner across the lobule of the ear with concavity upwards and backwards.
   C. *Posterior border*: It should be drawn by a straight line joining (c) and (d).

2. *Parotid duct*: 2 points
   a) 1st: A point on the lower border of the tragus of the ear.
   b) 2nd: A point midway between the ala of the nose and the red margin of upper lip. The middle third of the line joining (a) and (b) will be the surface line of parotid duct.
3. *Pituitary gland*: Join nasion and inion and depression at a distance of 7cm from nasion.
4. *Submandibular gland*: 4 points
   a) 1st: A point 1.5cm above the lower border of the mandible.
   b) 2nd: A point on the greater cornu of the hyoid bone.
   c) 3rd: A point on the angle of mandible.
   d) 4th: A point on the midpoint between symphysis of the mandible and its angle.

   An oval area is to be drawn in such a way that upper convexity reaches point (a) and lower convexity will reach point (b) and it will extend from point (c) to (d).
5. *Palatine tonsil*: An oval area is to be drawn just above and in front of angle of mandible and also on the lower part of masseter muscle. (Fig. 21.11)
6. *Thyroid gland*:

   A. *Isthmus*: 2 points
   a) 1st: A point 1cm below cricoid on 1st tracheal ring. Draw a horizontal line about 1.5cm which is the upper border of isthmus.

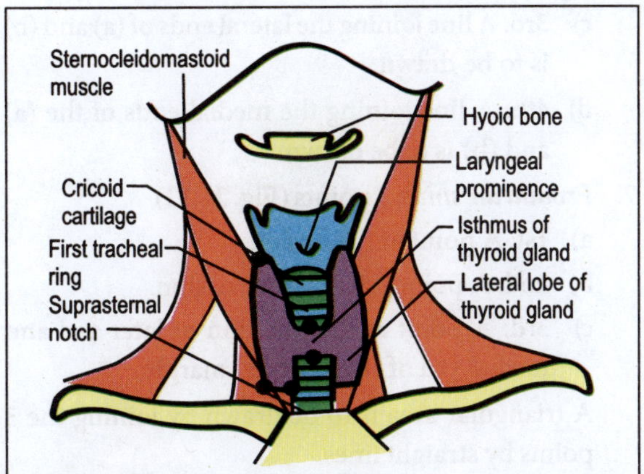

Fig. 21.11: Surface anatomy of the thyroid gland

b) 2nd: Take another point about 1.25cm below (a) and draw a horizontal line about 1.5cm which is lower border of isthmus.

Two parallel horizontal lines (upper and lower border of isthmus) are to be drawn along point (a) and (b), respectively.

B. *Lateral lobe*: 3 points

a) 1st: A point 1.2cm below lateral end of lower border of isthmus.

b) 2nd: A point 2.5cm away or lateral to (a).

c) A point on the anterior border of sternocleidomastoid at the level of prominence of thyroid cartilage.

Join the (a), (b) with a convexity below. It represent base of the lateral lobe.

Join: (i) lateral ends of upper border of isthmus with B(c);

(ii) B(b) with B(c);

(iii) lateral ends of lower border of isthmus with B(a)

which will represent whole of lateral lobe.

6. *Maxillary sinus*: (Antrum of Highmore)

Four lines are to be drawn.

a) 1st: A line along infraorbital margin (upper limit or roof).

b) 2nd: A line is drawn at the level of lower border of ala of nose opposite the premolar and molar teeth across the alveolar process of maxilla.

c) 3rd: A line joining the lateral ends of (a) and (b) is to be drawn.

d) 4th: A line joining the medial ends of the (a) and (b) is to be drawn.

7. *Frontal air sinus*: 3 points (Fig. 21.12)

a) 1st: A point at the nasion.

b) 2nd: A point 2.5cm above nasion.

c) 3rd: A point at the junction of later $\frac{2}{3}$rd and medial $\frac{1}{3}$rd of supraorbital margin.

A triangular area is to be drawn by joining the 3 points by straight lines.

8. *Naso-lacrimal duct*: 1 point

Inner canthus of eye will be marked.

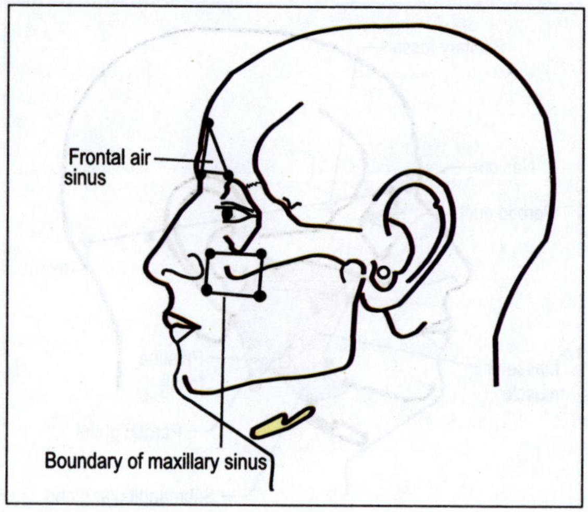

Fig. 21.1: Surface markings of frontal and maxillary air sinuses

A line about 1.5cm is to be drawn downwards and laterally from the point.

9. *Pituitary body*: A point on the nasion (It is about 6.2cm deep).

10. *Oesophagus in the neck*: 2 points

a) 1st: A point just below cricoid in the midline of the neck.

b) 2nd: A point about 1.25cm to left of midline of the neck at the lower border of left clavicle.

A 2.5cm broad line (2 lines 2.5cm a part) is to be drawn.

11. *Trachea*: 2 points

a) 1st: A point on the lower border of cricoid in the midline of the neck.

b) 2nd: A point on the sternal angle just right of midline.

2 parallel lines 2.5cm apart in the midline of the neck joining the 2 points are to be drawn.

RADIOLOGICAL ANATOMY OF HEAD AND NECK REGION

Two views of plane skiagram of skull are usually taken—

I. Lateral

II. Posteroanterior.

Readings of skiagrams of skull

I. **Value of skull (Lateral view)**: This is a lateral view of vault of skull showing.

1. Shape and size whether normal or abnormal (anomalous skull will be in case of hydrocephalus, anencephaly, oxycephaly and microcephaly etc.).
2. *Structure of cranial bones*:
   a) One lamella: 1st 3 years of life.
   b) 2 tables and appearance of dipole: 4th year.
   c) Markings of diploe vein: 35 years of age.
   d) Thicker part of skull: Occipital and frontal region.
   e) Thinner part: Squamous part of temporal and upper part of occipital bone.
   f) Generalised thickening: Paget's disease of bone.
   g) Thickening and characteristic sun ray appearance: Thalassaemia.
   h) Localised hyperostosis: Meningioma.
   i) Large punched out areas: Secondary deposits of malignancy.
   j) Fractures are usually in inner table.
3. *Sutures*:
   a) Commonly visible sutures are coronal (directed downwards and forwards in front part) and lambdoid (in the posteromedial part of skull).
   b) Obliteration of suture (usually on the inner table) occurs at the age of 30 to 40 years and on outer table after the 40 years of age.
   c) Early obliteration of suture takes place in craniostenosis (hereditary disease) and gaping opening of sutures take place due to increased intracranial pressure.
4. *Marking of blood vessels:*
   a) Shadow of anterior branch of middle meningeal: Slightly behind coronal suture. Shadow of posterior branch at a lower level directed upwards, and backwards and crossing the upper part of shadow of auricle.
   b) Shadow of transverse sinus: A curved dark shadow with convexity upwards from internal occipital protuberance to petrous part of temporal.
   c) Shadows of diploic veins: Irregular worm like shadows which are more prominent in cases of intracranial tension.
5. *Shadow of brain*: Normal impressions of cerebral gyri and copper beaten or silver beaten appearance due to pronounced impression when intracranial tension is increased.
6. *Arachnoidal granulation*: Shadows of indentation on each side of sagittal suture.
7. *Calcification (normal)*: Such as brain sand (pineal body calcification) at the age of about 17 yrs. It will be found about 2.5cm above and 1.2cm behind the shadow of external acoustic meatus. Besides, calcification may occur in choroid plexuses, arachnoid granulations, falx cerebri and other processes of dura mater.
8. *Auricle*: Shadow of curved margin of auricle may be seen above petrous part of temporal bone and meatus in the bone.
9. *Frontal sinus*: Shadow of frontal sinus in the outer inferior part of the vault of skull.

II. **Base of skull – (Lateral view)**: Lateral view of base of skull showing:

1. *Floor of anterior cranial fossa*: Shadow of backward and downwards sloping of fossa on each side and irregular markings of cerebral gyri
2. *Hypophyseal fossa*: It will be formed in the middle cranial fossa, it may be enlarged in tumours of pituitary gland.
3. *Sphenoidal air sinus* will be seen in front and below the hypophyseal fossa.
4. *Shadows of orbits, nasal cavities, ethomoidal and maxillary sinuses* will be found superimposed with each other below anterior cranial fossa.
5. *Petrous part of temporal bone*: Shadow of it will be found below and behind the hypophyseal fossa. The other features will be

a) Shadow of external acoustic meatuses of 2 sides (2 dark areas).

b) Internal acoustic meatus dark shadows.

c) Mastoid air cells – honey comb shadow in the posterior part.

6. *Mandible*: Shadow of it will be found in front of skull.

7. *Cervical vertebrae*: Pillar like shadow in the posterior part.

III. ***PA view for paranasal sinuses***

Process: Skiagrams should be taken in Water's portion i.e., head extended with chin to the palate and nose raised from it.

Reading of PA view of the skull

Skiagram shows:

1. *Frontal sinus*: Will be above the nose and medial parts of orbits.
2. *Nasal cavities*: On each side between orbits above and maxillary sinus below.
3. *Maxillary sinuses*: On each side below orbit and lateral to nasal cavity. Sinuses normally will cast black shadows (due to air) but the shadows will be hazy or opaque in case of sinusitis.

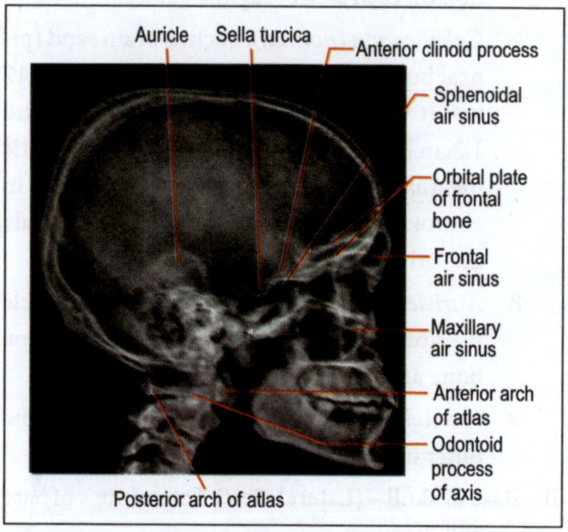

Fig. 21.13: Lateral view of the skull

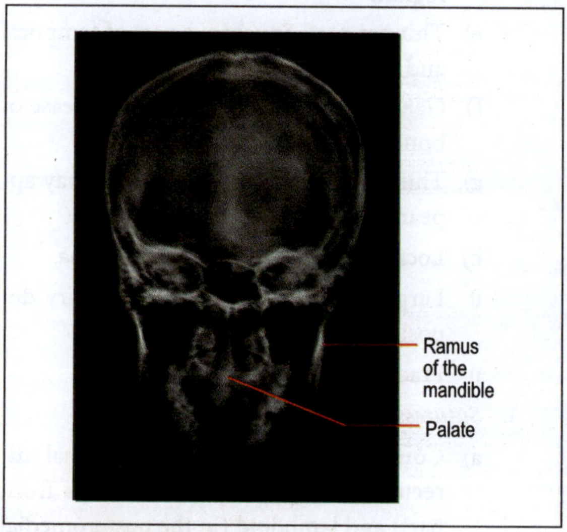

Fig. 21.14: AP view of the skull

APPENDIX OF CHAPTER 1

TABEL 1.30: Some points in this chapter

Name of parts of bone or foramen or fissures etc.	Structures attached or related or passing through
1. External occipital protuberance	1. At the junction of had & neck in the midline — An elevation in the occipital bone — Structures attached: a) Origin of trapezius (from upper part) b) Ligamentum nuchae (in the lower part)
2. Highest nuchal line	2. A faint line above the superior nuchal line Structures attached: a) Epicranial aponeurosis (medial 1/3rd) b) Origin of occipital belly of occipitofrontalis (lateral 2/3rd)
3. Superior nuchal line	3. A line passes laterally to the external occipital protuberance below the highest nuchal line — Structures attached: a) Origin of trapezius (medial 1/3rd) b) Insertion sternocleidomastoid & splenius capitis (lateral 1/3rd) c) Middle 1/3rd form the apex of posterior triangle
4. External occipital crest	4. Extend from external occipital protuberance up to margin of foramen magnus in the midline — Ligamentum nuchae attached
5. Areas between superior & inferior nuchal line	5. Insertion of a) Semispinalis capitis (medially) b) Obliquus superior (laterally)
6. Area below inferior nuchal line	6. Insertion to a) Rectus capitis posterior minor (medially) b) Rectus capitis posterior major (laterally)
7. Supraorbital margin	7. Lateral 2/3rd sharp, medial 1/3rd round
8. Supraorbital foramen	8. Supraorbital nerve & vessels passes through
9. Temporal lines	9. It starts from posterior margin from frontal process of zygomatic bone. It curve superolaterally splits into superior & inferior temporal lines. Superior temporal line give attachment of temporal fascia. Inferior temporal fascia gives attachment.
10. Zygomatic arch	10. Inner surface: Origin of the masseter muscle Upper border: Temporal fascia is attached Lower border: Origin of the masseter Outer surface: Subcutaneous.
11. Pterion	11. Meeting point of 4 bones: frontal, parietal, greaterwing of the sphenoid and temporal bone. It is a bony landmark for anterior branch of middle meningeal artery and start of lateral sulcus of the brain.
12. Suprameatal triangle	12. A triangular depression situated posterosuperior to external auditory meatus. It correspond to mastoid antrum.
13. Mastoid process	13. A projected part of just behind the external acoustic meatus. Three muscles attached: a) Sternocleidomastoid; b) Splenius capitis and c) Longissimus capitis
14. Styloid process	14. Three muscles attached: a) Styloglossus (at the tip) supplied by hypoglossal nerve b) Stylohyoid (midway posteriorly) supplied by facial nerve c) Stylopharyngeal (at the base) supplied by glossopharyngeal nerve Two ligaments are attached: a) Stylohyoid: at the tip; b) Stylomandibular (lateral aspect of tip)

Contd.........

Name of parts of bone or foramen or fissures etc.	Structures attached or related or passing through
15. Incisive canal	15. It is present in the anterior part of hard palate. It transmits nasopalatine (long sphenopalatine) nerve and greater palatine vessels.
16. Greater palatine foramen	16. It lies in the posterolateral part of hard palate through which greater palatine vessels and nerve passes.
17. Lesser palatine foramina	17. Those foramina situated behind greater palatine foramen and transmits lesser palatine nerve vessels.
18. Posterior nasal spine	18. Gives attachment of musculus uvulae
19. Palatine crest	19. It is near the posterior margin of the hard palate (horizontal plate of the palatine and gives attached to aponeurosis of tensor veli palatini.
20. Palatovaginal canal (Formed by palatine bone and vaginal process of medial pterygoid plate)	20. Transmit a) Pharyngeal branch of 3rd part of the maxillary artery b) Pharyngeal branch of pterygopalatine ganglion.
21. Pterygoid fossa	21. – Behind the fused part of pterygoid processes (upper part) – Contain tensor veli palatini and medial pterygoid.
22. Scaphoid fossa	22. Posterior border of medial pterygoid plate bifurcate to form the fossa – Gives origin of tensor veli palatini.
23. Spine of the sphenoid	23. Attachments: a) Sphenomandibular ligament b) Origin of tensor veli palatini c) Anterior ligament of malleus Relations: Medially: Chorda tympani & auditory tube. Laterally: Auriculotemporal nerve
24. Foramen ovale	24. Transmits: a) Mandibular nerve; b) Accessory meningeal artery; c) Lesser petrosal nerve; d) Emissary vein
25. Foramen spinogum	25. Transmits: a) Middle meningeal artery b) Nervous spinosus (meningeal branch of mandibular nerve).
26. Petrotympanic fissure	26. Transmits: a) Anterior ligament of malleus b) Anterior tympanic branch of maxillary artery
27. Foramen magnum	27. Alar ligament divide the foramen into smaller anterior part & larger posterior part (Fig. 1.20) **Structures passing through** anterior part: a) Apical ligament b) Upper band of cruciate ligament c) Membrane tectoria Structures passing through posterior part: a) Lower end of medulla oblongata with meninges b) Spinal accessory nerve c) Vertebral artery (4th part) d) Anterior spinal artery e) Posterior spinal arteries f) Sometimes tonsil of cerebellum
28. Hypoglossal canal	28. Transmits: a) Hypoglossal nerve b) Meningeal branch of ascending pharyngeal artery c) emissary vein

Contd.........

Name of parts of bone or foramen or fissures etc.	Structures attached or related or passing through
29. Jugular foramen	29. Three compartments: **Through anterior part transmits** a) Inferior petrosal sinus b) Meningeal branch of ascending pharyngeal **Through middle part transmits**: a) IXth, Xth, XIth cranial nerves. **Through posterior part transmits**: a) Sigmoid sinus continue as internal carotid artery b) meningeal branch of occipital artery (Fig. 20.21)
30. Carotid canal	30. Transmits: a) Internal carotid artery b) Sympathetic plexus around it.
31. Tympanic canaliculus	31. Transmits: a) Tympanic branch of glossopharyngeal nerve
32. Ganglia of glosso-pharyngal nerve	32. It lies in between carotid canal & jugular fossa
33. Jugular fossa	33. Superior bulb of internal jugular vein is related.
34. Mastoid canaliculus	34. Transmit auricular branch branch of the vagus nerve.
35. Stylomastoid foramen	35. Transmit facial nerve and stylomastoid branch of posterior auricular artery.
36. Mastoid notch	36. a) Medial to mastoid process b) Origin of posterior belly digastric muscle
37. Superior orbital fissure	37. Within the sphenoid bone. It is divided into three parts (middle, lateral & medial part) by common tendinous ring. **Structures transmitted**: a) Middle part (with common tendinous ring) i) Superior & inferior divisions of oculomotor nerve ii) Nasociliary nerve in between the divisions of oculomotor nerve. iii) Abducent nerve – Lateral to inferior division of oculomotor nerve. b) Lateral part: (Outside the common tendinous ring) i) Trochlear nerve; ii) Frontal nerve; iii) Lacrimal nerve; iv) Recurrent meningeal branch of lacrimal artery; v) Superior ophthalmic vein. c) Medial part (outside of common tendinous ring) — Inferior ophthalmic vein. (Fig. 1.26)
38. Foramen rotundum	38. Transmit maxillary nerve.
39. Pterygoid canal	39. Transmits: a) Nerve to pterygoid canal (greater petrosal nerve + deep petrosal nerve) b) Artery of pterygoid canal
40. Crista galli	40. Attachment of falx cerebri.
41. Anterior clinoid process	41. Attachment of free margin of tentorium cerebelli.
42. Sella turcila	42. A depressed area behind tuberculum sellae **Hypophyseal fossa**: Deepest part of sella turcica. It lodges hypophysis cerebri
43. Posterior clinoid process	43. A conical projection at the superior angle of dorsum sellae. — Gives attachment to fixed or attached margin of tentorium cerebelli
44. Groove for superior petrosal sinus at the superior border of petrous part of temporal bone	44. Attachment of attached margin of tentorium cerebelli & lodges superior petrosal sinus
45. Transverse sulcus	45. a) Attachment of attached margin of tentorium cerebelli b) Lodges transverse sinus
46. Jugular tubercle	46. Related to 9th, 10th & 11th cranial nerve.

Contd.........

Name of parts of bone or foramen or fissures etc.	Structures attached or related or passing through
47. Internal acoustic meatus	47. Transmits: a) Motor & sensory root of facial nerve b) Vestibulocochlear nerve c) Labyrinthine branch of basilar artery.
48. Internal occipital crest	49. Attached falx cerebelli containing occipital sinus
49. Foramen caecum present in relation to frontal crest	50. Transmit emissary vein from nasal cavity to joining superior sagittal sinus
50. Sulcus tubae	51. At the junction of sphenoid & petrous part (inferior surface) of temporal bone — Lodges cartilaginous part of auditory tube.

INDEX